BRAIN *and*
CONSCIOUS
EXPERIENCE

BRAIN *and* CONSCIOUS EXPERIENCE

Study Week September 28 to October 4, 1964,
of the Pontificia Academia Scientiarum

Edited by
JOHN C. ECCLES

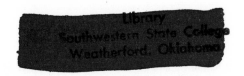
SPRINGER-VERLAG NEW YORK INC.
1966

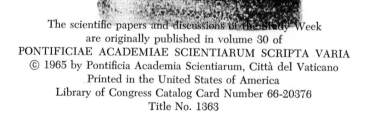
The scientific papers and discussions of the Study Week
are originally published in volume 30 of
PONTIFICIAE ACADEMIAE SCIENTIARUM SCRIPTA VARIA
© 1965 by Pontificia Academia Scientiarum, Città del Vaticano
Printed in the United States of America
Library of Congress Catalog Card Number 66-20376
Title No. 1363

Dedicated to the memory of two eminent Pontifical Academicians who contributed so much to the scientific and philosophical concepts that are the theme of this Study Week: C. S. Sherrington (1857–1952), E. Schrödinger (1887–1961).

Preface

The planning of this Study Week at the Pontifical Academy of Science from September 28 to October 4, 1964, began just two years before when the President, Professor Lemaitre, asked me if I would be responsible for a Study Week relating Psychology to what we may call the Neurosciences. I accepted this responsibility on the understanding that I could have assistance from two colleagues in the Academy, Professors Heymans and Chagas. Besides participating in the Study Week they gave me much-needed assistance and advice in the arduous and, at times, perplexing task that I had undertaken, and I gratefully acknowledge my indebtedness to them.

Though there have been in recent years many symposia concerned with the so-called higher functions of the brain, for example with perception, learning and conditioning, and with the processing of information in the brain, there has to my knowledge been no symposium specifically treating with brain functions and consciousness since the memorable Laurentian Conference of 1953, which was later published in 1954 as the book, "Brain Mechanisms and Consciousness." It was therefore my purpose from the beginning not only to bring together for the Study Week those who had contributed significantly to a wide range of problems related to the theme of the Study Week, but also to have their Contributions and particularly their Discussions published for world distribution, and not merely in a limited edition for private circulation, as has recently occurred with two Study Weeks of the Academy. I must express my gratitude and deeply felt appreciation to the publishers, Springer-Verlag, and particularly to Dr. Heinz Götze, for their cooperation and tenacity in bringing this project eventually to a successful conclusion.

I should mention that I was not able to invite any professional philosophers to the Study Week. Early in the planning I was instructed by the Chancellor that "the Academy by its constitution has for aim to promote the study and progress of the physical, mathematical and natural sciences and their history. Thus the discussion of philosophical questions is excluded." I replied, "I fear that some of your concern derives from the different linguistic usages that we have. For example, to me all sciences

vii

have a philosophical basis and it is generally agreed that there is a philosophy of science which is in fact basic to all scientific investigations and discussions. Certainly when one comes to a Study Week devoted to brain and mind it is not possible to exclude relations with philosophy, though I agree that there are certain philosophical questions which the Academy would be well advised to avoid. I do not think that any of the proposed subjects fall into this category."

After this somewhat inauspicious beginning I am happy to state that there has never been any attempt to change any Contributions and Discussions during the Study Week, which was conducted with the complete freedom customary in all scientific symposia.

It must be admitted that the subject matter of this Study Week raises the most important questions that man can ask about himself and his relation to the material world. It is for the reader to judge if we have contributed significantly to a clearer understanding of these questions and in any way aided in their solution. Besides the published lectures, I would refer the reader to the discussions that I think have a special merit because in the five days of meeting under excellent and convivial (in the best sense!) conditions many of us were prepared to talk with an unusual ease and freedom. This book therefore serves as a record of an intimate disputation between scholars of quite different approaches to the central theme, and in this respect it was an occasion that I think we can all remember with appreciation because we learned so much in this mutual interplay of ideas. I therefore recommend the Discussions as providing a good model of "symposium behaviour" if I may use such an expression!

I think it is important to appreciate the excellent convivial arrangements under which this symposium was held. The Academy building itself stands in the most delectable spot in the Vatican gardens, being built in 1561 as a Casino for Pius IV. The room in which we met had still the lovely tiled floor and the frescoed walls and ceiling of that period, and outside there was always the sound of the fountains in the marble paved court. Then we all lived (most of us with our wives who were also guests of the Academy) in the stately Hotel Reale, where we were magnificently entertained. We returned there between the sessions of each day for a sumptuous lunch with time even for a brief siesta before the late afternoon session. And in the evenings there were the pleasant social occasions of dinner and gatherings thereafter. From a rather large experience of symposia in the last decade I am convinced that the most fruitful have been the most enjoyable, because it is under these conditions that the human spirit (if I may use this phrase!) operates most creatively in debate.

It is in this belief that I as editor present for world circulation this volume as the conjoint creative effort of my colleagues during this most enjoyable Study Week that was devoted to the greatest scientific and philosophic problem confronting man: Brain and Conscious Experience.

JOHN C. ECCLES

January 10, 1966.

Contents

List of Participants

Lord Adrian of Cambridge, Master of Trinity College, Cambridge, England.

Dr. P. O. Andersen, Anatomical Institute, University of Oslo, Oslo, Norway.

Professor F. Bremer, Professor of General Pathology, Université Libre de Bruxelles, Bruxelles, Belgium.

Professor C. Chagas, Professor of Biophysics, University of Brasil, Rio de Janeiro, Brasil.

Dr. M. L. Colonnier, Department of Physiology, University of Montreal, Montreal, Canada.

Priv. Doz. Dr. O. Creutzfeldt, Abteilung für Experimentelle Neurophysiologie, Max-Planck-Institut, 8 München 23, Germany.

Sir John Eccles, Institute for Biomedical Research, American Medical Association, Chicago, U.S.A.; formerly Professor of Physiology, Australian National University, Canberra, Australia.

Dr. A. Gomes, Instituto de Biofisica, Universidade do Brasil, Rio de Janeiro, Brasil.

Professor R. A. Granit, Nobel Professor of Neurophysiology, Karolinska, Stockholm, Sweden.

Professor C. Heymans, Director, Instituut J. F. Heymans, Farmakologisch and Terapeutisch Laboratorium der Rijksuniversiteit, Gent, Belgium.

Professor Sir Cyril Hinshelwood, Chemistry Department, Imperial College, London, England.

Professor H. H. Jasper, Department of Physiology, University of Montreal, Montreal, Canada.

Professor B. Libet, Department of Physiology, University of California, San Francisco, U.S.A.

Professor D. MacKay, Professor of Communications, University of Keele, Keele, England.

Professor G. Moruzzi, Professor of Physiology, Istituto di Fisiologia dell' Universita, Pisa, Italy.

Professor V. B. Mountcastle, Professor of Physiology, Johns Hopkins University, Baltimore, U.S.A.

Professor W. Penfield, Honorary Consultant, Montreal Neurological Institute, McGill University, Montreal 2, Canada.

Dr. C. G. Phillips, Reader in Neurophysiology, Oxford University, Oxford, England.

Professor Hans Schaefer, Professor of Physiology, University of Heidelberg, Germany.

Professor R. W. Sperry, Professor of Psychobiology, California Institute of Technology, Los Angeles, U.S.A.

Professor H. L. Teuber, Professor of Psychology, M.I.T., Boston, U.S.A.

Dr. W. H. Thorpe, Director of Sub-Department of Animal Behaviour, University of Cambridge, England.

Introduction

by JOHN C. ECCLES

Mr. President and participants in this Study Week, let me first join with the President of the Pontifical Academy of Science in welcoming you to participate in this Study Week on this most challenging theme, Brain and Conscious Experience. Though we differ widely in our philosophical beliefs, each of us I think would regard the theme of this symposium as raising challenging and fundamental scientific problems. We would not range ourselves as agreeing with those obscurantist philosophers who classify problems relating to brain and mind as pseudo-problems arising from so-called category mistakes. Already professional philosophers (e.g., Kneale, 1962) and psychologists (Beloff, 1962) have reacted against such dogmatic strictures; and scientists, particularly physicists and what we may call neuroscientists, have continued to struggle with this most baffling of all scientific problems confronting man, namely the subject of this Study Week—Brain and Conscious Experience. In this context it is particularly appropriate to refer to two distinguished scientists, C. S. Sherrington and E. Schrödinger, who were both elected as Pontifical Academicians in the refounded Pontificia Academia Scientiarum on October 28th, 1936. They were then both Fellows of Magdalen College, Oxford, as was also I, and they greatly admired each other's contributions to the formulation and elucidation of the problems being discussed in this Study Week. I refer particularly to Sherrington's classic book, "Man on His Nature" (1940) and to Schrödinger's two books: "Science and Humanism" (1951) and Mind and Matter (1958). For example in the former book, Schrödinger states: "I consider science an integrating part of our endeavour to answer the one great philosophical question which embraces all others, the one that Plotinus expressed by his brief: τίνες δὲ ἡμεῖς;—who are we? And more than that: I consider this not only one of the tasks, but *the* task, of science, the only one that really counts."

I now come back to more detailed considerations of this Study Week. There have been criticisms that the programme is too physiological in its orientation, and that psychology is not adequately represented. But many of us are psychologists and will be presenting fundamental psychological discoveries, as, for example, Bremer, Penfield, Sperry, Teuber and Libet, though not usually classified as professional psychologists. Again there is perhaps inadequate representation from the fields of cybernetics and computers, which certainly are importantly related to the theme of this Study Week. However MacKay and Gomes are experts in this field. The absence of professional philosophers is a more serious deficiency, which I have referred to in the Preface. It is unfortunate that of the three physical scientists and philosophers who were invited, only Sir Cyril Hinshelwood was able to be with us: Professor W. Heisenberg and Professor E. Wigner were precluded by prior engagements.

As a prelude to the Study Week, I would like to read a passage from a paper of a most distinguished neuroscientist, Dr. R. Lorente de Nó (1934), because, though it refers particularly to neuroanatomical problems, it conveys so well the general atmosphere that will prevail during this Study Week. "A theoretical discussion of the conduction of nerve impulses through the cerebral cortex will follow. There is no doubt that new anatomical and physiological studies will prove the hypotheses I put forward to be insufficient and perhaps fundamentally wrong, but there is no doubt either that the problem must be taken up. No problem will be solved without having been proposed. At any rate, the following discussion will have the value of remembering that in the nervous system many different kinds of cells are present and that, therefore, in every attempt to explain the mechanism of any nerve activity, be it a spinal reflex or a high cerebral function, the presence of numerous kinds of cells with short axis cylinder and of neuron chains of determined composition must be accounted for. The spinal cord, the medulla, the cerebellum, the thalamus, the cerebral cortex, in short the whole nervous system have the same fundamental structure."

In conclusion I would like to say how much we are indebted to the Pontifical Academy for the excellence of arrangements made on our behalf; not only to the Chancellor and his staff, but also to Professor Sergio Cerquiglini and Dr. Renato Lazzari who generously will be devoting so much of their specialist knowledge to the deciphering and editing of the immense amount of recorded discussion that there will be over the five days of the Study Week.

REFERENCES

J. BELOFF. *The Existence of Mind*. London: Macgibbon and Kee (1962).

W. KNEALE. *On Having a Mind*. London: Cambridge University Press (1962).

R. LORENTE DE NÓ. Studies on the structure of the cerebral cortex. II. Continuation of the study of the ammonic system. *J. Psychol. Neurol.*, Leipzig, *46*, 113–177 (1934).

E. SCHRÖDINGER. *Science and Humanism*. London: Cambridge University Press (1951).

E. SCHRÖDINGER. *Mind and Matter*. London: Cambridge University Press (1958).

C. S. SHERRINGTON. *Man on His Nature*. London: Cambridge University Press (1940).

The Audience and Address by Pope Paul VI

Gentlemen,

Now that the study week organized by the Pontifical Academy of Sciences on the theme "Brain and Conscious Experience" is about to conclude, We have desired to bring you personally Our greetings and Our thanks and to express anew the interest with which We follow the development and the progress of your scientific activities.

1. First of all We greet with pleasure the President and the members of the Academy here present, and We also welcome most cordially the scientists of various nations who have accepted the invitation to attend this session. Their very presence in this place calls for lively gratitude on Our part, all the more when we consider the erudite communications which they have presented at this scientific meeting. Their many learned papers serve as an inspiration to the Pontifical Academy of Sciences, reflecting credit not only on the Holy See, but, We humbly dare to assert, for it is Our conviction, on the world of science itself.

We have had before Our eyes the series of researches already published in the official collection of the "*Commentarii*" of the Pontifical Academy of Sciences, as well as the three volumes of "*Miscellanea Galileiana*" which have been presented to Us in your name. These many signs of the vitality of your Academy are a source of deep joy to Us. The merit is yours, and with all Our heart We congratulate you and thank you.

2. Our intention, as you will surmise, is not to comment on the theme which you have been discussing during these days with such competence and scientific rigor. May We be permitted simply to underline in a word its importance, and to bring out its relationship—if one may use the term—with those domains in which the essential part of Our own activity is exercised, We refer to the moral and religious sciences.

"Brain and Conscious Experience": seeing these words associated suffices to make clear that there you touch on that which is most specifically human in man, on that which approaches most nearly the mechanisms of his psychology, the problems of his soul. To be sure, when you speak of "consciousness," you do not refer to the moral conscience: the very rigor of your methods ensures that you do not leave that strictly scientific domain which belongs to you. What you have in mind exclusively is the faculty of perceiving and of reacting to perception, that is to say, the psychophysiological concept which constitutes one of the accepted meanings of the word "conscience."

But who does not see the close connection between the cerebral mechanisms, as they appear from the results of experimentation, and the higher processes which concern the strictly spiritual activity of the soul?

3. Your labors are valued by Us, as you see, because of the domain in which they are pursued, because of their close affinities with that which is of supreme interest to a spiritual power such as Ours—the domain of the moral and religious activities of man.

But, widening Our field of view, We would like to profit by the occasion thus presented to Us to reaffirm before you the Church's attitude of esteem and confidence with regard to scientific thought in general.

The Church does not fear the progress of science. She undertakes willingly a dialogue with the created world and applauds the wonderful discoveries that scientists are making in that world. Every true scientist is for her a friend, and no branch of learning is shunned by her. The very variety of the subjects treated during the study weeks of the Pontifical Academy of Sciences is in itself a proof of this cultural "ecumenism" of the Church, of her readiness to welcome every true and real progress in the domain of the sciences, of every science.

The Church follows this progress with close attention, as she does also the spiritual expressions which accompany the scientific effort. These expressions have varied according to time and place, and their evolution is for the Church an object of great interest.

The scientific world, which adopted in the past a position of autonomy and of self-confidence, from which flowed an attitude of distrust, if not of contempt, for spiritual and religious values, is today, on the contrary, impressed by the complexity of the problems of the world and of mankind, and feels a sort of insecurity and fear when faced with the possible evolution of a science left, without any control, to follow its own driving force. Thus the fine self-confidence of early days has for many given place to a salutary unease, so that the soul of the scientist today is more easily open to religious values, and glimpses, beyond the prodigious achievements of science in the material domain, the mysteries of the spiritual world, and the gleams of the divine transcendence.

How can the Church not rejoice at this happy evolution? She is beside you in your labors, Gentlemen, you may be sure, and always ready to offer you the help of the lights of which she is the trustee, whenever your learned researches bring you to the threshold of those grave questions which transcend the domain of science and which from all time have presented themselves to the consciences of men: questions of the origin and of the destiny of man and of the world.

Receive from Us, Gentlemen, these too brief thoughts, which are meant simply as a cordial affirmation of Our esteem for your persons and your work, and of the profound interest with which the Church follows the evolution of scientific progress in the modern world. We wish complete success for the present session, and we invoke for you, and for the happy continuation of your learned activities, the most abundant divine favors.

1

The Structural Design
of the Neocortex

by M. L. COLONNIER [*]

University of Montreal, Montreal, Canada

The cerebral cortex is a sheet of gray matter usually described as composed of layers of cells tangential to the pial surface. The lamination is obvious even to the inexperienced eye, but the individual layers and their subdivisions are not always clear (Fig. 1.1). In fact, different schemes of lamination have been described by different investigators. The scheme which has gained widest acceptance is perhaps that of Vogt and Brodman into six layers [Sholl, 1956].

A six layered subdivision is used in this review (Fig. 1.3). Layer I designates the lamina, relatively poor in nerve cell bodies, found immediately under the pia. Layers II and III correspond to the layer of small and medium-sized pyramids and the layer of large pyramids as defined by Cajal [1911]. Layer IV is the zone of stellate cells and does not include Cajal's IV-*c* subdivision, containing small pyramidal cells with arciform axons. These [O'Leary, 1941] are preferably included in layer V, the layer of giant pyramidal cells. Layer VI, between layer V and the white matter, is mainly characterized by the presence of fusiform cells.

The neurons of the neocortex have been extensively studied and, for example, as many as 60 cell types have been described by Lorente de Nó [1922] in the rat. Sholl [1956] has found it more convenient to classify them into 7 cell types.

On the basis of the dendritic arborizations, there is a first basic sub-

---

* The author is a grantee of the Medical Research Council of Canada. The work was done at the University of Ottawa, Ottawa, Canada.

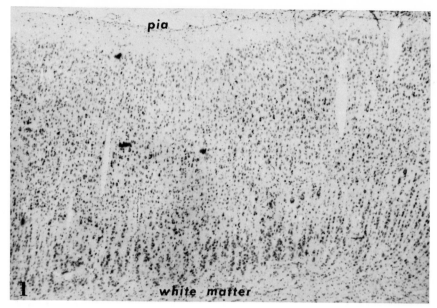

Fig. 1.1. Transverse section of the interhemispheric gyrus of the cat stained by the Nissl method.

division into pyramidal and stellate cells. The pyramidal cells (Fig. 1.4, pc) have a conical perikaryon from the summit of which a large process, the apical dendrite, ascends towards the pia to end in layer I by dichotomous branching. Thick but short dendrites leave the base of the cell to branch into numerous segments. All these dendrites possess a great number of spines, shown by Gray [1959] to be sites of synaptic contact.

The second type of neuron, on the basis of the dendritic pattern, is the stellate cell (Fig. 1.4, sc). It has an oval or circular perikaryon from which thin dendrites arise abruptly and soon divide into their component branches. The dendrites of many of these cells are beaded on Golgi preparations and possess virtually no spines. Others do possess spines but usually in smaller number than pyramidal cell dendrites.

A study of sections of visual cortex cut tangential to the pial surface [Colonnier, 1964b] has shown that the basal dendritic trees of pyramidal cells may spread as a circle, as a cross, or as an elongated figure in the tangential plane. The dendritic fields of the bushy terminals of the apical dendrites may also be elongated or circular. Most stellate cell dendritic trees are in the form of disks or cylinders elongated in the tangential plane. Their long axes may be orientated in all directions but in the cat they tend to be orientated mainly in the anteroposterior direction of the gyrus lateralis [Colonnier, 1964b and unpublished data].

The branching pattern of the dendritic trees was analyzed in great detail by Sholl [1953]. He was able to show that there is no simple law relating length of dendrites to position and size of perikaryon, although there is a relationship between the number of branches and the length of dendrites. By counting the number of dendrites crossing imaginary concentric shells at successive distances from the cell body, he found that the number of intersections per unit area of shell falls off exponentially with the distance of the shell from the cell body. This led to the suggestion that dendrites grew and ramified according to some mechanical principle of growth rather than according to specific circuits (Cragg and Temperley, 1954). Thus axons in the cortex would not have established connections with specific cells but rather with any cells which happened to fall within the fields of their branching terminals.

On the basis of axonal arborizations, Sholl [1956] subdivided pyramidal and stellate cells into four and three types respectively. There are pyramidal cells whose axons go to the white matter without giving off collateral branches. Axons of other pyramidal cells possess horizontal or recurrent or both horizontal and recurrent collaterals. Stellate cells may

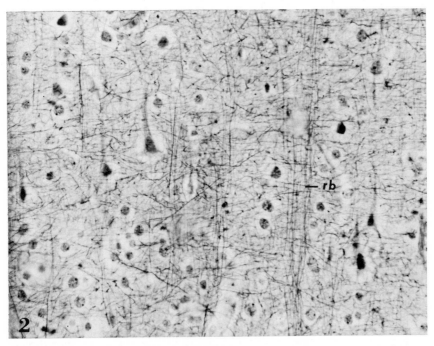

Fig. 1.2. Transverse section through the interhemispheric gyrus of the cat stained by the Holmes method. *rb*: radial bundle of axons.

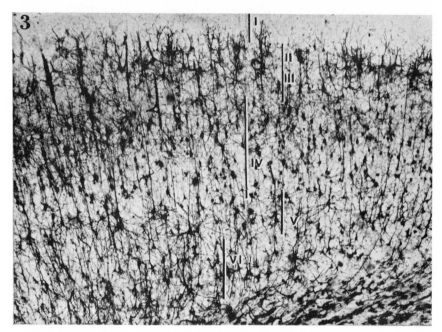

Fig. 1.3. Transverse section of the interhemispheric gyrus of the cat stained by the Golgi Cox method.

have axons distributed within their own dendritic fields, going to the white matter or ascending to the outermost cortical zone.

Sholl maintained that if fusiform or inverted pyramidal cells are considered as modified pyramidals, only 2.5 per cent of all cells do not fall within these categories. He showed quantitatively that pyramidal cells whose axons do not give recurrent collaterals are numerous in layers II, III, V, and VI, while those with recurrent collaterals are found mainly in layers V and VI. His tables show that stellate cells predominate in layer IV.

Specific afferents in a primary sensory area of neocortex end mainly in this stellate zone. They ascend obliquely through the deeper layers to end by spreading tangentially in the fourth layer. Cajal [1911] says that no fibers go above layer IV and that they do not establish contact with small and medium-sized pyramids of the second and third layers. He adds that this is not absolute and that he sometimes sees fine ascending collaterals leave the horizontal (tangential) branches in the fourth layer. These penetrate the border of the third layer where they articulate with pyramidal cells. Degeneration experiments have confirmed this description of the site of termination [Nauta, 1949] and the branching pattern (Szentágothai, personal communication) of specific afferent fibers.

Their tangential spread in layer IV is approximately 650 μ according to Sholl [1956].

Association fibers from other cortical areas ascend to all cortical layers except the uppermost [Nauta, 1949]. Their tangential spread is limited to 150 μ [Sholl, 1956].

If layer I does not receive specific afferent or association fibers, what is the source of its axons? Sholl said that they were in part branches of his stellate cells with ascending axons, adding that unfortunately he had been unable to determine what other cells contribute to the axonal population of this zone. In order to do this Szentágothai [1962, 1964a] undercut slabs of cortex at different levels through the layers and permitted the animals to survive until the distal ends of the cut axons were completely degenerated and the debris cleared from the tissue.

If the undercut is just below layers I and II, practically no fibers can be stained in layer I by the Bielchowsky technique (Fig. 1.6), indicating that cells in these two layers are not the main source of its axons. After undercutting below layers III and IV a few more fibers survive (Fig. 1.7), but it is not until the undercut has been made below layers V and VI (Fig. 1.8) that the axon concentration of layer I appears any-

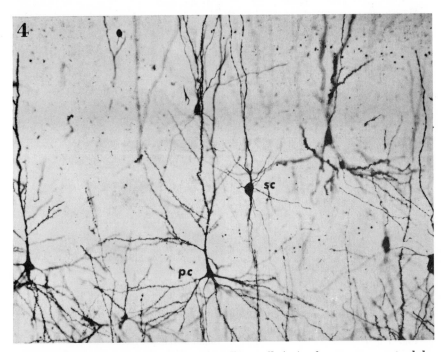

Fig. 1.4. Pyramidal cell (*pc*) and stellate cell (*sc*) of cat cortex stained by Ramon-Moliner modification of the Golgi method.

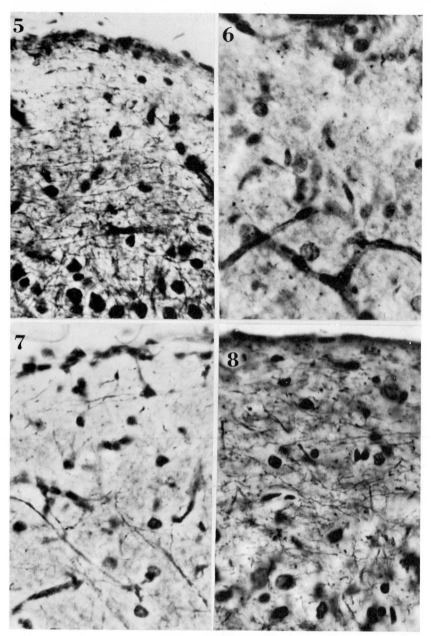

Fig. 1.5. Zonal layer of a normal gyrus lateralis stained by the Reumont modification of the Bielchowsky technique.

Fig. 1.6. Zonal layer of a chronically isolated slab of gyrus lateralis undercut through layer III. Reumont stain.

Fig. 1.7. Zonal layer of a chronically isolated slab of gyrus lateralis undercut through layer IV. Reumont stain.

Fig. 1.8. Zonal layer of a chronically isolated slab of gyrus lateralis undercut below layer VI. Reumont stain.

where near normal (Fig. 1.5). Axons in layer I are thus mainly derived from ascending intracortical axons originating from cells in the deeper layers of the immediately underlying cortex. This is the site of greatest concentration of pyramidal cells with recurrent axon collaterals [Sholl, 1956].

The fibers of the first layer may spread for several millimeters in the tangential direction according to both Sholl and Cajal. Neither of these authors mention a spread of this magnitude in other layers. Sholl's scale drawings rather suggest that in subzonal layers axons never spread out tangentially for more than a few hundred microns.

Szentágothai [1962, 1964a] has approached the problem of the tangential spread of fibers in the cerebral cortex by making cuts perpendicular to the pial surface and observing the extent of degeneration, on each side, with the Nauta technique. Terminal degeneration was found to extend for several millimeters in layer I, but for not more than a few hundred microns to each side, in other layers. If long axons measuring one or more millimeters are present in the subzonal layers, they must be extremely few in number.

Thus the geometrical spread of axons in the cerebral cortex suggests that the main pattern of connections between neurons is in the vertical direction. Fiber spread is more restricted tangentially. The overall organization is thus in the form of "vertical" or "radial" columns. A Holmes preparation of cat visual cortex gives a good visual impression of this organization (Fig. 1.2) in the form of a gridlike pattern of radial and tangential axons. In fact, the radial axons are mainly efferent axons of superimposed pyramidal cells. They group together into fascicles as they course towards the white matter.

Sholl [1956] speaks of vertical columns when discussing his results, but, probably influenced by the physiological data available to him, he refuses to consider these columns as some kind of cortical unit. He does state, however, on the basis of his anatomical investigation that the axons of any column have branches "leading not only to impulses leaving the cortex almost immediately but also to activity above, below and *to a more limited extent*, laterally to this region of primary excitation."

The work of Mountcastle [1957] and Hubel and Wiesel [1962] has now clearly shown functional columnar organization within the cortex. The columnar organization demonstrated by an analysis of the branching pattern of dendrites and axons may therefore well be considered as a basic cortical unit.

A detailed analysis of cell types and of the synaptic organization of the cortex shows the anatomical column more conclusively. Sholl's description of neuron types, though extremely valuable in the context of

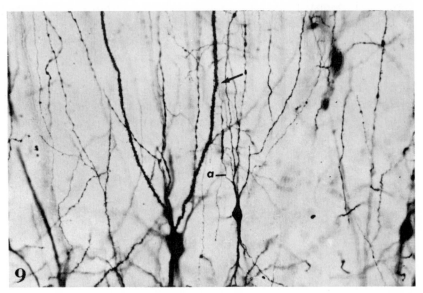

Fig. 1.9. *Cellule fusiforme à double bouquet dendritique* with its axon (*a*) ascending to approximate a large apical dendrite (at arrow). Ramon-Moliner modification of the Golgi technique.

his problem formulation, is perhaps a bit oversimplified. Cajal [1911] has described many stellate cell types not taken into account by Sholl.

There is in particular his *cellule fusiforme à double bouquet dendritique* (Fig. 1.18,a). This is a stellate cell with two bouquets of beaded dendrites sprouting from the upper and lower poles of the cell body. It is found in layers II, III, and IV. Cajal describes its axon in the following manner: "Le cylindre-axe très fin part du corps ou d'une dendrite monte ou descend radialement, c'est-à-dire dans une direction perpendiculaire à la surface des circonvolutions et se résout d'ordinaire à une grande distance du corps de la cellule en un faisceau de filaments, fins et délicats. Auparavant et pendant son trajet il émet à angle droit de nombreuses collatérales qui se décomposent elles-mêmes en faisceau parallèles et flexueux de fibrilles jaunes, variqueuses et descendantes ou ascendantes." In short, the *cellule à double bouquet dendritique* possesses an extremely ramified, vertically orientated axonal arborization. These radial arborizations are so long that they may extend for the whole thickness of the cortex including layer I. Their number is so great, especially in man, that on Golgi preparations staining them successfully, adjoining axonal arborizations touch each other, forming together a long vertical fringe. Cajal adds that when the parallel fascicles formed by the axons are carefully examined, empty vertical spaces can be seen between the fibrils, and the size of the space corresponds to the volume of the apical dendrites of large and medium-sized pyramidal cells. He presumes multiple synaptic contacts between them. As the axon forms many fascicles, it can establish connections with many pyramidal cells.

Figure 1.9 is a section of cat cortex stained by the new Ramon-Moliner [1963] modification of the Golgi technique showing this type of cell. The double bouquet of dendrites is clearly seen as well as the axon (*a*) ascending, branching and continuing to approximate a large apical dendrite (arrow). The Ramon-Moliner technique does not stain axons particularly well and the axonal arborization does not appear as extensive as suggested by Cajal. With the Golgi Kopsch technique and double impregnation, a method which stains axons more completely, extensive arborizations can be seen (Fig. 1.10,a) and they appear identical to Cajal's drawings.

In layer II there is a subvariety of these cells *à double bouquet dendritique* (Fig. 1.18,b). Its axon leaves the cell to bifurcate not far from its origin. It gives rise to a series of nests or plexuses around the bodies of smaller pyramidal cells.

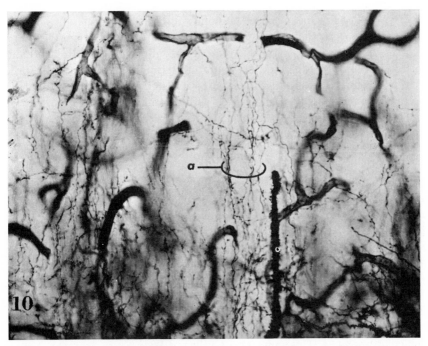

Fig. 1.10. Extremely ramified vertically orientated axonal arborization (*a*). Double impregnation Golgi Cox technique.

Layers III and IV possess a remarkable cell which Cajal describes in detail, stressing its similarity to the basket cells of the cerebellum (Fig. 1.18,c). It has a star-shaped dendritic tree and an ascending or descending axon immediately bifurcating into many horizontal or oblique branches of great length. He does not say how long the spread actually is, but he later refers to long horizontal axons as being two hundred to several hundred microns in length. It is safe to assume a spread of this order and indeed his drawings suggest this. The axonal branches end into tightly knit arborizations closely embracing the bodies and adjacent large dendritic segments of pyramidal cells.

Other cell types are a typical "neurogliform" cell whose axon arborizes within its own dendritic tree (Fig. 1.18,d); a small cell with short axon ascending to arborize into a dense feltwork (Fig. 1.18,e); and a large variety of cells with ascending, descending or horizontal branches (Fig. 1.18,f,g,h,i).

This short review shows quite clearly the extent of Sholl's oversimplification. Not only do axons go selectively to certain areas of cortex but they also may be specific for certain cells or parts of cells. Synapses may then still be considered random only insofar as they are established on all cell bodies or all dendrites or all pyramidal or all stellate cells that they meet in a specific layer or at a specific distance from the cell of origin. Axons do not contact randomly in the sense that they synapse indiscriminately with any neuronal surface along their course.

It is difficult to clarify the synaptic organization further with the light microscope. Both normal and degenerating terminals are difficult to stain in this region [Colonnier, 1964a]. Electron microscopy has fortunately permitted a more detailed analysis. Synaptic contacts in the normal cortex are identified as elsewhere in the central nervous system by the asymmetrical thickening of two apposed membranes and the presence of "synaptic" vesicles in the presynaptic cytoplasmic profile [Gray, 1959]. Two types have been described (Fig. 1.11) [Gray, 1959]. Type 1 is found on dendritic spines and dendritic trunks and is characterized by a widened synaptic cleft containing a plaque of extracellular material and by its very thick, dense, and extensive postsynaptic membrane. Type 2 is found on cell bodies and dendritic trunks and it has a narrower synaptic cleft usually devoid of extracellular material. Its postsynaptic membrane thickening is neither as dense nor as extensive as that of type 1.

These two synapses are the only synaptic types in the cerebral cortex. The synaptic morphology of the neocortex is therefore essentially very simple and does not possess the elaborate synaptic arrangement found in other regions of the central nervous system, for example, in the lateral geniculate nucleus [Colonnier and Guillery, 1964].

Electron microscopy also permits the identification of degenerating

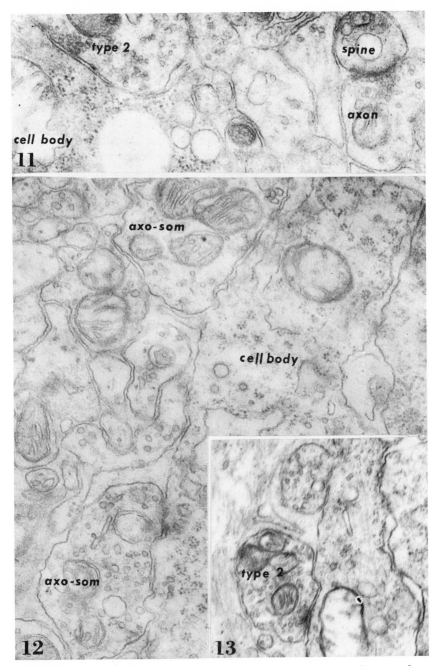

Fig. 1.11. Type 2 axosomatic and type 1 axon-spine contact in the normal cat neocortex.

Fig. 1.12. Two axosomatic type 2 synapses in chronically isolated cortical slab.

Fig. 1.13. One axosomatic type 2 synapse still intact in spite of surrounding gliosis in chronically isolated cortical slab.

terminals. After the cortex is undercut, many axon terminals become intensely electron opaque and are rapidly phagocytosed by glial cells. Adhering postsynaptic cytoplasm is also engulfed by the phagocytes [Colonnier, 1964a]. The synaptic organization is thus undergoing a dramatic upheaval immediately after the lesion and its study is correspondingly difficult. Later, when the degenerated endings have been phagocytosed, only intracortical axon synapses remain intact. Szentágothai [1964b] has used this experimental situation to study the synaptic organization of intracortical axons. He found that the majority of type 2 synapses survive on cell bodies and dendritic trunks.

Fig. 1.12 shows two axosomatic type 2 synapses from undercut cortex after a two-month survival period. Another contact of the same type is seen in Fig. 1.13. It was present in long survival cortex in spite of surrounding gliosis.

Some type 1 contacts are still present in the neuropil but they are significantly fewer than in normal material. Indeed, the very number of dendritic spines seems diminished (Fig. 1.17), suggesting that the pieces of postsynaptic cytoplasm phagocytosed with degenerating terminals in the acute stage were in fact small spines, harvested from the main dendritic trunk without damage to the postsynaptic cell. This may be considered as a kind of restricted transneuronal degeneration.

The study of long survival undercut cortex therefore suggests that afferent fibers to the cortex synapse mainly on dendritic spines and trunks with type 1 synapses. A large number of intracortical fibers contact cell bodies and dendritic trunks as type 2 synapses. The latter are probably, in great part, terminals of those intracortical axons which end as pericellular nests, for example, those of the basketlike cells described above. Similar neurons have been shown to be inhibitory in nature in the cerebellum [Andersen, Eccles, Voorhoeve, 1963] and in the hippocampus [Andersen, Eccles, Loyning, 1963, 1964]. It is tempting to assume that they may have a similar function in the cortex.

Surviving type 1 synapses would be from intracortical axons without pericellular endings. Golgi studies do show rather convincing pictures of intracortical axon collaterals contacting dendritic spines in normal material (Fig. 1.16). Such contacts can also be seen in long survival undercut cortex (Fig. 1.14). Axons climbing parallel to an apical dendrite can also be seen in isolated slabs (Fig. 1.15). The latter observation supports Cajal's contention that some of the fibers which acquire this type of climbing relation to the dendrites are truly intracortical axons. In the cerebellum Eccles, Llinás, and Sasaki [1964] have shown that the climbing fibers provide an extremely powerful excitatory mechanism, and again it is tempting to assume a similar function in the cortex for the axons climbing parallel to the apical dendrites.

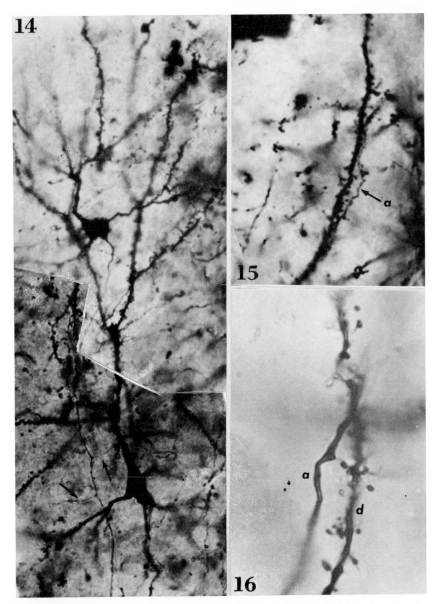

Fig. 1.14. Two surviving cells in chronically isolated cortical slab stained by the Golgi Rapid technique. The upper cell is a "star pyramid" with its axon running downwards and having two collaterals (arrows).

Fig. 1.15. "Climbing contact" in chronically isolated cortical slab stained by the Golgi Rapid technique.

Fig. 1.16. Synapse between pyramidal cell axon and pyramidal cell dendritic spine in normal cortex stained by the Golgi Cox technique.

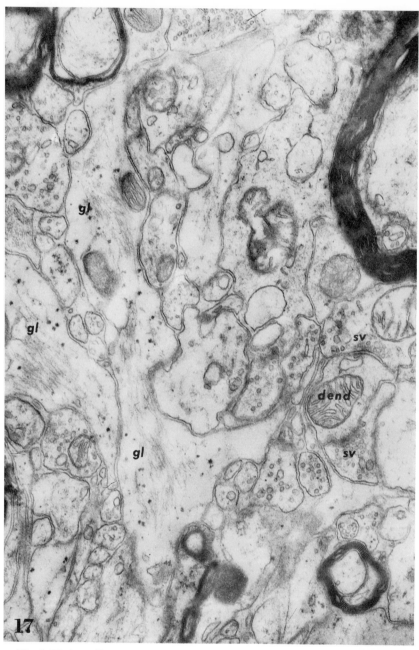

Fig. 1.17. Overall picture of the neuropil in chronically isolated cortical slab with strong gliosis and heavy reduction of spines.

The detailed synaptic organization of the cortex could thus be conceived as follows. The fusiform stellate cells with their intensely ramified vertical axons have "climbing" contacts with the apical dendrites of pyramidal cells (Fig. 1.19). If the repeated contacts established by these "climbing fibers" are as powerful a means of synaptic transmission as in the cerebellum, impulses set up by specific afferents in the third and fourth layers of the cortex are transmitted to all layers, activating many cells above and below the focus of excitation. The radial axons presumably also activate other fusiform stellates whose vertical arborizing axons would potentiate the radial spread of activity. Simultaneously the basket-like cells of layers II and IV (Fig. 1.19), if they behave like their counterpart in the hippocampus and cerebellum, inhibit cells to the sides

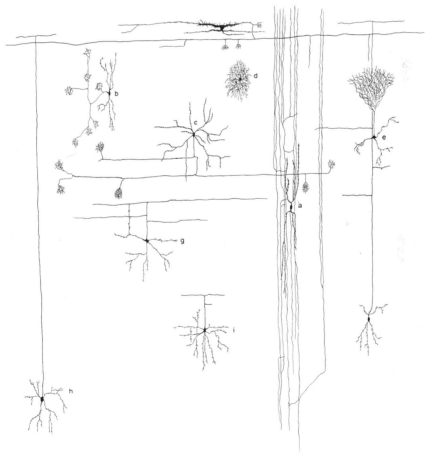

Fig. 1.18. Free-hand composite drawing of stellate cells described by Cajal (for explanation, see text).

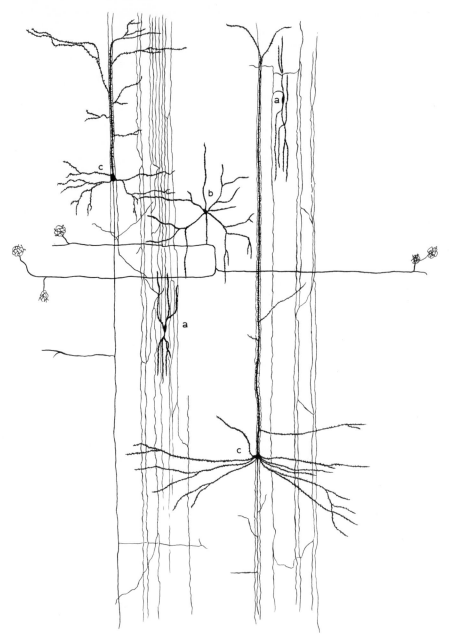

Fig. 1.19. Free-hand drawing summarizing some aspects of the structural design of the cerebral cortex. (*a*) *Cellules à double bouquet dendritique.* (*b*) Basket cell. (*c*) Pyramidal cells.

of this vertical activity through their pericellular terminals. Thus the anatomical organization would give rise to functional vertical columns with an inhibitory periphery.

The anatomical columns are not distinct, separate morphological entities. The tangential overlap is considerable. This need not impede the functioning of the columns as distinct physiological units. The principle of partially shifted overlapping as defined by Marshall and Talbot [1942] may convert a group of overlapping cells into effective columns through the input convergence. The physiological column results from a focus of effective stimulation of a number of definite units by the input, coupled with the inhibition of surrounding units through the "basket" cell axons.

How this could work in a sensory area is perhaps best exemplified by the work of Hubel and Wiesel [1962]. These investigators have shown that all cells of the visual cortex may be activated by visual impulses if the stimulation is of the proper type. Most significant is the spatial orientation of the stimulus. Cells within the same radial column respond to the same orientation. Thus the specific modality of this "physiological" column is the stimulus orientation. The authors have postulated a convergence of afferent fibers, representing an orientated series of retinal points, upon the cells of the cortex.

The anatomical organization shows that this convergence need only be to the stellate cells of layers III and IV. The extensive vertical and narrow tangential projection of these cells transmits the stimulus to overlying and underlying cells, producing a column of cells responding to the same orientation stimulus. Another stimulus pattern activates a different group of afferent fibers and thus another group of stellate cells which in turn project the activity to another column. The column exists because of vertically orientated axons; its modality depends on the tangential synaptic articulation between specific afferents and the receptor cells—probably stellate cells.

It has been suggested that this patterned convergence of specific afferents upon the neurons of the visual cortex may be served morphologically by the patterned tangential elongation of the dendritic trees of the stellate cells in layer IV [Colonnier, 1964b]. Whether or not this is the morphological mechanism underlying the specific modality of the columns, the essential point is that the convergence of specific afferents in the cortex is such that specific modalities are ascribed to the primary receptor cells of the cortex and that these project the modality to a whole column of cells within the cortex.

What the significance and modality of the columns would be in an association or motor area of cortex is more difficult to imagine, but the anatomical similarity of all parts of the neocortex suggests that a functional counterpart is present in all areas. The structural design of the whole neocortex is such that it should be conceived as a mosaic of overlapping columns each possessing its own functional specificity on the basis of its tangential articulation with incoming fibers and each processing this information up and down within the column for a significant output.

ACKNOWLEDGMENTS

I wish to thank Professor J. Szentágothai for his help and advice in the preparation of this text and for supplying Figs. 1.5–1.8 and 1.11–1.17. Figures 1.4 and 1.9 were obtained from preparations lent by Dr. E. Hall. I also wish to thank Professor J. Auer for reading the text, and Mr. K. C. Watkins for his technical assistance.

DISCUSSION

Chairman: PROFESSOR PENFIELD

CHAIRMAN: Thank you for this beautiful demonstration. I would like to say in initiating the discussion that I was a former pupil of Ramón y Cajal and Hortega. I can only tell you that they would have been delighted with your preparations and with the additions made by the electron microscope.

MOUNTCASTLE: This is certainly an admirable piece of work. Perhaps it might be appropriate to add some of the physiological correlates of this anatomical work. The physiological evidence for the columnar organization is based upon three observations: first, that the cells in such a column normal to the cortex are related to identical peripheral receptive fields; second, that all the cells in such a column in the somatic sensory cortex are activated by the same quality of stimulation from the identical set of peripheral receptors; and third, that the initial pattern of discharge of these cells is nearly identical from the top to bottom of such a column. The evidence in the visual cortex is slightly different and I raise the question of whether the second line of evidence for columnar organization there might eventually turn out to be color as the parallel to quality in the somatic sensory system. The evidence for that point, I think, is not yet available. It is of interest to me, from the physiological point of view, that the evidence for columnar organization is not nearly so clear in the auditory cortex as elsewhere, and I wonder if you have had an opportunity to look at that? Of course, the physiological experiments in that region are not as complete as they have been in the somatosensory and the visual cortex.

There is some evidence that the association cortex is organized in a similar way. We have found this to be true in areas 5 and 7, and I have seen in manuscript a paper from Hubel and Wiesel which describes a beautiful columnar organization in areas 18 and 19 of the visual cortex which parallels in extent that which they described earlier for area 17.

The function of the fusiform stellate cell is a revelation to me because I think it explains some other findings. If one is careful to orient the stimulus to the center of a peripheral receptive field, in all peripheral receptive fields encountered in such a penetration normal to the cortex, one finds that all the cells of the cortex make their initial discharge within 2 msec of the earliest discharge. This gives time for two synaptic transmissions, and fits very well with the connections that you describe for the fusiform cells.

There is one other matter I would like to raise here. We are faced with extraordinarily difficult problems in pursuing this any further; what one would like to do is to look at the relation between cells in different layers in sequential epochs of time. If we wish to know the total translation of activity between input and output within a column, one would like to record, of course, simultaneously from all these layers. Now, to do this—and we have tried this so far with electrodes with three leads—is extraordinarily difficult and we come up against the problem of the presence of the recording instrument modifying what one is seeing. Ideally, one would like to record from cells simultaneously in all layers from a tangential orientation, which is equally difficult, and I would like to know whether any physiologist in the room has any suggestions to make in this regard.

The last question I would like to put to you is whether or not we must include in this total picture of synaptic organization in the cerebral cortex the very clear dendritic connections which have been described by van der Loos and other people, and whether we have to include in our thinking what one might call an interaction between dendrites. I am committed on this myself, but I would like to know whether you have observed this very close relation of one dendrite to another, in the visual cortex.

COLONNIER: First in relation to the auditory cortex, I would like to say that it is interesting that in this region, Cajal has described an extremely large stellate cell possessing no spines and which he describes as typical of the auditory cortex. He calls it a "cellule géante spéciale." These cells are found through all layers of the auditory cortex, except layer I. The axon goes down to the white matter emitting horizontal and ascending collaterals on the way. They could conceivably mask the columnar organization in this area. I only say this because I am struck by the fact that you immediately choose to mention this one area where a "special" cell of large dimension is present.

With respect to the dendritic contacts, I am afraid that I am quite conservative in my criteria for identifying contacts on electron-micrographs. Let us not forget that we believe that the asymmetrical thickening of two apposed membranes and the presence of synaptic vesicles serve us to identify sites of synaptic contacts, because they were found at those sites where classical neuroanatomy had described synapses: in these circumstances the presynaptic bags containing the vesicles had the expected size and shape. Before we interpret simple contiguity as synaptic in nature, I think we should be very careful. If simple contiguity is sufficient evidence of synaptic contact, one could speak of glial contacts, of contacts on myelin sheaths, one could in fact say just about anything. I therefore rather take exception to this view until some definite proof is forthcoming.

MOUNTCASTLE: I would like to add other evidence that may fit very well with your findings: the measurement of the diameter of a column determined by tangential microelectrode penetrations, varies from the smallest diameter, as one goes across it, up to somewhere, I think, between 300 and 500 μ. I wonder if that would fit?

COLONNIER: Yes, that is in excellent agreement.

MOUNTCASTLE: And it varies a good bit, of course, because one hits this column at different angles.

BREMER: There are many things one would like to ask Dr. Colonnier after this beautiful presentation. I should like to ask him only one question. It concerns the synaptic organization between the thalamocortical afferent specific fibers and fusiform stellate cells of layers III and IV. Has one direct evidence of monosynaptic relation between the afferent fibers streaming from a thalamic relay nucleus, let us say, from the lateral geniculate to stellate cells? Or should this connection always involve short axon cells?

COLONNIER: The evidence that the specific afferents contact stellate cells of the fourth layer is indeed only indirect. The only method that I can think of which might give direct evidence would be degeneration experiments with the electron microscope, if one could find ultrastructural criteria to distinguish between pyramidal and stellate cells: That such criteria exist is a matter of pure speculation.

SPERRY: I did not understand your description of the reason for the oblique orientation of the synaptic relations there. You were speaking of the visual cortex and you referred to the tilt detectors described in the work of Hubel and Wiesel.

COLONNIER: Hubel and Wiesel have postulated that if a cell in the cortex responds to a slit in the visual field, this slit must be projected first on a linear series of points on the retina; these must be projected to a specific group of cells in the lateral geniculate and these in turn must then project to a cortical cell.

This projection of lateral geniculate cell axons to one cell of the cortex may be dependent exclusively upon the axonal trajectory. On the other hand, it could be the result of both axonal and dendritic orientation. The lateral geniculate axons are known to project in a rather strict topographical pattern to the cortex. If they are coming in this way into the fourth layer of the cortex, and the receptive cells have elongated dendritic trees in the plane of the projection, each cell may receive fibres which have such a spatial relation to each other that they represent the original linear series of points on the retina.

SPERRY: I was thinking you said that the oblique orientation corresponds to the orientation of the gyrus in which it is found.

COLONNIER: The point I wanted to make was that the long axis of the tangentially elongated stellate cells of the IVth layer of the visual cortex tend to be orientated mainly along the vertical axis of the cortical retina. This is the difficulty when one tries to relate these elongated fields to the work of

Hubel and Wiesel. They do not find that the slit-like visual fields of the cortical cells have a preferential orientation. The visual fields are orientated in all directions. I don't mean to imply that morphologically all dendritic fields are orientated only in one direction: they are also in all directions but they do tend to be more along the vertical axis than along other axes.

SPERRY: We tend to explain these relationships in terms of chemical gradients, of course, and that is why I was interested in your alternative explanation. The other question I was wondering about is: have you ever asked yourself to what extent this picture of cortical organization that you are working with is a product of growth and inheritance and to what extent it may be modified by use—that is, to what extent experience may add to the organization?

MOUNTCASTLE: There is a direct investigation done by Hubel and Wiesel on this point in which they examined the columnar organization in new-born animals, and in animals at different periods after birth which were exposed to normal patterned visual input, and those which were not allowed patterned visual input. They found that the highly organized columnar picture exists at birth but that it disappears unless the animal is continually exposed to patterned vision, which suggests that not only is the columnar organization given automatically, but also that it depends upon continued activation of these synaptic contacts.

PHILLIPS: The columns, of course, are very closely related to the input to the cortex where it actually enters; once the input has got into the cortex and been spatially segregated and organized within the columns, it then no doubt has to leak away from the columns if it is going to have any effect on any other part of the cortex or the central nervous system. It may be more difficult to detect activity spreading away from the column itself than to detect it within the column, where the input is very highly localized and very highly spatially organized in this vertical system.

Would you like to say something about how activity can escape from the columns? The recurrent and horizontal collaterals of pyramidal cells may be able to spread excitation.

You say that the stellate cells are probably inhibitory. Would you like to say a little more about the problem of horizontal spread of excitation?

COLONNIER: The influence would presumably be through association fibres which are going down towards the white matter and going up into another column. There may also be some axons coursing tangentially in layers other than I, which link columns together: very long axons of this type must be rather rare for the reasons I have presented today. For action at a great distance therefore it is safe to assume that the U fibres are probably most important.

REFERENCES

ANDERSEN, P., J. C. ECCLES, and Y. LØYNING. Recurrent inhibition in the hippocampus with identification of the inhibitory cells and its synapses, *Nature*, *198*, 541–542 [1963].

22 / M. L. Colonnier

ANDERSEN, P. Location of postsynaptic inhibitory synapses in hippocampal pyramids, *J. Neurophysiol.*, *27*, 592–607 [1964].

———, J. C. ECCLES, and P. E. VOORHOEVE. Inhibitory synapses on somas of Purkinje cells in the cerebellum, *Nature*, *199*, 655–656 [1963].

BOK, S. T. *Histonomy of the Cerebral Cortex*. Amsterdam: Elsevier [1959].

CLARK, W. E., LE GROS. Deformation patterns in the cerebral cortex, *Essays on Growth and Form*. Oxford: Clarendon Press, pp. 2–22 [1945].

COLONNIER, M. L. Experimental degeneration in the cerebral cortex, *J. Anat.*, *98*, 47–53 [1964*a*].

———. The tangential organization of the visual cortex, *J. Anat.*, *98*, 327–344 [1964*b*].

———, and R. W. GUILLERY. Synaptic organization in the lateral geniculate nucleus of the monkey, *Z. Zellfornschug*, *62*, 333–355 [1964].

CRAGG, B. G., and H. N. V. TEMPERLEY. The organization of neurones: A co-operative analogy, *Electroenceph. Clin. Neurophysiol.*, *6*, 85–92 [1954].

ECCLES, J. C., R. LLINÁS, and K. SASAKI. Excitation of cerebellar Purkinje cells by the climbing fibres, *Nature* (London), *203*, 245–246 [1964].

GRAY, E. G. Axosomatic and axodendritic synapses of the cerebral cortex: An electron microscopic study, *J. Anat.*, *93*, 420–433 [1959].

HUBEL, D. H., and T. N. WIESEL. Receptive fields, binocular interaction and functional architecture in the cat's visual cortex, *J. Physiol.* (London), *160*, 106–154 [1962].

LORENTE DE NÓ, R. La corteza cerebral del raton, *Trab. Lab. Invest. Biol.* (Univ. Madrid), *20*, 41–78 [1922].

MARSHALL, W. H., and S. A. TALBOT. Recent evidence for neural mechanisms in vision leading to a general theory of sensory acuity, *Biol. Symp.*, *7*, 117–164 [1942].

MOUNTCASTLE, V. B. Modalities and topographic properties of single neurons of cat's sensory cortex, *J. Neurophysiol.*, *20*, 408–434 [1957].

NAUTA, J. H. Terminal distribution of some afferent fiber systems in the cerebral cortex, *Anat. Record*, *118*, 333 [1954].

O'LEARY, J. L. Structure of area striata of the cat, *J. Comp. Neurol.*, *75*, 131–164 [1941].

RAMON MOLINER, E. Personal communication [1963].

RAMÓN Y CAJAL, S. *Histologie du Système Nerveux de l'Homme et des Vertébrés*. Vol. 2. Madrid: Consigno Superior de Investigaciones Cientificas. Instituto R. y Cajal, 1952; Paris [1911].

SHOLL, D. A. Dendritic organization in the neurons of the visual and motor cortices of the cat, *J. Anat.*, *87*, 387–406 [1953].

———. *The Organization of the Cerebral Cortex*. London: Methuen [1956].

SZENTÁGOTHAI, J. On the synaptology of the cerebral cortex (Russian; ed. by S. A. Sarkissov), *Structure and Function of the Nervous System*. Moscow: State Publishing House for Medical Literature, pp. 6–14 [1962].

———. The use of degeneration methods in investigation of short neuronal connexions (ed. by M. Singer and J. P. Schadé), *Progress in Brain Research*. Amsterdam: Elsevier, Vol. 14, pp. 1–30 [1964].

SZENTÁGOTHAI, J. Short connexions of the cerebral cortex, *Symposia Hungarica* (ed. by J. Szentágothai). Volume in honor of the 100th anniversary of the birth of v. Lenhossek. Budapest: Akadémiai Kiado [1965].

————. The synapses of short local-neurons in the cerebral cortex, *Symp. Biol. Hung.* 5, 251–276 [1965].

2

Cerebral Synaptic Mechanisms

by J. C. Eccles

*Institute for Biomedical Research, Education and
Research Foundation, American Medical Association,
Chicago, Illinois; formerly Professor of Physiology,
Australian National University, Canberra, Australia*

Introduction

Classical neurohistology revealed that the cerebral cortex is composed of nerve cells resembling in their essential features nerve cells at lower levels of the nervous system, but differing from these lower levels in the immense complexity of neuronal organization. We have just heard from Dr. Colonnier that the much finer structural features of synapses observed with electron microscopy have also shown a remark-able similarity through the whole nervous system; and this is particularly the case with chemically transmitting synapses. The presynaptic component contains synaptic vesicles and mitochondria and the 200 Å synaptic cleft is bounded by membranes displaying patches of thickening that may be assumed to be the active zones for chemical synaptic transmission. It would therefore be expected that physiological mechanisms of synaptic action would be comparable at all levels of the nervous system. There is as yet no evidence of electrical synaptic transmission at the higher levels of the central nervous system.

Until a decade ago electrophysiological investigations were restricted to the extracellular recording of spike potentials and field potentials in the cerebral cortex. It was generally postulated that the excitatory synapses acted by depolarizing the surface membranes of nerve cells and that spike potentials were generated when this depolarization reached a critical level. It was also postulated that inhibitory postsynaptic potentials were responsible for the suppression of impulse discharge that was observed under many conditions, Jung in particular being one of the

24

first to emphasize the importance of inhibitory synapses at the cerebral level [Jung and Baumgartner, 1955]. From 1955 onwards cortical neurons have been examined by the intracellular technique, so that in this present symposium we have the advantage of many systematic studies of cortical neurons, not only of the spike responses and the excitatory and inhibitory postsynaptic potentials, but also of biophysical properties of cortical pyramidal cells. As yet all this intracellular investigation has been restricted to the large pyramidal cells, for only these large cells tolerate microelectrode puncture. Those large pyramidal cells projecting into the pyramidal tract have been most intensively studied, but their responses are generally found to be not significantly different from the other large cortical pyramidal cells.

Biophysical Properties of Cortical Pyramidal Cells

There is agreement among the many investigators in this important field (Phillips, Li, Purpura, Klee, Lux, Creutzfeldt, Stefanis and Jasper, Kubota, and their various associates) that, so far as membrane and spike potentials are concerned, cortical neurons resemble those at the lower levels of the nervous system. In relatively uninjured pyramidal cells, recorded membrane potentials are between -50 and -70 mV and spike potentials range from 60 to 100 mV.

As in Fig. 2.1,A, antidromic potentials sometimes show an initial segment spike with an inflection leading on to the soma-dendritic spike. This inflection is accentuated during the relative refractory period (second response, Fig. 2.1,A), or as in the second response of B there may even be blockage of transmission into the soma and dendrites. Creutzfeldt, Lux, and Nacimiento [1964] did not find any sign of IS-SD separation with spike potentials generated either by depolarizing currents or by excitatory synapses. However, with deteriorated or strongly depolarized pyramidal cells (Fig. 2.1,E, the last two spikes) there appears to be evidence of blocked transmission into the soma-dendrite membrane.

By taking rigid precautions to exclude stimulation of fibers in adjacent tracts, Jabbur and Towe [1961] showed that a pyramidal tract volley evoked only a double positive wave on the surface of the motor cortex, an initial spike, and a later slower and smaller wave. All other potentials that have been described, as for example by Chang [1955], are due to afferent impulses evoking specific and nonspecific responses in the motor cortex. These results of Jabbur and Towe certainly show that antidromic impulses do not propagate all the way up the apical dendrites to their surface efflorescence.

Creutzfeldt, Lux, and Nacimiento [1964] have just completed a remarkable study of the effects produced by intracellular application of

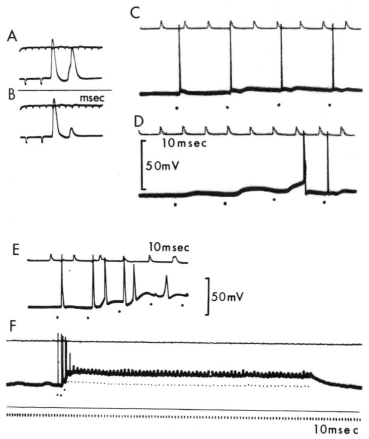

Fig. 2.1. Intracellular records of responses evoked in neocortical pyramidal cells in response to repetitive stimulation of the pyramidal tract. (A,B) Two antidromic impulses at 2.4 msec interval. In A there is a clear inflection on the rising phase indicating a delay in antidromic transmission between the initial segment (IS) and somadendrite (SD) components of the pyramidal cell, while in B the SD response failed. As indicated, the membrane potential was −49 mV. (C,D) Another cell with repetitive stimulation at 48 per sec, the stimulation being above threshold for the axon of the impaled cell in C, and below threshold for all but the last response in D. Time line is at zero potential. (E,F) Another cell with repetitive stimulation at 78 per sec to show build up of synaptically induced depolarization to a level at which antidromic spikes failed partially and then completely [Phillips, 1961].

currents to cortical pyramidal cells. In Fig. 2.2 electric currents of 200 msec duration and of the specified intensities were applied to a pyramidal tract cell. The responses very closely resemble those obtained by Granit, Kernell, and Shortess [1963] with the tonic variety of rat and cat motoneurons. The higher the applied current the greater the frequency of discharge, and it is also evident that during the first 70–100 msec there is a rapid decline of frequency (adaptation), which thereafter remains fairly stable. As shown in the lower curves of Fig. 2.3,A,B the adapted frequency is almost linearly dependent on current strength, just as reported by Granit et al [1963] for spinal motoneurons. All investigated cortical neurons gave similar responses with well-maintained discharge during the depolarizing currents, there being no examples of phasic-type responses as observed with spinal motoneurons. With linearly rising currents, the onset of discharge appeared at much the same current intensity over a wide range of steepness of rise, accommodation thus being negligible.

The responses of neurons to applied current enabled Creutzfeldt et al [1964] to measure the time constants of the neuronal membrane as seen by the intracellular electrode. For example, in Fig. 2.4,A there are tracings of the rise and decline both with subthreshold depolarizing (cf. Fig. 2.2,A) and with hyperpolarizing steady currents. It will be noticed that there is even an indication of a small accommodative recovery of membrane potential during continued current flow, as has

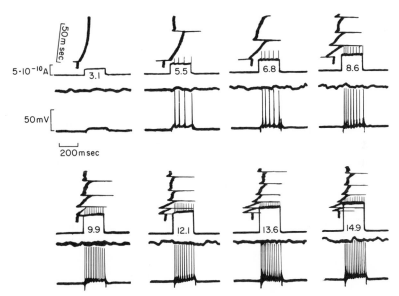

Fig. 2.2. Responses evoked in a pyramidal tract cell by the passage of brief rectangular current pulses through the intracellularly recording microelectrode. There are four traces for every current application, which are from above downwards: a fast intracellular potential on a vertical base line (below-upwards) shown by 50 msec time scale; the current pulse with intensity given in 10^{-10}A; the surface EEG record; the intracellular potential at a slower sweep and lower amplification than the vertical traces [Creutzfeldt, Lux, and Nacimiento, 1964].

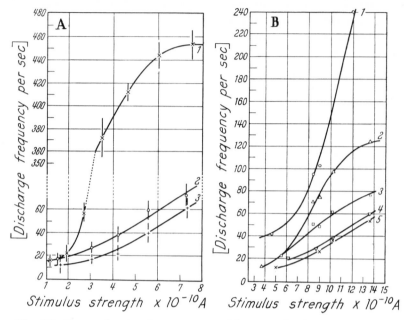

Fig. 2.3. Curves showing for two pyramidal tract cells the relationship of frequency of discharge to strength of applied intracellular current. In A, the interval between the first and second discharges is expressed as frequency in curve 1, while in curves 2 and 3 the respective frequencies are calculated from the intervals between two discharges at 30–40 msec and 160–200 msec after the onset of the applied current. In B, curve 1 is plotted for the latency of the first discharge expressed as a frequency, while curve 2 is for interval between the first and second discharges, and curves 3, 4, and 5 for two discharges at 30–40 msec, 80–100 msec, and 140–180 msec after the onset of the applied current [Creutzfeldt, Lux, and Nacimiento, 1964].

been described by Araki, Ito, and Oshima [1961] for cat motoneurons. The plottings in Fig. 2.4,B,C show that the potential changes at the onset and cessation of the currents follow approximate exponential curves from which time constants can be calculated, the mean value of the membrane electrical time constant as so determined being 8.5 msec. The potentials produced by subthreshold depolarizing currents and by hyperpolarizing currents enable the neuronal resistance to be calculated, the mean value being 28 megohms. The threshhold depolarization for impulse generation had a mean value of about 6 mV and the mean rheobasic current was 2.6×10^{-10} amp.

These biophysical investigations reveal that the large cortical pyramidal cells have many resemblances to spinal motoneurons. The 20-fold larger resistance can be accounted for in part by the much smaller surface area of the soma and proximal dendrites of pyramidal cells, which are the areas that would transmit the greater part of an electric current injected through an intrasomatic microelectrode. However, the time constant is about three times longer than with spinal motoneurons [Coombs, Curtis and Eccles, 1959], and presumably this is mainly due to a higher specific resistance of the surface membrane. The other important difference from spinal motoneurons consists in the small or

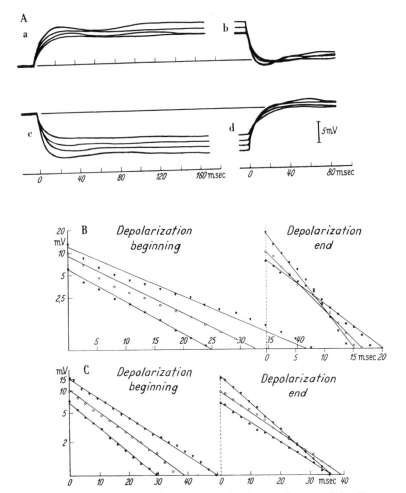

Fig. 2.4. Time courses of membrane potentials of cortical pyramidal cells at onset and cessation of rectangular current pulses of various intensities. (A) Superimposed tracings of onset and cessation of depolarizing pulses (*a, b*) and of hyperpolarizing pulses (*c, d*). (B,C) Semilogarithmic plottings of onset and cessation of three different intensities of depolarizing current for two different cells [Creutzfeldt, Lux, and Nacimiento, 1964].

negligible after-hyperpolarization that follows the spike [cf. Stefanis and Jasper, 1964a], as may be seen in Figs. 2.1 and 2.2. Earlier investigations employing antidromic activation of pyramidal cells showed spikes followed by a large hyperpolarization [Phillips, 1956a], but this has now been recognized as an inhibitory postsynaptic potential (IPSP). Because of the small size of the after-hyperpolarization, cortical pyramidal cells are able to fire at much higher frequencies than motoneurons, as may be seen in Fig. 2.3, where the highest maintained adapted frequencies were about 60 per sec. A high specific membrane resistance would be important in ensuring a more effective electrotonic transmission along the dendrites of pyramidal cells, though it has yet to be shown that the more peripheral zones of the dendritic membranes have such a high specific resistance.

SYNAPTIC ACTIONS ON CORTICAL NEURONS

The Synaptic Action of Axon Collaterals of Pyramidal Tract Cells

Besides the antidromic responses, stimulation exclusively applied to the pyramidal tract produces later potentials that are attributable to excitatory and inhibitory synaptic action [Phillips, 1959, 1961; Stefanis and Jasper, 1964a; Armstrong, 1965; Kubota and Takahashi, 1965; Kubota, Sakata, Takahashi, and Uno, 1965]. I will not consider the earlier investigations on the cortical responses evoked by pyramidal tract stimulation because, as already stated, adequate precautions were not taken to prevent the stimulation of afferent pathways, which themselves produce large cortical responses.

In Fig. 2.1,C depolarizing potentials can be seen following all antidromic spike potentials except the first. In Fig. 2.1,D the first three stimuli were below the threshold of the axon so that the excitatory postsynaptic potentials (EPSP's) with a latent period of about 5 msec were uncomplicated by antidromic spikes, though the third EPSP itself generated a spike discharge. With Fig. 2.1,E,F, still larger EPSP's were produced when the pyramidal tract stimulation was at the high frequency of 78 per sec. The EPSP's rapidly built up to a plateau of depolarization (20 mV) that was high enough partially to inactivate the spike mechanism of the last two spikes of Fig. 2.1,E, and thereafter suppressed all spikes (Fig. 2.1,F). Kubota and Takahashi [1965] found that the EPSP's were graded in size and had a duration of up to 70 msec, closely resembling EPSP's of motoneurons except for their slower time course.

In recent studies of synaptic action by antidromic pyramidal tract volleys, Armstrong [1965] found that, when measured from pyramidal stimulation in the brain stem, the latency of the EPSP ranged from 2.1

to 5 msec (mean 3 msec); and an almost identical mean value (3.2 msec) was found by Stefanis and Jasper [1964a]. Since this EPSP followed frequencies up to 200 per sec, Armstrong concluded that the initial component is monosynaptic, though presumably there are later polysynaptic additions. Thus it is envisaged that the axon collaterals from pyramidal cells give excitatory synapses directly to adjacent pyramidal cells as well as to interneurons, which would be a variety of the cortical stellate cells that were originally described by Ramón y Cajal [1911] and later by Sholl [1956] and Colonnier [1966]. Often brief repetitive pyramidal stimulation is required for evoking the EPSP's, hence Stefanis and Jasper [1964a] conclude that the pathway from the axon collaterals is usually via one or more interneurons. On the other hand, Kubota and

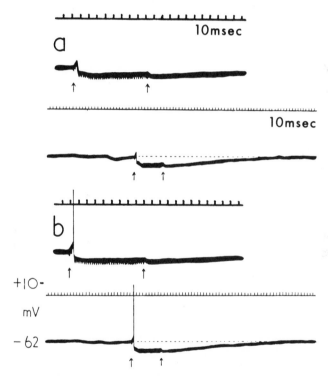

Fig. 2.5. Intracellular records of inhibitory postsynaptic potentials evoked by repetitive pyramidal tract stimulation that did not stimulate the axon of the impaled cell. In *a* are fast and slow records of the same response to repetitive stimulation at 420 per sec applied between the two arrows. Note the brief initial EPSP. In *b* this initial EPSP was larger and evoked a spike discharge just at onset of the IPSP. Note the very slow recovery of the IPSP after the stimulation in the slow traces of both *a* and *b*. In *b*, membrane potential of −62 mV was reversed to +10 V at summit of the spike [Phillips, 1959].

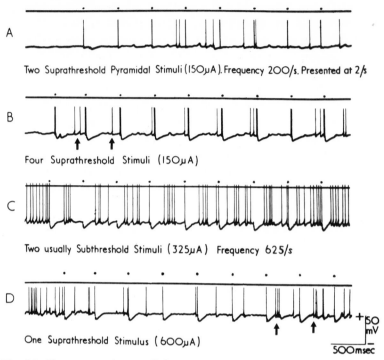

A

Two Suprathreshold Pyramidal Stimuli (150μA). Frequency 200/s. Presented at 2/s

B

Four Suprathreshold Stimuli (150μA)

C

Two usually Subthreshold Stimuli (325μA) Frequency 625/s

D

One Suprathreshold Stimulus (600μA)

+50 mV

500 msec

Fig. 2.6. Slow traces of intracellular responses evoked in pyramidal tract cells by repetitive stimulation of the pyramidal tract. The tract stimulation was repeated every 500 msec at the times indicated by the dots above each tracing. This stimulation was repetitive in A (two at 5 msec), in B (four at 5 msec) and in C (two at 1.6 msec), and subthreshold or suprathreshold (as indicated) for the axon of the impaled cell. In C and D the cell was spontaneously rhythmic [Armstrong, 1965].

Takahashi [1965] ascribe the long latency to the slow conduction velocity in the pyramidal tract fibers that were responsible for evoking the EPSP, there being as a consequence only time for monosynaptic action in the cortex.

Antidromic pyramidal tract volleys also produce large and prolonged IPSP's of pyramidal cells [Phillips, 1961; Stefanis and Jasper, 1964a, 1964b; Armstrong, 1965; Kubota, Sakata, Takahashi, and Uno, 1965]. In Fig. 2.5, brief repetitive stimulation below the threshold for the axon of a pyramidal cell produced an IPSP of about 0.5 sec duration. Actually in Fig. 2.5,B an initial synaptic excitation generated a spike. In Fig. 2.6 there are examples of IPSP's produced in several pyramidal tract cells by 1, 2, or 4 antidromic volleys. These IPSP's have a duration of 100–200 msec and are produced by stimulation that is either subthreshold or suprathreshold for the axon of the impaled pyramidal cell. Single stimuli failed to produce an IPSP in many units, but with brief repetitive stimulation IPSP's were always produced. Evidently synaptic facilitation is required for the effective production of IPSP's. The latency of action of the IPSP's is 4–7 msec for single volleys, but shortens considerably with repetitive stimulation so that there is time for no more than one interpolated interneuron. Comparable results have been reported by Stefanis and Jasper [1964a]. These several investigators have further presented evidence derived from laminar field analysis that the inhibitory synapses are concentrated on the soma of the pyramidal cells, which makes them comparable with the inhibitory synapses of basket cells on hippocampal pyramidal cells. One can envisage that the axon collaterals of pyramidal cells are only sparsely distributed to inhibitory interneurons and that most of the inhibitory action is due to polysynaptic paths, probably through excitatory stellate cells. With repetitive stimulation

NEOCORTEX
RECURRENT INHIBITION

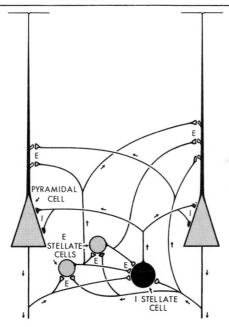

Fig. 2.7. Diagram showing postulated synaptic connections of axon collaterals of pyramidal cells. The single inhibitory interneuron together with its inhibitory synapses on the somata of the pyramidal cells are shown in black. All other stellate cells and the pyramidal cells are assumed to be excitatory and are shown open. The arrows indicate directions of impulse propagation. Note that, as suggested by the experimental evidence, both the excitatory and inhibitory pathways can include interpolated excitatory interneurons.

the residual facilitation at the various synapses results in a shortening of the inhibitory pathway. Stefanis and Jasper [1964a] and Armstrong [1965] found that IPSP's as large as 10 mV were produced in pyramidal cells with a resting potential of -50 to -60 mV, and the duration of the IPSP's varied from 50–200 msec, sometimes, as in Fig. 2.6, terminating in what appears to be a small rebound discharge which is indicated by arrows.

Evidently, as shown diagrammatically in Fig. 2.7, axon collaterals of pyramidal cells have very complex pathways leading to excitatory and inhibitory synaptic actions on pyramidal cells. These pathways become particularly effective at relatively high frequencies of repetitive activation. However, it will be realized that pyramidal cells often fire at frequencies giving such potentiated synaptic action. Hence these experiments demonstrate the existence of important positive and negative feedback controls of pyramidal cell activity.

Specific Responses of the Somatosensory Area of the Cerebral Cortex

Nerve Stimulation

An afferent volley from a peripheral nerve evokes a diphasic potential on the surface of the somatosensory cortex, an initial positivity and a later negativity [Adrian, 1941; Marshall, Woolsey, and Bard, 1941; Amassian, 1952]. By recording intracellularly from pyramidal cells in this area [Li, 1961], it has been shown that the initial positive wave is concurrent with an EPSP that often rises to generate one or two spike discharges (Fig. 2.8,A,B). The EPSP has a characteristic very long time course of about 80 msec, which can be particularly well seen when the cell deteriorates so that there is eventually no complicating spike discharge (Fig. 2.8,C,D,E). Thus pyramidal cells behave in a typical manner to synaptic stimulation. Probably the initial phase of the EPSP is generated monosynaptically by the specific thalamocortical impulses. The slow rise and long time course of the EPSP in part may be due to a large temporal dispersion in transmission from the periphery and to the relatively long time constant of the neuronal membrane [Creutzfeldt et al, 1964], but it may be necessary also to postulate a prolonged transmitter action, as with many synapses in the central nervous system [Eccles, 1964]. Another factor delaying the decline of the EPSP could be electrotonic transmission from remote dendritic synapses [Rall, 1959, 1960; Eccles, 1961].

A laminar field analysis with penetrating microelectrode recording [Amassian, Patton, Woodbury, Towe, and Schlag, 1955] shows that the

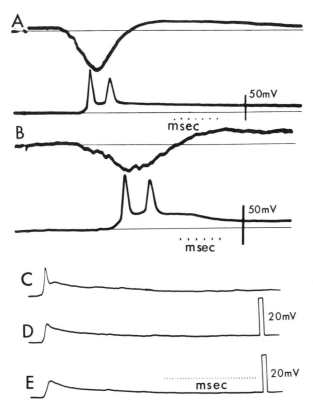

Fig. 2.8. Responses evoked by single stimulation of the superficial radial nerve. In A, B the upper traces are from the surface of the somatosensory cortex, showing the typical diphasic (positive-negative) response, while the lower traces are the simultaneously recorded intracellular potentials from two pyramidal cells in the same area. C, D, E are intracellular responses similarly evoked in a pyramidal cell during progressive deterioration that eventually resulted (E) in failure of the spike response [Li, 1961].

initial surface positivity is in fact attributable to the excitatory synaptic action of the pyramidal cells in the region of the fourth layer, where there are the profuse branches and brushes of the thalamocortical fibers and a wealth of synaptic endings deep on the apical dendrites of the pyramidal cells [Ramón y Cajal, 1911; Chang, 1952]. Depolarization at this level gives an active sink with a passive source from the more superficial levels of the apical dendrites. There is still much unresolved difference of opinion in regard to the exact level of the active sinks [cf. Amassian, 1961], some observers [Mountcastle, Davies, and Berman, 1957] locating the depolarizing synaptic action more superficially, at 200

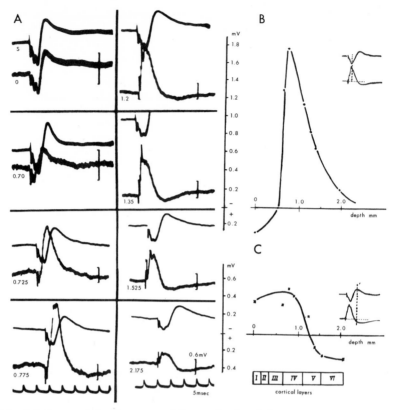

Fig. 2.9. Potential distribution in different depths of the somatosensory cortex in response to a single stimulation of the ventralis posterior nucleus of the thalamus. In A the upper traces give the potential at the cortical surface, while the lower traces were recorded by a microelectrode at the indicated depths below the surface. In B is the depth profile measured for a series of such traces at the time of the peak of the surface positive potential (see inset). In C is the depth profile similarly plotted, but at the time of the peak of the surface negative potential. The rectangles below indicate the cortical layers for the depth scales in B and C [Li, Cullen, and Jasper, 1956a].

to 250 μ. It is possible that deterioration of the superficial layers of the cortex may result in a deeper location of the sinks as suggested by Mountcastle et al [1957]. However, the superficial depolarization that they observed has a longer latency than the surface positive wave which is the counterpart of the deep negativity in Fig. 2.9. Hence the findings of Mountcastle et al may be interpreted as arising because there is a later extension of synaptic excitation to more superficial levels of the cortex, presumably on account of interneuronal activity.

Stimulation of Specific Thalamic Nuclei (nucleus ventralis posterolateralis, nucleus ventralis posteromedialis, nucleus ventralis lateralis: VPL, VPM, and VL; and the lateral geniculate nucleus)

A single stimulation of the specific thalamic nuclei produces surface potentials localized to the ipsilateral somatosensory area. Just as with peripheral nerve stimulation, the surface potential has a diphasic (positive-negative) configuration (Fig. 2.9,A, upper traces). Intracellular recording (Fig. 2.10); [Li, 1963; Klee and Offenloch, 1964; Purpura, Shofer, and Musgrave, 1964; Nacimiento, Lux, and Creutzfeldt, 1964] shows that, concurrent with the surface positive wave, there are EPSP's of pyramidal cells with superimposed spike discharges resembling responses to peripheral nerve stimulation (Fig. 2.8). Likewise, the initial components of these EPSP's are probably monosynaptic.

By using laminar field analysis, Li, Cullen, and Jasper [1956a] showed that a single thalamic stimulation produces a large negative field potential in the fourth layer of the cortex (maximum at 0.8–1.2 mm in Fig. 2.9), which is synchonous with the initial surface positivity. A similar potential profile was found by Spencer and Brookhart [1961], who show in addition spike discharges superimposed on the negative potential wave in the fourth and fifth layers of the cortex. It can certainly be concluded therefore that synaptic excitatory action on the pyramidal cell dendrites at the level of the fourth layer causes the initial phase of the laminar field, namely, a superficial positivity and a deep negativity, exactly as with nerve stimulation. The laminar field further shows that the later superficial negativity reverses to a deep positivity at a depth of about 1 mm (Fig. 2.9,C). Possibly there are two synaptic mechanisms producing this wave, namely, excitatory synapses at the superficial levels of the apical dendrites and inhibitory synapses at the level of the pyramidal cell bodies. A further analysis is required in order to assess the relative contributions of these two mechanisms.

When the specific thalamic nuclei are repetitively stimulated at about 6–10 a sec (Fig. 2.10,D), there is the so-called "augmenting response" of these specific thalamic actions, as first described by Dempsey and Morison [1943] and Morison and Dempsey [1943]. By a careful comparison of intracellular potentials and surface potentials, Klee and Offenloch [1964] showed that the augmenting response was compounded of two EPSP's of pyramidal cells (Figs. 2.10,D; 2.11,A,B,D,E), usually separated by a trough of repolarization and followed by an IPSP, and similar observations have been made by Nacimiento, Lux, and Creutzfeldt [1964]. These three components, particularly the second EPSP, increased during repetitive stimulation at frequencies up to 10 per sec.

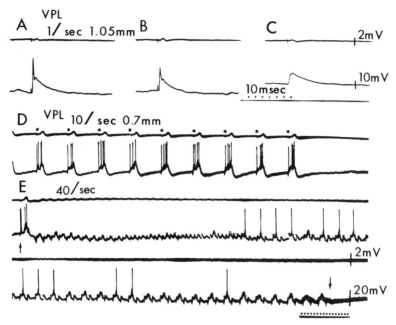

Fig. 2.10. Potentials evoked in the somatosensory cortex by stimulation of the VPL nucleus of the thalamus. (A–C) Lower traces are intracellular records from a pyramidal cell at a depth of 1.05 mm, while upper traces are the potentials at the cortical surface. The membrane potential declined from −50 mV in A to −40 mV in C and correspondingly there was failure of the spike potentials as in Fig. 2.8, C to E. D, E are similar traces from another pyramidal cell (depth 0.7 mm) evoked by repetitive stimulations at 10 per sec and 40 per sec respectively. In E the arrows signal beginning and end of the repetitive stimulation. In D the initial EPSP with superimposed spikes is followed by a prolonged IPSP, while in E the IPSP is maintained during the whole duration of the stimulation [Li, 1963].

The earliest EPSP is, of course, the specific response observed with single stimulation. Klee and Offenloch [1964] suggest that the later EPSP and the IPSP are due to more complex pathways recruited into action by the repetitive stimulation and really correspond to the recruiting responses produced by the nonspecific thalamic stimulation that will be considered below. Similar suggestions had already been made by Jankowska and Albe-Fessard [1961] and also for the visual pathway by Bishop, Clare, and Landau [1961]. Probably, in addition to the direct sensory pathway, there is a separate polysynaptic afferent path from the thalamus with more superficial excitatory synapses on the pyramidal cells giving the negative surface potential that becomes so prominent a feature with augmenting responses.

The intracellularly recorded IPSP's (Figs. 2.10,D; 2.11,A,B) have a relatively late onset (latent period 5–10 msec) and a long duration 80–200 msec [Li, 1963; Lux and Klee, 1963; Klee and Offenloch, 1964; Nacimiento et al, 1964]. There is excellent correspondence between the time courses of this directly observed IPSP and of the depressed excitability of pyramidal tract cells observed by Brookhart and Zanchetti [1956]. Sometimes this IPSP seems to be followed by a rebound spike discharge (Fig. 2.11,B) that somewhat resembles the observation with single and repetitive stimulation of thalamocortical relay cells [Anderson, Eccles, and Sears, 1964]. It will be recognized that such rebound thalamic

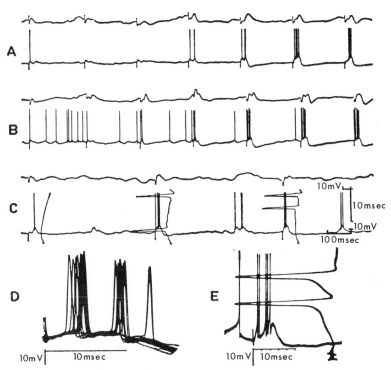

Fig. 2.11. Intracellular recordings of two neurons in the motor cortex showing different stages of the developing postsynaptic potentials during augmenting responses. Stimulus frequency of the specific thalamic nucleus: 2 per sec in C, 4.5 per sec in the other recordings. In A to C the upper trace shows the EEG (negativity upward), and the lower trace shows the intracellular potential; C shows the first 15 msec of the stimulus responses, also vertically, in a large time scale; D shows the relative constancy of the discharges of the first spike group; ten single traces are superimposed. (E) Postsynaptic potentials and spike pattern of fully developed augmenting response with clear repolarization after about 10 msec. The vertical sweep in larger time scale shows only the first two discharges [Klee and Offenloch, 1964].

discharges could contribute to the delayed discharges observed in pyramidal cells.

When the specific thalamic stimulation is at a relatively high frequency, for example, 50 a sec (Fig. 2.10,E), [Li, 1963], there is a prolonged IPSP of the pyramidal cells and suppression of all discharges. At the same time there is a prolonged surface negative potential. Certainly these results suggest that in part the surface negative potential of the specific response arises because of the passive superficial sinks relative to the deep active sources produced by the IPSP's. It remains to be discovered how far the IPSP's of specific thalamic responses are due to the recurrent collaterals acting on pyramidal cells, presumably via interneurons (Fig. 2.7), and how far they are due to the afferent fibers acting via polysynaptic paths. In Fig. 2.10,E the IPSP is maintained despite cessation of pyramidal cell discharge, so presumably it is produced by afferent collateral pathways. Purpura and Shofer [1964a] have applied hyperpolarizing pulses to the intracellularly recorded pyramidal cells in order to define more effectively the precise relationship of inhibitory and excitatory synaptic actions. The IPSP is, of course, identified by its inversion to a depolarizing potential by a sufficiently large hyperpolarizing pulse. There was a great variability in the EPSP-IPSP relationship of different pyramidal cells, but the IPSP always had a much longer latent period—usually it was more than 10 msec.

When antidromic activation from the pyramidal tract is used in identification of pyramidal tract cells, Purpura, Shofer, and Musgrave [1964] have shown that these cells respond very effectively to specific thalamic stimulation. This provides direct evidence for the fast pathway from specific thalamic nuclei to the pyramidal tract via the cerebral cortex [Brookhart and Zanchetti, 1956; Purpura and Housepian, 1961; Towe and Zimmermann, 1962]. However, those pyramidal cells not projecting down the pyramidal tract respond similarly to the tract cells, and presumably are the means of distribution of sensory information within the cortex.

Nacimiento et al [1964] have examined the time course of the EPSP and IPSP in relation to the measured membrane time constant of the same pyramidal cell. The time course of the VPL EPSP is very little slower than would be expected with passive decay of a potential across the membrane. For example, in Fig. 2.10,C the time constant of decay of the EPSP is longer, but not greatly so, than the mean time constant (8.5 msec) determined by Creutzfeldt et al [1964]. On the other hand, the time constant of decay of the IPSP (cf. Figs. 2,10,D; 2.11,B) is always many times longer than the membrane time constant, mean values being 56 and 8.5 msec respectively. Evidently there is a very prolonged action of the inhibitory synaptic transmitter, a possible ex-

planation being the limitation imposed by perisynaptic barriers on its
diffusion out of the synaptic cleft. There is a similar large discrepancy
between the time constants of decay of the IPSP and of passive polarizations of the hippocampal pyramidal cells [Kandel, Spencer, and Brinley,
1961; Spencer and Kandel, 1961].

Stimulation of Nonspecific Thalamic Nuclei (usually nucleus centrum
medianum (CM), but also the intralaminar nuclei and nucleus reuniens)

Stimulation of nonspecific thalamic nuclei gives rise to potentials
widely dispersed over the cortical surface [Morison and Dempsey, 1942;
Bremer, 1958; Albe-Fessard, 1957]. These potentials are small or negligible for single stimuli, but recruit with repetitive stimulation, and
characteristically there is a long latency negative wave with little or no
preceding positivity (Fig. 2.12,A,B); [Dempsey and Morison, 1942a,
1942b; Li, Cullen, and Jasper, 1956b; Li, 1963]. With intracellular recording from pyramidal cells (Fig. 2.12), [Li, 1963] there is an EPSP of

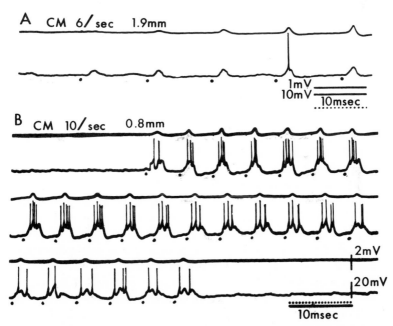

Fig. 2.12. Potentials evoked in the somatosensory cortex by stimulation of the
CM nucleus of the thalamus. (A) Upper trace is surface potential and the lower is
intracellular record from a cortical pyramidal cell at 1.9 mm depth. The interval
between the two horizontal lines gives 1 mV for upper trace and 10 mV for lower
trace. Dots signal stimuli at 6 per sec. (B) Similar to A, but in another pyramidal
cell at 0.8 mm depth and with stimulation at 10 per sec. The tracings are continuous
in the three successive bands [Li, 1963].

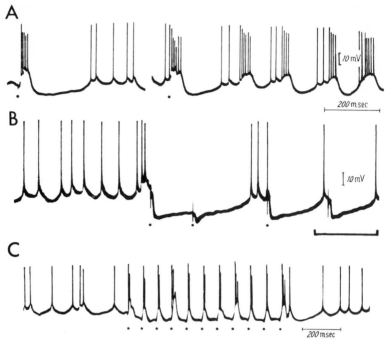

Fig. 2.13. Intracellular recording from a pyramidal cell in the neocortex with stimulation of the unspecific thalamus (centre median, CM). In A to C the dots signal the stimulations. Same potential scale for all traces [Lux and Klee, 1963].

irregular configuration synchronous with the surface negatively, and on it there may be spikes superimposed (Figs. 2.12,B, 2.13), [Albe-Fessard and Buser, 1955; Lux and Klee, 1963]. Following this EPSP and spikes, there is often a prolonged and large IPSP (Fig. 2.13,A,B). This deep IPSP contributes to the later phases of the large surface negativity of the recruiting responses [Li, 1963]. There is also evidence in Fig. 2.13 of a rebound discharge following each IPSP, and in A there is even a sequence of IPSP's and rebound discharges just as with the thalamus [Andersen, Eccles, and Sears, 1964; Andersen and Sears, 1964]; hence it can be presumed that the repetitive sequence of responses is actually generated in the thalamus, the cortex merely responding to the thalamic burst discharges.

Purpura and Shofer [1964a] use a hyperpolarizing current pulse in order to identify IPSP's. In this way it is shown that the relationship of EPSP to IPSP is much more variable than with specific thalamic stimulation and, of course, the latencies are much longer. Evidently very complex neuronal pathways are involved.

Using a laminar field analysis, Spencer and Brookhart [1956a] show

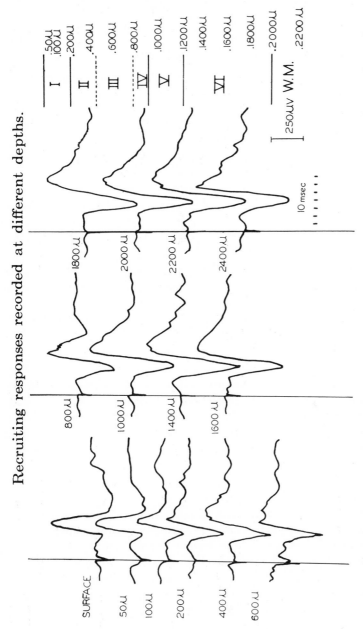

Fig. 2.14. Recruiting responses evoked by repetitive stimulation of the nucleus reuniens at 6 per sec and recorded at the specified depths in the anterior sigmoid gyrus. To the right there is a scale showing the depth profile for the various cortical layers [Spencer and Brookhart, 1961a].

that there is reversal of the superficial negative wave at a depth of 100–400 μ (Fig. 2.14). Deeper than this it is replaced by a large positive wave of similar time course. Li, Cullen, and Jasper [1956b] described a somewhat similar laminar field except that in their Fig. 3 there is an enormous positive wave at about 1 mm depth. Possibly this is due to injury, as it was only observed on a few occasions.

This laminar field analysis together with the intracellular recording indicates that the nonspecific cortical response begins with EPSP's of apical dendrites at a very superficial level. This depolarization may give rise to a discharge of impulses that are observed, however, only at greater depths, being then superimposed on the positive wave at these depths [Li, Cullen, and Jasper, 1956b, Fig. 6]. When pyramidal cells in the motor cortex are subdivided according to whether they do or do not have axons in the pyramidal tract, it is found that the tract cells are much more excited by nonspecific afferents than are the non-tract cells [Purpura, Shofer, and Musgrave, 1964]. Thus recruiting responses also will lead to pyramidal tract discharges, and these have been recorded by several investigators [Arduini and Whitlock, 1953; Purpura and Housepian, 1961; Spencer and Brookhart, 1961b]. These pyramidal tract discharges have long latency and the duration of burst responses; they recruit *pari passu* with the negative potentials led from the cortical surface.

Creutzfeldt and Lux [1964] have investigated the effect of membrane potential changes on the specific and nonspecific intracellular potentials. They find that specific EPSP's are increased by hyperpolarization and decreased by depolarization in an approximately linear manner, which suggests that the excitatory synapses are close to the location of the microelectrode in the pyramidal cell soma. By contrast, the nonspecific potentials are but little changed by polarizing currents and, in particular, hyperpolarization does not increase them. It therefore seems likely that nonspecific EPSP's are generated remotely from the soma, which is in good accord with the laminar field studies. Chang [1952] recognized two zones of thalamocortical terminals in the cerebral cortex superficial and at layer IV.

In conclusion one can state that specific afferents from the thalamus have excitatory synapses on pyramidal cells close to the soma, presumably on the apical dendrites and in layer IV of the cortex, as illustrated in Fig. 2.15. At least some of this excitatory action is monosynaptic. On the contrary, nonspecific afferents have a complex polysynaptic pathway and form synapses much more superficially on the apical dendrites. However, it has now been recognized that these two types are not sharply differentiated [cf. Buser, 1964]; and, particularly with the augmenting responses produced by repetitive specific thalamic stimulation, there is much contamination by polysynaptic pathways resembling those re-

NEOCORTEX

AFFERENT COLLATERAL INHIBITION

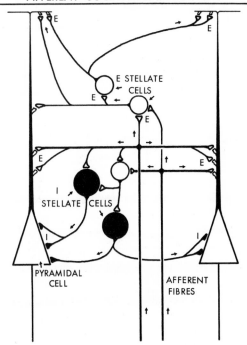

Fig. 2.15. Diagram with same convention as in Fig. 2.7, but showing postulated connections of specific afferent fibers to the neocortical pyramidal cells. Note that the inhibitory path is through inhibitory cells that are activated either directly by the afferent fibers or by mediation of excitatory interneurons. Also note the various degrees of complexity of the excitatory pathways to the pyramidal cells.

sponsible for nonspecific effects. The pathways for inhibition are not yet identified, but seem to act mainly but not entirely in the region of the soma. It seems that some of the pathway is via afferent collaterals, but pyramidal axon collaterals presumably also exert an inhibitory action via interneurons.

Surface Stimulation of Cerebral Cortex

Surface stimulation of the cerebral cortex gives rise to the surface negative wave that spreads for as far as 5 mm from the site of stimulation [Adrian, 1936; Burns, 1950; Chang, 1951; Brooks and Enger, 1959]. Intracellular recording (Fig. 2.16,A,D) shows that this surface negative wave is associated with an EPSP and often with superimposed spike potentials [Phillips, 1956b; Li and Chou, 1962]. Also, if the stimulus is strong there is a later IPSP with a latency as brief as 7.5 msec after the

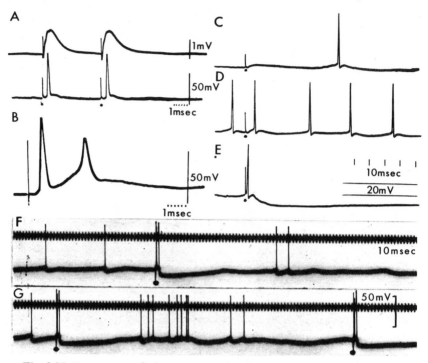

Fig. 2.16. Responses evoked in neocortex by direct stimulation of the cortex by a surface electrode within 3 mm of the recording electrode. (A) Two stimuli evoked surface negative waves (upper trace) and also intracellular spike potentials of a subjacent pyramidal cell (lower trace). (B) Intracellular potential similarly evoked in another pyramidal cell. (C,D,E) Intracellular responses of a pyramidal cell to graded surface stimulation by a stimulus of 1 msec duration. The interval between the parallel lines gives 20 mV [Li and Chou, 1962]. (F) Intracellular responses evoked in a pyramidal cell by surface stimulation (focal cathodal stimulus, 10 msec in duration, 1.0 mA) 4.5 mm away. Stimuli are signaled by dots and produce an initial spike discharge, as in Fig. 2.16A,B,D,E, followed by a large prolonged IPSP as in E [Phillips, 1961].

local stimulus (Fig. 2.16,E,G). During the IPSP there is suppression of spontaneous firing, but there may be a rebound discharge as the IPSP declines (Fig. 2.16,G).

Laminar field potentials show that this EPSP is generated by a synaptic excitatory action that is relatively superficial on the apical dendrites and that there is a deep source to this superficial sink. The EPSP's have such a short latency that they must be monosynaptically generated by nerve fibers that are directly excited. Possibly the principal presynaptic components are those axons of stellate cells that run a superficial course of several millimeters [Sholl, 1956]. When not cut short by an IPSP, the

EPSP has a long duration which, however, need not imply a prolonged transmitter action; the relatively long time constant of the membrane [Creutzfeldt et al, 1964], together with a synaptic action on dendrites remote from the soma, may provide an adequate explanation. Presumably, as with specific thalamic responses, the IPSP's are produced both by transmission via the axon collaterals of pyramidal cells acting via interneurons, and by activation of inhibitory interneurons through interneuronal paths.

Excitatory Synaptic Action and Dendritic Local Responses

It has been suggested [Clare and Bishop, 1955; Bishop, 1958] that in the apical dendrites of cortical cells the synaptically induced depolarization may evoke partial spike responses that greatly aid the electrotonic spread of the depolarization to the soma or adjacent axon where the propagated impulse is initiated. This suggestion is particularly valuable because it provides a mechanism whereby the remote synapses on the apical dendrites of a pyramidal cell can contribute effectively to the generation of an impulse at the axon-soma region. With intracellular recording from the pyramidal cells of the hippocampus, Spencer and Kandel [1961b] have shown that synaptic excitation of the apical dendrites generates local responses which propagate to the soma and may produce sufficient depolarization to initiate the discharge of an impulse, just as occurs with chromatolysed motoneurons [Eccles, Libet, and Young, 1958].

In Fig. 2.17, local responses can be seen in cortical pyramidal cells [Purpura and Shofer, 1964a]. For example, in A and B the arrows show either a local response on its own or a local response later generating a full spike potential. Isolated local responses can also be seen when the membrane is hyperpolarized in E and F, whereas otherwise they can be seen preceding the full spike potentials. More recently Purpura and Shofer [1964b] have shown that these local responses, presumably arising in the dendrites, are much more common in kittens (Fig. 2.18); and, in fact, the spontaneous discharges of all sizes of partial responses as well as the full spike potentials can be seen, the inflections indicating the transitions being marked in G by the horizontal arrows. They assume that spike potentials such as *b* are responses of the initial segments, whereas in *e* there is a transition from an IS to a SD spike. In *d* the lower arrow points to the transition from a local response to a full spike.

Purpura and Shofer [1964b] state that such partial spike potentials are much rarer in neocortical pyramidal cells in adult animals. However,

I would suggest that possibly these spike potentials may be in dendrites so remote from the soma that with intracellular recording they are not recognizable as local responses because of their great slowing by electrotonic distortion, and may well be regarded as elements of excitatory synaptic potentials. If there are no local responses along the apical dendritic tree, it is difficult to see how excitatory synaptic actions exerted at a distance as great as 2 mm from the soma can have any appreciable influence on the generation of an impulse discharge, though according to Pappas and Purpura [1961] there are relatively few synapses on the terminal efflorescence of an apical dendrite. Before concluding that, in the adult, dendritic local responses are of little significance in the generation of pyramidal cell discharge, it is certainly desirable to test for their existence by a more appropriate technique than the intracellular recording from the distant somas of the pyramidal cells. The existence of local and propagated spike potentials in the dendritic branches of Purkinje cells has been revealed by extracellular recording at a very superficial level of the molecular layer of the cerebellum [Eccles, Llinás, and Sasaki,

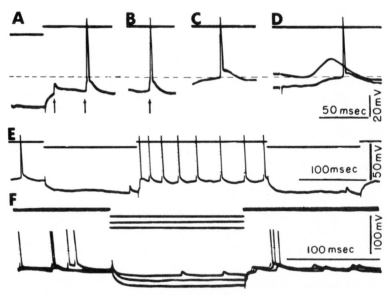

Fig. 2.17. Intracellularly recorded spike potentials in pyramidal cells of the anterior sigmoid gyrus of cats to show partial spike responses that may trigger full spike potentials. In A, B the arrows show partial spikes often leading onto full spikes, but this was not observed in C and D. In E a weak hyperpolarizing current blocked the full spikes, but during each current pulse there was one partial spike. In F, superimposed traces illustrate blockage of spikes and then of partial spikes with hyperpolarizing current pulses of increasing strength (0.25 to 0.6 μA) [Purpura and Shofer, 1964a].

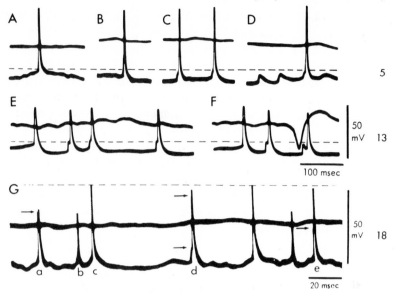

Fig. 2.18. Intracellularly recorded spike potentials in pyramidal cells of the sensorimotor cortex of kittens. A to D, 5 days old; E and F, 13 days old; G, 18 days old. Note the various sizes of partial spike responses either alone or preceding the full spike potentials. Inflections are indicated by horizontal arrows in G [Purpura and Shofer, 1964b].

1966], and a similar technique should be employed to test for local spike potentials in the dendrites of cortical pyramidal cells.

POSTSCRIPT

This brief survey of cerebral synapses has been focused onto the somatosensory and motor areas of the cerebral cortex, but it will be generally agreed that the synaptic mechanisms of other areas of the neocortex are essentially similar, and Dr. Andersen will next be reviewing the archicortex. As a generalization it can be stated that the excitatory and inhibitory synapses resemble in their essential features the synapses in the spinal cord. For example, the inhibitory synaptic transmitter may be assumed to act by increasing the permeability of the subsynaptic membrane to potassium and chloride ions. However, it differs from the inhibitory transmitter at many locations in the spinal cord in that its action is not blocked by strychnine [Crawford, Curtis, Voorhoeve, and Wilson, 1963]. There has as yet been no evidence for the existence of presynaptic inhibition in the cerebral cortex: electron microscopy has not revealed any axo-axonic synapses (Gray, personal communication);

and there is no physiological evidence for presynaptic inhibition, though admittedly further investigation is desirable.

I have endeavored to give an account of the elementary components of brain action—of synapses, of nerve cells, and of some simple patterns of neuronal interconnection. With remarkable insight Sherrington grasped the essential character of the neuronal mechanism of the brain, namely, power of integration beyond all imagining; and has inspired many neurophysiologists of this generation, notably Bremer and Fessard. In this present symposium we will be searching for new insights in our efforts to understand the nervous system. We can envisage this task as an effort to put together an enormous jigsaw puzzle. I have outlined some elementary functional components as they are at present understood, neurons linked by excitatory and inhibitory synapses into simple patterns that appear to have functional meaning.

DISCUSSION

Chairman: PROFESSOR PENFIELD

CHAIRMAN: Dr. Phillips would you like to open this discussion?

PHILLIPS: I just want to know how convinced Eccles really is about the partial responses of dendrites in the neocortex. As I remember, when Kandel and Spencer described the fast prepotential in some pyramidal cells of the hippocampus, they distinguished the fast prepotential as something that did not form part of an antidromic impulse, but occurred in response only to orthodromic stimulation. It was not, therefore, an impulse in the axon (M spike) and so was probably a spike which arose at a bifurcation of the apical dendrite of the pyramidal cell. In that picture of Purpura's that you showed, there was no antidromic impulse for comparison, and I wonder if you have more evidence on this point.

ECCLES: I don't know any more about the neocortex, but I do know about the Purkinje cells in the cerebellum, where, in the great branching dendritic tree, local responses may be generated at many sites. These impulses may grow up to propagate, and they can be inhibited at their site of initiation in the dendritic tree. Dr. Andersen will be giving evidence for propagated impulses in the dendrites of hippocampal pyramidal cells, which can be so much more easily investigated than in the neocortex, because there you have the cell bodies all at one level and the apical dendrites all in parallel. I agree with you that we should try much harder with the neocortex to look for local responses.

CREUTZFELDT: I should like to add some new observations to the material that has been presented by Dr. Eccles. With regard to the IPSP, we have done experiments now on undercut cortex, and after a survival time of two to four weeks we observed IPSP's after epicortical stimulations. These observations would fit very well, of course, with the proposed recurrent inhibitory pathway. I hope to present tomorrow some work on the visual system where we even think that inhibition in the higher levels is mainly by collaterals.

A question which we have not yet been able to decide is whether inhibition always goes through interneurons. I think Dr. Phillips is able to say something more about this, but it is not necessary from the physiological point of view to postulate interneurons in order to explain all inhibitory potentials. We could explain almost all findings by just assuming a recurrent loop making synaptic contacts with the neighboring cells. As far as I know the literature, there has been no clear bimodal distribution of latency after specific thalamic stimulation in the cortical neurons of the motor cortex. If there is an interneuron on the inhibitory pathway, one would expect two peaks, first that due to the direct excitation both of the pyramidal cells and of the interneurons, and then one synaptic delay later, the IPSP's of the pyramidal cells. I would also like to enquire further about the proposed correlation between the function and the fine structural details revealed by electron microscopy.

ECCLES: The evidence is, I think, quite good with the hippocampus, where the basket cells form synapses around the bodies of the hippocampal pyramidal cells that are of Gray type 2, while the endings on the dendritic spines, which we believe to be excitatory, are all Gray type 1. I refer to Hamlyn's excellent paper [1963] in this respect. It is true I think, too, in the cerebellum that the synapses of the basket cells on the bodies of the Purkinje cells are all of Gray type 2. I would not go so far as to say that Gray type 2 synapses were always inhibitory, but I would say that probably all type 1 synapses are excitatory. I don't know whether Dr. Colonnier would like to add to that.

COLONNIER: All our evidence about the function of these synapses is derived from the work that you have been doing on the hippocampus and cerebellum, and it is only by extrapolation that we believe that they may have a similar function in the cerebral cortex.

ECCLES: But you do find a pericellular nest around the bodies of neocortical pyramidal cells; and these synapses are all type 2, aren't they? *

COLONNIER: Yes, of course.

ECCLES: So it looks as though some generalizations can be put up. The other point in reply to Dr. Creutzfeldt's question is that the latencies of the postsynaptic inhibitory potentials were always longer than for the postsynaptic excitations, whether these synaptic actions are produced by antidromic impulses from the pyramidal tract, or by the specific afferents from the thalamus.

SCHAEFER: I think that Dr. Eccles has beautifully described what, for the moment, we may perhaps name the network properties of the several structures, and I wonder whether there are other properties which I would like for the moment to name single membrane properties. I come to this question from our completely different approach to the behavior of membranes in cardiac cells. When I looked at your pictures, I had the impression that the positive wave following a depolarization could perhaps be related to the positive wave

---

* (Note added later): Evidence for the inhibitory action of the pericellular synapses on neocortical pyramidal cells has recently been presented by K. Kubota, H. Sakata, K. Takahashi, and M. Uno. *Proc. Jap. Acad.,* 41, 195–197 [1965].

following the discharge of a cardiac cell and which is only a property of the membrane itself. My question is: Have you evidence of any such hyperpolarization following a single discharge of the cell, just as occurs with the sinus cell of the heart? The second question is: Of course one could doubt whether there is any similarity between a cardiac cell which is so simple to investigate and these very complicated neuronal networks; but I saw in these very fine records of Dr. Creutzfeldt's, as in many other tissues, the same behavior of the electrotonic curve. During anodal polarization, you always find that the potential comes first to a rather deep point and then swings back into the steady state. I found this many years ago and described it as the *Anodenschwung* of the electrotonic potential. This seems to be quite the same in these central cells as well as in cardiac cells. A third question: We found in recent unpublished experiments in our department that, if you clamp cardiac cells at a very low membrane potential, there is an extreme lability of the resistances of the membranes (Dr. Haas). It could be that in the same moment when the potentials of neocortical cells are going down by some process, you come to such-a lability too, which may play an important role in the networks as well. These are the three points concerning possible differences between network properties and single membrane properties. Then I have a fourth question: Would you agree with me that the inversion point of the negativity and positivity of a potential field is simply a matter of statistics, so that the majority of impulses moving to the exploring electrode will give a positive wave, while the majority moving away from the electrode must give a negativity?

ECCLES: I will try to answer your first question, but I think Dr. Andersen will have more to say about it in regard to hippocampal pyramidal cells. There are very interesting membrane properties of pyramidal cells. First, the large hyperpolarizing potentials may certainly be identified as inhibitory postsynaptic potentials because they have the expected inversion potential, and are to a considerable extent due to chloride permeability. We can therefore be confident that these hyperpolarizations are true inhibitory postsynaptic potentials comparable with those elsewhere in the nervous system. During recovery from these inhibitory potentials you often observe a rebound discharge, and it is this that may be linked with some of your heart observations, there being some fundamental membrane property common to these two very different types of cell. I illustrated a succession of hyperpolarizing waves and later rebound discharges with the intracellular recordings of Klee and Lux, and we have found it to be very well developed with thalamic neurons. With regard to the depth of the inversion point for the extracellular potentials that you mentioned, it is of course statistical, the sources and sinks of thousands of pyramidal cells being involved.

BREMER: One thing in the very elaborate and impressive survey which Eccles has given us disturbs me a little, and my question has some relation to Professor Schaefer's. I am struck once more by the fact that these hyperpolarizations are so often preceded by a high frequency discharge of the cell. One could wonder if they could not be explained sometimes by a sequence of that discharge rather than by a dual causality, involving an inhibitory process. Furthermore, we don't have for the cortex the pharmacological test which is provided for the motoneuron by the blocking of the inhibition by strychnine. Therefore, the evidence, in spite of the biophysical and other arguments which we shall hear, seems to me somewhat uncertain still, and I ask if it would not be possible to get a pure hyperpolarization not preceded by any discharge, and having besides a clear functional meaning. That is not an impossibility. I suggest, for example, the repetition, with intracellular recordings, of Hubel and Wiesel's binocular interaction experiments on the visual area. There, one could get pure inhibition unpreceded by any axonic discharge of the nerve cell and that would be very convincing.

ECCLES: This distinction is very easy with the hippocampus and Dr. Andersen has a slide which we will see shortly, showing you a pure inhibitory potential. Kandel and Spencer have published similar observations and I illustrated records of Dr. Phillips, which showed only an initial EPSP without spike followed by a large hyperpolarization. In all these cases the true inhibitory potentials are not depressed by strychnine.* All inhibitions above the foramen magnum seem to be resistant to strychnine, and these strychnine-resistant inhibitions are moreover very large and have a much slower decay than you expect from the time constant of the membrane. Dr. Creutzfeldt finds about 58 msec on the average for the time constant of decay of inhibitory potentials of pyramidal cells as against 8.5 msec for the electric time constant of membrane, so you can see there must be a long lingering of the inhibitory transmitter.

BREMER: Indeed, but don't you think, nevertheless, that it would be important to demonstrate electrophysiologically in the neocortex a pure, and functionally significant, inhibitory process?

ECCLES: I agree, but still I am not worried too much, because we have all the analogs in the hippocampus.

MAC KAY: In order to determine the information-processing function of these networks which Professor Eccles has described, it would be important to know the time relationships as well as the space relationships of the signals. To specify inhibition and excitation as such would not be enough; one has to say, for example, "A inhibits B provided that it comes within a certain time interval." In particular, I wonder what is known about the time-resolving power of the dendritic system. If a dendritic synapse sends a relatively slow signal down to the cell body, do we know whether the resulting facilitation or depression lasts for milliseconds, or tens of milliseconds, or what?

ECCLES: I should make it clear at this stage that I was presenting crude physiological experiments. They were crude because they were the results of massive synchronized inputs. This technique is appropriate for investigations into the physiological properties of these systems. The real physiological

---

* (Note added later): Stefanis and Jasper [*Int. J. Neuropharmacol.,* 4, 125–138, 1965] and Pollen and Ajmone Marsan [*J. Neurophysiol.,* 28, 342–358, 1965] have reported that inhibitory potentials in the cerebral cortex are greatly depressed and even inverted by strychnine, but it should be pointed out that extremely high concentrations of strychnine were employed—the direct application to the cortical surface of 1.0 per cent solutions of strychnine—whereas inhibitions in the spinal cord are greatly depressed by intravenous injections of 0.1 to 0.2 mg/kg. See literature in these reviews: D. R. Curtis. *Internat. J. Neuropharmacol.,* 1, 239 [1962]; and J. C. Eccles. *Brit. Med. Bull.,* 21, 19 [1965].

situation is that there are repetitive discharges at various frequencies along the many fibers that converge on the synapses of a particular neuron, so that one has to envisage a randomized bombardment of both the excitatory and inhibitory synapses. There is an estimated total of ten thousand synapses on a single cortical pyramidal cell. When the dominance of excitation causes such a cell to fire impulses, it in turn will be feeding back via interneurons both positively and negatively to itself and to other cells in the neighborhood. The whole of this complex performance has to be integrated into the communication system. It is much more complicated, but at least it is important to realize what are the basic elements that are built into this system and that are operated not only by synchronized inputs but also by the immense number of repetitive discharges at all kinds of frequencies that normally converge onto any part of the cortex. So we have to, as it were, put your question into storage until we have much more knowledge about the behavior of cortical neurons under these much more complex conditions of input.

Your other question concerns the mode of action of synapses on dendrites. The dendritic tree is so long that, even if there is quite good electrotonic transmission of postsynaptic potentials, there would be very little information coming from synapses on the superficial dendritic efflorescence down to an impulse-firing zone at the soma or axon hillock. But, if you have local responses generated in the apical dendrites and transmitting even in a decremental manner, there will be a much more effective transmission of synaptically induced depolarization down the apical dendrites, and summation with other local responses of the dendrites of that cell, eventually to generate the discharge of a full-sized impulse. All this facilitation could occur in a fraction of a millisecond. As already mentioned, these local responses can be observed in cortical pyramidal cells and they also occur in hippocampal pyramidal cells.

REFERENCES

ADRIAN, E. D. The spread of activity in the cerebral cortex, *J. Physiol.*, 88, 127–161 [1936].

———. Afferent discharges to the cerebral cortex from peripheral sense organs, *J. Physiol.*, 100, 159–191 [1941].

ALBE-FESSARD, D. Activités de projection et d'association du néocortex cérébral des mammifères. I. Les projections primaires, *J. Physiol.* (Paris), 49, 521–588 [1957].

———, and P. BUSER. Activités intracellulaires recueillies dans le cortex sigmoide du Chat: participation des neurones pyramidaux au "potentiel evoqué" somesthétique, *J. Physiol.* (Paris), 47, 67–69 [1955].

AMASSIAN, V. E. Interaction in the somatovisceral projection system, *Res. Publ. Ass. nerv. ment. Dis.*, 30, 371–402 [1952].

———. Microelectrode studies of the cerebral cortex, *Int. Rev. Neurobiol.*, 3, 67–136 [1961].

———, J. W. PATTON, A. T. WOODBURY, and J. E. SCHLAG. An interpretation of the surface-response in somatosensory cortex to peripheral and interareal afferent stimulations, *Electroenceph. Clin. Neurophysiol.*, 7, 480–482 [1955].

ANDERSEN, P., J. C. ECCLES, and T. A. SEARS. The ventrobasal complex of the thalamus: types of cells, their responses and their functional organization, *J. Physiol.*, 174, 370–399 [1964].

——, and T. A. SEARS. The role of inhibition in the phasing of spontaneous thalamo-cortical discharges, *J. Physiol.* (London), 173, 459–480 [1964].

ARAKI, T., M. ITO, and T. OSHIMA. Potential changes produced by application of current steps to motoneurones, *Nature* (London), 191, 1104–1105 [1961].

ARDUINI, A., and D. G. WHITLOCK. Spike discharges in pyramidal system during recruitment waves, *J. Neurophysiol.*, 16, 430–436 [1953].

ARMSTRONG, D. M. Synaptic excitation and inhibition of Betz cells by antidromic pyramidal volleys, *J. Physiol.*, 178, 37P–38P [1965].

BISHOP, G. H. The dendrite: Receptive role of the neurone, *Electroenceph. Clin. Neurophysiol.*, Suppl. 10: 12–21 [1958].

——, M. H. CLARE, and W. M. LANDAU. The equivalence of recruiting and augmenting phenomena in the visual cortex of the cat, *Electroenceph. Clin. Neurophysiol.*, 13, 34–42 [1961].

BREMER, F. Cerebral and cerebellar potentials, *Physiol. Rev.*, 38, 357–388 [1958].

BROOKHART, J. M., and A. ZANCHETTI. The relation between electro-cortical waves and responsiveness of the corticospinal system, *Electroenceph. Clin. Neurophysiol.*, 8, 427–444 [1956].

BROOKS, V. B., and P. S. ENGER. Spread of directly evoked responses in the cat's cerebral cortex, *J. Gen. Physiol.*, 42, 761–777 [1959].

BURNS, B. D. Some properties of the cat's isolated cerebral cortex, *J. Physiol.*, 111, 50–68 [1950].

BUSER, P. Thalamic influences on the EEG, *Electroenceph. Clin. Neurophysiol.*, 16, 18–26 [1964].

CHANG, H. T. Dendritic potential of cortical neurons produced by direct electrical stimulation of the cerebral cortex, *J. Neurophysiol.*, 14, 1–21 [1951].

——. Cortical and spinal neurons. Cortical neurons with particular reference to the apical dendrites, *Cold Spr. Harb. Symp. Quant. Biol.*, 17, 189–202 [1952].

——. Cortical response to stimulation of medullary pyramid in rabbit, *J. Neurophysiol.*, 18, 332–352 [1955].

CLARE, M. H., and G. H. BISHOP. Dendritic circuits: The properties of cortical paths involving dendrites, *Amer. J. Psychiat.*, 111, 818–825 [1955].

COLONNIER, M. L. The structural design of the neocortex, in: *Brain and Conscious Experience*, New York, Springer-Verlag [1966].

COOMBS, J. S., D. R. CURTIS, and J. C. ECCLES. The electrical constants of the motoneurone membrane, *J. Physiol.*, 145, 505–528 [1959].

CRAWFORD, J. M., D. R. CURTIS, P. E. VOORHOEVE, and V. WILSON. Strychnine and cortical inhibition, *Nature*, 200, 845–846 [1963].

CREUTZFELDT, O. D., and H. D. LUX. Zur Unterscheidung von "spezifischen" und "unspezifischen" Synapsen an corticalen Nervenzellen, *Naturwissenschaften, 51,* 89–90 [1964].

———, and A. C. NACIMIENTO. Intracelulläre Reizung corticaler Nervenzellen, *Pflüg. Arch. Ges. Physiol., 281,* 129–151 [1964].

DEMPSEY, E. W., and R. S. MORISON. The production of rhythmically recurrent cortical potentials after localized thalamic stimulation, *Amer.`J. Physiol., 135,* 293–300 [1942a].

———. The interaction of certain spontaneous and induced cortical potentials, *Amer. J. Physiol., 135,* 301–308 [1942b].

———. The electrical activity of a thalamocortical relay system, *Amer. J. Physiol., 138,* 283–296 [1943].

ECCLES, J. C. Membrane time constants of cat motoneurones and time courses of synaptic action, *Exp. Neurol., 4,* 1–22 [1961].

———, B. LIBET, and R. R. YOUNG. The behaviour of chromatolysed motoneurones studied by intracellular recording, *J. Physiol., 143,* 11–40 [1958].

———, R. LLINAS, and K. SASAKI. Intracellularly recorded responses of the cerebellar Purkinje cells, *Exp. Brain Res., 1,* 161–183 [1966].

GRANIT, R., D. KERNELL, and G. K. SHORTESS. Quantitative aspects of repetitive firing of mammalian motoneurones, as caused by injected currents, *J. Physiol., 168,* 911–931 [1963].

HAMLYN, L. H. An electron microscope study of pyramidal neurons in the Ammon's Horn of the rabbit, *J. Anat. Lond., 97,* 189–201 [1963].

JABBUR, S. J., and A. L. TOWE. Analysis of the antidromic cortical response following stimulation at the medullary pyramids, *J. Physiol., 155,* 148–160 [1961].

JANKOWSKA, E., and D. ALBE-FESSARD. Sur l'origine et l'interprétation de la seconde phase du potentiel évoqué primaire de l'aire somatique, *J. Physiol.* (Paris), *53,* 374–375 [1961].

JUNG, R., and G. BAUMGARTNER. Hemmungsmechanismen und bremsende Stabilisierung an einzelnen Neuronen des optischen Cortex, *Pflüg. Arch. Ges. Physiol., 261,* 434–456 [1955].

KANDEL, E. R., W. A. SPENCER, and F. J. BRINLEY. Electrophysiology of hippocampal neurons. 1. Sequential invasion and synaptic organization, *J. Neurophysiol., 24,* 225–242 [1961].

KLEE, M. R., and K. OFFENLOCH. Postsynaptic potentials and spike patterns during augmenting responses in cat's motor cortex, *Science, 143,* 488–489 [1964].

KUBOTA, K., H. SAKATA, H. TAKAHASHI, M. UNO. Location of the recurrent inhibitory synapse on cat pyramidal tract cell, *Proc. Japan Acad., 41,* 195–197 [1965].

———, and H. TAKAHASHI. Recurrent facilitory pathway of the pyramidal tract cell, *Proc. Japan Acad., 41,* 191–194 [1965].

LASHLEY, K. S. In search of the engram, *Symp. Soc. Exp. Biol., 4,* 454–482 [1950].

LI, C.-L. Cortical intracellular synaptic potentials, *J. Cell. Comp. Physiol., 58,* 153–167 [1961].

LI, C.-L. Cortical intracellular synaptic potentials in response to thalamic stimulation, *J. Cell. Comp. Physiol.*, *61*, 165–179 [1963].

————, and N. CHOU. Cortical intracellular synaptic potentials and direct cortical stimulation, *J. Cell. Comp. Physiol.*, *60*, 1–16 [1962].

————, C. CULLEN, and H. H. JASPER. Laminar microelectrode studies of specific somato-sensory cortical potentials, *J. Neurophysiol.*, *19*, 111–130 [1956].

LUX, H. D., and M. R. KLEE. Intracelluläre Untersuchungen über den Einfluss hemmender Potentiale im motorischen Cortex. 1. Die Wirkung elektrischer Reizung unspezifischer Thalamuskerne, *Arch. Psychiatrie Z. Ges. Neurologie*, *203*, 648–666 [1963].

MARSHALL, W. H., C. N. WOOLSEY, and P. BARD. Observations on cortical somatic sensory mechanisms of cat and monkey, *J. Neurophysiol.*, *4*, 1–24 [1941].

MORISON, R. S., and E. W. DEMPSEY. A study of thalamo-cortical relations, *Amer. J. Physiol.*, *135*, 281–292 [1942].

————. Mechanism of thalamocortical augmentation and repetition, *Amer. J. Physiol.*, *138*, 297–308 [1943].

MOUNTCASTLE, V. B., P. W. DAVIES, and L. BERMAN. Response properties of neurons of cat's somatic sensory cortex to peripheral stimuli, *J. Neurophysiol.*, *20*, 374–407 [1957].

NACIMIENTO, A. C., H. D. LUX, and O. D. CREUTZFELDT. Postsynaptische Potentiale von Nervenzellen des motorischen Cortex nach elektrischer Reizung spezifischer und unspezifischer Thalamuskerne, *Pflüg. Arch. Ges. Physiol.*, *281*, 152–169 [1964].

PAPPAS, G. D., and D. P. PURPURA. Fine structure of dendrites in the superficial neocortical neuropil, *Exp. Neurol.*, *4*, 507–530 [1961].

PHILLIPS, C. G. Intracellular records from Betz cells in the cat, *Quart. J. Exp. Physiol.*, *41*, 58–69 [1956a].

————. Cortical motor threshold and the thresholds and distribution of excited Betz cells in the cat, *Quart. J. Exp. Physiol.*, *41*, 70–84 [1956b].

————. Actions of antidromic pyramidal volleys on single Betz cells in the cat, *Quart. J. Exp. Physiol.*, *44*, 1–25 [1959].

————. Some properties of pyramidal neurones of the motor cortex. *Ciba Symposium. The Nature of Sleep* (ed. by G. E. W. Wolstenholme and M. O'Connor). London: Churchill, pp. 4–24 [1961].

PURPURA, D. P., and E. M. HOUSEPIAN. Alterations in corticospinal neuron activity associated with thalamocortical recruiting responses, *Electroenceph. Clin. Neurophysiol.*, *13*, 365–381 [1961].

————, and R. J. SHOFER. Cortical intracellular potentials during augmenting and recruiting responses. 1. Effects of injected hyperpolarizing currents on evoked membrane potential changes, *J. Neurophysiol.*, *27*, 117–132 [1964a].

————, R. J. SHOFER, and F. S. MUSGRAVE. Cortical intracellular potentials during augmenting and recruiting responses. II. Patterns of synaptic activities in pyramidal and nonpyramidal tract neurons, *J. Neurophysiol.*, *27*, 133–151 [1964].

Purpura, D. P., R. J. Shofer, and T. Scarff. Personal communication [1964b].

Rall, W. Branching dendritic trees and motoneuron membrane resistivity *Exp. Neurol.*, *1*, 491–527 [1959].

———. Membrane potential transients and membrane time constant of motoneurons, *Exp. Neurol.*, *2*, 503–532 [1960].

Ramón y Cajal, S. *Histologie du Système Nerveux de l'Homme et des Vertébrés.* Paris: Maloine, Vol. II, 993 pp. [1911].

Sholl, D. A. *The Organization of the Cerebral Cortex.* London: Methuen [1956].

Spencer, W. A., and J. M. Brookhart. Electrical patterns of augmenting and recruiting waves of depths of sensorimotor cortex of cat, *J. Neurophysiol.*, *24*, 26–49 [1961a].

———. A study of spontaneous spindle waves in sensorimotor cortex of cat, *J. Neurophysiol.*, *24*, 50–65 [1961b].

———, and E. R. Kandel. Electrophysiology of hippocampal neurons. III. Firing level and time constant, *J. Neurophysiol.*, *24*, 260–271 [1961a].

———. Electrophysiology of hippocampal neurones. IV. Fast prepotentials, *J. Neurophysiol.*, *24*, 272–285 [1961b].

Stefanis, C., and H. H. Jasper. Intracellular microelectrode studies of antidromic responses in cortical pyramidal tract neurons, *J. Neurophysiol.*, *27*, 828–854 [1964a].

———. Recurrent collateral inhibition in pyramidal tract neurons, *J. Neurophysiol.*, *27*, 855–877 [1964b].

Towe, A. L., and I. D. Zimmerman. Peripherally evoked cortical reflex in the cuneate nucleus, *Nature, 194*, 1250–1251 [1962].

3

Correlation of Structural Design with Function in the Archicortex

by P. O. ANDERSEN

Nevrofysiologisk Laboratorium, Oslo, Norway

In the study of cortical function, one line of investigation is to seek information on the individual elements of the cortex, most often the pyramidal cells. However, the complexity of the cerebral cortex presents a great difficulty in the investigation of single pyramidal neurons. The main reason for this situation is the histological arrangement, as is evident from Fig. 3.1. In particular, there is a scarcity of information on synaptic activity of the neocortical pyramidal cells. However, in the archicortex, a simpler arrangement is found. In Fig. 3.1 the neocortex is to the left, with its six cell layers. The pattern changes as we enter the enthorinal area (R.e.), part of the hippocampal gyrus. Even simpler is the picture, when we look at the hippocampus proper (CA1, CA2, CA3). Here, virtually all cells are arranged with their cell bodies, or somata, in a single and compact layer. Golgi staining of these cells reveals that the dendritic pattern is also very uniform (Fig. 3.2). From the cell bodies, the apical dendrites go towards the hippocampal fissure. All neighboring apical dendritic shafts are lying parallel to each other, and the branching is moderate in CA1 until a point some 500 μ from the soma. At this depth, the branching of the apical dendrites gets profuse and the diameter of the branches tapers rapidly off. At the other side of the soma, the basal dendrites make a finely meshed network. Closer to the ventricular surface, are the myelinated thin axons constituting the alveus. Paradoxically, this cortex is usually seen upside down by the physiologist. The alveus represents the white matter under the cortex, and the hippocampal fissure represents the surface.

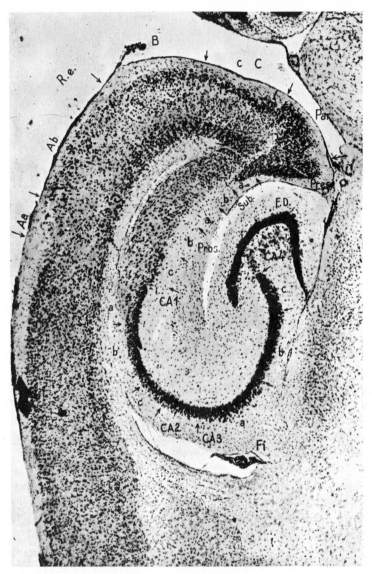

Fig. 3.1. Photomicrograph of a horizontal section of the hippocampal region of a mouse stained with thionin. Following the cortex clockwise from the lower left corner, the neocortex ends at Aa, where the entorhinal area begins. The hippocampus proper has four main subdivisions, CA1, CA2, CA3, and CA4. Fi is the fimbria [from Lorente de Nó, 1934].

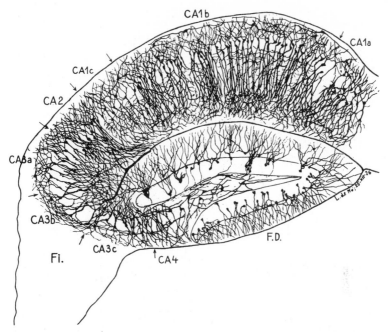

Fig. 3.2. Sagittal section of the hippocampus of a mouse stained with the Golgi-Cox method [from Lorente de Nó, 1934].

We owe to Cajal [1911] and Lorente de Nó [1934] most of our knowledge on the normal histology of this region. Figure 3.3 is taken from the work of the last author, and shows how in this uniform cortex one can discern several functionally different layers. Thus a microelectrode, advancing parallel to the apical dendrites of the pyramidal cells, penetrates one laminar section after the other, each with a particular afferent inflow. Since all the pyramidal cells are lying parallel to each other, and at the same depth, each cell will be inpinged upon by one given set of synapses on a certain stretch of its extension. For example, in CA1 the most peripheral parts of hippocampal apical dendrites are activated from the enthorinal area. The next section receives information through the Schaffer collaterals, and the following part is synaptically influenced by the commissural pathway. The soma itself is exclusively affected by the basket cell terminals. In addition to these afferent systems, there are several others.

In this presentation I would like to focus attention on two of these afferent systems, in which it is possible to demonstrate a clear correlation between the structure and the function. These two systems are first the basket cell terminations on the pyramidal cell bodies, and, secondly, the

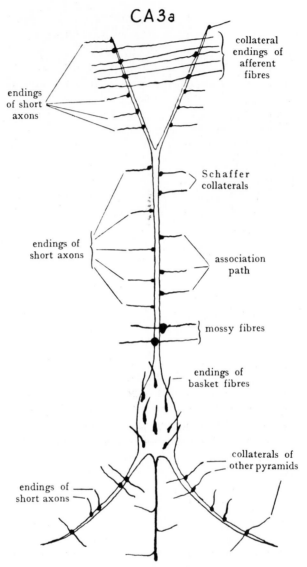

Fig. 3.3. Diagrammatic representation of a CA3 pyramidal cell (bordering CA2) with the laminar arrangement of the various afferent systems [from Lorente de Nó, 1934].

Schaffer collateral synapses ending peripherally on the apical dendritic shafts.

As shown by recording with an intracellular microelectrode in the cell body, all afferent systems so far tested produce large and long-lasting inhibitory postsynaptic potentials (IPSP's) in the hippocampal pyramids (Fig. 3.4,A) [Andersen, Eccles, and Løyning, 1964]. Increasing strengths of stimuli given to three afferent pathways, the commissural (C), the septal (S), and the local (L), produce augmenting hyperpolarization of the cell. The hyperpolarization is so large that it may bring the membrane potential up to -80 mV, which, presumably, is very close to the equilibrium potential for the IPSP. This fact suggests that the current generating the hyperpolarization must flow across the membrane very close to the impaling microelectrode. In Fig. 3.4,B, a local stimulus produces an antidromic invasion of the cell. However, even when such autidromic invasion fails, there appears a hyperpolarization, showing that this response is an IPSP and is not due to an afterhyperpolarization [Kandel, Spencer, and Brinley, 1961]. Similar results were obtained with stimulation of a deafferented fimbria [Spencer and Kandel, 1961]. Because all orthodromically conducting fibers were degenerated, the IPSP's were due to impulses conducted antidromically along the axons and their collaterals and, thus, generated by a recurrent inhibitory pathway. The latency of this IPSP is always longer than that of the antidromic spike, the latency difference being about 2 msec (Fig. 3.4,B). With synaptic activation, there was a similar latency difference between the excitatory spike response and the IPSP.

Such IPSP's have been recorded in virtually all the impaled hippocampal neurons. Much more seldom, spikes were encountered. The consistent latency difference between the excitatory responses recorded from a population of cells and the onset of the IPSP, and the more frequent occurrence of IPSP's as compared to spikes, favor the notion that there is a distributing element involved in the production of the IPSP. This element is presumably one, or a set of interneurons.

When the electrode is withdrawn from the cell, an extracellular positive wave is recorded from the region of the cell bodies. This wave has a time course that makes it possible to correlate it with the intracellular IPSP. By recording the amplitude of this positive wave at various layers and plotting the amplitude against the recording depth, a laminar profile can be constructed, as shown in Fig. 3.5. To the left are records, taken at the indicated depths in mm, in response to stimulation of the commissural (C), septal (S), and local (L) pathways. In B, the amplitude of the positive wave at various depths is measured at the time indicated by the stippled lines in A. It is evident that there is a maximum positivity in response to all three pathways at a depth of 0.35–0.4 mm. As indicated

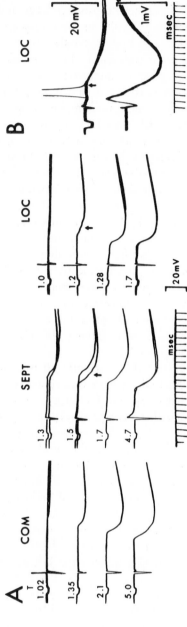

Fig. 3.4. (A) Inhibitory postsynaptic potentials (IPSPs) recorded intracellularly from a CA3 pyramidal cell in response to increasing strengths of stimulation of three afferent pathways, the commissural (COM), the septal (SEPT), and the local (LOC). The numbers give the stimulus strength in multiples of threshold, T. The arrows point at wavelike increments of the IPSP. (B) Intracellular record from a CA3 pyramid in response to a local stimulus of a strength just at the threshold for production of an antidromic spike. The arrow points at the onset of the IPSP that occurred irrespective of whether the cell was firing or not [from Andersen, Eccles, and Løyning, 1964].

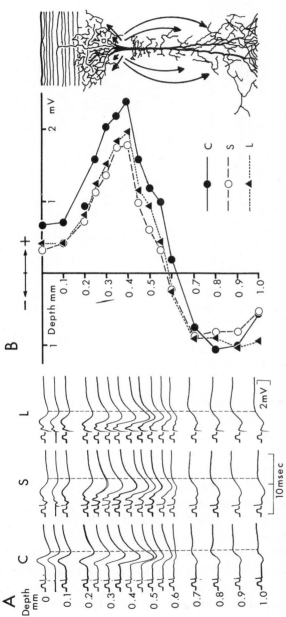

Fig. 3.5. (A) Extracellular records obtained at the indicated depths of the field CA3 of the hippocampus in response to an afferent volley in three pathways, C, commissural; S, septal; and L, local. (B) Graph in which the amplitude of the records measured at the stippled lines in A is plotted against the recording depth. The cell to the right is a CA3 pyramidal cell, drawn to scale to facilitate comparison with the graph. The extracellular positivity has a definite maximum corresponding to the cell body layer. The arrows indicate the current flow at the time given by the stippled lines in A [from Andersen, Eccles, and Løyning, 1964].

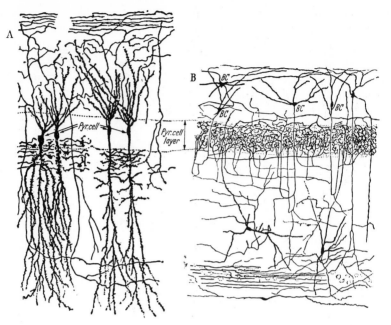

Fig. 3.6. (A) Two CA3 pyramids (left) and two CA1 pyramids (right) drawn from a Golgi section. Note the extensive axonal collaterals being distributed in the layer between the cell bodies and the white matter, alveus. (B) Basket cells (BC) with their extensive axonal ramifications ending exclusively around the cell bodies of the pyramidal neurons. The magnification of B is matched to A, and mounted so that the layers in A and B correspond to each other [from Cajal, 1911].

to the right, this depth corresponds to the cell body layer. The slope of the profile of the potential graph in B indicates that at the time indicated by the stippled lines there is a current flowing from the depth of 0.4 mm towards the surface as well as towards the depth of the cortex. Since this current is associated with a marked hyperpolarization of the cell, no alternative is left but the conclusion that the current is flowing owing to a synaptic hyperpolarization of the cell body.

Turning to histology, the synapses located at the cell body belong exclusively to one type, namely those of the basket cell terminals. One basket cell (Fig. 3.6B, BC) sends its axon into the apical dendritic layer, where it branches extensively, turns back and ends among a great number of pyramidal neurons. From the drawings of Cajal [1911] and Lorente de Nó [1934], it is possible to calculate that one basket cell may make synaptic contact with between 200 and 500 pyramidal cells. Figure 3.6A shows two sets of pyramidal neurons. The dendritic pattern is extensive, but I would like to draw attention to the distribution of the axons. In both sets of neurons, the axons are coursing towards the alveus. However, before reaching that far, they send off a great number of collaterals, which, according to Cajal [1911] and Lorente de Nó [1934], end in the layer between the cell bodies and the alveus, the stratum oriens. In this layer the main cellular elements besides the pyramidal basal dendrites are the cell bodies and dendrites of the basket cells.

This recurrent inhibitory system accounts for the latency difference between the initially activated cells and the onset of the IPSP as well as for the wide distribution of these IPSP's.

Since the basket cell terminals form the only afferent system known to impinge upon the pyramidal cell bodies, it is possible to study morphologically a cortical cell synapse that is identified as inhibitory in function. Figure 3.7 is an electron micrograph taken from the cell body synapses in the CA3 of the hippocampus [Blackstad, 1964, personal communication]. To the right in the picture is the cell body cytoplasm with its abundance of Nissl substance and mitochondria. Along the cell membrane one can see three synapses bordering each other. All of these synapses belong to the type 2 of Gray [1959]. To the left, it is possible to identify thin axons making up the plexus of the basket fiber terminals. A formidable

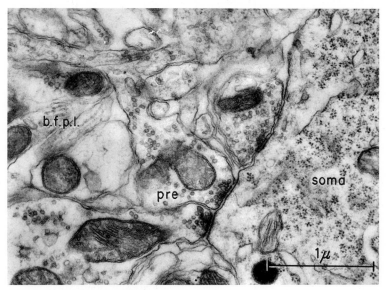

Fig. 3.7. Electron micrograph from the pyramidal layer of CA3 of a rat. To the right is the cell body of a pyramidal cell on which three synapses make contact of the type 2 of Gray [1959]. To the left is seen part of the plexus made of the basket cell terminals. b.f.pl., basket fiber plexus; pre, presynaptic terminal. (Courtesy Dr. Blackstad.)

number of synapses impinge upon the cell bodies of these cells, 40 per cent of the soma membrane being covered with basket cell terminals. The concentration of the synapses is so large that, presumably, their activity very effectively can change the conductance across the soma membrane.

The evidence at hand suggests that these synapses are inhibitory. Therefore, we have the first example of a recurrent inhibitory system in mammals where the synapses and the pathway are histologically identifiable.

Little is known about the neurochemistry of these synapses. However, some information can be gathered by experiments such as those in Fig. 3.8. A section of the brain has been stained for cholinesterase (ChE). Control sections with inhibition of the butyryl cholinesterase indicate that the cholinesterase in the nervous elements is acetyl-cholinesterase (AcChE). The amount of AcChE in the hippocampal region is much greater than that in the neocortex. However, the enzyme is not evenly distributed, but aggregated in certain layers [Storm Mathisen, and Blackstad, 1964]. Cells that most likely are basket cells contain AcChE, and this enzyme is also found between the pyramidal cell bodies. Thus, it is a possibility that acetylcholine is the inhibitory transmitter substance in this region. This possibility rests upon the assumption that neurons with intracellular AcChE also produce ACh at their synaptic terminals.

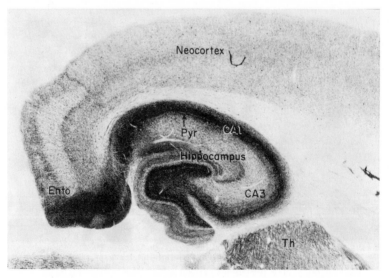

Fig. 3.8. Section of the hippocampal formation with the adjoining neocortex, stained for cholinesterase. Ento, area entorhinalis; pyr, pyramidal cell body layer; Th, thalamus [from Storm Mathisen and Blackstad, 1964].

Perfusion of the lateral ventricles with tubocurarine produces abnormal discharges in the hippocampus [Feldberg and Fleischhauer, 1962, 1963]. It may be that this effect could be linked to an interference with inhibitory action on hippocampal pyramidal cells, tubocurarine blocking a cholinergic mechanism.

In the next part of my talk I will deal with another synaptic system, the so-called Schaffer collaterals. These collaterals emanate from the axons of the CA3 pyramids, turn backwards, and end with synapses on the apical dendrites of the CA1 pyramids some 400–500 μ from the cell bodies. The Schaffer collaterals can be activated indirectly by stimulation of the entorhinal area. By recording the activity at various depths in response to such stimulation, a large negative wave is recorded extracellularly with a maximum at a depth of 0.8 mm [Fujita and Sakata, 1962; Andersen, Holmqvist, and Voorhoeve, 1966], (Fig. 3.9). This wave is indicated with an open square in A, and with open squares and a stippled line in the graph in B. The crosses give the magnitude of the spike at various depths. The extracellular negative wave is confined to a relatively small part of the pyramidal cells, corresponding exactly to the layer of the Schaffer collateral synapses. On the top of the wave, a small spike is seen, which is larger on recording closer to the soma (crosses). It is the sign of the synchronous discharge of a number of pyramidal cells. The extracellular negative wave has a considerable amplitude. The morphological basis for this can possibly be sought in the electron micrographs in the following figures. These are taken by the late Dr. Hamlyn of London. Figure 3.10 is a cross section of an apical dendrite at the Schaffer collateral level, being completely surrounded by synapses, almost all of them having active sites on to the dendrite and leaving no space for other types of neuronal elements to cover the dendritic membrane. The synapses are of the type 1 of Gray [1959]. In the upper part of Fig. 3.11 the same area is seen in longitudinal section; the density of the synapses is equally large. Coupled with the information from Fig. 3.10, it can be concluded that the synapses form a cuff of considerable length and density around the dendrites at this level of the cortex. When these synapses are synchronously activated, as they were in our experiments, they are expected to produce a considerable conductance change across the dendritic membrane, and thus explain the development of the large extracellular wave, as a sign of depolarization of the pyramidal apical dendrite.

If the Schaffer collateral synapses are excitatory, they would be expected to produce cell discharges. This is exactly what can be recorded. In Fig. 3.12A the inset is a CA1 cell of an adult rabbit stained with the Golgi-Cox method. The neuron has its apical dendrite to the left and its basal dendrites to the right. The records were taken by

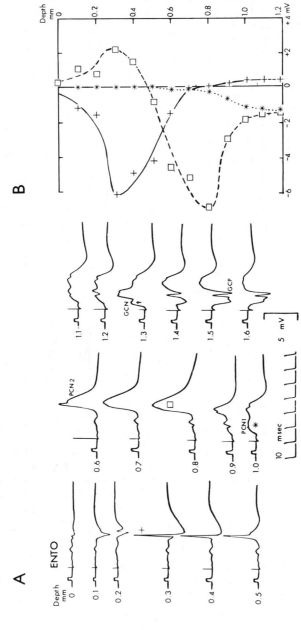

Fig. 3.9. (A) Extracellular records obtained from a microelectrode penetrating the field CA1, in response to entorhinal stimulation. The numbers give the recording depth in mm. The large negative wave at 0.6–0.8 mm (PCN2) is produced by the Schaffer collateral synapses. (B) Graph in which the amplitudes of the spike (crosses) and the large negative wave (open squares) are plotted against recording depth [from Andersen, Holmqvist, and Voorhoeve, 1966].

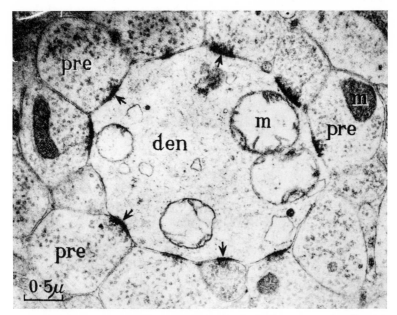

Fig. 3.10. Electron-micrograph showing a transverse section of an apical dendritic shaft at the level of the Schaffer collaterals. The dendrite (den) is completely surrounded by presynaptic structures (pre), almost all of which form active sites onto the dendrite. The synapses are of the type 1 of Gray [1959]. [From Hamlyn, 1963.]

a microelectrode, being inserted parallel to the CA1 apical dendritic shafts at the depths indicated by the arrows [Andersen and Lømo, 1965]. In each assembly of three records, the upper line gives the microelectrode recording on ordinary sweep, the middle and the lowest traces are the microelectrode and surface records, respectively, both taken with an expanded sweep. The thick portion of the upper trace indicates the part of the signal being expanded in the two lower traces. Each record consists of five superimposed traces. In the records from 0.9 and 0.8 mm depth, the spike appears as a positive notch only. At 0.7 mm a small negative deflection is seen, and from 0.6 to 0.4 mm a definite negative spike occurs. Further superficially the spike is diphasic, positive/negative.

Because of spontaneous, slight shifts in the excitability of the cortex, it is necessary to record any latency difference of the spike from a reference point in the surface potential. In Fig. 3.12A, this point is taken as the peak positivity and marked with a stippled line in each set of records. The arrows point at the peak of the negativity of the spike. As shown by the relation of the arrows to the stippled line, the latency of the spike is shortest at the deepest point it can be detected, hence this is its point of origin.

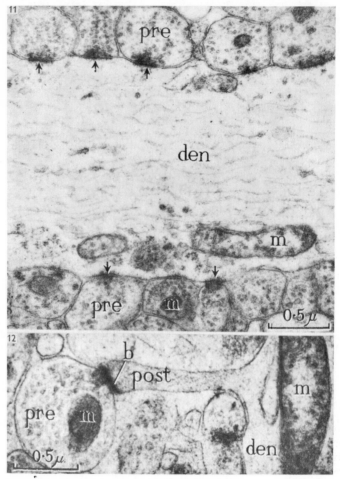

Fig. 3.11. The upper part is an electron-micrograph of a longitudinal section through an apical dendrite at the level of the Schaffer collaterals. Throughout the length shown, the dendrite (den) is completely covered with synapses (pre), almost all having type 1 contact. The lower part shows the way in which a presynaptic swelling (pre) makes contact with a dendritic spine (post). This is the most usual contact between afferent axons and dendrites [from Hamlyn, 1963].

By plotting the latency of the spike against the recording depth, the graph in Fig. 3.12B was drawn. The slope of the graph gives the conduction velocity of the spike propagated along the apical dendritic shaft, starting at about 0.4 m per sec and sinking to about 0.2 m per sec when the cell body is passed, where presumably the spike invades the basal dendrites. Two reasons can be given for assuming that the spike recorded between the cell body layer and the alveus (stratum oriens) is due to

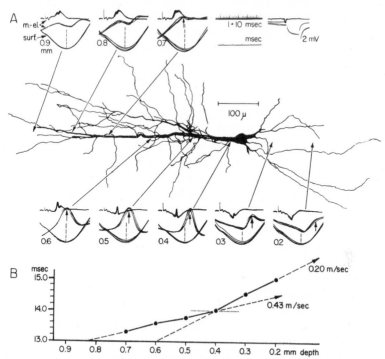

Fig. 3.12. (A) Extracellular records obtained from various depths of the field CA1 of the rabbit hippocampus in response to entorhinal stimulation. The recording depths are given in mm by the number under the records, and also indicated by the arrows. The inset is a drawing of a CA1 pyramidal cell, drawn from a Golgi-Cox section of an adult rabbit. In each assembly of three traces, the upper is the micro-electrode record, normally displayed. The middle trace is the microelectrode signal, and the lower is the surface potential, both shown on expanded sweeps. The portion of the sweep being expanded is indicated by the thick portion in the upper trace. The peak positivity of the surface record is indicated with a stippled line. The peak negativity of the spike recorded by the microelectrode is labeled with an arrow. A large negative wave is recorded at the 0.7 and 0.8 mm depths. The peak latency of the spike, as measured in relation to the peak surface positivity, is increasing as the microelectrode was withdrawn towards the ventricular surface. The surface record was similar to the 0.2 mm microelectrode record. (B) Graph in which the peak latency of the spike is plotted against the recording depth. The stippled lines are drawn to facilitate calculation of the conduction velocity of the spike. The dotted line indicates a latency of 14 msec. The conduction velocity is smaller in the thin basal dendrites than in the thick apical dendritic shaft [from Andersen and Lømo, 1965].

propagation along the basal dendrites and not along the axons. First, the axons are myelinated and very small—few are thicker than 1 μ. Hence, the magnitude of the potential produced by the axonal volley propagating in the volume conductor would be much smaller than that due to excitation of the large area of the unmyelinated dendrites. Secondly, the speed of propagation of alvear axons in rabbit is 6–7 m per sec [Andersen, 1960], which is considerably higher than that observed for the spike in stratum oriens.

The propagation of the dendritic spike cannot be due to a passive electrotonic spread because both the rising and the falling phases of the spike are increasing as the recording is made closer to the soma; and, according to the cable theory, the opposite would be the case if the spike was passively conducted towards the soma.

The evidence at hand suggests that the spike is generated in that part of the dendritic membrane in close proximity to the very effective Schaffer collateral synapses. At the level of the synapses themselves the conductance increase is presumably high. This conductance change will prevent both the initiation of the spike at the synaptic level of the apical dendrite, as well as the somatofugal conduction of the spike along the thinner apical dendritic branches.

Thus, the peripherally located Schaffer collateral synapses seem to be able to discharge the cell through a propagated dendritic spike. We may ask whether this is the physiological mode of operation, or just an experimental curiosity. Can these synapses depolarize the soma sufficiently to make the cell discharge through the cable properties of the apical dendrites?

An answer to this question may be sought in an experiment like the one illustrated in Fig. 3.13. In A are extracellular records taken at the indicated depths in response to direct stimulation of the Schaffer collaterals [Andersen, Holmqvist, and Voorhoeve, 1966]. B, C, and F show the usual response as recorded intracellularly. In none of 25 cells impaled at the soma level were we able to detect any excitatory postsynaptic potential (EPSP), in spite of a large extracellular spike potential signaling that a number of the pyramidal cells were in fact excited.

Only in one instance did we detect an EPSP (D, E), but this penetration was abnormally deep (0.2 mm below the pyramidal layer), and was associated with an extracellular negativity. There is a possibility that the thick portion of the apical dendrite of the neurone was impaled.

During the last few months we have extended these studies [Andersen and Lømo, 1965]. In order to get the most favorable conditions for excitation, the stimulating electrode has been placed on the border between the fimbria and the hippocampus, so as to excite as many afferent fibers to the CA3 area as possible. In about 40 neurons, we have

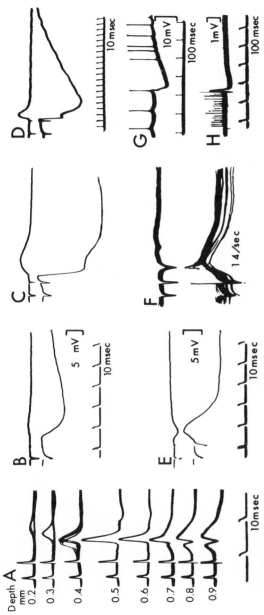

Fig. 3.13. (A) Extracellular records obtained at the indicated depths of CA1 in response to direct stimulation of the Schaffer collaterals in cat. B, C, and F are intracellular records (lower traces) from a pyramidal cell, showing IPSPs as the only response to such stimulation. Upper traces are the extracellular records. D and E are records obtained as in B, C, but at a greater depth. This result may be due to an impalement of the apical dendritic shaft, or of a cell not being a pyramidal cell, since it was recorded 0.2 mm below the pyramidal layer. G and H are records showing cessation of spontaneous discharge following the same stimulation as in A to F [from Andersen, Holmqvist, and Voorhoeve, 1966].

not been able to detect any EPSP, in spite of the fact that extracellular records revealed a well-developed excitation and a considerable number of the cells showed antidromic spike invasion, and some also synaptically induced spikes. These spikes took off from the baseline without any readily detectable prepotential. Our conclusion is that the excitatory synapses impinging upon these neurons exert their effect too far away from the soma to be detectable by an intrasomatic electrode.

In trying to bring together these physiological data and the histology, reference is made to Fig. 3.14. A shows the soma and initial part of the apical dendrite, both having a smooth membrane. The diameter of the apical dendrite at the base is 6.5 μ without allowance for shrinking due to the histological procedure. In B is the apical dendrite some 500 μ from the soma. This is the region of branching of the dendrites, and where the Schaffer collaterals make their synaptic contacts. At this site the diameter of the apical dendritic shaft is 2.8 μ. The membrane shows now a few spines, but very many less than on the secondary dendritic branches. All of these are so much thinner (0.5–1.0 μ), that it is possible to talk about two classes of dendrites: the thick and relatively straight apical dendrite, and the thin and twisted secondary dendritic branches. The latter have an initial smooth portion of about 10 μ. Distal to this

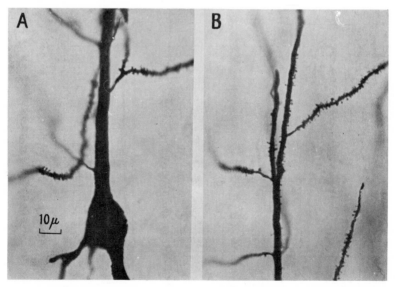

Fig. 3.14. Photomicrograph of a CA1 pyramidal cell of an adult rabbit, stained with the Golgi-Cox method. A shows the soma and the initial part of the apical dendrite; B is taken from the level of the Schaffer collaterals. Note the smooth membrane of the soma and the thick apical dendritic shaft. The spines are located predominantly on the thinner dendritic branches.

part, the secondary dendrites carry a large number of spines. By far the largest majority of the synaptic terminals make synaptic contact with such spines (Fig. 3.11, lower part). Thus, excitatory synapses are found mostly upon the thin dendrites, even to their finest extensions.

Based upon the evidence presented above, the following hypothesis on the mode of operation of hippocampal pyramidal cells is presented, referring to Fig. 3.15, taken from Cajal's work [1911]. Excitatory synapses act largely by depolarizing the thin dendritic twigs by a synaptic action on their spines. Following a sufficiently intense release of transmitter substance, an action potential is produced which is propagated along the dendrites towards the apical dendritic shaft, or towards the soma if the synapses are located on the basal dendrites. Particularly efficient synaptic action can be made by synapses located on the thinner portion of the apical dendritic shaft itself. The safety factor for propagation of the action potential along the dendrites is, presumably, low for the thinnest branches. Propagation is particularly difficult when the action potential arrives at a branching point where there is an increase in the area of the membrane to be invaded. In such circumstances, conduction is greatly facilitated if both of the joining branches are synaptically depolarized. Such confluence of depolarizing activity may give synapses, located remotely on the dendritic tree, a say in the integration of excitatory influence upon the neuron. The striking lack of EPSP's in spite of an effective synaptic excitation and the occurrence of spikes in a neuron with a healthy membrane potential indicate that the length constant for the pyramidal dendrites is smaller than the figure of 350 μ calculated for the motoneurons [Coombs, Curtis, and Eccles, 1959]. Without the possibility of influencing the initial segment of the axon electrotonically, the remotely located excitatory synapses, which are far more numerous than the synapses on the trunks of the large dendrites, seem to be able to influence the probability of discharge of the cell only through the initiation and propagation of action potentials along the dendrites. Thus, this hypothesis is remarkably similar to the concept which Cajal [1911] had about the operational activity of the hippocampal cortex, although arrived at with a different technique.

Finally, in assessing the role of the remotely located synapses, one has to bear in mind the great power of facilitation of the synaptic transfer by frequent stimulation. In this way the efficiency of a given afferent volley can be increased manyfold, as measured by the number of neurons it can bring to discharge, by increasing the stimulus rate from 1 per sec to 10 per sec. Frequency potentiation of cortical synapses may well be one of the most significant factors in regulating the integrative behavior of the pyramidal neurons.

The location of inhibitory synapses at the soma makes it possible to

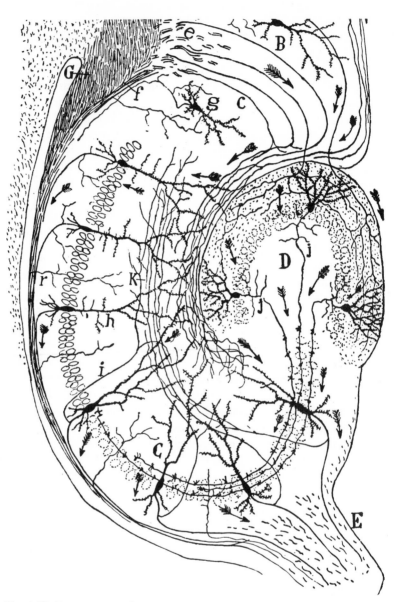

Fig. 3.15. Diagram over the cells and main connections of the hippocampal formation. The arrows indicate the direction of propagation of the nervous activity along the dendrites, as envisaged by Cajal [1911].

suppress all discharges that arrive from the dendrites on their way through the soma towards the axon. This braking action is most impressive, and seems to work through an increase of the membrane potential as well as through an augmented conductance of the soma membrane. Although no evidence is available on this point, it is possible that inhibitory synapses could be located at other parts of the pyramidal cells. A strategic site would be just somatopetal to the Schaffer collateral synapses. Interestingly, there are a few synapses of the type 2 on the apical dendritic shaft at this level.

By stressing the importance of the majority of the excitatory synapses that are located on thin dendritic branches, the great capability that the neuron has for a differentiated response is underlined. This differentiated response to various magnitudes of synaptic inputs will be reflected by the frequency of discharge of the pyramids. It is the great flexibility of response of the cortical pyramidal cell that is likely to be the basis for the versatility of its performance.

This investigation was supported by a PHS research grant, NB 04764, from the National Institute of Health, U. S. Public Health Service, which is gratefully acknowledged.

DISCUSSION

Chairman: PROFESSOR PENFIELD

JASPER: There are certainly many questions raised by this interesting analysis, which have a general bearing on organization of synaptic circuits in the brain. I would like to mention, even though unpublished, studies with the multibarrel microelectrode method that are being performed on hippocampal pyramidal cells by my colleague Stefanis. He finds them exquisitely sensitive to acetylcholine in an excitatory manner; in fact, they are the most sensitive of cells he has tested, and he has studied many in the cerebral cortex and elsewhere. This raises difficulties for your suggestion of a cholinergic inhibition of these pyramidal cells. Stefanis also finds these cells extremely sensitive to inhibitory action by gamma aminobutyric acid, which acts in lower concentration even than acetylcholine.

ANDERSEN: Of course, acetylcholine producing inhibition was only meant as a suggestion. We don't even know what intracellular cholinesterase means; it may not mean that the cell itself is able to produce acetylcholine.

With regard to the passing out of drugs through the multibarrel electrode in the hippocampus, Dr. Curtis and I tried this in Canberra. We gave it up because we could not get rid of all the inhibition. When you start passing out current you certainly get cells fired. So there are cholinoceptive elements in the cortex, but we were never able to identify them as pyramidal cells. This is, of course, crucial, because when you put out your drug it is diffusing out among all kinds of cellular elements, including the basket cells. The complexity of the pattern was such that we abandoned this work, and I do not know whether we shall ever be able to return to it. My final comment is that it is important to identify the responding units before we can say anything about the cholinoceptive mechanism on pyramidal cells.

JASPER: Dr. Stefanis feels confident they are pyramidal cells. They can be excited to the level of sustained epileptic discharge by small quantities of ACh.

ECCLES: Is there any evidence for positive feedback in the hippocampus, that is for an excitatory action of axon collaterals of pyramidal cells onto pyramidal cells such as occurs in the neocortex?

ANDERSEN: No, we have never been able to see any positive feedback at all. There is one mechanism, however, whereby you can break down inhibition, and this is by frequency potentiation. If you increase the stimulus rate from, say, 1 per sec, which is rather high anyway for the hippocampus, to about 10 or 20 per sec, you decrease the efficiency of inhibition. Recording intracellularly you can see that the IPSP's diminish, and although you can, so to speak, clamp the cell at the higher potential for a short time, you cannot keep it there for a long time; the membrane potential slowly attains the level it had before; and then the frequency potentiation of the excitatory synapses seems to take over. This is a kind of an avalanche: high frequency stimulation increases the efficiency of the excitatory synapses; at the same time the cells seem to break away from the inhibition, so you force your excitation upon the cells.

CREUTZFELDT: Also in the motor cortex it can be observed that IPSP's do not follow above a frequency of 6–8 per sec [Nacimiento et al, 1964 *]. During repetitive stimulation of n. ventrolateralis thalami, for example, you only get an IPSP in cortical pyramidal cells with the first stimuli. The IPSP's then fade away and only pure EPSP's are produced, which are "augmented" during medium frequencies (5–10 per sec). This suggests a very slowly recovering transmitter mechanism for cortical IPSP's. The situation here seems indeed to be very similar to that in the hippocampus.

ECCLES: The fading away of inhibition with repetitive stimulation fits in very nicely with the idea of there being an interneuron on the pathway as distinct from it being monosynaptic. At the higher frequencies, monosynaptic actions of the nervous system are often potentiated by repetition. Could Dr. Andersen make any suggestions about the flow of information through the hippocampus, that is, about the input and the output under conditions of natural functioning?

ANDERSEN: No, I don't think we can. This is a big riddle, of course, and I think at present there is absolutely no evidence what exactly this piece of cortex does. There have been, of course, a lot of investigations done, and certainly the hippocampus does affect certain properties of the total animal. Its activity influences the behavior of the animal in many ways. Still, I don't think a clear-cut picture of its effect has been produced.

* A. C. Nacimiento, H. D. Lux, and O. D. Creutzfeldt. Post-synaptische Potentiale von Nervenzellen des motorischen Cortex nach elektrischer Reizung spezifischer und unspezifischer Thalamuskerne, *Pflügers Arch., 281,* 152–169 [1964].

I would like to ask Dr. Creutzfeldt about his reduction of the IPSP's—whether or not this was done on DC recording or AC recording. We can certainly see a reduction of the IPSP in the AC records, but this could be due to DC clamping as you approach the equilibrium potential for the IPSP's.

CREUTZFELDT: Yes, it is done with DC amplification. By changing the membrane potential with intracellular stimulation you can prove that during repetitive stimulation the IPSP's really are abolished after a while, and that their disappearance is not simply due to a polarization of the membrane. May I just ask you a short question relating to the possible function of the hippocampus? In recent papers of Adey and collaborators, it was shown that under certain behavioral conditions the direction of the slow waves traveling across the hippocampus may change. Can these observations be correlated to your findings in that excitation sometimes may come from the entorhinal area across the Schaffer collaterals, but under other conditions may travel the other way from the hippocampus towards the entorhinal area? Or is it not yet possible to correlate the findings observed under different experimental conditions?

ANDERSEN: I think we have to say the latter. There is still a rather great gap between the two sets of observations.

MAC KAY: Have you done any experiments in which you have varied the rhythm of a constant mean frequency of stimulating impulses? For example, have you used a combination of two pulse trains of the same frequency with a variable phase relationship? I ask partly because the map you showed suggests a system that could be sensitive to interval ratios in the pulse train; and also because, in some experiments at Keele using flash excitation of the visual system, we find that changing the ratio of intervals, keeping the mean frequency constant, changes the direction of the evoked potential vector on the scalp.

ANDERSEN: In fact you can show quite nicely, I think, that there is a preferred frequency at which you can drive the cells. This seems to be around 5 per sec. If you increase the stimulation rate, there is a brief period of enhanced activity, this soon gives place to a deep and prolonged depression. Also you have another puzzling type of response, the postanodal rebound. We don't know whether it is a normal or a pathological phenomenon in the hippocampal cells. It can cause an enormous increase of the output from the system if you time your stimuli so that the next is coming just at the onset of the postanodal rebound. This would be about 3 per sec.

MAC KAY: I was not thinking about changing the frequency, but rather, with a given mean frequency, varying the ratio of successive intervals. This is what we found to have a marked effect on the evoked potential in man.

ANDERSEN: We have done somewhat similar experiments, but I cannot yet report anything definite.

JASPER: May I suggest that our Chairman make some comments about Professor Eccles' question about the functional significance of the hippocampus. He has good opportunity to observe in man the effects of electrical stimulation, and this investigation has been continued by Dr. Rasmussen and colleagues with electrical recordings simultaneously of the effects of stimulation not only from the hippocampus itself but from the neocortex, which has given us some ideas of its function in conscious human subjects.

CHAIRMAN: This takes us into another field. From the point of view of stimulation of the human brain it seems clear that direct stimulation of the hippocampus itself does not produce recall of previous experience, no recall of the past. If the amygdaloid nucleus and the hippocampus play an active role in memory recordings, I would not expect the electrode on the hippocampus to do anything but interfere with recall. Activation of the memory record can only come when gray matter at a distance is stimulated by the electrode. Then normal neuronal activation may occur.

Furthermore, removal of the hippocampus on both sides inevitably interferes with memory. The interference is most marked for events of recent years and, for some strange reason, memory for more distant years is less disturbed. I was sorry that you did not throw any light on the amygdaloid nucleus as well as the hippocampus. The amygdala is certainly of importance in the same area.

I don't know whether what I am about to say is what Dr. Jasper had in mind—but I think we can state with certainty that there is a neuronal record of conscious experience. In my opinion this record is not situated in the neocortex although it can be activated by applying an electrode to the neocortex in the areas we have described.

COLONNIER: I was fascinated to see that the most effective synaptic contacts in the hippocampus were those cuff-like arrangements of type 1 synapses directly on the dendritic trunks and not on spines.

Szentágothai has some evidence that in the cerebellum the climbing contacts may also be directly upon the Purkinje cell dendritic trunks and not on spines: the latter seem to be synaptically related to the parallel fibres. The climbing fibres of the cerebellum, as we have seen, were also shown to be a very powerful mechanism of synaptic transmission and excitation.

If we can extrapolate that contacts on dendritic trunks are universally more effective than those on dendritic spines, it may be noteworthy that cortical stellate cells have very few spines and that most contacts must therefore be on the dendritic trunk itself. We might infer that the contacts on these cells are probably more effective than those found on the spines of pyramidal cells.

It is interesting in this respect that Hubel and Wiesel have shown that there are cells in the visual cortex with simple fields i.e., responding to individual points of light, and others with complex fields i.e., responding only to larger luminous slits. The cells with simple fields are found distributed through the layers of the cortex in approximately the same ratio as the stellate cells. If the stellates are those cells which possess simple fields, the fact that most contacts are on the dendritic trunk itself may be related to the fact that these cells respond to fewer afferents i.e., react to individual points of light.

PHILLIPS: Have you ever seen a case in which activation of the Schaffer synapses caused an impulse which apparently started with an A or IS impulse? I ask because my colleague Shepherd worked on the mitral cells of the olfactory bulb; unfortunately neither he nor I was able to get good intracellular records from these, but we were readily able to get giant extracellular spikes, in which the A and B impulses were clearly distinguishable.

When recording from such cells he stimulated the olfactory nerve filaments, which form their synapses in the olfactory glomeruli which are at least half a millimetre away from the soma and axon of the mitral cell; in some cases one could see that the impulse began with an A impulse which then invaded the B membrane. As he increased the size of the presynaptic volley, this hesitation between the A and the B impulse got less and eventually disappeared, so that with a large presynaptic volley you could see no A-B inflexion. Have you ever seen an A impulse initiating the impulse that you get from stimulating the Schaffer collaterals?

ANDERSEN: We have not been looking for this event. What we have been concerned with so far is just to see if we could get impulses at all.

TEUBER: I have two questions. Do you have any observations on hippocampal recordings from very young animals? Dr. Joseph Altman and his colleagues in our department have gained the impression that this structure differentiates rather late and that there are curious changes that go on after birth, particularly in the rodent. The second question is a related one: Do you have any comments relating to the peculiar chemical affinities of the structures for various injected substances besides this question of whether or not they are cholinergic? Dr. Altman and his colleagues in our department have recently come across a large uptake of radio-labeled, tritiated thymidine all along the hippocampus and have found a similar affinity for labeled steroids.

ANDERSEN: We have so far done all our experiments in adult animals. However, it is striking to see the Cajal and Lorente de Nó pictures from newborn animals in which, as you know, the dendritic apparatus is much more diversified with very many more spines. I wonder if it could be that the apical dendritic shaft at least seems to lose some of its spines during the development to leave the excitation to the thinner dendrites and perhaps to take over more of the dendritic conduction. With regard to the second question on drugs acting upon the cell, I don't know very much about that. The striking thing is that in CA3 you have synapses containing a huge amount of zinc, and it is possible to block conduction in these synapses by interfering with the zinc metabolism. In further answer to Dr. Phillips's question, I can say that Kandel, Spencer, and Brinley certainly saw an A-B break in the pyramidal cells of the hippocampus, although I don't think they ever stimulated afferents that impinge peripherally upon the neurons.

CHAIRMAN: If there is no further discussion, may I say, as Chairman, that this has been a brilliant beginning of this symposium, thanks to Eccles, Colonnier, and Andersen. We are still at the level of the single cell. There is a long way to go in our effort to throw light on the nature of consciousness.

REFERENCES

ANDERSEN, P. Interhippocampal impulses. IV. A correlation of some functional and structural properties of the interhippocampal fibres in cat, rabbit and rat, *Acta Physiol. Scand.*, 48, 329–351 [1960].

———, J. C. ECCLES, and Y. LØYNING. Location of postsynaptic inhibitory synapses on hippocampal pyramids, *J. Neurophysiol.*, 27, 592–607 [1964].

ANDERSEN, P., B. HOLMQVIST, and P. E. VOORHOEVE. Excitatory synapses on hippocampal apical dendrites activated by entorhinal stimulation, *Acta Physiol. Scand.* (In press) [1966].

——, and T. LØMO. Excitation of hippocampal pyramidal cells by dendritic synapses, *J. Physiol.* (Lond.), *181*, 39–40P [1965].

BLACKSTAD, T. W. Personal communication [1964].

COOMBS, J. S., J. C. ECCLES, and P. FATT. The electrical properties of the motoneurone membrane, *J. Physiol.* (London), *130*, 291–325 [1955].

FELDBERG, W., and K. FLEISCHHAUER. The site of origin of the seizure discharge produced by tubocurarine acting from the cerebral ventricles, *J. Physiol.* (London), *160*, 258–283 [1962].

——. The hippocampus as the site of origin of the seizure discharge produced by tubocurarine acting from the cerebral ventricles, *J. Physiol.* (London), *168*, 435–442 [1963].

FUJITA, Y., and H. SAKATA. Electrophysiological properties of CA1 and CA2 apical dendrites of rabbit hippocampus, *J. Neurophysiol.*, *25*, 209–222 [1962].

GRAY, E. G. Axo-somatic and axo-dendritic synapses of the cerebral cortex; An electron microscope study, *J. Anat.* (London), *93*, 420–433 [1959].

HAMLYN, L. H. An electron microscope study of pyramidal neurones in the Ammon's horn of the rabbit, *J. Anat.* (London), *97*, 189–201 [1963].

KANDEL, E.R., W. A. SPENCER, and F. J. BRINDLEY, Jr. Electrophysiology of hippocampal neurons. I. Sequential invasion and synaptic organization, *J. Neurophysiol.*, *24*, 225–242 [1961].

LORENTE DE NÓ, R. Studies on the structure of the cerebral cortex. II. Continuation of the study of the Ammonic system, *J. Psychol. Neurol.* (Leipzig), *46*, 113–177 [1934].

RAMÓN Y CAJAL, S. *Histologie du Système Nerveux de l'Homme et des Vertébrés.* Paris: Maloine, Vol. 2, 993 pp. [1911].

SPENCER, W. A., and E. R. KANDEL. Hippocampal neuron responses to selective activation of recurrent collaterals of hippocampofugal axons, *Exp. Neurol.*, *4*, 149–161 [1961].

STORM MATHISEN, J., and T. BLACKSTAD. Cholinesterase in the hippocampal region, *Acta Anat.*, *56*, 216–253 [1964].

4

The Neural Replication of Sensory Events in the Somatic Afferent System[1]

by V. B. MOUNTCASTLE

Johns Hopkins University, Baltimore, Maryland

The investigator interested in the neural mechanisms of sensation and perception wishes first to define the neural activities which compose the central reflection of sensory events—the neural replication of the external world seen across sheets of sensory receptors. This leads him inevitably to what I believe is one of the major problems with which we are concerned in this symposium. On the one hand is the commonly held idea that there is represented in neural space and time an isomorphic phantom of the real world, a phantom then surmised to be interfaced with some other process of uncertain nature which, deriving input from this conjunction, evolves an activity of its own which is regarded as a basically mental or psychic thing, as perception, consciousness, and the other concomitant aspects of the inner life of man.

On the other hand is the set of assumptions, composing the *modus labori* of many neurophysiologists, which may be summarized under the term *psychoneural identity* [Feigl, 1958; Pepper, 1960]. That is, that the neural activity set in motion by sensory stimuli, successively transformed through successively interconnected populations of neurons, complexed against stored information, contributing to and conditioned by those neural locales and activities concerned with set or affect—that these neural activities do themselves lead to and are in fact the very essence

[1] The research described in portions of this paper was supported by grant number NB-1045, from NINDB, NIH, U. S. Public Health Service.

of the private event of perception, and, at choice, its public expression in the form of a discrimination, a localization, an estimated magnitude, or a description of quality. Both private and public happening are considered the results of the same chains of neural events. While this concept proves to be a useful one for the experimentalist, I know that all of you will agree with me that the matter is not finally settled, and should be left open for modification in the light of future discoveries.

Following the idea of a psychoneural identity, the task of the neurophysiologist is greatly amplified and made more complex, for nothing less is envisaged than an explanation in neural terms of the totality of behavior, public and private, including the phenomena labeled as mental or psychic, even though it is clear to everyone that our understanding of these things in these terms is presently very primitive indeed.

One way to approach these goals is to begin with studies of sensory systems, that is, to learn how it is that impinging energy from the external world, falling upon sheets of nerve endings, evokes in them patterns of nerve impulses which provide for central detectors a neural counterpart or paradigm, a description couched in neural language, of peripheral stimuli—a transform in neural space and time of the stimulus object qualities.

We wish to know how the qualities of form, contour, locus, intensity, and temporal movement are transduced into neural patterns, how these are further relayed centralward, and which aspects of this neural activity are likely to be critical for an interpretative and decision mechanism itself composed of neurons. This is a large order indeed, and from what I shall now say you will see that detailed information in terms of neural actions is limited and is largely confined to the input and the output links between the brain and the external world.

Studies of the somatic afferent system, which links the skin and other peripheral tissues with the brain, have in the last few years been passing through a period of very rapid change, which is true I believe for all of central neurophysiology. A great deal of knowledge has now accumulated concerning the detailed topography of sensory systems. This knowledge has come from the study of humans and animals with brain lesions, from continuing anatomical studies, and particularly from electrophysiological studies in anesthetized animals, using both the evoked potential method and that of single-unit analysis. More recently the evolution of new conceptual and methodological approaches for dealing with the dynamic aspects of neural activity have opened an era in which the aim is to elucidate mechanism, to answer questions which begin with the interrogative *how*, as well as *where*. Notable success has been achieved in understanding synaptic action and I believe that our major immediate task, using this new knowledge about singular events, is to try to understand some of the emergent aspects of the action and interactions of large populations of elements.

Concerning the somatic afferent system, I should like to summarize briefly without documentation the results of the geographic era, and to enumerate the general principles which have evolved, and some of the problems which they pose. Then I shall present the results of a new study of neural activity at the input level of the system and I shall attempt to correlate these findings with some psychophysical findings in man.

The input stage of the somatic afferent system comprises first-order fibers responsive to mechanical stimulation of the skin and subjacent tissues, to joint rotation, to temperature changes, and to noxious stimuli. How differentially sensitive (how "specific") each fiber is, until recently has been a matter of considerable disagreement. The controversy led to a re-examination of the properties of first-order fibers. The results have been summarized in other places [Mountcastle, 1961a, 1961b; Rose and Mountcastle, 1959], and it is perhaps sufficient to say that the overwhelming majority of both myelinated and unmyelinated fibers are differentially sensitive for quality, and that this is true both for those fibers which innervate hairy skin and for those ending in glabrous skin. One group of myelinated fibers, and a companion one of unmyelinated, are sensitive to both mechanical stimulation and to temperature changes. However, the differential sensitivity is so overwhelmingly in favor of mechanoreception as the adequate stimulus for these fibers, and the response to temperature changes so irregular and the response curve so flat, that they can also, I believe, be regarded as quality specific. In fact, they are so exquisitely sensitive to mechanical stimulation that I have chosen them for the quantitative studies which I shall describe.

First-order fibers enter the nervous system over dorsal roots and cranial nerves. Their distribution to various body parts is not uniform, but varies with the function of the parts as sentient organs. Thus the pattern of representation of the body form is even at this early stage a distorted one, arranged in terms of innervation density rather than bodily geometry. This distorted replica is faithfully repeated at each level of the system where synaptic transfer occurs, and in the postcentral gyrus of the cerebral cortex. This specificity for place has been fully confirmed by studies of single neurons of the system, in both deeply anesthetized and in unanesthetized animals [Poggio and Mountcastle, 1963]. Each cell of the system subtends a highly restricted peripheral receptive field, and together these fields compose the holistic pattern. This pattern is rich in intrinsic detail, is set, and apparently unchanged in normal life.

This rather rigid isomorphism at one time provoked a highly deterministic model of the representation of the external world in the nervous system. However, the elegant sensory performance of humans can scarcely be explained in terms of a system of insulated parallel lines; the grain is not sufficiently fine. Further, studies of the relation between periphery and center, both with the evoked potential method and with that of single-unit analysis, show that the two are arranged in a mutually convergent and divergent relation: a single central neuron receives impinging activity from a considerable number of first-order fibers. Reciprocally, a stimulus to a restricted peripheral locale activates a population of central cells. Activity is graded across this population from most to least intense, from its center to its fringe.

In addition to this remarkable specificity for place, there exists in the lemniscal component of the somatic system an equally precise spec-ificity for quality. Within a population of cells related to a peripheral locus there are some elements restricted to activation by one quality, such as touch; and others by another, such as joint position; all inter-digitated in a common topography.

Thus we are faced with an important problem: how is it that a central detector, itself composed of neurons, reads with such accuracy the location of neural activity in a related group of cells, and reads the sign of the quality of the stimulus as well? This is the problem of the meaning of place in the nervous system, one with which neurologists have long been concerned. It is not enough to say that activity in one portion of a population evokes activity in a linked portion of the next population in line. How this might occur is obvious, but only postpones the questions. At some stage in the long chain of events from stimulus to introspective evaluation the signs of place and quality must be coded in some more efficient way. The mechanism eludes us; there are not even—to my knowledge—reasonable models for experimental test. I cite this as one of the emergent properties of populations of neurons, one which I see no way of understanding as a simply additive property of the function of single cells, so far as we presently know them.

These specifics of place and quality are set by the static or continually renewed details of neural connections. Another of these static properties is afferent inhibition, which is thought to play an important role in spatial discriminations [Mountcastle, 1957; Mountcastle and Powell, 1959]. The phenomenon is this. A peripheral stimulus not only evokes the profiled pattern of excitation in central cells. Via relays impinging both pre- and postsynaptically the input set up by the stimulus also inhibits some cells. The important point is that these two synaptic actions are not randomly distributed across the neural field engaged by the stimulus. Cells at its center receive strong excitation and weak in-hibition, and the proportion of these opposing effects changes gradually from center to fringe, for cells at the latter will be strongly inhibited and only weakly excited. This has the effect of restricting the spread of excitation, of funneling it along narrow channels, and thus helps preserve at higher levels local areas of excitation, in spite of the successively additive divergence across synaptic relays. The phenomenon is thought to be important for a central detector sensing position in neural space.

Thus there is available at the present time some understanding of how stimulus-evoked neural activity is channeled through successive relays of this system, and into the postcentral gyrus of the cerebral cortex—at least as far as those aspects which are solely structure-determined. We have only faint glimmerings of what events occur at the cortical level, those which lead to behavioral reaction. Single neuron studies have revealed that at least through the cortical input stage the specificity for place and quality is preserved. They have also indicated what the plan of functional organization there may be. It appears that this is not one related transversely in accord with the layers of classical cytoarchitecture. The functional unit is a vertical column of cells extending across the cortical layers, for each cell of such a vertical column is related to nearly identical receptive fields, and all are excited by stimuli of the same quality, and at least in the initial stage of response these cells all discharge nearly identical patterns of impulses [Mountcastle, 1957; Powell and Mountcastle, 1959]. The overall representational pattern within the postcentral gyrus is thus composed of an intricately fitted mosaic of vertical units. That this is a more general plan for cortical action is shown by the recent work of Hubel and Wiesel [1962, 1963b] on the visual cortex, for they have elucidated in considerable detail a similar organization there.

I have said that this highly structured and specific representation of the external world depends upon static synaptic connections. The important question arises of whether these connections are absolutely set and unchanging. Is the plan genetically determined and functionally mature at birth, or does it represent an ontogenetic maturation determined by experience? Wiesel and Hubel have addressed themselves to this problem, in experiments dealing with the visual system. They found that the specific relations of central cell to restricted peripheral receptive fields, and the columnar plan of functional organization, are present in the mature form in the new-born cat [Hubel and Wiesel, 1963a]. Moreover, they discovered that the preservation of these patterns depends upon continued input from the periphery, for the highly ordered relations disappear in the visual cortex of a kitten deprived of patterned visual input for two or three months after birth [Wiesel and Hubel, 1963], and the cortical cells are then largely unresponsive to light delivered to the deprived eye. The implication of this important finding is that the panorama of synaptic connections in the nervous system is, to a certain extent, a labile affair depending upon a genetically given plan and the dynamics of afferent activity, and that the details of synaptic connections are modifiable by life experience.

Thus from the researches of the geographic era, certain general principles governing function within the somatic afferent system are clear. Synaptic connections specified genetically and maintained by experience provide an elegant specificity for place and quality. Even this degree of specificity is thought to be not sufficient to account for the niceties of spatial and quality discriminations, for the system is reciprocally linked from input to cerebral cortex in a mutually divergent-convergent array.

The problem of the action of populations of neurons is posed, and the role of afferent inhibition in sharpening spatial localization is suggested. Above all, a pressing problem is to discover the mechanisms of certain emergent aspects of population action: for one, how a neural detector reads position in neural space.

I must emphasize one further fact; namely, that what I have said pertains only to the lemniscal component of this system. However, at the level of entry this system divides, and another portion, the spino-thalamic system, feeds neural activity to a widely dispersed group of subcortical nuclei. The properties of this component are quite different: specificity for place and quality is negligible; convergence within this and with other sense systems is widespread [Poggio and Mountcastle, 1963]. In my opinion this does not mark an example of a higher order integration of neural activity, but that this system is concerned with the maintenance of general levels of awareness, and perhaps with those aspects of sensation subsumed under the words "set" and "affect." Thus we are led much closer to the ideas of Head, transferred to a central setting, than many would have thought possible a few years ago.

All that I have said is concerned with what I term the static properties of the nervous system, those set by the specifics of neural connections. Yet beyond static connection neural action is a dynamic thing, and in particular is a function of the variable time. Investigations of these time-bound aspects of neural activity now compose a large share of neurophysiology, and I should like to cite in some detail a specific example.

The Dynamic and Quantitative Aspects of Neural Input

Recently evolved concepts and methods for study of the dynamic and quantitative properties of neural activity make it possible to pursue certain aspects of an area of investigation first explicitly formulated in the second half of the nineteenth century, mainly by von Helmholtz [1954]. That is, one might relate the subjective phenomena of human sensory experience to objectively measured sensory processes and, further, compare this human experience with the neural events evoked in the sensory systems of experimental animals by sensory stimuli.

Following this line of thought, we have chosen to study a class of mechanoreceptive fibers which innervate the hairy skin of cats and monkeys, and which terminate there in highly specialized endings.[2] These fibers and their endings have been studied in detail by Iggo [1963a, 1963b]. He recognized as "touch spots" certain hemispheric, domelike elevations of the skin which are commonly situated between the hairs, are raised from the surrounding skin by about 150 μ, receive afferent fibers of the A-beta class, and are highly sensitive to mechanical stimuli. Figure 4.1 shows a reconstruction of this ending from electron microscopic studies by Iggo and Muir [1963]. These endings have been shown by Hunt and McIntyre [1960], Iggo [1963b] and Tapper [1964] to be exquisitely sensitive to mechanical stimulation, and to discharge at more or less regular rates for some seconds when stimuli are maintained steadily.

We wished to measure the stimulus-response relation across this receptor, and to compare certain derived aspects of this measurement with similar quantitative studies of the relation between tactile stimuli and the subjective sensory experiences evoked by them in humans; namely, the size of the discriminable stimulus increment at different levels of intensity, and the capacity for information transmission. The aim is to discover to what extent the subjective sensory experience may be determined by peripheral mechanisms, and if the S-R relation and its derived aspects remain invariant in the passage of neural activity through successive central stages of the afferent system; or, if not, what transformations are there impressed upon it.

Aims such as these require a precise control of the stimulus, and this we have achieved within an accuracy of ± 2 μ skin indentation. Automatic computation has allowed rapid analysis of the large quantity of experimental data obtained, and a general purpose digital computer has been used on-line during the experiments to provide for programing of stimulus sequences and for immediate calculations of certain response parameters which determined the future course of the experiments. Recordings have been made from single nerve fibers isolated by dissection of the saphenous nerve, in both cats and monkeys.

[2] The studies referred to were made with my colleague Dr. Gerhard Werner, and are described in greater detail in the *Journal of Neurophysiology, 28,* 359–397 [1965].

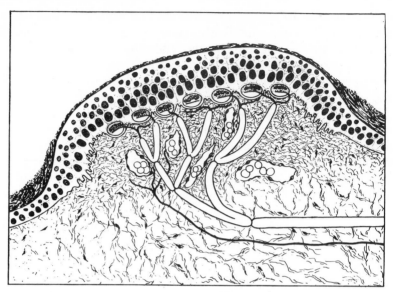

Fig. 4.1. Diagram of a "touch spot" in the hairy skin of the cat, based on optical and electron microscope studies [Iggo and Muir, 1963], very kindly provided by Dr. Ainsley Iggo, and published here with his permission. The myelinated axon branches in the outer layers of the dermis, and is accompanied by one or more unmyelinated axons. The myelinated axon branches lose their myelin preterminally, and end in expanded disks which resemble Merkel's bodies. When the living skin is examined with a dissecting microscope (16×) using incident light, these touch corpuscles appear as raised, partially translucent "bleebs," most commonly situated between the hairs. Occasionally a guard hair is seen exiting from the skin through such a touch corpuscle. The corpuscles range in diameter from 100 to 250 μ, and are raised from the surrounding skin surface by as much as 150 μ. They have been identified in the hairy skin of cats, dogs, and monkeys.

NATURE OF THE RESPONSE: THE EARLY STEADY STATE

Figure 4.2 shows, in the two columns to the left, the responses of a mechanoreceptive fiber to a series of successively stronger stimuli. It is apparent from these records that at about 100 msec there is a change from the early transient to a discharge which is highly periodic in nature, and that the frequency of this discharge is sensitively determined by the intensity of the stimulus. I wish to define this period of the discharge as an early steady state; I shall document this definition in a moment. The five records to the right in Fig. 4.2 were evoked by five stimuli of the same intensity, delivered at intervals of 3 sec. They indicate the metronomelike quality of the response of these fibers, and suggest the very high degree of accuracy with which the mean value of the

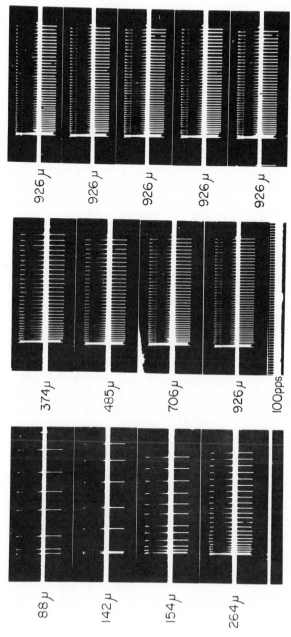

Fig. 4.2. Nerve impulses evoked in a single afferent fiber of the saphenous nerve of a cat by mechanical stimulation of its corpuscular ending in the skin of the lower leg. Net skin indentation in microns is shown to the left of each record. Stimulus duration was 450 msec. The stimulus onset, arrival at plateau, and offset are indicated by the three code signals of the record to the lower left. Time line is 100 pps. The five records to the right display responses to stimuli of a single intensity, delivered at intervals of 3 sec.

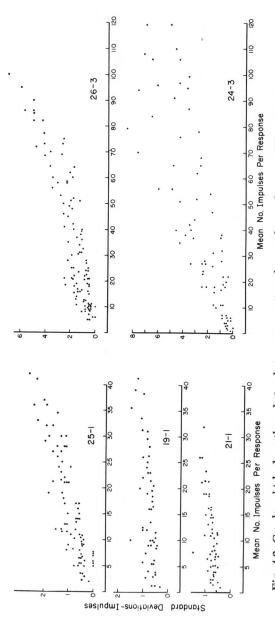

Fig. 4.3. Graphs which show the relation between mean impulse number and its variability, for five mechanoreceptive fibers activated by brief mechanical stimuli delivered to their corpuscular endings in the skin. Each data point plots the estimate of the mean for the number of impulses evoked by 30–50 identical stimuli, for different intensities and observation times. Stimuli delivered at rate of 1 in 3 sec. The variability in response number is, for some fibers, nearly constant from the least to the highest counts; for others it increases at a flat slope. The low values of the standard deviations illustrate the metronome-like nature of the response of first-order fibers to stimuli of equal strength.

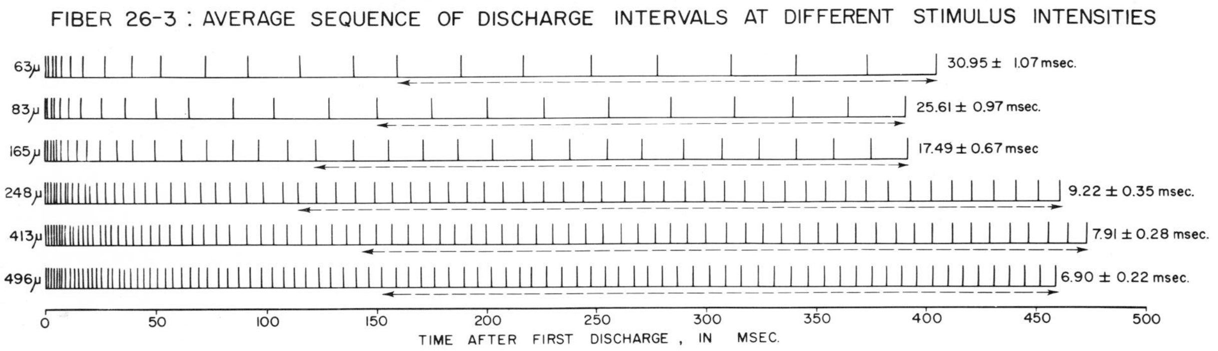

Fig. 4.4. Graphical display of the averaged sequence of discharge intervals in 30 consecutive responses to skin stimuli at each of the intensities given to the left of each sequence. The intervals between the short vertical lines represent the means of the 1st, 2nd, 3rd, . . . *n*th intervals throughout the trains of nerve impulses, until firing indices fell below 100 per cent, which occurred just as the stimulus was removed. The portions of the averaged discharge sequences indicated by the dashed lines are those periods of time after stimulus onset during which the cumulative post-stimulus histograms are linear. Mean interval and standard error (in msec) over these portions are given to the right of the discharge displays.

discharge rate can be estimated, in the early steady state. The data given in Fig. 4.3, in which the mean response numbers are plotted against their standard deviations when estimated from populations of 30–50 responses, support the contention that the true mean number can be estimated with considerable precision.

Figure 4.4 presents the results of a serial position analysis of the trains of impulses evoked by mechanical stimuli. For each intensity, 30 such responses were obtained. Each vertical line represents the mean post-stimulus time at which each serially numbered impulse occurred. The dashed lines with arrows bracket the early steady states, and the numbers to the right give the mean impulse intervals during these periods, and their standard errors. Thus both in terms of impulse counting and in terms of the temporal ordering of impulses, the value of the response can be estimated with considerable accuracy.

This remarkable regularity of response, both within a single response and from one trial to the next, promised that the stimulus-response relation could be measured with precision. Some attention should be given, however, to the scale along which the stimulus is measured. There are some experimental observations which suggest that this ending is particularly sensitive to direct pressure, rather than to distortion or stretch of the skin, and that an optimal stimulus metric would be force. While we have been able to measure both force and indentation for long-lasting stimuli, we have been unable to measure accurately the force produced by stimuli of less than one sec. duration—which interested us the most. Nevertheless, the use of indentation as a metric has yielded monotonic relations, and it has the advantage that this is the stimulus scale used in many experiments in humans.

THE STIMULUS-RESPONSE RELATION

Figure 4.5 depicts the stimulus-response relation for a single mechanoreceptive fiber. The fitted curve is the best fitting power function of the general form

$$R = K \cdot S^n.$$

The graph to the right of the figure plots these same data in log-log coordinates. We have found similarly excellent fits of power functions for the S-R relation for 18 of the 21 fibers for which this particular experiment was carried to completion. For several of these, analysis was also made of the relation when sequentially lengthening portions of the early state were taken for measurement. The power function relation

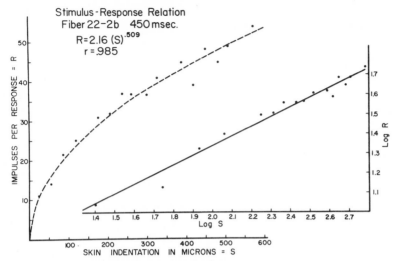

Fig. 4.5. (*To the left*): Graph illustrating the stimulus-response relation for a mechanoreceptive fiber ending in an Iggo corpuscle of the skin on the inner surface of the leg of a monkey. The single afferent nerve fiber was isolated for study by dissection of the saphenous nerve in the thigh. The dependent variable is plotted as the net skin indentation produced by the mechanical stimuli; the zero point for this scale (contact of stimulating probe with skin surface) was determined with an error of no more than ±10 μ. For each intensity 30 identical stimuli, each 450 msec long, were delivered at intervals of 3 sec. The mean numbers of impulses for each of these response populations are plotted as data points. Standard errors for their estimations varied from 0.34 to 0.95 impulses. The fitted curve is the best-fitting power function: $R = 2.16 \cdot S^{0.509}$; correlation coefficient of the regression, $r = 0.985$; $p < 0.005$.

(*To the right*): Log-log transformation of the data presented in the graph to the left. The fitted straight line is the power function given above; its slope is equal to the value of the exponent.

holds for each of these observation periods, the exponents for the series of functions are nearly identical, and the proportionality constant increases monotonically with longer observation times. Detailed results for one of these fibers are given by the graphs of Fig. 4.6. The near constancy of the exponent n predicts that upon logarithmic transformation these curves will appear as a series of nearly parallel lines, as illustrated in Fig. 4.7.

A more general impression of the behavior of a population of fibers is obtained by converting all values to percentile scores, as shown for 10 fibers on the graph of Fig. 4.8. This procedure eliminates the constants, and the exponent n becomes a weighted exponent for the entire population. The log-log plot to the right indicates the goodness of fit and, what is important, that the deviations of the data around the fitted function are random. This graph is reproduced at the top of Fig.

4.9, for comparison with that below on which the data are plotted in the Fechnerian semilogarithmic relation. The non-random deviation of the data points in this lower graph is obvious.

Now the form of the best-fitting function describing the stimulus-response relation is intrinsically of little interest. It becomes of great interest, however, when compared with the results of somewhat similar studies in man. As most of you know, it has become clear in the last few years that when humans are asked to make subjective estimations of the magnitude of sensory stimuli, the resulting relation is best described by a power function. The exponent for tactile sensibility is very close to that obtained for these mechanoreceptive fibers [Jones, 1960; Stevens, 1957].

I believe this near identity of the S-R relation for human observers and first-order fibers is of some importance. It suggests that the neural transforms intervening between input and a final verbal description of an introspective magnitude estimation of the strength of tactile stimuli

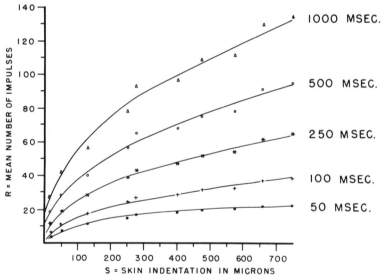

Fig. 4.6. Stimulus-response relations for a mechanoreceptive fiber ending in an Iggo corpuscle of the skin of the inner side of the leg of a monkey. Single afferent fiber isolated for study by dissection of the saphenous nerve in the thigh. The fitted curves plot the S-R relations for a series of observation times, each of which begins with stimulus onset. All correlation coefficients of regression better than 0.991; all p's < 0.005. Thirty stimuli delivered at each intensity, at repetition rate of one in three seconds; variability of response number shown by the graph to the lower right in Fig. 4.3. Standard errors of the estimates of mean values varied from zero to 1.46 impulses.

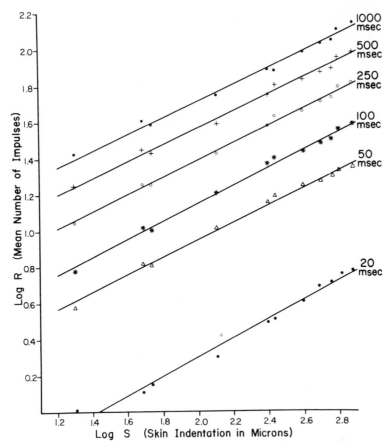

Fig. 4.7. Replot of the data given in Fig. 4.6, here on log-log coordinates, with best-fitting functions hence given as straight lines. The nearly parallel positions of the lines illustrates the near constancy of the value of the exponent n in the series of power functions; from below upwards, $n = 0.479$, 0.536, 0.479, 0.499, 0.474, 0.458, 0.448, 0.444.

must be linear for the intensive continuum. This does not imply, of course, that those intervening transforms must all be linear, but that the sum of their serial superposition must be so. Whether they are all linear can of course only be settled by the results of future experiments.

What Is the Neural Discriminandum?

Early studies of stimulus discrimination in man led to the formulation of Weber's law, that the size of the discriminable stimulus increment

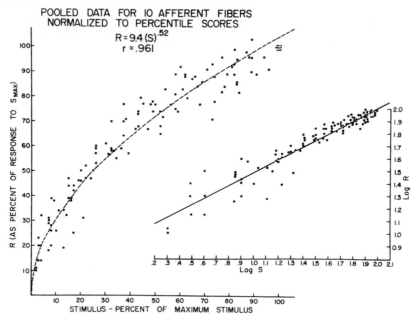

Fig. 4.8. Graph to the left shows stimulus-response relation for 10 mechanoreceptive fibers, on normalized scales. The relation for each fiber was fitted by a power function of the form $R = K \cdot S^n$, with n's less than unity, with a high degree of certainty (p's < 0.005). Data for each fiber normalized by conversion of stimulus values, measured in microns of skin indentation, to per cents of the maximal indentation, and response number values to per cents of the response evoked by that maximal stimulus. In this procedure, variations in value of the constant K from fiber to fiber are eliminated, and the trend of the entire population is revealed. The graph to the right replots these same data on log-log coordinates.

at any level of stimulus intensity is a constant fraction of that intensity, $\Delta S/S = C$. Further study revealed, however, that the Weber function for man deviates markedly from Weber's law, particularly for stimuli in the weaker range. Knowledge of the precise S-R relation for mechanoreceptive fibers has allowed us to test certain assumptions about the nature of the least increment in neural input which may be discriminable by a central detector. In this way we have constructed Weber functions, and have sought for and lent credence to that one most closely resembling the Weber function for man. We have done this both by calculation from the S-R relation, and directly in experiments using automatic computation, by a method which I shall not detail here [Werner, 1965].

We have tested two of the many possible assumptions about the nature of the discriminable neural increment. The first is that no matter

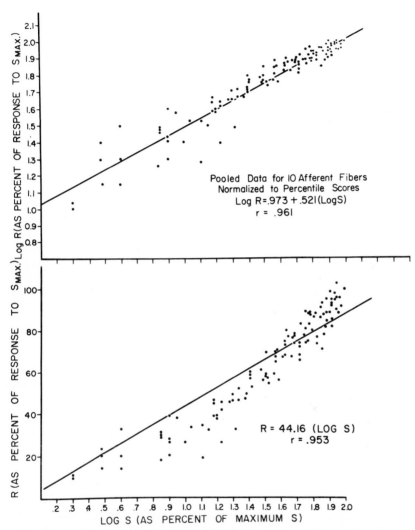

Fig. 4.9. The graph above is a duplicate of that shown to the right of Fig. 4.8, and plots on log-log coordinates the stimulus-response relation for 10 mechanoreceptive fibers, on normalized scales. The same data are shown on the graph below plotted as real percentile response number against the logarithm of the percentile stimulus value. The steady deviations from the Fechnerian relation are apparent.

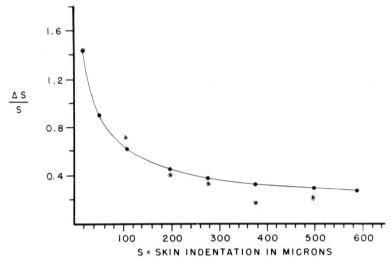

Fig. 4.10. Graph of the Weber function $\Delta S/S = f(S)$ for a mechanoreceptive fiber. The points connected by the drawn curve are calculated from the stimulus-response relation for this fiber: $R = 2.161 \cdot S^{0.502}$, assuming that the least discriminable response increment $R = 7$ impulses per response, at any stimulus intensity. The asterisks mark points of the Weber function which were experimentally determined, as described in Werner and Mountcastle [1965], using the same least discriminable response increment of 7 impulses.

what the intensity of the comparison stimulus, or the level of the response to it, the discriminable neural increment above that comparison response is a constant number of impulses, in a given period of time. The graph of Fig. 4.10 shows the results obtained for one fiber, with the assumption that the discriminable neural increment is 7 impulses, in the response to a 400 msec mechanical stimulus. The filled dots represent results obtained by calculation, the asterisks the results of direct experiment. Figure 4.11 shows a series of Weber functions for another fiber, here calculated for a series of different observation times, with the assumption for each that the discriminable neural increment is 5 impulses. The curves shown in these two figures closely resemble the Weber function which holds for tactile sensibility in man: they do not resemble Weber's law. A function identical to Weber's law is obtained, however, if one assumes that the just discriminable neural increment is a constant fraction of the comparison response. The contrasting functions obtained on the basis of these two different assumptions are indicated by the curves of Fig. 4.12. These results imply, but of course do not prove, that a central detector discriminates equal rather than fractional increments in neural activity, across the full range of neural response.

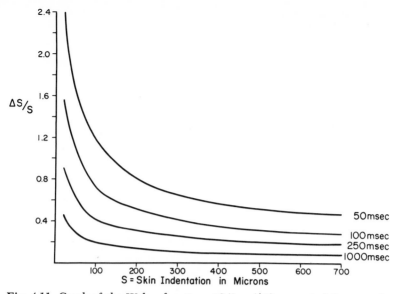

Fig. 4.11. Graph of the Weber functions $\Delta S/S = f(S)$ computed for a mechanoreceptive fiber on the basis of the stimulus-response relations determined for different observation times (in msec, to the right of the curves). The least discriminable response increment was assumed to be 5 impulses per response at any stimulus intensity.

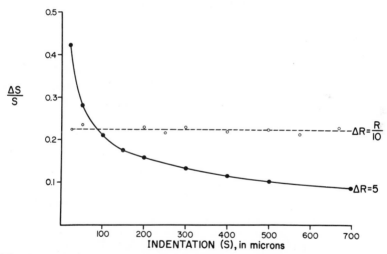

Fig. 4.12. Graph of two Weber functions $\Delta S/S = f(S)$ computed for a mechanoreceptive fiber on the basis of the stimulus response relation determined for an observation time of 1000 msec: $R = 7.004 \cdot (S)^{0.444}$. The solid points connected by the curve were obtained by assuming that the least discriminable response increment $\Delta R = 5$ impulses per response, at any stimulus intensity. The empty circles connected by the dashed line were obtained by assuming that ΔR is a constant fraction (in this case $\frac{1}{10}$) of the response at any stimulus intensity.

The Capacity of Afferent Touch Fibers to Transmit Information

In preceding sections I have compared the general form of the S-R relation and the derived Weber function for first-order neural activity with their respective counterparts for tactile sensation in man. What seems to me to be a remarkable similarity exists; and from it we can, I believe, propose reasonable conjectures about the neural transformations which link the two — hypotheses which can be tested experimentally. However, it was not possible to compare directly the numerical parameters for the two cases. In the first place, sensation magnitude cannot be equated directly with any one measure of neural activity, precise though that may be; and secondly, some uncertainty remains as to the proper stimulus metric, though the actual magnitudes used in our experiments were quite similar to those used in psychophysical experiments in man.

One way of circumventing the problem of the specific of stimulus and response metrics, which allows one to compare events occurring in the quite different experimental situations, is provided by a very simple application of some methods and concepts of information theory [Garner, 1962]. This has been done for a number of sense continua in man, and we have applied this method to the stimulus-evoked activity in mechanoreceptive fibers, for comparison.

Consider a number of stimuli composing a set of different discrete stimuli of different intensities. There then exists some uncertainty about the identity of any given stimulus, depending upon the frequency with which it occurs in the set. That stimulus uncertainty is given by

$$U(S) = -\Sigma[p(S) \cdot \log_2 p(S)].$$

All the responses to all the stimuli of such a set can be grouped in an S-R matrix such as that shown for one fiber in Fig. 4.13. A simple transformation of such a matrix is to convert the individual values to their probabilities. One can then calculate the joint uncertainty which exists between the two variables:

$$U(S, R) = -\Sigma[p(S, R) \cdot \log_2 p(S, R)].$$

Similarly, a matrix can be constructed with the same marginal probabilities, but now on the assumption that there is no dependent relation between the two variables. The probability terms in such an orthogonal matrix can be used to calculate an uncertainty,

$$U_{\max}(S, R) = -\Sigma[p(S, R \cdot \log_2 p (S,R)],$$

STIMULUS CATEGORIES — maximal = 30

Fiber 25-1, Random Series — Stimulus-Response Matrix

Response Categories–Impulses Per Response

Response	4	5	6	7	8	9	10	11	12	13	14	15	16	17	18	19	20	21	22	23	24	25	26	27	28	29	30	Σ
0-1	29	15	3																									47
2-3	3	11	3																									17
4-5		5	2	1																								8
6-7			8	1																								9
8-9			6	7																								13
10-1			1	10	1																							12
12-3				7	7																							14
14-5				1	7	1																						9
16-7					4	10	3																					17
18-9						8	9	2	1		1		1															22
20-1							2	16	3	2	1	1																25
22-3									5	8	7	7	11	6	4		1											49
24-5										3	9	6	4	5	9	2	4	2										44
26-7											4	3	5	7	5	8	6	2	5	4								49
28-9											1		1	2	8	2	2	5	6	9	4							40
30-1												1			5	6	7	4	6	7	5	7	3		1			52
32-3																2	4	2	6	7	11	9	7	8	5	1		62
34-5																	2	1	5	2	5	9	11	4	3	4	3	49
36-7																		1		1	3	4	6	11	9	4	8	47
38-9																		1			1	5	7	6	7	4		31
40-1																						1	2	5	8	3		19
42-3																								1	3	1		5
44-5																									2	1	1	4
Σ →	32	31	23	27	19	20	34	16	24	18	23	20	27	17	21	21	20	26	23	19	24	24	31	30	27	27	20	644

Fig. 4.13. Stimulus-response matrix for a mechanoreceptive fiber activated by light mechanical stimuli delivered to its corpuscular ending, which lay in the skin of the inner side of the leg of a monkey. The afferent nerve fiber was isolated for study by dissection of the saphenous nerve in the thigh. The maximal movement of the stimulus probe was 690 μ, which was divided into 30 equal steps. Threshold lay between steps 4 and 5 throughout study of this fiber. The stimulus duration was 500 msec, and stimuli were delivered once in three seconds. Stimuli of different intensities were delivered in a random order until 644 were given; numbers of stimuli of different intensities are indicated by the lower horizontal row of numbers. Responses to each of the stimuli categorized by the number of impulses, in steps of 2 impulses. Maximal and contingent uncertainties calculated from the matrix in the manner described in the text.

which is the maximal joint uncertainty of Garner and McGill [1956]. The difference between these two values,

$$U_c(S, R) = U_{max}(S, R) - U(S, R),$$

is termed the contingent uncertainty, and is a measure of the amount by which the receiver's uncertainty — his doubts about the identity of a stimulus when he inspects the response evoked by it — is reduced by virtue of the dependent relation between S and R. It is thus a measure of the information received. The procedure is analogous in many ways to an analysis of variance.

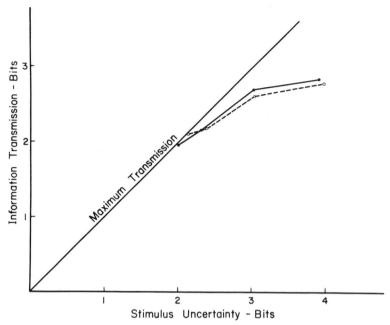

Fig. 4.14. Graph plotting information transmission per stimulus for a mechano-receptive fiber. For the experiment represented by the dashed line the stimuli were delivered in a random order until all stimuli of all intensities selected had been given; the S-R matrix was then constructed, and information transmission calculated as described in the text. For the experiment represented by the solid line all stimuli of any given intensity were delivered *ad seriatim,* then all those of another, etc., and the calculation procedure repeated. The results are not significantly different. Information transmission per stimulus levels off at something less than 3 bits, that is, by inspection of the responses a receiver could divide the stimulus continuum into only seven or eight categories.

The graph of Fig. 4.14 plots this reduction in uncertainty as information transmission in bits, on the ordinate, against stimulus uncertainty, which of course increases as the number of steps into which the stimulus continuum is divided is increased. The graph shows that information transmission is perfect (that is, identification of the stimulus by inspection of its response is perfect) up to a stimulus uncertainty of 2 bits (four categories). As the stimulus uncertainty increases to 3 bits (eight categories) and to 4 bits (sixteen categories) the information transmitted gradually levels off towards a maximum of something less than 3 bits; that is, that by inspection of all responses a receiver could place them into no more than about seven categories. Figure 4.15 shows the results of similar calculations for each of 14 mechanoreceptive fibers. The maximum information transmitted is, on the average, about 2.5 bits per stimulus.

Figure 4.16 shows the results obtained when the hypothetical receiver is allowed to inspect the first 20 msec of the response, then 100 msec, etc. A maximum transmission is reached at about 400 msec, and continuation to 500 or beyond did not produce further increases beyond the 2.5 bit peak, that is, beyond six or seven categories.

Now this rather tedious procedure turns out, at least to me, to be of some interest. The reason is this. When human observers are presented with a series of stimuli of different intensities and asked to place them in categories, they are able to divide the intensive continuum into no more than about seven categories — what Miller [1956] has called the "magic number 7, plus or minus 2!" The implication for an understanding of the neural basis of the human performance is that, at least in principle, information about stimulus intensity could be provided by a single nerve fiber! The recent finding of Hensel and Boman [1960] that a single impulse in a single or each of a very few cutaneous afferents is sufficient to evoke a sensation in conscious humans makes this idea less preposterous than it appears at first glance.

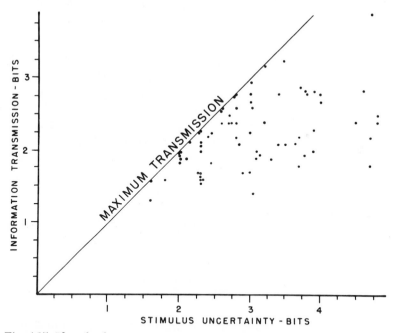

Fig. 4.15. Plot of information transmission calculated from S-R matrices for each of 14 mechanoreceptive fibers, as described in the text. In each case, transmission was calculated, at different degrees of stimulus uncertainty, for only the maximal observation times, which varied from 250 to 500 msec for 13 fibers, and was 1000 msec for 1 fiber. The mean maximum value of transmission is about 2.5 bits per stimulus.

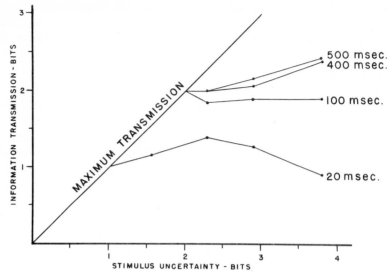

Fig. 4.16. Information transmission calculated from a series of S-R matrices constructed for a mechanoreceptive fiber, for a series of successively longer observation times. Transmission increases little beyond 400 msec of observation. Stimulus duration for this fiber 500 msec.

Now, what contribution is made by the fact that cutaneous afferent fibers innervate peripheral fields in the skin which overlap one another, and converge centrally upon second-order neurons? In this regard it is important to note, I believe, that the limits of categorization of stimulus intensities by man indicated by the magic number seven do not set his limits for comparative judgments. Everyone knows that two stimuli can be discriminated to a very fine degree when only two are considered. In this regard the distribution of activity across a population of fibers, and across the population of central neurons upon which they impinge, must certainly be of importance. This neural profile is also of importance in sensing the locus, the contour, the spatial extent, and the rate and direction of movement, of peripheral stimuli.

Summary

In the beginning I made the statement that from the philosophical standpoint the idea of a psychoneural identity is for me the most suitable. It eliminates distinctions between brain and mind, between neural and psychic, and sets forth the proposition that those more complex aspects of brain function, including introspective aspects of the life of man, may be regarded as more complex aspects of a neural activity with which, at simpler levels, we are now familiar. I then summarized what has been learned during the era of geographical exploration of the somatic afferent system, emphasizing the specificity for space and quality which it displays, the highly organized functional plan of the cerebral cortex, the importance of considering neural matters in terms of the action of populations, with their as yet mysterious emergent properties, and the important role afferent inhibition is likely to play in spatial discrimination.

In the major part of this paper I presented the results of a new study at the first-order level, the input stage of the nervous system, of a certain class of mechanoreceptive fibers which innervate the hairy skin and which end there in highly organized receptor organs. These endings respond to brief stimuli with trains of impulses which quickly reach a stage of a remarkably periodic discharge, which replicates most precisely from one stimulus to the next. The stimulus-response relation could then be determined with some precision, and is accurately described by a power function quite similar in form and constants to that descriptive of the S-R relation for humans, when making introspective estimations of the magnitudes of tactile stimuli. Certain derived aspects of this relation were then considered. It was found that Weber functions resembling those for man could be constructed on the assumption that the least increment in neural activity discriminable by a central detector is a constant number of impulses, and not a fractional increase.

Finally, calculations of information transmission across the skin to these fibers resulted in values almost exactly comparable to those found for man when performing magnitude estimations. The implication for neural processes is that the central nervous system can preserve intact, from input to output, all the information it receives.

DISCUSSION

Chairman: PROFESSOR HEYMANS

ECCLES: You spoke about the power function of the single afferent unit, and you showed experimentally that there was a power relationship. How was this related to Stevens' work on the power relationship as tested for perceptual judgment of the same sensation? There is actually a very wide range of the power functions for different sensory systems.

MOUNTCASTLE: Yes, it is true that the power function for first-order mechanoreceptors is quite similar in the value of the exponent to the power functions which Jones found to describe adequately the relation between the deformation (indentation) of the skin in humans and the subject's subjective estimation of the intensity of the stimulus. This is true even though the stimulating tips used in the two cases differed in diameter by a factor of three. The significance of this identity is, I believe, that the sum of all intervening transformations must be very close to one, though the finding is surprising.

ECCLES: It is important in this connection that, where it has been tested by Granit, Creutzfeldt, and their colleagues, the depolarization produced by an intracellularly applied current is linearly related to the frequency of firing of a neuron.

MOUNTCASTLE: In this connection it would be very exciting indeed if, in the experimental situation, central cells of a sensory system could be brought under complete input control. One could then test different frequencies and avenues of input and measure frequency of output, to determine whether synaptic transmission across the relay is actually linear, in this sense.

TEUBER: Those of us who have been concerned with proving these power functions purely psychophysically feel tremendous relief that you can show them so directly and elegantly. I think the parallelism between the results of your experiments and those of Stevens is more than a coincidence. We have made similar observations, using a much cruder method, namely the recording of computer-averaged potentials from the human scalp to flashes of light of different intensities. Dr. Herbert Vaughan in our laboratory found that the latencies of these evoked potentials can be arranged as a function of the different intensities of the flash and that this plot conforms to a simple power law with an exponent of 0.3. This happens to be exactly the exponent which is yielded by Stevens' method of brightness estimation. Thus, although we are dealing here with a different sensory modality, and a rather different physiological technique, we still get a rather good correspondence between the power law of Stevens and the electrophysiological results.

Subjective estimates of magnitudes of sensation increase much more rapidly if one uses electrical shock to the finger rather than light flashes to the eye. It might be worthwhile to examine whether evoked potentials would again reflect this more rapid increase, since for direct electrical shock to the finger the exponent is around 3.

MOUNTCASTLE: I did not emphasize to any considerable extent the remarkable similarity between the values of exponents we have found for evoked neural activity and those observed in psychophysical measurements. True, they are similar, but the chance remains (I believe at long odds) that this is coincidental, for the stimulus situation has been different in the two cases. It would be ideal if neurophysiological experiments on animals and psychophysical experiments on humans could be carried out using the same stimulators.

CREUTZFELDT: It may be mentioned that in the visual system the exponent of the power function which relates intensity and reaction (of single neurons or in psychophysical tests) seems to be always relatively low (between 0.1 and 0.4). Such a power function, however, is hardly distinguishable from a logarithmic function over a wide range. By expressing the intensity-reaction relation in the visual system by a power function, therefore, the classical Weber-

Fechner relation is not ruled out. But since both functions are not more than a formal description of a systematic relation without giving a clear hint as to the transform mechanism at the receptor site, the argument, exponential versus power function, within the visual system seems to me to be merely academic.

MAC KAY: When Dr. Mountcastle speaks of overall linear transmission from "input" to "output," what output is in question?

MOUNTCASTLE: The output in question is the final behavioral response, that is, the verbal expression of a subjective estimation of magnitude. Of course, any number of nonlinear transformations might intervene between first-order neural input and that output. All I wish to imply is that, in sum, they are likely to be linear. Of course, as you know, Stevens has gone further and asked his subjects to express the value of that subjective magnitude estimation in terms of the strength of hand squeezing, measured with a dynamometer. Certainly some of those intervening transfers may be nonlinear, but the final output (motor in this case) is very nicely matched, value for value, with the subjective estimation described verbally.

MAC KAY: I am thinking of the possibility that, in the estimation of subjective intensity, the subject's information system is "backing off" the intensity of input by generating something internally.* In that case, nonlinearity in transmission could be tolerated, provided that the backing off activity suffered a similar transformation. It should be noted, too, that if we chose to define the stimulus by some parameter other than displacement, not related to it by a power law, the overall law could not be a power law.

MOUNTCASTLE: Yes, it did occur to us that the use of a different physical scale along which to measure the intensity of the stimulus might result in a stimulus-response relation of another form. For the late steady state period of the response, we were able to test this possibility, for then we could measure both the extent of skin indentation and the force produced by it. We found that when force is used as the independent variable, the relation is fitted by a power function, with only a slight change in value of the exponent. The value shifted a bit closer to one, and in one case actually reached a linear relation. In another test of the possibility you mention, we have studied the relation of the transient onset phase of the response to the *rate* of skin indentation. Once again, the relation is best described by a power function with an exponent slightly less than one.

Even assuming, on your hypothesis, that the subject estimates stimulus magnitude by generating some neural activity which matches that evoked by the stimulus—the backing off process—surely for each stimulus magnitude the degree to which he must generate this backing off process to reach a null point must be exactly determined by the degree of neural activity evoked by the stimulus. I know of no direct evidence that such a process takes place, and the very short intracortical times required for discriminations make it unlikely, I believe.

MAC KAY: With regard to the interpretation of the informational rate of two or three bits per stimulus, it is true that, where the input is *randomly* dis-

* D. M. MacKay. *Science, 139,* 1213–1216 [1963].

tributed, this would correspond to an assumption of seven categories; but in the typical biological situation, in which there is a high degree of correlation between successive stimuli, does not this interpretation become questionable?

MOUNTCASTLE: Your point is a good one, and the results which I describe pertain only to the experimental situations in which the responses to successive stimuli can be shown to be independent events. A point which interested us is that when stimuli are delivered to the skin at rates more rapid than once in 3 sec the temporal dependency seems to be determined by the properties of the skin much more than by neural refractoriness, or unresponsiveness. Upon observing the skin at 16× magnification during a stimulus, one sees that the skin rebounds along a two-phased time course. One of these, and much the greater, occurs very rapidly; the second and smaller is much slower, and the skin does not rebound to its prestimulus position in space for nearly 3 sec. What we must do now is to determine the information transmission when stimuli are delivered more rapidly. We know that when the somatic system is performing most elegantly, as in the reading of Braille, spatial discriminations are made at a very rapid rate indeed. Whether intensity discriminations can be made at such rapid rates, I do not know. What is certain from its physiological properties is that this system is most potently organized for spatial discriminations.

ECCLES: Has Stevens himself or his pupils ever attempted to change the power factor by repeated application over a long time of the same input? Such an experiment would be relevant to learning or habituation. Has this been tried quantitatively?

MOUNTCASTLE: Not to my knowledge. Perhaps Dr. Teuber can provide this information, but I believe the result of most of the psychophysical experiments has been just the opposite.

TEUBER: The initial emphasis in all of these experiments, of course, has been the converse—to avoid corrective changes of the kind that Creutzfeldt hints at. It should be noted that there is a general tendency in assessing intensity of sensory information to utilize a power function, as, for example, in estimating the magnitude of weights.

MOUNTCASTLE: I do know of one experiment which may be relevant to Dr. Creutzfeldt's suggestion. It is reported that an intellectually gifted person was able, with prolonged practice, to increase the number of categories from 7 or 8 to 9 or 10.

CREUTZFELDT: Yes, and this "differential judgment" seems to be the most important point.

SCHAEFER: May I add a word to the problem of Creutzfeldt? As far as I remember, the exponential functions in the temperature sensation are nearly the same as you demonstrated. Hensel showed this, and as far as I know, the subjective scale of our information, which we get subjectively, is as accurate as we have it in the touch sense, though in the temperature senses we know it is an unconscious function which only serves the balance of heat production and heat delivery. So far, the whole problem could be some sort of a sham problem because behind the story is some sort of statistical effect which only informs the animal of such a very general thing as the temperature on its surface.

JASPER: I seem to remember that Dr. Stevens has reported that it requires a great deal of training on the part of the subject as a preliminary to these experiments on numerical assessment of sensory experiences.

MOUNTCASTLE: No, I do not believe that is correct. In fact, the most regular results were obtained when the observers were given no instruction whatsoever, not even a single stimulus of stated value as a scalar orientation. The subjects were simply told that they would receive certain stimuli, and were asked to assign numbers to them.

I would like to make one general comment. I believe that the importance of making quantitative estimations of these relations for sensory receptors and for central neural relays is independent of whether or not they should match the relations observed in psychophysical studies, though whether or not the two are similar is of predictive value for the further neural processes interposed between input and behavioral response. When such measurements are available one can then make some derived measures which are of great importance.

JASPER: The second question I would like to ask is: What is the relation between the quantitive alterations in first-order afferent discharge and discharge of thalamic units? Are these not some important modifications at first- and second-order synapses? Would you be willing to tell us more of your observations at higher levels along the pathway?

MOUNTCASTLE: Dr. Werner and I do already have similar measures for a few thalamic neurons which are linked only to these receptors (a remarkable example of specificity!). The exponents determined hover around one, or slightly below. So we can say, on the basis of these preliminary studies, that transfer across the two intervening synaptic relays is linear.

MAC KAY: But you would agree, would you not, that in cases where Stevens demonstrates an overall power law and physiology demonstrates a receptor logarithmic law, there need be no incompatibility? You are not suggesting that it was necessary for *both* to give power laws? In the visual system, for instance, you would not have any particular stake in proving that the response of photoreceptors was a power law function and not a logarithmic one?

MOUNTCASTLE: Certainly not; but it is of considerable interest, at least to me, when the two are similar.

REFERENCES

FEIGL, H. The "mental" and the "physical," in: *Concepts, Theories and the Mind-Body Problem; Minnesota Studies in the Philosophy of Science.* Vol. II (ed. by H. Feigl, G. Maxwell, and M. Scriven). Minneapolis: Univ. Minnesota Press, pp. 370–497 [1958].

GARNER, W. R. *Uncertainty and Structure as Psychological Concepts.* New York: Wiley [1962].

114 / V. B. Mountcastle

GARNER, W. R., and W. J. McGILL. Relation between information and variance analyses, *Psychometrika, 21,* 219–228 [1956].

VON HELMHOLTZ, H. L. F. *On the Sensations of Tone as a Physiological Basis for the Theory of Music.* New York: Dover, 2nd English ed. [1954].

HENSEL, H., and K. K. A. BOMAN. Afferent impulses in cutaneous sensory nerves in human subjects, *J. Neurophysiol., 23,* 564–578 [1960].

HUBEL, D. H., and T. N. WIESEL. Receptive fields, binocular interaction and functional architecture in the cat's visual cortex, *J. Physiol., 160,* 106–154 [1962].

——. Receptive fields of cells in striate cortex of very young, visually inexperienced kittens, *J. Neurophysiol., 26,* 994–1002 [1963a].

——. Shape and arrangement of columns in cat's striate cortex, *J. Physiol., 165,* 559–568 [1963b].

HUNT, C. C., and A. K. McINTYRE. Properties of cutaneous touch receptors in cat, *J. Physiol., 153,* 88–98 [1960].

IGGO, A. New specific sensory structures in hairy skin, *Acta Neurovegetativa, 24,* 175–180 [1963a].

——. An electrophysiological analysis of afferent fibers in primate skin, *Acta Neurovegetativa, 24,* 225–240 [1963b].

——, and A. R. MUIR. A cutaneous sense organ in the hairy skin of cat, *J. Anat., 97,* 151 [1963].

JONES, F. N. Some subjective magnitude functions for touch, in: *Symposium on Cutaneous Sensibility* (ed. by G. R. Hawkes). Report No. 424. Fort Knox, Ky.: U. S. Army Med. Res. Lab. [1960].

MILLER, G. A. The magical number seven, plus or minus two: Some limits on our capacity for processing information, *Psychol. Rev., 63,* 81–97 [1956].

MOUNTCASTLE, V. B. Modality and topographic properties of single neurons of cat's somatic sensory cortex, *J. Neurophysiol., 20,* 408–434 [1957].

——. Duality of function in the somatic afferent system, in: *Brain and Behavior* (ed. by M. A. B. Brazier). Washington, D. C.: Amer. Institute Biol. Sci., pp. 67–93 [1961a].

——. Some functional properties of the somatic afferent system, in: *Sensory Communication* (ed. by W. A. Rosenblith). Cambridge, Mass.: MIT Press, Chapt. 22, pp. 403–436 [1961b].

——, and T. P. S. POWELL. Neural mechanisms subserving cutaneous sensibility, with special reference to the role of afferent inhibition in sensory perception and discrimination, *Bull. Johns Hopkins Hosp., 105,* 201–232 [1959].

PEPPER, S. C. A neural identity theory of mind, in: *Dimensions of Mind* (ed. by S. Hook). New York: New York Univ. Press, pp. 45–61 [1960].

POGGIO, G. F., and V. B. MOUNTCASTLE. The functional properties of ventrobasal thalamic neurons studied in unanesthetized animals, *J. Neurophysiol., 26,* 775–806 [1963].

POWELL, T. S. P., and V. B. MOUNTCASTLE. Some aspects of the functional organization of the cortex of the postcentral gyrus of the monkey: A correlation of findings obtained in a single unit analysis with cytoarchitecture, *Bull. Johns Hopkins Hosp., 105,* 173–200 [1959].

ROSE, J. E., and V. B. MOUNTCASTLE. Touch and kinesthesis, in: *Handbook of Physiology*. Washington, D. C.: Amer. Physiological Soc., Vol. 1, Chapt. 17, pp. 387–429 [1959].

STEVENS, S. C. On the psychophysical law, *Psychol. Rev.*, *64*, 153–181 [1957].

TAPPER, D. N. Cutaneous slowly adapting mechanoreceptors in the cat, *Science*, *143*, 53–54 [1964].

WERNER, G., and V. B. MOUNTCASTLE. A study of neural activity in mechano-receptive cutaneous afferents: Stimulus-response relations, Weber functions, and information transmission, *J. Neurophysiol.*, *28*, 359–397 [1965].

WIESEL, T. N., and D. H. HUBEL. Single-cell responses in striate cortex of kittens deprived of vision in one eye, *J. Neurophysiol.*, *26*, 1003–1017 [1963].

5

Sensory Mechanisms in Perception

by Ragnar Granit

The Nobel Institute for Neurophysiology, Stockholm, Sweden

It may be necessary at the outset to emphasize that my theme is taken to be physiological mechanisms in perception, as elucidated by reasonably precise experimentation. Many participants are laymen in this field and may like to know how far into psychology we can penetrate by the analysis of cell properties, impulses, and circuitry and I shall try to provide an answer to this question by selecting suitable cases. Clearly we cannot explain the existence of conscious modalities such as sight, smell, and hearing, though we can trace their pathways. Probably the physiologist in the past has done best when studying the sense organs purely as measuring instruments, quantifying his findings, and going on to look for equivalents in perception. There is, for instance, in vision and acoustics the threshold in terms of impulses per unit energy in different wavelengths which determines thresholds as perceived. Thus the rhodopsin distribution of spectral sensitivity can be measured photochemically, physiologically, and psychologically (as perceived threshold), and the values obtained by these different methods lie on the same curve (after correction in the last case for slight selective absorption in the ocular media). The information from the transducer has thus been relayed without distortion.

Nevertheless, it is not any more the main problem of sensory physiology to define transducer properties of end organs at the various places where their message can be intercepted in order to compare with psychophysical experiences. On the contrary, physiology is chiefly engaged in finding out how simple transducer properties are played upon by the nervous system in order to produce a representation of the world around us and of the state of our own body. Our science may, in the course of this work, often have to stop and be satisfied with generalizations which cannot immediately be interpreted in terms of sensory experience. This need cause no worry. If the generalizations are good, they tell us something about the properties of the central nervous system and sooner or later this knowledge will come in handy.

A very simple example will show how important it is that the sensory input should be subjected to restraining influences. You have all heard about the fabulous sensitivity of our sense organs. If mechanisms for attenuating, organizing, and distributing the impulses from the periphery did not exist, there would be a continuous and formidable bombardment of the central nervous system by this barrage which would be fatal for the organism. The really challenging problem of sensory physiology of this day is to study the nervous system as an instrument for transmitting, selecting, and reorganizing the peripheral messages. This is where circuit analysis comes in and holds out a promise to those feeling that it is worth their while hunting for general principles. After all, the central circuits are not exceptionally complicated and in suitable places can be isolated for study. The complexity lies in the multiplication of them and this in turn will be a mathematical problem, provided we first have given the mathematicians something to work on in the way of first principles.

Let us begin with the simplest problem of a straightforward set of relays transmitting, as we know, a message with little distortion. A good example is the lemniscal pathway for touch, intercepted by Mountcastle [1961] and his colleagues at various places and all along found to exhibit much the same properties in terms of impulse frequency. We are on relatively firm ground in evaluating the factors concerned in relaying quantity or intensity of a message. Impulse frequency was established as such a factor long ago by Adrian [1928], and Adrian and Bronk [1929] showed that total number of activated fibers also determines the effect. We should add synaptic density. A sufficient number of synaptic knobs is necessary or else the system becomes too facultative, depending too much on other influences playing upon the relay cell. Impulse frequency at the next cell is translated into depolarizing current, often recordable intracellularly as the postsynaptic potential of Eccles [1957, 1964] and his colleagues. The depolarizing current in its turn makes that cell fire off impulses. By injecting current through the tip of the intracellular electrode we [Granit, Kernell, and Shortess, 1963] have recently tried to establish the quantitative relationship between impulse frequency and current strength (Figs. 5.1 and 5.2). It is seen to be one of direct proportionality, the proportionality constant being high for a brief initial discharge and rapidly diminishing, owing to adaptation at the membrane. These results have been independently confirmed [Shapovalov, 1963]. The finally adapted constants in motoneurons are of the order of 2.5

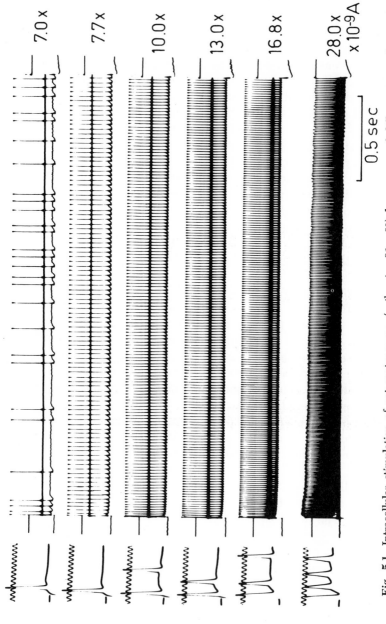

Fig. 5.1. Intracellular stimulation of rat motoneuron (spike size 81 mV) by currents of different strength. On the left, initial spikes recorded on fast sweep circuit with time in msec. Note change of sensitivity of current-recording beam of oscillograph between 7.0 and 7.7×10^{-9} A. For the strongest current, spike size has diminished (cf. Fig. 5.2 for plot) [from Granit, Kernell, and Shortess, 1963, p. 913].

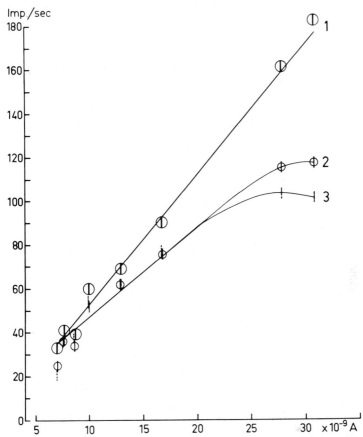

Fig. 5.2. Frequency of discharge plotted against current strength for motoneuron of Fig. 5.1. Curve 1, slope constant 5.9 impulses per sec per nA derives from ⅓ sec following first interval; curve 2, same after 1.3 sec; curve 3, same after 2.6 sec, measuring time extended to ½ sec. Slope constant of 2 and 3 is 4.1 impulses per sec per nA. The rectilinear portion of these curves was calculated by the method of least squares [from Granit, Kernell, and Shortess, 1963, p. 914].

impulses per sec per nA. The large majority of the cells in the spinal cord and elsewhere are much smaller internuncial cells or interneurons, and in them we have found proportionality constants ten to twenty times higher (Granit and Kernell, unpublished), which means that they can serve as efficient amplifiers, a point to be returned to.

Do the nerve impulses also deliver current in proportion to their frequency? Indirect evidence from the *Limulus* eye [Hartline and Ratliff, 1956] and from Renshaw cells [Granit and Renkin, 1961] suggest this to be the case. If in relay after relay direct proportionality prevails in the alternating transition from impulse frequency to depolarizing current to impulse frequency, then freedom from distortion is explained. Depending upon the proportionality constants, the message can be stepped up or attenuated.

Having begun with the relatively simple case of a pure relay function, let us now proceed to design an elementary nervous center, making use of postsynaptic inhibition which the intracellular method showed to be caused by hyperpolarizing currents across the cell membrane [Brock, Coombs, and Eccles, 1952], often recordable as an inhibitory postsynaptic potential. There is little one can do with only one end organ and one relay cell if that end organ has inhibitory synapses on the latter, unless this cell is fired from elsewhere. The message simply comes to an end and communication is prevented. We need a minimum of two end organs, A and B, and if B were inhibitory on the relay cell of excitatory A, then something could be done. This gives us two signaling directions, and if A and B differed spatially, or with respect to sensitivity to wavelength or in some other way, then the relay could dispatch a message consisting of a comparison of the effect from A with that from B. While convergence of two or several end organs upon the same cells is quite common, I am not aware of any proven case in vertebrates for which the first synapses had been shown to be of different sign, one $+$, the other $-$. I shall discuss recurrent inhibition later.

The basic organization seems, in fact, to be a little more complicated. As far as we now can conclude from present evidence, the simplest working center would be the one shown in Fig. 5.3 (left). A and B are two end organs, both excitatory on their own relay cells, R_A and R_B, as well as on their internuncial cells I_A and I_B. This is marked by $+$. The internuncial cell of A is inhibitory on B and that of B is inhibitory on A, marked by $-$. Now we have inhibition working against excitation to modulate or stop it. A can, for example, exclude B, and B can exclude A. The classical example is reciprocal reflex innervation of a flexor and its antagonist extensor from muscle receptors, long ago elucidated by Sherrington. Eccles and his coworkers have laid down a great deal of hard work in proving that inhibition needs an internuncial cell and he will, no doubt, at this meeting present his evidence for it. The internuncial cells are a kind of biasing device on which some other influence, say, from a higher station, can be made to work. Their high amplification factors, mentioned above, make them very potent in control. In Fig. 5.3 (right) I have indicated control of the interneuron for I_B by an inhibitory line. Assume that the organism encounters a situation in which flexors and extensors have to work together, a quite common case. Then the internuncial cells can be inhibited from some other

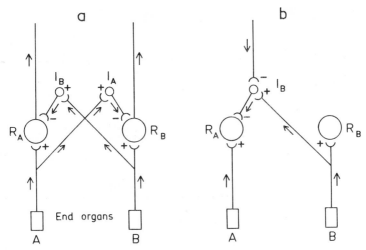

Fig. 5.3. Diagram of simplified afferent centers. (a) From two end organs, A and B, excitatory ($+$) impulses run to relay cells R_A and R_B as well as to internuncial cells I_A and I_B. From the latter, inhibitory ($-$) impulses to the relay cells. (b) Part of center as in a provided with centrifugal control ($-$) from elsewhere.

station in the brain or elsewhere, and A and B will now initiate contractions in both flexors and extensors.

As I shall use the visual pathway for many illustrations of first principles, let us already at this stage look at the behavior of a retinal ganglion cell in which the characteristic effect of illumination [Hartline, 1938] is a discharge at onset and cessation of illumination (Fig. 5.4), the so-called on- and off-effects. Light inhibits the off-effect [Granit and Therman, 1935; Hartline, 1938]. It has also been shown that the on- and off-discharges are mutually exclusive [Granit, 1949, 1951; Kuffler, 1953]. The retinal message dispatched upwards along the optic nerve fibers from the retinal ganglion cells are thus organized on the principle of reciprocal innervation. We should perhaps recall that the message from a retinal receptor runs to a bipolar cell and from there to the ganglion cell, and that there are two strata of interneurons in this organ, the so-called horizontal and amacrine cells. Thus what the muscle receptors achieve in the spinal cord, the retina can do already in the eye itself.

I have been niggardly in using only two end organs and two relay cells in designing an elementary center that can illustrate—as we shall see—most of the fundamental principles discovered by microrecording. For the time being I have also left out recurrent fibers, which deliver the feedback effects, to be discussed briefly below. As to the rest, I maintain that we can get very far with our design by merely multiplying end

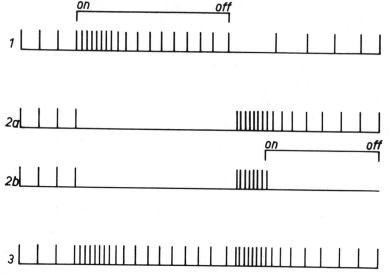

Fig. 5.4. Diagram illustrating three fibers in the optic nerve firing spontaneously and their responses to illumination [from Granit, 1955, p. 34].

organs, relay cells, and interneurons, the way the central nervous system has done in order to go about its business.

The simple center designed to illustrate first principles also emphasizes a principle so far only tacitly introduced. This is the principle of comparison. The message from A is compared with that from B. Thinking of vision, if A were strongly illuminated and the nearby B weakly illuminated, the relays would operate in one way; if both received the same amount of illumination they would work in another way. The basis of comparison is that A and B, which differ in some way or another in the end, are connected anatomically and functionally are capable of cross talk. Comparisons will operate at all stages and sensory messages can be compared in many different ways with events elsewhere. Adding memory, we can ultimately, for example, see that an orange is soft. I shall show later how space is organized as piecemeal comparisons by groups of cells within anatomical maps.

In the first center that we designed, A and B were connected to the same relay cells and this arrangement was neglected temporarily because it did not take care of inhibition. It was assumed that convergence of this kind at the first relay carries excitation only. Massive convergence of receptors at the first relay is very common. In the peripheral retina, hundreds of rods and several cones run to the same bipolar cell and several bipolars converge towards the same ganglion cell. Measuring thresholds at the level of the optic nerve in different wavelengths in order optimally to isolate the excitatory effects, one finds a broad curve, called the dominator [Granit, 1947], which gives the average distribution of light sensitivity without wavelength specification. This is best obtained from the large ganglion cells which collect information of this general type. The dominator corresponds well with the psychophysical function called brightness distribution and shifts its point of maximum sensitivity with state of adaptation the way the psychophysical curves do. Convergence has only served to improve sensitivity. There are also fibers in the optic nerve which dispatch narrow-banded messages, obviously far more useful for color specification. These are called modulators and represent a discrimination of wavelength for which it has been necessary to introduce the action of retinal inhibitory cells cutting down band width by a process of interaction whose basis is spectral overlap of sensitivity of, say, red A and green B in the scheme of Fig. 5.3 (left).

It is a little surprising that for the sense of smell, convergence at the first relay should be as high as 20,000 receptors per one cell in the olfactory bulb, which in spite of this is capable of very high discrimination. From the comparison with the retina, one would be inclined to think of excitatory convergence merely as an organization for ensuring a general background of olfactory depolarization, but let us see what we can do, assuming the number of elementary odors to be very much larger than those of elementary receptors to wavelengths of light. These are not likely to be more than three, and four if rhodopsin rods be included. To illustrate this idea, let us take six specific receptors, which is likely to be much too small a figure. Let the six organs A–F be combined in groups of three. This would give twenty combinations. The number of combinations would be very much greater if the combinations also represented different proportions, say, $2A + 1B + 3C$, etc. If such combinations at higher relays were compared by making use of excitation and inhibition, much as elsewhere in the central nervous system, good discrimination would be possible, and no unknown principles need be invoked.

The discussion of first principles would be deficient if discrimination by mapping were not considered in some detail. This is the very foundation stone for all work on sensory mechanisms of perception. A century of anatomical and histological study has provided us with a great deal of fundamental knowledge as to where impulses go, expanded during the last three decades by the method of electrophysiological localization employing "evoked potentials." These are electrical responses elicited from some point in the afferent pathway and recorded as evoked at another point to which that pathway has access. Discrete pathways deliver messages to discrete patches of cells. One speaks of somatotopic specificity and it seems that anything that can be spatially discriminated actually is found laid out on a somatotopic map of its own. I leave to Professor Mountcastle the task of considering the tactile maps of the body surface and take as my example the visual projections which we have known in considerable detail long before the electrophysiological era introduced testing by evoked potentials. In this field we owe our basic knowledge to a large number of first-rate anatomists and pathologists. A good historical review of their work has been given by the late Stephen Polyak [1957].

The visual maps from the two eyes are laid out with great precision both on the geniculate body and on the cortical surface. Crossed and uncrossed portions of the optic tract are represented in separate juxtaposed layers. Impulses serving binocular vision are thus taken to separate layers in the geniculate body, and the field of vision is mapped out on the cortical striate area with a degree of magnification that reaches a maximum for the foveal area of optimal visual acuity. Talbot and Marshall [1941] with six monkeys found a peripheral magnification at 5° averaging 18 min of visual angle per mm increasing centrally to 2 min per mm.

Impulse recording at various sites in the visual pathway has led to greater clarity than in any other sensory pathway and for this reason deserves to be singled out for a presentation of what can be achieved by this technique. Beginning at the retinal ganglion cells sending their fibers into the optic nerve, let us recall that each of them takes off from a miniature center consisting of a number of receptors, bipolars, horizontal and amacrine cells, all of which contribute to the properties of the receptive field represented in one ganglion cell. This varies in size with type of retina and location, but we can think of it as being of the order of 0.5 to 1.0 mm in diameter. Hartline's [1940] analysis of the receptive fields of the frog eye showed them to overlap and to be most sensitive in the middle, some firing in response to light "on," some to light "off" and some to both "on" or "off." In the cat, Kuffler [1953] found fields whose centers were either on- or off-centers, while in each case the surrounds were of opposite type so that the on-off antagonism, as it were, was incorporated into the spatial analyzer which the receptive field represents. In this general manner, receptive fields have since been found to be organized in the goldfish retina [Wagner, MacNichol, and Wolbarsht, 1960], in the retina [Barlow and Hill, 1963] and geniculate body [Arden, 1963] of the rabbit, in the geniculate body of the cat [Hubel and Wiesel, 1961], in the cortex of the cat [Hubel and Wiesel, 1959, 1961] and the monkey [Hubel and Wiesel, 1964]. To speak of on-impulses to illumination and off-impulses to cessation of illumination has become customary, but it

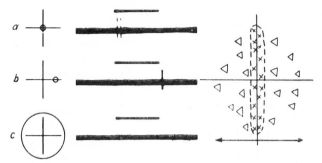

Fig. 5.5. Responses of a unit in the cat's striate cortex to stimulation with circular spots of light. Receptive field located in area centralis of contralateral eye. (This unit could also be activated by the ipsilateral eye). (a) 1° spot in the center region; (b) Same spot displaced 3° to the right. (c) 8° spot covering entire receptive field. Stimulus intensity 1.65 log mc, background illumination 0.17 log mc [from Hubel and Wiesel, 1959, p. 578].

should be realized that increase of illumination and some darkening suffice to elicit the on- and off-discharges respectively.

The question now arises of what role this apparently fundamental organization into receptive fields, based on reciprocal antagonism between center and surround, plays in the visual act, since it is so well maintained up to the final station. In vertebrates, the fields increase in size upwards and we have to think of several retinal fields being incorporated in one larger cortical field organized in the same manner. The cortical receptive fields often turn out to be elongated in shape and also the antagonism between center and surround increases upwards. While most retinal receptive fields respond with on- and off-effects even when the whole receptive area is filled out so as to give the antagonistic forces full play, the cortical fields under similar circumstances tend to be silent because of the mutual inhibition between their on- and off-components. This is shown in Fig. 5.5 from the paper by Hubel and Wiesel [1959]. A small spot in the on-center gives a discharge (a) and there is an off-effect to the same spot in the surround of the receptive field (b). The large area illuminated (c) elicits no response. Nor do we have to assume that a primitive function such as "light-on" or "light-off" across a large portion of the retina need be corticalized.

Now, looking at the behavior of the same field to a rectangular light patch placed at different angles (Fig. 5.6), it is clearly capable of responding to "form" by summation of excitation or inhibition or by utilizing their antagonism, depending upon how the rectangle is located within the field. And, as to movement, a spot moving along the on-center would

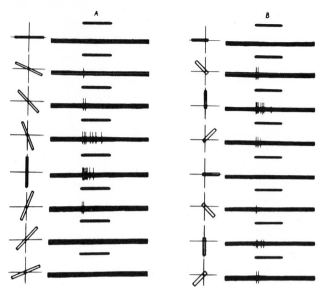

Fig. 5.6. Same unit as in Fig. 5.5. (A) Responses to shining a rectangular light spot 1° × 8°; center of slit superimposed on center of receptive field; successive stimuli rotated clockwise, as shown to left of figure. (B) Responses to a 1° × 5° slit oriented in various directions, with one end always covering the center of the receptive field: note that this central region evoked responses when stimulated alone (Fig. 5.5a). Stimulus and background intensities as in Fig. 5.5; stimulus duration 1 sec [from Hubel and Wiesel, 1959, p. 579].

be a stimulus very different from one moving across it and eliciting an off-on-off alternation.

The cortical fields are lying at different angles and this may be a mechanism of labeling visual events spatially. Apparently some fields are also organized in a more complex manner, yet to be investigated. They need not necessarily be circular or oblong and provided with on- or off-centers merely in the manner depicted in Figs. 5.5 and 5.6 [Grüsser et al, 1964]. Recent work has shown that directional sensitivity to movement also occurs in the retina of the rabbit [Barlow and Hill, 1963], and not only in its lateral geniculate body [Arden, 1963]. The fields which record movement in one but not in the opposite direction seem to be on/off-fields in which center and periphery fail to be differentiated in the manner described above.

Having now become more familiar with the retinal organization, it is not surprising that interaction should be capable of producing the narrow bands of color sensitivity from different regions of the spectrum that have been known as the modulators [Granit, 1945, 1947]. At the time (1939–1945), one had to be cautious in propounding an explanation in terms of interaction because it seemed possible that photochemical substances might exhibit such narrow curves. The considerably greater experience of today in the field of retinal photochemistry, for which Dartnall's [1962] summary may be consulted, makes it unlikely that primary photochemical absorption curves of receptors ever are as narrow as the modulator curves. Still narrower are the color bands recorded by De Valois et al [1958] in the geniculate body of the macaque, and by Hill [1962] in that of the rabbit. The principle of sharpening up specificity as to quality by inhibitory interaction also recurs in the auditory system. Tasaki [1954] succeeded in recording the primary response from auditory fibers. This is characterized by a high-frequency cut-off and a broad expansion of tonal sensitivity at the lower frequencies. In the cochlear nucleus there appears a low-frequency cut-off, most clearly present when two tones are active as simultaneous stimuli. Rose, Galambos, and Hughes [1959] point out that the auditory units are of two types: one giving tonal bands which remain narrow when stimulus strength is increased, another which under similar circumstances greatly expands so as to cover most of the tonal spectrum below their best frequency.

The on- and off-components in the retina have been found by Wagner, MacNichol, and Wolbarsht [1960] to be connected to receptors with different wavelength sensitivity within one and the same receptive field (in the eye of the goldfish), meaning, for instance, that an off-center may have a spectral sensitivity different from its on-surround. It would, however, carry us too far to enter upon the explanations of color contrast that such experiments suggest.

Let us summarize this all too brief review by stating that the evidence presented has shown that functional and anatomical differentiation closely cooperate to provide an efficient analyzer of visual space, and we shall, no doubt, hear more about similar analyzers of the surface of the body from Professor Mountcastle. In the future it will be necessary to pay more attention to anatomical structures which suggest definite spatial organizations, such as the dendrites of the cerebellar Purkinje cells which form a trellis structure in a definite plane. They may have an equally definite function in interpreting space. J. Z. Young [1960, 1962], in his thorough studies of visual learning in the octopus, noticed that the dendrites of the cell surface of the optic lobe do not take a random course in all directions, but tend to run straight for distances as long as half a millimeter. The majority of them run horizontally relative to the normal posture of the animal, many run vertically, and fewer obliquely. He has suggested that the organized dendritic field is a central space receptor, a reasonably probable notion in view of what has been mentioned above about the vertebrates. We do not yet know enough about the orientation of dendritic fields in the visual cortex of higher animals because tangential sections have not attracted much interest.

It should be added that vision with a moving eye, as in man, profits from the on-off-organization in a manner which has been elucidated by Riggs, Ratliff, Cornsweet, and Cornsweet [1953] and Ditchburn [1958]. I do not merely refer to the slow drift of an eye across the visual surroundings but also to the small irregular oscillations dependent upon minute twitches and tetani of the eye muscles. In fact, the eye is never quiet, and if the image is artificially stabilized by compensatory optics, it tends to fade out. Continuous sampling goes on and we can imagine the lively play of on-off impulses across contours separating spatial differences of brightness and wavelength.

Enough has been said to justify my initial remark that, as no other sense organ, the eye has served as an eye opener in sensory physiology, demonstrating how far analysis can be carried by physiological methods. We are beginning to understand how such an instrument as our visual pathway can handle information dealing with form, movement, direction of movement, and wavelength. These, after all, are perceived entities. Our examples show the physiologist as a kind of bioengineer who, instead of designing a space analyzer, operates in the reverse: he has been given a space analyzer which one could call a black box (if it did not deal with light) and has tried to find out how it works. Engineers, let us remember, have also designed space analyzers such as the chromatic photographic plate and the color television set, excellent in themselves but neither up to the standard of the eye as an all-round instrument.

The recurrent inhibition which we now turn to has been best analyzed in the lateral eye of the horseshoe crab (*Limulus polyphemus*), but the idea, once conceived deep down in the phylum millions of years ago, the organisms have clung to tenaciously and also improved upon. In the *Limulus* facette eye, consisting of ommatidia, the lateral inhibition, as Hartline [1949] called it, is organized by recurrent fibers possessing axo-axonic synapses on the afferent fibers coming from the excentric cell of each ommatidium. This apparently is a random distribution in every sense, except that distance naturally plays a role. Ommatidia sufficiently far apart do not influence one another's firing. Nearby ommatidia inhibit each other's discharge. This has been very fully analyzed by Hartline and Ratliff [1956], who have shown that the discharge from ommatidium A inhibits the firing of the adjacent ommatidium B in strict proportion to the frequency of discharge of the inhibiting ommatidium. The value of the proportionality constant depends upon distance between them. A record of the lateral or recurrent inhibition is shown in Fig. 5.7.

A simple example will show the usefulness of lateral inhibition in the facette eye. If a patch of light be projected onto the ommatidia, some

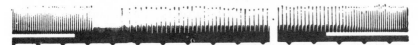

Fig. 5.7. Inhibition of the activity of an ommatidium in the eye of *Limulus* produced by illumination of a nearby retinal region. Oscillogram of action potentials in a single optic nerve fiber. See text for description. Time in ⅕ sec [from Hartline, Wagner, and Ratliff, 1956, p. 656].

of them will be in focus and deliver impulses at a rate considerably higher than that of ommatidia in the surround, which merely receives stray light. Since the inhibitory effect is in proportion to rate of discharge, the focal ommatidia will inhibit their weakly illuminated neighbors more efficiently than the latter can inhibit them. This means that the image will be sharpened by contrast. As it is possible with this preparation, which lasts for hours, to work out the constants for a number of combinations, it has also proved possible to substitute a number of simultaneous equations, solve them, and return to experimentation for a check on the result. A complex but naturally occurring process of inhibitory control has thus been resolved into components and made accessible to a simple mathematical treatment.

Ramón y Cajal [1900] pointed out that recurrent fibers are found in most nervous centers also in mammals, but only one instance has so far been subjected to a quantitative analysis. This is the recurrent circuit of the motoneurons which incorporates an interneuron, the Renshaw cell. In this system, too, a constant inhibition always removed the same number of impulses from a firing motoneuron, whatever the rate of discharge of the latter, and the inhibitory effect was proportional to the rate of the discharge elicited in an assembly of Renshaw cells [Granit and Renkin, 1961]. In spite of the intercalated internuncial cell, the rules thus were identical with those valid for the eye of the horseshoe crab, and it is interesting, too, that frequency of discharge is the parameter that in both cases leads to simple equations. But it also proved possible to excite or inhibit the interneuron from supraspinal sources [Granit, Haase, and Rutledge, 1960; Haase and van der Meulen, 1961] and thus to bias the potency of recurrent inhibition. This is very characteristic of the central nervous system. There is check upon check; a system with feedback is regularly provided with accessory feedbacks. It may not be an unsurmountable task to develop mathematics for such circuits, but what about going back to experimentation with the theories thus produced!

Recurrent circuits have been discovered experimentally—and in keeping with anatomical knowledge—in the olfactory bulb [Green, Mancia, and von Baumgarten, 1962; Phillips, Powell, and Shepherd, 1963], in the hippocampus [Kandel, Spencer, and Brinley, 1961], and in the sensory gracilis nucleus [Gordon and Jukes, 1962]. Understanding of their role in mammals is at an advanced level only for motoneurons, but beyond the few facts mentioned above it is not intended to branch off into the motor field with further explications. Surround inhibition in the somato-sensory path may well be based on recurrent fibers, but this is a theme that is better left to Professor Mountcastle.

Hitherto I have tacitly assumed that whenever a message or part of it is rejected by the central nervous system, this is an effect caused by active inhibition. In our recent work on the projections of the muscular afferents upon the spinal motoneurons in the cat, we [Granit, Kellerth, and Williams, 1964] have been struck by a mode of behavior on the part of these cells which illustrates the importance of "bias" or "setting" in a particularly clear manner. We were studying by the intracellular tech-nique the afferent response to muscle stretch which is a complex natural stimulus evoking activity from two types of end organs within the muscle spindle and in addition from the Golgi tendon organs. Assume that the tip of the microelectrode is inside a motoneuron belonging to an ankle extensor. In extensor motoneurons, pull on the muscle would, in the decerebrate cat and in a spastic patient, cause a stretch reflex, in spite of the fact that only one of the muscular sense organs is excitatory, the other two inhibitory. Neither man nor cat normally has a stretch reflex.

Looking at the recipient motoneuron from the inside, one sometimes finds a variety of signs indicating that something has happened. There may or may not be definite depolarization in response to stretch, a mono-synaptic test response may or may not be influenced, there may or may not be visible synaptic activation noise apparently depending upon how near to the active source of such noise within the neuron the tip of the microelectrode happens to be. But if the motoneuron then is depolarized by current from the tip of the intracellular electrode, the cell delivers a clear reply to pull on its muscle and this is always an increase of the rate of firing (Fig. 5.8a,b).

Pull on an antagonist should elicit inhibition. Nevertheless, one may or may not see a clear indication of this effect, just as above with pull on the protagonist. There may be little or no synaptic activation noise, and testing excitability by a monosynaptic postsynaptic potential may prove equivocal. But, no sooner is the cell depolarized from the intra-cellular electrode so as to discharge impulses, then pull on the antagonist regularly stops this discharge or reduces its frequency (Fig. 5.8a) by postsynaptic inhibition. In Fig. 5.9 the motoneuron belongs to ankle flexors. On them, both the antagonist extensor (*triceps surae*) and the upper flexor, semitendinosus, exerted strong inhibitory effects, provided

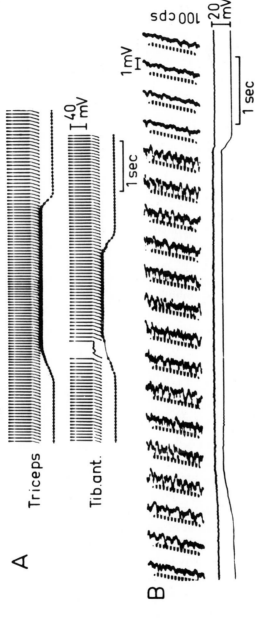

Fig. 5.8. Cat. Popliteal spike (spike height 100 mV). (a) Motoneuron fired by injected current. Influence on this discharge of loading muscles, indicated along records, with weight of 500 g. (b) Synaptic activation noise of same motoneuron during pull on triceps surae (500 g) [from Granit, Kellerth, and Williams, 1964, p. 453].

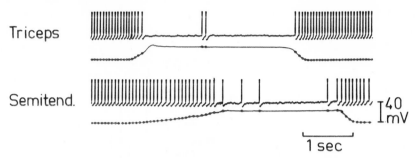

Fig. 5.9. Cat. Ventral roots L_7 and S_1 cut. Peroneal motoneuron (spike height over 70 mV). Motoneuron fired by injected current and discharge inhibited by muscle stretch. Weight 500 g in both cases [from Granit, Kellerth, and Williams, 1964, p. 453].

that the cell was kept firing by intracellular stimulation from the tip of the microelectrode. Since it is the cell membrane itself that has been made to fire by intracellular stimulation, the inhibitions are postsynaptic, and this is one of the advantages of this method of attacking problems of inhibition. One need not worry about presynaptic effects.

Clearly, therefore, depolarization of a motoneuron reveals effects of postsynaptic excitation and inhibition which in the nonactivated cell would often have been impossible to trace. To put it differently, unless there be some biasing organization of interneurons depolarizing the cell membrane, imitated in our experiments by transmembrane depolarization, the afferent energy is dissipated as synaptic activation noise. Unless biased, the cell refuses to take notice of the afferent input caused by muscle stretch. Thus no special inhibitory mechanism is necessary for rejection of the message from the muscle receptors. This it does unless specially activated. What is required, therefore, is a correct setting or bias of the motoneuron from cells capable of depolarizing it. We believe that these cells are the interneurons—mentioned above—which we found to have very high amplification factors, defined as large proportionality constants in a plot of impulse frequency against current strength. Then and only then does muscle stretch become a "meaningful" stimulus.

I shall end my presentation of sensory mechanisms here. The theme is far too large to be discussed by any single participant of this meeting. My self-imposed restrictions have made circuit analysis by micromethods of the fate of the afferent input the focus of my talk. I have left out every reference to the diffuse or nonspecific afferent input feeling that others present at this meeting, in particular Professors Moruzzi and Jasper, are more competent to deal with this large field of research. But, clearly, the experiments on muscular afferents, just reviewed, support and add precision to a notion which I have tried to propound [Granit, 1955], namely, that the nonspecific afferents serve as specific energizers, meaning, in physical terms, that they provide the basic depolarization necessary for forcing the cell to take notice of inhibition and excitation.

DISCUSSION

Chairman: PROFESSOR HEYMANS

ECCLES: Professor Granit referred to the Purkinje cells and the planar organization of these cells at right angles to the length of the cerebellar folia. The cerebellum provides the best organized geometry in the central nervous system, and recently there is anatomical and physiological evidence by Szentágothai and our Canberra group suggesting that a localized input via the mossy fibers to the cerebellum is transformed into a long narrow strip of excitation compressed in on each side by inhibition. This mossy fiber input would activate the granule cells that send their axons, the parallel fibers, for about 3 mm along the cerebellar folium and so excite the Purkinje cells and the basket cells that have their dendrites in this long strip. These basket cells send their axons transversely from the central zone of activation, strongly inhibiting the Purkinje cells on each side, so this single small stream of localized mossy fiber excitation not only activates Purkinje cells in the strip, but also at the same time activates the inhibitory basket cells that give an inhibited zone of Purkinje cells for about 500 μ on either side. I would suggest that there might be a comparable arrangement in the visual cortex, which would account for the observations of linear excited zones, and we have today heard from Dr. Colonnier that there is an organization in the cerebral cortex that might form the anatomical basis, namely, the stellate cells with their axonal branches on each side.

GRANIT: What Eccles says seems to me quite likely. I believe that we have far too much neglected such points of view. We have been, perhaps, too "psychological" about it, instead of thinking in terms of special organizations as we know them. The properties of special analyzers need to be considered in anatomical terms, that is why I mentioned Dr. Young's fascinating experiments.

MOUNTCASTLE: Is there any evidence that the descending system which regulates transmission across nuclear relays does so in a simple way by changing the proportionality constant for that relay, which you describe? It seems to me reasonable to think it might operate as well for descending systems which regulate transmission across relay nuclei. Could they operate simply by changing the proportionality constant and preserving the linearity of transmission?

GRANIT: Dr. Kernell was one of the coworkers in this work on the proportionality constant and he has been going on with it. Kernell stimulates at high frequency in the brain stem and he can bring about changes of the proportionality constants.

MOUNTCASTLE: I would like to ask about the classification of neurons, as being either movement or form sensitive. Do you believe that different receptors are actually sensitive in a direct manner to direction of movement; or is it, as seems to me more likely, the result of a complex series of convergences of excitation and inhibition?

GRANIT: We are not speaking about a cell alone, we are speaking about a receptive field consisting of several cells projected onto one cell.

MOUNTCASTLE: Do you think that the directionality, for example, is due in each case to a particular type of excitation and inhibition, resulting from the directionality?

GRANIT: What the great wonder is, to my mind, is not that you have directionality in the cortex on the basis of the picture of oblong receptive fields at different angles. That is what one would expect. The greater wonder is that you have it already in the retina of the rabbit for certain receptive fields. This means that when the object moves in a field in one way, there must be a wake of inhibition that does not work the other way round, and how that is done I think no one knows, but we want from many points of view a full description of such fields. We have become a little bit stationary now in thinking of all fields in terms of center-surround antagonism, but these fields do not have it, so we have to think of new types of receptive field which still require to be analyzed.

MOUNTCASTLE: May I raise just one more problem, which perhaps others here may wish to discuss at a later stage of the symposium. Do you think it possible that at the higher levels of sensory systems it will be possible, or profitable, to seek explanations of the actions of large populations of neurons as the simply additive result of those single elements? Or is it possible that we should look for what I shall term the "emergent properties of neural populations," properties which may be not at all evident in the action of any single member of a population?

REFERENCES

ADRIAN, E. D. *The Basis of Sensation. The Action of Sense Organs.* London: Christophers, 122 pp. [1928].

———, and D. W. BRONK. The discharge of impulses in motor nerve fibers. Part II. The frequency of discharge in reflex and voluntary contractions, *J. Physiol., 67,* 119–151 [1929].

ARDEN, G. B. Complex receptive fields and responses to moving objects in cells of the rabbit's lateral geniculate body, *J. Physiol., 166,* 468–488 [1963].

BARLOW, H. B., and R. M. HILL. Selective sensitivity to direction of movement in ganglion cells of the rabbit retina, *Science, 139,* 412–414 [1963].

BROCK, L. G., J. S. COOMBS, and J. C. ECCLES. The recording of potentials from motoneurones with an intracellular electrode, *J. Physiol., 117,* 431–460 [1962].

DARTNALL, H. J. A. The photobiology of visual processes, in: *The Eye* (ed. by H. Davson). New York: Academic Press, pp. 323–553 [1962].

DeValois, R. L., C. J. Smith, S. T. Kitai, and A. J. Karoly. Response of single cells in monkey lateral geniculate nucleus to monochromatic light, *Science*, 127, 238–239 [1958].

Ditchburn, R. W. Eye-movements in relation to perception of colour, in: *Visual Problems of Colour*. London: H.M. Stationery Office, Vol. II, pp. 417–427 [1958].

Eccles, J. C. *The Physiology of Nerve Cells*. Baltimore: Johns Hopkins Press, 270 pp. [1957].

———. *The Physiology of Synapses*. Berlin: Springer, 316 pp. [1964].

Gordon, G., and M. G. M. Jukes. Correlation of different excitatory and inhibitory influences on cells in the nucleus gracilis of the cat, *Nature*, 196, 1183–1185 [1962].

Granit, R. The electrophysiological analysis of the fundamental problem of colour reception. 14th Thomas Young Oration. *Proc. Physical Soc. London*, 57, 447–463 [1945].

———. *Sensory Mechanisms of the Retina*. London: Oxford Univ. Press, 412 pp. 1947. Reprinted Ed. Hafner Publ. Co., New York [1963].

———. The effect of two wave-lengths of light upon the same retinal element, *Acta Physiol. Scand.*, 18, 281–294 [1949].

———. The antagonism between the on- and off-systems in the cat's retina, *L'Anné Psychol.*, 50, 129–134, Vol. jubil. H. Piéron [1951].

———. *Receptors and Sensory Perception*. New Haven: Yale Univ. Press, 367 pp. [1955].

———, J. Haase, and L. T. Rutledge. Recurrent inhibition in relation to frequency of firing and limitation of discharge rate of extensor motoneurones, *J. Physiol.*, 154, 308–328 [1960].

———, J. O. Kellerth, and T. D. Williams. "Adjacent" and "remote" postsynaptic inhibition in motoneurones stimulated by muscle stretch, *J. Physiol.*, 174, 453–472 [1964].

———, D. Kernell, and G. K. Shortess. Quantitative aspects of repetitive firing of mammalian motoneurones caused by injected currents, *J. Physiol.*, 168, 911–931 [1963].

———, and B. Renkin. Net depolarization and discharge rate of motoneurones, as measured by recurrent inhibition, *J. Physiol.*, 158, 461–475 [1961].

———, and P. O. Therman. Excitation and inhibition in the retina and in the optic nerve, *J. Physiol.*, 83, 359–381 [1935].

Green, J. D., M. Mancia, and R. von Baumgarten. Recurrent inhibition in the olfactory bulb. I. Effects of antidromic stimulation of the lateral antidromic tract, *J. Neurophysiol.*, 25, 467–488 [1962].

Grüsser, O.-J., U. Grüsser-Cornhels, and T. H. Bullock. Functional organization of receptive fields of movement detecting neurons in the frog's retina, *Pflügers Arch. Ges. Physiol.*, 279, 88–89 [1964].

Haase, J., and J. P. van der Meulen. Effects of supraspinal stimulation on Renshaw cells belonging to extensor motoneurones, *J. Neurophysiol.*, 24, 510–520 [1961].

HARTLINE, H. K. The response of single optic nerve fibers of the vertebrate eye to illumination of the retina, *Amer. J. Physiol.*, *121*, 400–415 [1938].

————. The receptive field of the optic nerve fibers, *Amer. J. Physiol.*, *180*, 690–699 [1940].

————. Inhibition of visual receptors by illuminating nearby retinal areas in the *Limulus* eye, *Fed. Proc.*, *8*, 69 [1949].

————, and F. RATLIFF. Inhibitory interaction of receptor units in the eye of *Limulus*, *J. Gen. Physiol.*, *40*, 357–376 [1956].

HILL, R. M. Unit responses of the rabbit lateral geniculate muscles to monochromatic light on the retina, *Science, 135*, 98–99 [1962].

HUBEL, D. H., and T. N. WIESEL. Receptive fields of single neurons in the cat's striate cortex, *J. Physiol.*, *148*, 574–591 [1959].

————. Integrative action in the cat's lateral geniculate body, *J. Physiol.*, *155*, 385–398 [1961].

————. Lecture at Symposium in Honour of Lord Adrian. Cambridge, March [1964].

KANDEL, E. R., W. A. SPENCER, and F. J. BRINDLEY. Electrophysiology of hippocampal neurons. I. Sequential invasion and synaptic organizations, *J. Neurophysiol.*, *24*, 225–242 [1961].

KUFFLER, S. W. Discharge patterns and functional organization of mammalian retina, *J. Neurophysiol.*, *16*, 37–68 [1953].

MOUNTCASTLE, V. B. Some functional properties of the somatic afferent system, in: *Sensory Communication* (ed. by W. A. Rosenblith). New York: Wiley, Chapt. 22, pp. 403–436 [1961].

PHILLIPS, C. G., T. P. S. POWELL, and G. M. SHEPHERD. Responses of mitral cells to stimulation of the lateral olfactory tract in the rabbit, *J. Physiol.*, *168*, 65–88 [1963].

POLYAK, S. *The Vertebrate Visual System*. Chicago: Univ. Chicago Press, 1390 pp. [1957].

RAMÓN Y CAJAL, S. *Studien über die Hirnrinde des Menschen. 1. Sehrinde.* Leipzig: Barth, 77 pp. [1900].

RIGGS, L. A., F. RATLIFF, J. C. CORNSWEET, and T. N. CORNSWEET. The disappearance of steadily fixated visual test objects, *J. Opt. Soc. Amer.*, *43*, 495–501 [1953].

ROSE, J. E., R. GALAMBOS, and J. R. HUGHES. Microelectrode studies of the cochlear nuclei of the cat, *Bull. Johns Hopkins Hosp.*, *104*, 211–251 [1959]

SHAPOVALOV, A. I. Multiple discharges and rhythmical activity of spinal neurones evoked by intracellular microelectrode stimulation, *Sechenov Physiol. J. USSR*, *50*, 444–456 [1964].

TALBOT, S. A., and W. H. MARSHALL. Physiological studies on neural mechanisms of visual localization and discrimination, *Amer. J. Ophthal.*, *24*, 1255–1264 [1941].

TASAKI, I. Nerve impulses in individual auditory nerve fibers of guinea pig, *J. Neurophysiol.*, *17*, 97–122 [1954].

WAGNER, H. G., E. F. MACNICHOL, and M. L. WOLBARSHT. The response properties of single ganglion cells in the goldfish retina, *J. Gen. Physiol.*, 43, 45–62 [1960].

YOUNG, J. Z. The visual system of *octopus*. Regularities in the retina and optic lobes of *octopus* in relation to form discrimination, *Nature*, 186, 836–844 [1960].

———. How can the memory of the nervous system be studied? *Metodo Sperimentale in Biologia da Vallisneri ad Oggi*. Padova [1962].

6

Some Problems of Information Transmission in the Visual System

by O. Creutzfeldt, J. M. Fuster, A. Herz, M. Straschill

Max-Planck-Institut, Munich, Germany

As an addition to the review of Dr. Granit on the neurophysiology of the visual system, I should like to treat some special problems of information transmission in this system which might have some bearing on the general problems how the brain handles information. This presentation is based on material collected in our laboratory during the last years and which has been published recently.

It is well known to all workers in this field that the activity and re-activity of nerve cells in different levels of the central visual pathways change considerably. This is not only true for the organization of receptive fields, as the investigations of Baumgartner and Hakas [1962] and Hubel and Wiesel [Hubel, 1962] in the cat, and of Maturana et al [1960] in the frog have shown, but also in a more quantitative sense as far as the activity of single neurons is concerned [cf. Creutzfeldt, 1961]. We investigated these quantitative differences by looking at some statistical characteristics of nerve cell activity in different levels of the visual system during spontaneous and evoked activity [Herz et al, 1964; Fuster et al, 1965b; Straschill, 1965]. In addition, intracellular recording from neurons in the lateral geniculate body and the visual cortex of rabbits gave some hints relating to the mechanisms by which the observed quantitative and qualitative changes might come about [Fuster et al, 1965a].

Average Activity at Different Levels of the Visual System

If we count the spontaneous average activity of neurons at different levels of the visual system without external stimulation, that is, during darkness, we find that it decreases considerably at each level. This is shown in Table 1 where the average activity of representative groups of units in the tractus opticus, the lateral geniculate body, and the cortex is given. No general anesthetic was used in these experiments, the room was dark.

Table 1

Mean discharge rate of neurons in the optic tract, lateral geniculate body, and visual cortex during darkness. Discharges per sec during 3–22 min records. Mean values and S.E. (After Herz et al [1964].)

Location	No. of Neurons	Reaction to diffuse light stimuli on	off	on-off	A	Sum
Tractus opticus	13	39.2 ± 4	24.0 ± 6.0	34.2 ± 4.2		35.5
Lateral geniculate body	24	13.2 ± 3.7	9.8 ± 4.4	17.4 ± 5.8		14.0
Visual cortex	145	5.7 ± 1.3	2.8 ± 0.4	8.7 ± 2.0	4.5 ± 0.7	5.7

This decrease of activity at higher integrative levels is not only true for the "resting" state. Long-lasting light stimuli increase or decrease the activity of retinal as well as that of geniculate neurons in a systematic way according to their type of reaction to diffuse light. This is shown in Fig. 6.1, where the relation between the intensity of a light diffusely illuminating the retina and the activity of on- and off-neurons in the optic tract and in the lateral geniculate body is shown. Since it takes about 2–3 min to attain a steady state discharge rate after switching on or off the light [Kuffler et al, 1957; Straschill, 1966] there was a delay of at least two minutes after the beginning of the light stimulus before the activity was counted. It can be seen that in the steady state a logarithmic relation exists between light intensity and average discharge rate for both types of neurons, the on- and, in the reversed sense, the off-units. The regression line for off-units is identical in the optic tract and the lateral geniculate body, but the activity of geniculate cells is smaller at all intensities (the numbers in brackets on each diagram give the mean discharge rate of all investigated units at "100 per cent," which is the maximal activity to which the lower values are compared). On-units show about the same

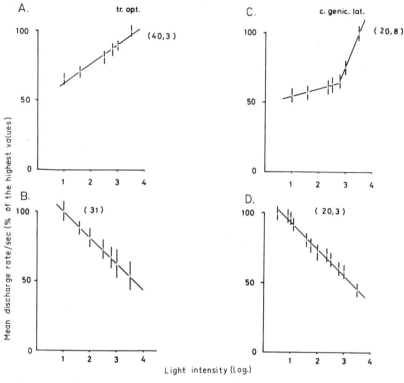

Fig. 6.1. Relation between logarithm of light intensity and average discharge rate of neurons of the optic tract (A and B) and of the geniculate body (C and D). The plots represent the average discharge rate of several units against the log of light intensity (diffuse light on a tangent screen). The activity was counted during the steady state discharge, that is, 1.5–2 min after the light was switched on. The values of discharge rate of each neuron are transformed into percentage of the discharge rate during the most intense (on-neurons) or weakest (off-neurons) light intensity before the means were calculated. The maximal mean discharge rate of all units in each group is given in brackets on each diagram. The vertical lines indicate the standard deviation. (A) Intensity versus discharge rate relationship of 5 on-neurons and on-off-neurons of the optic tract. (B) Of 9 off-neurons of the optic tract. (C) Of 6 on-neurons and on-off-neurons of the lateral geniculate body. (D) Of 8 off-neurons of the geniculate body [after Straschill, 1965].

difference in both levels, but in the geniculate, an inconsistent relation between discharge rate and intensity exists, at low and high intensities. This might be due to a decrease of surround inhibition at higher intensities [Kuffler, 1953]. A straight line drawn through all points would be again parallel to the regression of optic tract units.

These findings indicate that the driven activity in higher visual centers is reduced by a linear factor [see also Grüsser et al, 1962]. This would be comparable to the observations of Mountcastle et al, which are presented at this meeting and which, in the somatosensory system, also demonstrated an identical relation between stimulus intensity and neuron activity at different levels, but here too the activity at different stimulus intensities was reduced by a linear factor at the thalamic compared to the more peripheral levels. There is, however, a difference between the somatosensory and the visual system in as far as the relation between stimulus intensity and neuronal reaction in the somatosensory system seems to be best described by a power function [Mountcastle and coll., 1963], whereas in the visual system it can be expressed by a power as well as by a logarithmic function. This is mainly due to the fact that in the visual system power functions are found with an exponent between 0.2 and 0.4 which can be expressed almost as well by logarithmic functions. It is, therefore, not surprising that both functions can be fitted almost equally well to the observed data (see Table 2). It might be men-

Table 2

Fit of logarithmic and power functions to the relation between discharge activity and light intensity during the steady state. (After Straschill [1966].)

Neurone	Location	Reaction to Diffuse Illumination	Fit of Logarithmic Function		Fit of Power Function		
			P, %	T	P, %	T	n
9/1/1	Tr. opt.	off	98	-0.98	98	-0.99	-0.2
I/I/I	Tr. opt.	on	80	0.85	99	0.94	0.14
4/I/1	Tr. opt.	on	99	0.98	99	0.97	0.17
5/II/2	Tr. opt.	on-off	85	-0.86	95	-0.9	-0.26
5/I/2	Tr. opt.	on-off	98	0.96	99	0.96	0.23
11/I/I	Lat. gen.	off	99	-0.98	99	0.96	-0.15
11/III/I	Lat. gen.	on-off	93	-0.87	95	-0.89	-0.16

P = Probability according to χ^2-test; T = correlation coefficient; n = exponent of power function.

tioned in this context that Stevens [1962] in psychophysical experiments also found intensity-reaction relations according to a power function with an exponent of 0.15–0.3, which is almost identical with a logarithmic function over a wide range.

Interval Histograms of Neurons at Different Levels of the Visual System

Besides these quantitative differences of unit activity, qualitative ones exist between different levels of the afferent visual system. To a certain amount, some investigators were well aware of this, but the actual differences were not yet well analyzed until recently [Herz et al, 1964; Bishop et al, 1964; Fuster et al, 1965b]. Thus, Herz et al [1964] have shown that the interval histograms in the optic tract, the lateral geniculate body, and the visual cortex show conspicuous differences. In general it can be said that the interval distribution of optic tract neurons is almost random, that of geniculate neurons is mostly multimodal, whereas cortical units in general show a peak of short intervals flanked by a wide and unsystematic distribution of longer intervals. Certain interval distributions of cortical and geniculate units may look similar. Examples are given in the following figures. Figure 6.2 shows the interval distribution of an optic tract neuron in a linear (A), semilogarithmic (B), and logarithmic (C) plot. After an initial dead time, a peak appears at about 10–15 msec after which the frequency of longer intervals decays exponentially. This suggests that each discharge is independent from the foregoing or from the following. This has been tested in joint interval histograms which in fact have shown that the probability of an interval to be followed by any other regardless of its duration is equal for all intervals [Herz et al, 1964]. The initial dead time of the exponential distribution lies between 5 and 15 msec for the different units tested and is probably mainly due to relative refractoriness of retinal cells, but for long dead times an additional factor may be supposed (see discussion). During long-lasting illumination the type of interval distribution does not change, though the slope of the exponential decay may become steeper and—especially with transient stimuli—the initial dead time may shorten, approaching the absolute refractory period [Fuster et al, 1965b]. This is shown for the same unit in Fig. 6.3, where 1 per sec stroboscopic flashes produce a peak around 1 msec which is due to the short, high frequency initial reaction after each flash. The peak time is, to a certain extent, dependent on the flash intensity, though no systematic relation could be found in this investigation. This is due to the high intensity of the flashes used, which drove the unit to its maximal frequency already with the relatively weakest flash.[1]

[1] Since this lecture was given, interval distributions of a large number of optic tract units have been tested mathematically in this laboratory. Most distributions were best fitted by an exponential function though some could be fitted better by a γ function [see Kuffler et al, 1957]. It must be left open presently whether two different types of neurons are represented by this difference or whether these two distributions are only due to some statistical deviations.

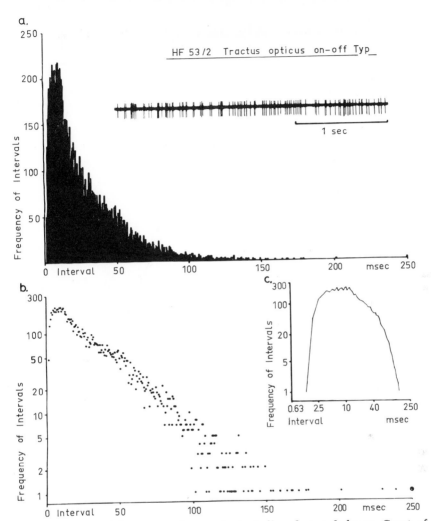

Fig. 6.2. Interval histogram of an optic tract fiber during darkness. Count of 10,542 intervals over 5 min. (A) Linear plot (inset: piece of original record). (B) Semilogarithmic plot in order to show exponential decay. (C) Logarithmic plot for comparison with interval histograms of geniculate (Fig. 6.5) and cortical (Fig. 6.6) activity [after Herz et al, 1964].

In contrast to the more uniform interval distributions of optic tract fibers, geniculate neurons show different forms, mostly bi- or trimodal distributions (see Fig. 6.4). This can best be shown in logarithmic plots. The first maximum was between 2 and 3.5 msec in most geniculate units, the second between 6 and 15 msec, and the third between 80 and 200 msec. The interval distributions of different geniculate units could show

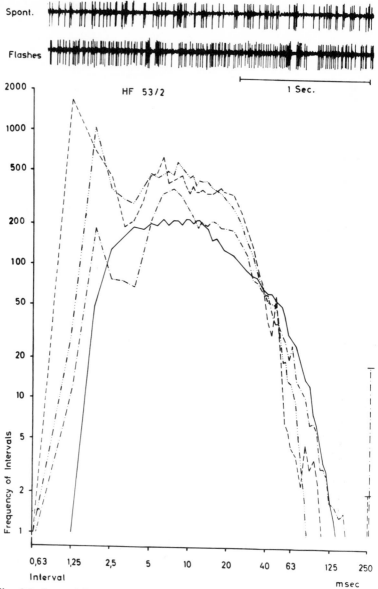

Fig. 6.3. Interval histogram (logarithmic plot) of an optic tract on-unit during spontaneous activity in darkness and during rhythmical light stimulation. Above: Original records of spontaneous activity (top) and of activity during 0.9 per sec stimulation with stroboscopic flashes (indicated by arrows). Below: Logarithmic plot of interval histograms based on equally long records of 5 min during spontaneous dark activity (————), during 0.9 per sec stroboscopic stimulation with intensity I (—·—·—·—·—), with intensity II (—·········—··—) and with intensity III (-----). Intensities I:II:III = 1:2:30. Bars on right represent all intervals longer than 250 msec. Pay attention to shortening of initial dead time during stroboscopic stimulation. The second mode is due to spontaneous activity in between stimuli and does not change considerably as compared with spontaneous dark activity [after Fuster et al, 1965b].

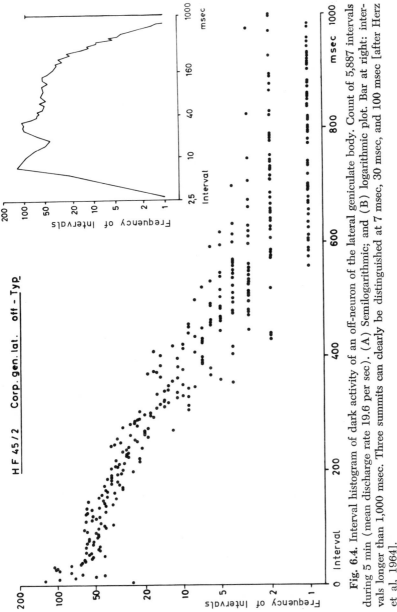

Fig. 6.4. Interval histogram of dark activity of an off-neuron of the lateral geniculate body. Count of 5,887 intervals during 5 min (mean discharge rate 19.6 per sec). (A) Semilogarithmic; and (B) logarithmic plot. Bar at right: intervals longer than 1,000 msec. Three summits can clearly be distinguished at 7 msec, 30 msec, and 100 msec [after Herz et al, 1964].

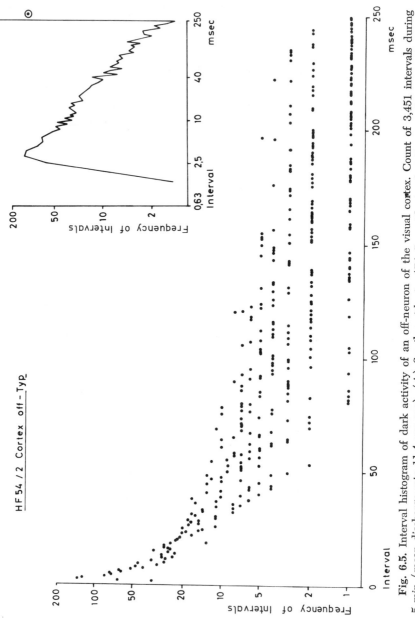

Fig. 6.5. Interval histogram of dark activity of an off-neuron of the visual cortex. Count of 3,451 intervals during 5 min (mean discharge rate 11.4 per sec). (A) Semilogarithmic. (B) Logarithmic plot. Bar at right: intervals above 250 msec. Summit at short intervals (3 msec), initially decaying exponentially until 12–15 msec, then flanked by slow decay with large distribution [after Herz et al, 1964].

some variations, especially between different experiments [see Herz et al, 1964; Bishop et al, 1964]. These differences mainly concern the relative heights of the different peaks, and, as in the experiments of Bishop et al [1964], are partly due to anesthesia.

In cortical units, finally, only the first peak is clearly discriminated (see Fig. 6.5). It is also located at very short intervals (3–5 msec) and may sometimes show a short exponential decay before it leads over in a broad flank of unsystematic distribution. Only in light anesthesia a second peak may come out clearly at 80–150 msec [see Herz and Fuster, 1964]. Joint interval histograms of cortical activity show that short intervals are more probably followed by short ones whereas long intervals by long ones [Herz et al, 1964]. This corresponds well to the well-known grouping of cortical activity during rest where clusters of several discharges (up to 4 and more) of high frequency can be observed.

INTRACELLULAR RECORDINGS IN THE LATERAL GENICULATE BODY AND THE VISUAL CORTEX

In order to get more knowledge of the transducer functions of the lateral geniculate body and the visual cortex, intracellular recordings from cells in the lateral geniculate body and in the visual cortex have been done [Fuster et al, 1965]. Such recordings give a better idea of the input-output relations of neurons at these different levels, which otherwise can only be deduced from statistical comparison of the neuronal reactions in both structures. The experiments have been performed on rabbits because of technical reasons. Though membrane potentials of up to 60 mV could be found in geniculate cells, they generally did not last long enough. For more systematic studies, therefore, cells with a stable membrane potential of 30–40 mV and a constant firing level were used. It is admitted that some of the records in the lateral geniculate body do not represent true intracellular activity but seem to be derived from an intermediate electrode position. They give, however, a clear picture of the postsynaptic activity of the cell with which the electrode is in contact. A systematic study of such "quasi-intracellular" records is in progress in our laboratory (McIlwain and Creutzfeldt, 1966) which will allow a better interpretation of such records. Intracellular records from cortical cells, on the other hand, are relatively more easy to obtain and more satisfactory from the biophysical point of view.

The difficulties of getting enough good and long-lasting intracellular records have as yet allowed an adequate investigation of only a few units with punctiform illumination of different parts of their retinal receptive fields. Therefore, here mainly the reactions to diffuse light at different intensities and to stroboscopic stimuli shall be described.

In the lightly anesthetized rabbit (nembutal anesthesia), two kinds of spontaneous postsynaptic activity can be discerned in geniculate cells (see Fig. 6.6). The first is characterized by more or less randomly distributed, distinct EPSP's of 2–5 mV and a duration of 20–60 msec (Fig. 6.6A,B). They may be clustered, so producing a stepwise depolarization, which might reach the firing level and thus lead to one or two discharges quickly following each other. No IPSP's are found in such resting records of spontaneous activity. The other kind of postsynaptic activity appears periodically and is only seen during complete rest, that is, without any external stimulation, especially during light barbiturate anesthesia. It is characterized by sequences of rhythmical membrane depolarizations on the background of increased polarization (see Fig. 6.6C). The depolarizations are topped by grouped discharges of high frequency (marked by a dot in Fig. 6.6C). Each polarization-depolarization sequence is about 100–200 msec long, the whole period lasts 1–2 sec. Single steps cannot be clearly distinguished on the depolarizations, though the beginning of the hyperpolarization may sometimes be recognizable as a small irregularity on the decaying phase of the depolarization. Similar sequences of polarization-depolarization can be produced by single afferent stimuli (flash or electrical stimulation of the optic nerve) as an "afterdischarge," though, in general, such units seem to be less sensitive to light stimuli than the first group.

In cortical records (Fig. 6.7), also two different types of spontaneous activity can be observed: those with more or less well distinguishable EPSP's *and* isolated IPSP's (Fig. 6.7A) and those with long-lasting de- and hyperpolarizing waves in a rhythmical sequence (Fig. 6.7C). The latter waves are mainly seen under light barbiturate anesthesia if rhythmical waves in the corticogram are present. Then, the slow waves of the corticogram are in phase with the slow cellular rhythm in such a way that depolarizations correspond to surface positive waves and vice versa. Under chloralose-urethane anesthesia, long-lasting depolarizations mostly leading to inactivation processes [Granit and Phillips, 1956] and accompanied by large and slow biphasic positive-negative waves are often observed, even though isolated synaptic potentials and single discharges may well be present between the inactivation processes (Fig. 6.7B).

Comparing spontaneous activity of geniculate and cortical cells, one comes to the conclusion that in geniculate cells in general, the PSP's appear more distinctly detached from the baseline, and steps of summated EPSP's are more sharply separated than in cortical cells. IPSP's in geniculate resting activity are only present during rhythmical activity.

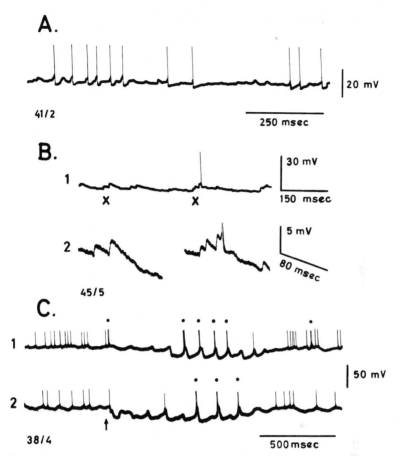

Fig. 6.6. Spontaneous postsynaptic activity of cells of the lateral geniculate body of the rabbit. Intracellular recordings from three different cells. (A) Flaxedilized animal. Resting potential 36 mV. Randomly distributed EPSP's of different steepness. No IPSP's, only afterhyperpolarizations after spike discharge. (B) Flaxedilized animal. Resting potential 55 mV. Cell with EPSP's well detached from the baseline and occasionally appearing in clusters which may reach the firing level. Two such EPSP groups (marked by cross) are shown with higher amplification and faster recording speed in B2. (C) Nembutal anesthesia. Resting potential 70 mV. (1) Phasic activity with long polarizing potentials (IPSP's) followed by broad EPSP's which lead to grouped spike discharges. The dots above the record indicate grouped discharges of two to four spikes. (2) Similar phasic activity elicited by an electric shock to the optic tract (arrow) as an "afterdischarge" [after Fuster et al, 1965a].

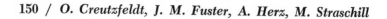

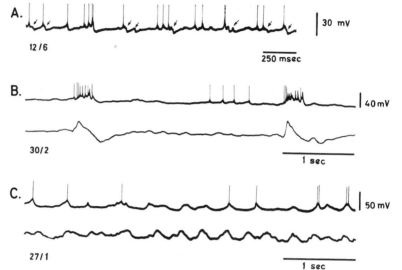

Fig. 6.7. Spontaneous postsynaptic activity of three different cells of the visual cortex of the rabbit. Intracellular recordings. (A) Resting potential about 37 mV. Nembutal anesthesia. Randomly distributed EPSP's with occasional spike discharges and well distinguishable IPSP's (arrows). (B) Resting potential about 44 mV. Urethane anesthesia. Grouped discharges with inactivation processes together with large biphasic slow waves in the EEG. In between normal PSP and spike activity. (C) Resting potential about 60 mV. Nembutal anesthesia. Phasic activity with more or less regular smooth polarizations and depolarizations, the latter occasionally reaching the firing level. Close phase relation to the EEG which shows the same sort of phasic activity (characteristic for the rabbits isocortical EEG during light nembutal anesthesia). In B and C the EEG is recorded with positivity upwards [after Fuster et al, 1965a].

Most cells in the lateral geniculate body and the striate cortex reacted to diffuse light stimuli to the contralateral eye. Principally two different types of reactions can be discriminated: those with a primary excitation (summated EPSP's) and those with a primary inhibition (polarizing IPSP's) (see Fig. 6.8). The primary event may be followed either by a reaction of reversed direction, that is, EPSP's followed by a polarization or a primary polarization followed by EPSP's, or may lead continuously into a steady state activity which is of the same direction as the primary response but less pronounced. Thus, sequences of EPSP's would appear during the steady state of a primarily excited neuron and a lack of excitatory potentials or even a long-lasting polarization with occasional IPSP's in primary inhibited cells. After "light-off," the reversed reaction to that at "light-on" appears in all cells. Using diffuse light, in general only the first

EPSP's of a reaction regularly reach the firing level, thus leading to a group of frequent discharges, whereas during the steady state, only occasionally the firing level will be reached. The degree of steady state spike activity depends upon the light intensity. Since most primarily inhibited cells show a secondary excitation with spike discharges, they would appear in extracellular records as on-off cells, but the latency of the on-discharge would be somewhat longer than that of a primary excitatory reaction (80–150 msec compared with 15–30 msec). The primary inhibition before the excitation corresponds to the well-known pre-excitatory inhibition of on-off cells described by Granit [1950] in retinal cells and confirmed in cortical cells by Jung and Baumgartner [1955]. On the other hand, many primarily excited cells will show a secondary excitation after light-off and would thus also give, with extracellular recording, the picture of an on-off reaction (with a long latency off-reaction). It is understandable, therefore, that with relatively short diffuse light stimuli, the majority of geniculate cells are classifiable as on-off-cells according to their extracellularly recorded reaction. Schematically, the two types of reaction to diffuse light may thus be represented by the

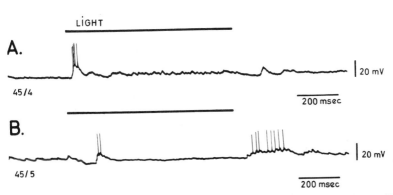

Fig. 6.8. Two typical reactions of geniculate cells to diffuse light stimulus. Rabbit, nembutal anesthesia. Intracellular recording. (A) Resting potential about 57 mV. At "light-on," primary activation with summated EPSP's and spike discharges followed by reduction of excitatory input, increased EPSP activity during "steady state." At "light-off" primary inhibition (slight polarization) followed by secondary summated EPSP (not reaching the firing level), leading over into reduced EPSP activity. (B) Resting potential about 55 mV. At light-on, primary reduction of EPSP activity and slight polarization, followed by secondary activation (grouped EPSP's with spike discharges), clear reduction of EPSP frequency and amplitude during steady-state (almost flat baseline). At light-off, summation of EPSP's which reach the firing level, followed by secondary reduction and finally leading into normal dark activity of EPSP's. Compare steady-state activity of EPSP's during darkness and light in cell A and B [after Fuster et al, 1965a].

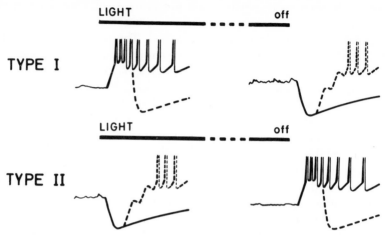

Fig. 6.9. Schematic representation of the two commonly found types of reaction of geniculate cells to a diffuse light stimulus. Rabbit. Type I: Primary activation leading smoothly into steady discharge and finally into steady state EPSP activity or interrupted by secondary reduction of excitatory input or even by IPSP's (indicated by broken line) before steady discharge. At light-off, strong primary reduction of excitatory input or even appearance of IPSP's, leading slowly into dark activity or interrupted by secondary activation (broken line). Type II: Reversed behavior with primary inhibition, mostly followed by secondary excitation (broken line), EPSP reduction during steady state at light-on; primary activation leading slowly into steady state dark activity, or temporarily interrupted by secondary inhibition (broken line) before steady dark activity [after Fuster et al, 1965a, slightly modified].

following schema (see Fig. 6.9). The type I reaction is represented by a primary excitation at light-on, occasionally followed by a secondary inhibition (indicated by the dashed line), the type II reaction by primary inhibition (polarization), occasionally followed by secondary excitation. At light-off the reversed reaction is observed.

In those few cells in which punctiform light to the functional center of the receptive field could be applied, it was observed that the reaction to such a stimulus was more uniform, that is, the primary reaction (excitation or inhibition) continued without interruption by a reversed potential, the adaptation to a steady state was slower and, during the latter, the activity was more intense or the inhibition more complete respectively. Examples for punctiform stimulation of the receptive field center of an on- and an off-center neuron are shown in Fig. 6.10. In the record Fig. 6.10B, the attention might be drawn to the fact that most EPSP's are topped by one to three discharges, an observation which might explain certain interval distributions of geniculate cells (see discussion).

With stroboscopic flashes (duration below 1 msec), biphasic reactions,

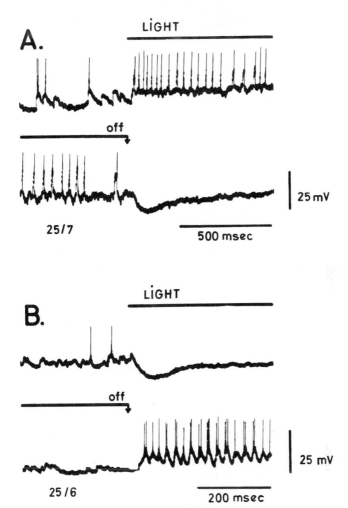

Fig. 6.10. Reaction of two geniculate cells to a spot of light (2°) into the center of their receptive field. Rabbit, nembutal anesthesia, intracellular records. (A) Resting potential about 35 mV. On-center cell. Long-lasting on-activation without interruption by secondary inhibition, clear reduction of excitatory input at off (IPSP). (B) Off-center cell. Resting potential about 30 mV. Strong inhibition (IPSP) at light-on and long-lasting reduction of excitatory input during whole length of stimulus, strong activation at light-off. See EPSP's at light-off topped by double and triple discharge [after Fuster et al, 1965a].

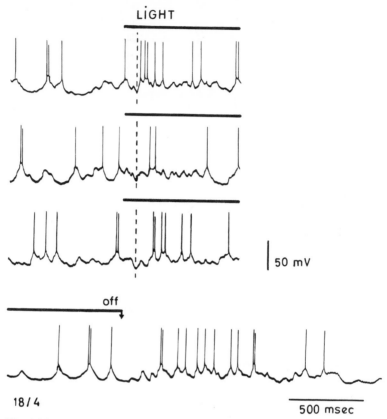

Fig. 6.11. Reaction of a cell of the visual cortex to light. Rabbit, nembutal anesthesia, resting potential about 72 mV, diffuse light shone onto a translucid screen. Shown are three on-reactions (a–c) and one off-reaction (d), c and d continuous record. At light-on, primary IPSP (connected with broken line in all records), followed by irregular sequence of EPSP's which inconsistently reach the firing level. Spontaneous rhythmical activity with activation-inhibition periods is resumed already 500–600 msec after light-on. At light-off, increased EPSP activity with increased discharge rate. This reaction could be classified as type II reaction if the classification for geniculate cells (see Fig. 6.9) would be adopted [after Fuster et al, 1965b].

that is, either excitatory-inhibitory or inhibitory-excitatory sequences, are always produced. In Fig. 6.12A an on-reaction (EPSP-IPSP sequence) is shown. Increasing the frequency of stimulation, it can be shown that in on-cells the primary excitation gets more and more delayed and less efficient when it falls on the secondary IPSP of the foregoing flash (see third line of Fig. 6.12A). The reduction of the "flicker fusion frequency" (FFF) in higher centers may thus partly be explained by such a mechanism of occlusion due to excitation—inhibition sequences which enhance the effect of decrease of retinal output relative to each flash at higher flicker frequencies [Enroth, 1952; Grüsser and Creutzfeldt, 1957], an effect which is probably mainly due to adaptation at the receptor levels.

In a number of cells it was possible to investigate sufficiently the reactions to diffuse light at different intensities. The amplitudes of summated EPSP's as well as of IPSP's showed a clear dependence from the light intensity. The relations could be described satisfactorily by power functions with exponents around 0.2–0.3, but could be expressed as well by simple logarithmic functions [Fuster et al, 1965]. The situation, therefore, is comparable to the spike activity versus intensity relationship of optic tract and geniculate units in the steady state.

In the visual cortex, generally the postsynaptic responses to diffuse light are less constant and smaller in a given cell compared to the lateral geniculate body. Furthermore, the spontaneous activity is resumed earlier after the beginning or the end of the stimulus (after a few 100 msec in general), so that the steady state activity during a long stimulus may not be different from the resting activity before the stimulus. The postsynaptic potentials frequently are subthreshold so that an obvious change of cell

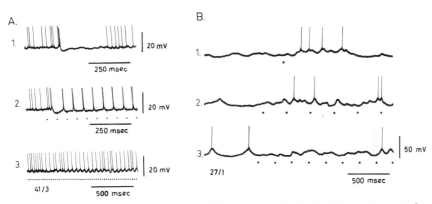

Fig. 6.12. Reaction of a geniculate (A) and a cortical cell (B) to short stroboscopic flashes. Rabbit, nembutal anesthesia. Flashes indicated by dots. (A) Geniculate on-center cell, resting potential 20–25 mV. (1) Single flash induces primary on-activation with grouped discharge, followed by long-lasting inhibitory potential. (2) 9 per sec; (3) 40 per sec stimulation. In 2, latency of on-reaction increases and only two instead of four discharges are elicited because of interaction with the IPSP of the preceding flash. In 3, only one spike is elicited during the first part of the record (about 0.4 sec after initiation of the flash series), later on, only every second flash leads to a discharge. (B) Cortical cell, primary visual area, resting potential about 60 mV. (1) Single flash; (2) 4 per sec; and (3) 6 per sec stimulation. Only irregular sequence of EPSP's is elicited by each flash, and already at low repetition frequencies no stimulus related driving can be recognized. Note the difference in reactivity of geniculate and cortical cells [after Fuster et al, 1965a].

firing may not be visible at each stimulus and is sometimes hard to detect even statistically. Such units would, in extracellular recordings, correspond to A neurons of Jung et al [Jung, 1961]. The presence of subthreshold postsynaptic potentials also in such cells explains, however, observations according to which A neurons may show distinct responses to light if activated otherwise, for example, by midline thalamic stimulation [Creutzfeldt and Akimoto, 1958]. In addition to these quantitative differences with more delicate reactions, in general the same responses as in the geniculate body can be seen in cortical units, that is, excitation-inhibition or inhibition-excitation sequences. An example is shown in Fig. 6.11.

The reaction of cortical cells to stroboscopic flashes is also weaker and more inconsistent than that of geniculate cells. A single flash may produce only a series of subthreshold or near-threshold EPSP's, and higher stimulation frequencies are not capable of driving consistently a stimulus-related postsynaptic reaction (see Fig. 6.12B). The contrast between geniculate and cortical reactions is well shown in this figure.

DISCUSSION

It was shown that the spontaneous as well as the light-induced activity in the ascending visual system decreases quantitatively at higher levels, and at the same time shows qualitative changes. The usually exponential interval distributions in optic nerve fibers can best be explained by being due to a trigger mechanism corresponding to a Poisson process. The relatively long dead time in some units, however, which cannot be explained alone by the refractory period of retinal neurons, makes it probable that some interaction of activity of different units may take place already in the retina [Herz et al, 1964]. This may also be the explanation for some interval distributions which are better described by a γ function than by an exponential function [Kuffler et al, 1957]. Compared to the bi- and multimodal interval distributions of central neurons, however, the little deviation of retinal activity from the exponential form must be emphasized. The "triggering" Poisson process may be sought in a spontaneous liberation of excitatory substances at the junction between the receptor and first-order neurons within the retina. The more complicated interval distributions of geniculate and cortical cells, on the other hand, indicate a considerable transformation of the incoming retinal activity and suggest also some interaction of the activity of several neurons at the geniculate level. Thus, it was assumed that inhibitory processes may play a role [Herz et al, 1964; Bishop et al, 1964]. Intracellular records from geniculate neurons have indeed confirmed that supposition and, furthermore, help to explain even more complicated (multimodal) interval distributions in the geniculate.[2] Two types of activity were found in geniculate cells with intracellular recording: (1) more randomly distributed EPSP's which might reach the firing level and thus lead to a discharge or to a short high-frequency group of discharges; and (2) rhythmical inhibitory-excitatory phasing at 5–10 per sec leading to high-frequency grouped discharges on top of the EPSP's. A mixture of this activity can be taken as the basis for a 3-modal interval distribution: the first peak is due to the high-frequency groups on top of EPSP's (cf. with the first peak of very short intervals in geniculate neurons); the second would be due to the mode of the afferent activity which elicits the EPSP's (it corresponds well to the mode of spontaneous optic nerve activity at 10–20 msec); and the third peak, finally, would correspond to the duration of the inhibitory period during phasic inhibitory-excitatory activity. The differing prominence of this last peak in different neurons and experiments is well understandable, because phasic activity may not always be present in all experiments and records since it depends upon the general state of activity (wakefulness, sleep, anesthesia, degree of external stimulation, etc.) and since not all units show this sort of activity. In addition to these different "trigger" mechanisms, an extravisual input into the lateral geniculate body must be supposed as it is suggested by experiments from Arden and Söderberg [1960]. This is especially the case in the cortex where, besides the already complicated input from the geniculate, nonspecific inputs from nonvisual centers or afferent systems are well established [Creutzfeldt and Akimoto, 1958; Baumgartner et al, 1961] and will, furthermore, complicate the picture. Hence, the less characteristic interval distributions of cortical neurons. The decrease of spontaneous and evoked activity at higher stations of the visual system also finds its explanation from intracellular records, with which it could be shown that the output (spike activity) of geniculate and cortical cells is only a fraction of its excitatory input recordable as EPSP's. This is partly due to the fact that a certain summation of EPSP's is necessary in order to reach the firing level, partly due to the presence of IPSP's under certain conditions. Since, however, the transfer function between pre- and postgeniculate activity has been found to be linear, at least during steady state conditions, no complicated transformation except a linear reduction at the input-output level has to be assumed.

It was an unexpected finding that IPSP's in the geniculate are almost absent during spontaneous dark activity except during the phasic activity.

[2] Hence, geniculate activity of the cat and the rabbit will be compared. This is possible, since in preliminary experiments which are now going on in our laboratory, it was observed that the intracellular activity of cells in the lateral geniculate body of rabbits and cats does not differ considerably. This, however, does not seem to be the case for the cortex.

In cortical neurons they are somewhat more frequent, though an exact analysis of Watanabe et al [1965] revealed that even in cortical nerve cells, spontaneous IPSP's constitute only a fraction of 5–15 per cent of all cortical PSP's during resting activity. On the other hand, quick transient light or optic nerve stimuli evoke in most geniculate cells an IPSP which might be preceded or not by an excitatory potential. Using electrical stimulation of the optic nerve, it was shown that the latency of IPSP's was always 1.5–3 msec longer than that of EPSP's (or spike discharges) [Fuster et al, 1965]. Using near-threshold stimulation for the afferent fibers to the cell from which the record was taken, it could be shown that the IPSP was present independently from a preceding EPSP or spike discharge of the recorded cell, whereas with suprathreshold stimulation, all geniculate cells first showed an excitation before the IPSP.

Such findings suggest the paucity if not the lack of direct inhibitory fibers from the retina, and suggest that inhibition of geniculate cells by afferent stimuli is probably mediated mainly by collateral connections within the geniculate. Histologically, there is a basis for this form of inhibition since recurrent collaterals as well as short axon cells, perhaps serving as interneurons, have been found in the geniculate [Cajal, 1955, pp. 390–391; O'Leary, 1940]. In the cortex, recent findings suggest that also here inhibition seems to be mainly due to collateral recurrent inhibition [Stefanis and Jasper, 1964; Creutzfeldt et al, 1965], even though in the visual cortex such a mechanism has not yet been confirmed convincingly.[3] Reduplication at every station of the visual pathway of a synaptic organization permitting collateral inhibition has been previously suggested [Baumgartner and Hakas, 1962; Jung, 1961a]. This type of inhibition, which appears to be a feature of all sensory projection systems, probably accomplishes the important purpose of enhancing contrast at central levels [Brooks, 1959]. Furthermore, it may be responsible for transformations which lead to different receptive fields of neurons at higher levels of the visual system [Hubel, 1962]. For the phasic activity a similar mechanism may be assumed as that proposed by Andersen et al [1964] for the correspondent activity in the ventrobasal nucleus of the thalamus.

The combination of findings gained with extra- and intracellular recordings has thus been shown to be of help to solve some problems of

---

[3] Since this lecture was given, intracellular records in the visual cortex of cats have shown that also here the latency of IPSP's after optic tract and radiation stimulation is in the average 1 msec longer than that of EPSP's. These findings and additional observations are in accordance with recurrent collateral inhibition in the visual cortex (Watanabe, S., Konishi, M., and Creutzfeldt, O. D.: Postsynaptic potentials in the cat's visual cortex following electrical stimulation of afferent pathways. *Exp. Brain Res.* (1966), in print).

information transmission in the visual system. The difficulty of intra-cellular recording in central parts of the visual system makes it difficult, however, to collect quickly enough sufficient data in order to keep pace with the wealth of extracellularly gained findings. It also has to be real-ized that much "information processing" (as form and movement detec-tion, simultaneous contrast, etc.) takes place already at the retinal level, especially in lower animals [Baumgartner and Hakas, 1962; Maturana et al, 1960; Barlow et al, 1964]. Repetition of many experiments in the visual system with intracellular records, especially those using stimulation of restricted parts of the receptive fields of single neurons, are necessary to definitely solve some of the problems touched during this presentation.

SUMMARY

1. Spontaneous and light-induced unit activity in the afferent visual system decreases at higher levels (tractus opticus > lateral geniculate body > visual cortex). The relation between discharge rate and light in-tensity can be expressed by exponential as well as by power functions with exponents of 0.2–0.3. This is due to the similarity of exponential and power functions with such exponents.

2. Interval analysis of spontaneous activity of neurons in the optic tract, the lateral geniculate body, and the visual cortex also shows characteristic differences. In the optic tract, mainly exponential interval distributions with an initial dead time of several msec and, correspond-ingly, a mode at 8–15 msec were found. Joint interval histograms con-firmed randomness of the discharges. With intermittent light stimulation, a shortening of the initial dead time can be produced. Bi- and trimodal interval distributions were found in the lateral geniculate body with peaks at 2–5, around 10, and between 80–200 msec. In the visual cortex, distributions with a peak at very short intervals (2–5 msec) flanked by a wide and unsystematic distribution of longer intervals are mostly found. During barbiturate anesthesia, bimodal distributions also in cortical units are frequently encountered, the second peak is located at 80–150 msec. Joint interval histograms of cortical units are typical for "grouped" dis-charging.

3. Intracellular records are described from neurons of the lateral geniculate body and the visual cortex of rabbits. In darkness, geniculate units showed random series of only EPSP's or rhythmical sequences of large hyperpolarizing potentials alternating with depolarizing ones, these producing grouped spike discharges. Cortical units showed both EPSP's and IPSP's either in irregular succession or in form of rhythmical waves.

These waves were most frequently observed in animals anesthetized with nembutal. Phase relationships were found between intracellularly recorded potentials of cortical cells and the surface EEG.

In geniculate as well as in cortical cells, intracellularly recorded responses to diffuse illumination of the retina were generally composite of EPSP's and IPSP's. Two main types of reactions were found: one characterized by primary EPSP at light-on and primary IPSP at light-off; the other characterized by the reverse primary reactions. A primary PSP is frequently followed by one or more PSP's of the opposite polarity. The magnitude of postsynaptic reactions of geniculate cells was seen to be related to intensity of light stimulation according to power as well as logarithmic functions.

Using repetitive brief flashes at various frequencies, interactions of EPSP's and IPSP's were found to determine the critical flicker frequency (CFF) of central units.

The reaction of geniculate and cortical cells to electric shock in the optic tract consisted of an EPSP followed by a large and long IPSP.

4. The findings are discussed and special attention is drawn to the mechanisms of transformation of the information flux at different stations of the ascending visual pathway.

DISCUSSION

Chairman: PROFESSOR HEYMANS

TEUBER: I wish to refer to the first part of Dr. Creutzfeldt's presentation where he showed logarithmic relations between stimulus intensity and frequency of discharge. After our discussion of Professor Mountcastle's presentation, it might seem as though there were a possible contradiction. I do believe that MacKay has a very cogent argument which shows that there is no contradiction whatsoever, and I wonder whether he can be stimulated into saying it now.

MAC KAY: Suppose we have a receptor whose response function is given by $f_1 = k_1 \log I$, and suppose that the process of perception, as I will be arguing later, can be likened to a process of "backing off" the input by means of internally generated activity, guided by some sort of comparison process. Suppose further that the "response function" of this internal generator is also logarithmic, say, $f_2 = k_2 \log \psi$, where ψ is a physical input to the generator analogous to the physical excitation of the receptor. Then, of course, on this basis, if the estimation of intensity requires the internal setting of $f_2 = f_1$ (to take the simplest possibility), we have $k_2 \log \psi = k_1 \log I$, or $\psi = I^\beta$, where $\beta = k_1/k_2$. In other words, a power law would relate I to ψ even though (or *because*) the receptor followed a log law. If the subject's estimate were linearly related to ψ, a psychophysical power law would follow.* In other words, like Professor Mount-castle, I would plead for open-mindedness here. We need not feel that finding a logarithmic receptor law in any way controverts belief in a psychophysical power law.

CREUTZFELDT: I should like to repeat that I do not want to question the power law whose applicability is well proven in different systems and by different methods. I only pointed to the fact that, in the visual system, logarithmic functions can mostly be applied as well as power functions because of the low exponent. The more important fact is that in the visual system the exponent in general seems to be smaller than in mechanical transducers where the exponent is closer to 1. It must be realized, however, that systematic studies in the visual system have not been done except with diffuse light. It is possible that the exponents will increase if only restricted parts of the receptive fields of single units are stimulated with punctiform light.

BREMER: I had the occasion to study with focal intranuclear recordings the inhibition at the geniculate level, which has two interesting points: first, as already shown by P. O. Bishop and his associates, its maximum is a very late one, about 30 msec, which is curious and which recalls the time course of a presynaptic inhibition. I realize that we have little evidence, but Professor Szentágothai told me by letter that there is evidence of axo-axonic contacts there. A second curious fact which I found concerning this binocular suppression at the geniculate level is that it affected more the corticopetal discharge than the field potential in the lateral geniculate. The radiation potential which is the expression of the discharge of the geniculate, can be suppressed or greatly reduced at a time when the field potential of the geniculate is almost unaltered. Your intracellular recording might clarify this problem.

CREUTZFELDT: With intracellular and quasi-intracellular records we have not found evidence for or against presynaptic inhibition in the geniculate. The long relative refractory period of geniculate cells is not due to a special property of the membranes of these neurons, but can be well explained by the large and long IPSP's which follow a synchronous afferent volley from the optic nerve. With supramaximal stimuli and with corresponding summation of excitatory potentials a more realistic picture of the refractory period of these cells can be gained. Its real time course, however, can only be investigated with antidromic stimulation, as has been done by P. O. Bishop and his group.

ECCLES: I would like to ask you why you chose to speak in terms of recurrent inhibition giving negative feedback, when alternatively you could have postulated afferent collateral inhibition with its feedforward orientation.

CREUTZFELDT: We interpreted the inhibition seen in the lateral geniculate as being due to recurrent collateral inhibition, since with suprathreshold optic nerve stimulation all cells showed first an EPSP with or without a spike discharge followed by an IPSP. IPSP's always had larger latencies than EPSP's. This is in agreement with the findings of Bishop and colleagues [Bishop, 1964] as well as of Gruesser-Cornehls and colleagues [1960] who, with extracellular

* See: Psychophysics of perceived intensity: a theoretical basis for Fechner's and Stevens' laws, *Science, 139,* 1213–1216 [1963].

recordings also always found primary excitation in geniculate cells after optic nerve stimulation. It may be suggested, however, that the invariably longer latency of IPSP's may be due to the intercalation of an inhibitory interneuron between inhibitory optic nerve fibers and geniculocortical neurons. This suggestion cannot be ruled out completely. But if it would be so, these interneurons also must receive "recurrent" inhibition, since with suprathreshold stimulation all neurons show an IPSP following the excitation. This might be conceivable but to me it sounds a bit complicated.

ANDERSEN: It was extremely nice to see these records, because they are so similar to what you can find in the somatosensory nucleus of the thalamus. First, large EPSP's in the somatosensory nucleus are produced just by straddling the threshold. Sometimes, only two of them are necessary in order to fire the cell, sometimes three, exactly like you find. The IPSP's are of the same shape, the same duration, the same size, and I think the maximum inhibition at 30 msec can be explained since you have the peak IPSP at 30 msec—a very slow rising phase of the IPSP. We have also seen spontaneous spindles in the V.P.L., and we have made a theory for their production. So, it is all very similar. I wonder if this could be a general phenomenon at the thalamic level, because we find very much the same principles also in the medial geniculate. However, all this has to be taken with certain reservations, I think. In your preparation, as well as in ours, we have an anesthetized animal, and the unanesthetized thalamus, I think, is very different. I am sure Mountcastle would agree with this. So what should be needed, I think, is to repeat all these experiments, if possible in an unanesthetized preparation, to see what inhibition means there. Finally, I should like to add that although we do not know much about presynaptic inhibition in the thalamus, we do know that we can produce presynaptic depolarization as tested with the method of Wall. So, there is at least one point of evidence that fits in with the morphological findings of Szentágothai.

REFERENCES

ANDERSEN, P., C. McC. BROOKS, J. C. ECCLES, and T. A. SEARS. The ventrobasal nucleus of the thalamus: Potential fields, synaptic transmission and excitability of both presynaptic and postsynaptic components, *J. Physiol.* (London), *174*, 348–369 [1964].

ARDEN, G. B., and U. SÖDERBERG. The transfer of optic information through the lateral geniculate body of the rabbit, in: *Sensory Communication* (ed. by A. Rosenblith). Cambridge, Mass.: MIT Press, pp. 521–544 [1961].

BARLOW, H. B., R. M. HILL, and W. R. LEVICK. Retinal ganglion cells responding selectively to direction and speed of image motion in the rabbit, *J. Physiol.* (London), *173*, 377–407 [1964].

BAUMGARTNER, C., O. D. CREUTZFELDT, and R. JUNG. Microphysiology of cortical neurons in acute anoxia and during retinal ischemia, in: *Cerebral Anoxia and the Electrencephalogram* (ed. by T. S. Meyer and H. Gastaut). Springfield, Ill.: C. C Thomas [1961].

BAUMGARTNER, G., and P. HAKAS. Die Neurophysiologie des simultanen Helligkeitskontrastes, *Pflügers Arch. Ges. Physiol.*, *274*, 489–510 [1962].

BISHOP, P. O., W. R. LEVICK, and W. D. WILLIAMS. Statistical analysis of the dark discharge of lateral geniculate neurones, *J. Physiol.* (London), *170*, 598–612 [1964].

BROOKS, V. B. Contrast and stability in the nervous system, *Trans. N. Y. Acad. Sci.*, *21*, 387–394 [1959].

CREUTZFELDT, O. D. General physiology of cortical neurones and neuronal information in the visual system, in: *Brain and Behavior* (ed. by M. Brazier). Washington, D. C. Vol. I, 299 pp. [1961].

———, and H. AKIMOTO. Konvergenz und gegenseitige Beeinflussung von Impulsen aus der Retina und den unspezifischen Thalamuskernen an einzelnen Neuronen des optischen Cortex, *Arch. Psychiat. Nervenkr.*, *196*, 520–538 [1958].

———. Propriétés biophysiques des cellules nerveuses de l'écorce cérébrale, in: *Actualités Neurophysiologiques* (ed. by A. M. Monnier). Paris: Masson [1965].

ENROTH, C. The mechanism of flicker and fusion. Studies on single retinal elements in the dark-adapted eye of the cat, *Acta Physiol. Scand.*, *27*. Suppl. 100, 1–67 [1952].

FUSTER, J. M., O. D. CREUTZFELDT, and M. STRASCHILL. Intracellular recording of neuronal activity in the visual system, *Z. Vergl. Physiol.*, *49*, 605–622 [1965a].

———, A. HERZ, and O. D. CREUTZFELDT. Interval analysis of cell discharge in spontaneous and optically modulated activity in the visual system, *Arch. Ital. Biol.*, *103*, 159–177 [1965b].

GRANIT, R. The organization of the vertebrate retinal elements, *Erg. Physiol.*, *46*, 31–70 [1950].

———, and C. G. PHILLIPS. Excitatory and inhibitory processes acting upon individual Purkinje cells of the cerebellum in cats, *J. Physiol.* (London), *133*, 520–527 [1956].

GRÜSSER, O. J., and O. D. CREUTZFELDT. Eine neurophysiologische Grundlage des Brücke-Bartley-Effektes: Maxima der Impulsfrequenz retinaler und corticaler Neurone bei Flimmerlicht mittlerer Frequenzen, *Pflügers Arch. Ges. Physiol.*, *263*, 668–681 [1957].

———, K. A. HELLNER, and U. GRÜSSER-CORNEHLS. Die Informationsübertragung im afferenten visuellen System, *Kybernetik*, *1*, 175–192 [1962].

HERZ, A., O. D. CREUTZFELDT, and J. M. FUSTER. Statistische Eigenschaften der Neuronaktivität im aszendierenden visuellen System, *Kybernetik*, *2*, 61–71 [1964].

———, and J. M. FUSTER. Beeinflussung der Spontanaktivität von Neuronen des visuellen Cortex durch Barbiturate und Amphetamin, *Naunyn-Schmiedebergs Arch. Exper. Path.*, *249*, 146–161 [1964].

HUBEL, D. H. Transformation of information in the cat's visual system, in: *Information Processing in the Nervous System* (ed. by R. W. Gerard and J. W. Duyff), *Excerpta Med.* Amsterdam, pp. 160–169 [1962].

JUNG, R. Neuronal integration in the visual cortex and its significance for visual information, in: *Sensory Communication* (ed. by W. A. Rosenblith). Cambridge, Mass. and New York: MIT Press and Wiley, 627–674 [1961].

———, and G. BAUMGARTNER. Hemmungsmechanismen und bremsende Stabilisierung an einzelnen Neuronen des optischen Cortex, *Pflügers Arch. Ges. Physiol.*, *261*, 434–456 [1955].

KUFFLER, S. W. Discharge patterns and functional organization of the mammalian retina, *J. Neurophysiol.*, *16*, 37–68 [1953].

———, R. FITZHUGH, and H. B. BARLOW. Maintained activity in the cat's retina in light and darkness, *J. Gen Physiol.*, *40*, 683–702 [1957].

MATURANA, H. R., J. Y. LETTVIN, W. S. McCULLOCH, and W. H. PITTS. Anatomy and physiology of vision in the frog (*Rana pipiens*), *J. Gen. Physiol.*, *43/2*, 129–175 [1960].

McILWAIN, J., and O. D. CREUTZFELDT. A microelectrode study of synaptic excitation and inhibition in the lateral geniculate nucleus of the cat, *J. Neurophysiol.* [1966]. (In press.)

MOUNTCASTLE, V. B., G. F. POGGIO, and G. WERNER. The relation of thalamic cell response to peripheral stimuli varied over on intensive continuum, *J. Neurophysiol.*, *26*, 807–834 [1963].

O'LEARY, J. S. A structural analysis of the lateral geniculate nucleus of the cat, *J. Comp. Neurol.*, *73*, 405–430 [1940].

RAMÓN Y CAJAL, S. *Histologie du Système Nerveux de l'Homme et des Vertébrés.* Madrid: Consigno Superior de Investigaciones Cientificas, Vol. II, pp. 309–391 [1955].

STEFANIS, C., and H. H. JASPER. Recurrent collateral inhibition in pyramidal tract, *J. Neurophysiol.*, *27*, 855 [1964].

STEVENS, S. S. Sensory transform functions, in: *Information Processing in the Nervous System* (ed. by R. W. Gerard and J. W. Duyff), *Excerpta Med.* Amsterdam, pp. 53–60 [1962].

STRASCHILL, M. Aktivität von Neuronen im Tractus opticus und Corpus geniculatum laterale bei langdauernden Lichtreizen verschiedener Intensität, *Kybernetik*, *3*, 1–8 [1966].

WATANABE, S., and O. D. CREUTZFELDT. Spontane postsynaptische Potentiale von Nervenzellen des motorischen Cortex der Katze, *Exp. Brain Res.*, *1*, 48–64 [1966].

7

Brain Stimulation and the Threshold of Conscious Experience

University of California Medical Center,
San Francisco, California

The subject of this paper stems out of a more general question which asks, what is the spatiotemporal configuration of neuronal activity which effectively elicits or is at least uniquely correlated with a conscious awareness of something? Now, to attempt a study of whole configurations of neuronal activities is obviously much too difficult and complicated. One would like to delimit severely the experimental approach to this question, and this we have done in two ways.

The first limitation consists in investigating only the simplest reportable elements of conscious experience, and for that we have chosen a primitive sensation or, as some philosophers (for example, Feigl) have termed it, a "raw feel." Lord Adrian has stated this position much more elegantly than I can. In his lecture in The Physical Basis of Mind series [1952] he said, "I think there is reasonable hope that we may be able to sort out the particular activities which coincide with quite simple mental processes like seeing or hearing. At all events that is the first thing a physiologist must do if he is trying to find out what happens when we think and how the mind is influenced by what goes on in the brain." In our work the simple sensations happen to be somesthetic ones, because of the regions of brain available to us for study.

The second limitation consists in studying the changes at the threshold level of awareness of a sensation. The general problem is then reformulated to ask, what are the critical events, within the whole necessary substratum of the dynamic and structural configuration, which are associated with bringing something into conscious experience? It is implied that there will be some unique general differences between the states that exist just below as opposed to just above this threshold level of awareness.

We must briefly define our usage of "threshold conscious experience of sensation." On the premise that the subjective or introspective feeling of a sensation is the primary criterion of conscious experience, it must be the report of such a feeling by the subject that is operational in such an investigation. Such a report, of course, includes processes of short memory, recall, and expression (verbal in our case) on the part of the subject. There may be a nonreportable type of immediate but ephemeral awareness, and I believe it probably does exist; to detect it for the purpose of study, however, is another matter. In any case, an ephemeral awareness would presumably not be of primary significance to the kind of human conscious experience which has continuity, although conceivably it would play a role in later unconscious processes and thus indirectly in conscious ones.

It should be noted that other criteria of threshold awareness of sensation have been employed by others in some psychophysical studies. These include (*a*) guessing by the subject as to whether he has or has not been stimulated, (*b*) an immediate unthinking motor reaction by the subject if he has any impression of a stimulus having been delivered, and (*c*) reaction times of such motor responses, taken as an index of the degree (or certainty) of such awareness. None of these involves a report of introspective awareness and may not represent the same phenomenon that we chose to study.

Indeed, significant differences in the behavior of the differently defined responses in certain experimental situations have already been observed. Using the report of subjective feeling as the criterion, we found relatively sharp thresholds for the intensity and the duration of the train of stimulus pulses, whether at the cortical somatosensory area or at the skin. There was at times uncertainty about the response in a narrow range of parametric values around the threshold level, but below this range level the subject never reported a sensation and above it he always did. In studies in which the subject was guessing as to whether he has been stimulated [for example, Eijkman and Vendrik, 1963], no definite thresholds were observable; instead the incidence of positive responses followed a probabilistic relationship over the whole range of parametric values. A second difference appears to be evident in the effects of a change in the procedure of alerting the subjects. Responsiveness may be studied in the condition of "EEG-arousal," when the alpha rhythm is "blocked" and replaced by a low voltage irregular activity, by asking the subject to keep his eyes open and by alerting him with a "ready" signal before the delivery of each stimulus. In the alternative procedure, alpha rhythm is present; the subject is asked to relax with the eyes closed, is given no "ready" signal and, in our study, was asked not to think about reporting any sensation that he might experience until requested to do so. These two different states of EEG activity have been thought to be associated with a difference in attentive responsiveness or alertness. Motor reaction times to a fixed stimulus have in fact been found to be considerably lower in the condition of blocked alpha rhythm which followed a ready signal [Lansing, Schwartz, and Lindsley, 1959]. Yet we found no significant differences between the two different alerting procedures, either in threshold intensities or train durations required of a stimulus, when using our criterion of conscious experience. This held true with stimuli at all points tested in the somatosensory pathway—skin, thalamic, and cortical.

It may be suggested, even more generally, that behavioral manifestations of attentiveness are not necessarily a reflection of responsiveness at the conscious, introspective level. A homely example may be cited in further support of this contention. You have no doubt had the experience of behaving as if you were listening to a conversation, even nodding correctly at appropriate cues in the conversation, and yet not consciously hearing a word of what is going on, as you are thinking of other things or of nothing at all. One should then be aware of a possible fundamental error in experimental approaches which assume that conscious experience of a reportable, continuous nature accompanies a particular motor response, even when the motor act is complicated and involves the making of decisions by the agent.

From this discussion of what it is we are attempting to study, we may proceed to our experimental questions. What is the unique nature of the input at cerebral levels which just reaches the threshold for eliciting a conscious sensory experience, as opposed to a subthreshold one which just fails to do so? Secondly, are there unique differences in the cerebral responses to these two classes of inputs? (We are only in the beginning stages of this second part of the study.) Peripheral sensory inputs do not appear to be very satisfactory for this experimental purpose, as the stimulus thresholds and the resulting discharges of sensory impulses are, in attentive subjects, generally rather close to the minimum physical or physiological quantities possible. Perhaps the most clear-cut experiment with somatic sensation in this regard has been carried out by Hensel and Boman [1960]. They exposed a small skin nerve in a human subject, and severed all the nerve fibers in it but one, whose electrical responses to mechanical stimulation of the skin innervated by it could be followed. The weakest stimulus that could be detected subjectively as a sensory experience (of touch) gave rise to one single conducted impulse in the one remaining nerve fiber. Such sensitivities mean that one can go from no input to some input at the threshold level, and thus the corresponding changes in cerebral activities may involve more than those which are unique to conscious experience.

Threshold stimuli applied to the somatosensory cortex are not, as we shall see further, of such a minimal character as are peripheral ones. There is the additional advantage that with stimulation at cerebral levels one has complete control of the immediate input here, instead of having to discover what complex alterations have been imposed on the nature of the original peripheral input by subcortical mechanisms. Much work has already shown that one can elicit simple sensations, usually paresthesia-like, by electrical stimulation of the postcentral gyrus in awake human subjects; Professor Penfield and his group [for example, Penfield and Rasmussen, 1950] have contributed greatly to this knowledge and have carried out elaborate topographical mapping of the representation of body sensibilities on the human cortex by this method. For our problem we have generally selected one responsive point in the postcentral gyrus and, with an electrode fixed at this position, have studied the nature of the adequate stimulus there for eliciting a conscious sensory experience. Such work is made possible by the cooperation of awake patients who are undergoing therapeutic surgical treatments of the brain which require that they be essentially non-medicated except for the local anesthetics injected into the scalp.

A number of parameters of the electrical stimuli applied to somatosensory cortex have potential physiological significance,[1] but I shall discuss chiefly those aspects which have turned out to be of special interest to the problem of conscious experience. The area of postcentral gyrus usually available to us produced sensation in the contralateral fingers or hand when suitably stimulated with rectangular current pulses, delivered generally through a unipolar surface electrode.

It is important to realize at the outset that the general nature of the threshold response to cortical stimuli can differ, depending on the combination of values for the different stimulus parameters, even though the electrode position is constant. The threshold cortical stimuli can thus be grouped into three parametric regions (Table 1). Those in parametric region A are characterized by the lowest or liminal threshold intensities, by relatively long durations of the train of repetitive pulses (0.5 sec or more), and by pulse repetition frequencies greater than about 10 per sec. These threshold stimuli elicit reports of the introspective experience of purely somatic sensations. The question of the control of the quality of the sensations by the input cannot be considered at length here; stimuli

---

[1] A fuller treatment of these may be found in the paper by Libet, Alberts, Wright, Delattre, Levin, and Feinstein [1964].

Table 1

Summary of Parametric Regions for Threshold Stimuli

	Region A	Region B	Region C
Intensity (peak current)	Liminal	2 or more times that in A	Intermediate range, between A and B
Train duration (T.D.)	>0.5–1 sec	<0.1–0.3 sec Single pulses	0.5–5 sec, at 8 pps; 0.1–0.5 sec at pulse frequencies ≧15 pps
Pulse frequency	≧15 pps (can get with 8 pps if T.D. >5–10 sec)	Any	Probably any, but best seen in low range (<15 pps)
Facilitation still evident after 30 sec or more	Usually none	Usually considerable	Usually present
Response at threshold	Purely somatosensory (no motor)	Observable muscular contraction	No observable contraction; sensation changes from that in A to one with aspect of motion (at <15 pps often has slow pulsatile quality)

in this parametric region may produce virtually all types, both paresthesia-like and more normally specific types of qualities. On the other hand, with stimuli in parametric region B, having threshold intensities two or more times the liminal ones in region A and very short train durations (<0.1–0.2 sec), the response at threshold levels was a localized muscular contraction. The sensation of a movement was presumably due to returning sensory information of it from the periphery, and no purely somatic sensations independent of this were reported. Single pulses all belong in region B. Those threshold stimuli which fell between the characteristics of regions A and B seemed to comprise an intermediate class, region C. The latter produced no visible motor response but often did elicit a sensation with an aspect of motion in it. The difference from the responses in region A could be seen best when changing from stimuli in parametric region A to those in C. At pulse frequencies of 8 per sec or less, the sensation usually had a pulsatile character, with pulsations being felt at a frequency (about 1 per sec) which was independent of the pulse repetition frequency of the stimulus.

Another differential feature of the parametric regions which deserves consideration relates to the long-persisting effects following a stimulus. Threshold stimuli in parametric region A were not, in general, followed by any long-lasting facilitatory effects; they could be delivered at intervals of 30 sec with no effect on the thresholds of succeeding stimuli. In regions B and C, however, in which threshold responses are, respectively, frankly motor or have motion aspects to the sensations, a long-lasting facilitatory effect on the thresholds of succeeding stimuli was commonly seen, for as long as several minutes after a stimulus. This may be a function of the higher intensity levels characteristic of such stimuli.

Following stimuli in parametric region A, on the other hand, an interesting long-lasting effect on the quality of sensations in succeeding responses could be demonstrated. For example, a threshold stimulus with a pulse frequency of 60 per sec might elicit a tingling sensation. If this was followed after a 30-sec interval by a threshold stimulus now employing an 8 per sec pulse frequency, the subject tended to report the same type of tingling sensation. If one waited for about 5 min, however, the 8 per sec stimulus elicited a pulsatory sensation, as described earlier, instead of the tingling one. We have no very good explanation to suggest for this enduring effect on sensory quality, recalling that it is not accompanied by a similarly long-lasting effect on threshold requirements. It is possible that a persistence of facilitation occurs in those parts of the responding neural apparatus other than the ones that set the threshold requirements of the surface stimulus. What significance this phenomenon may have for the problems of long-persisting alterations of cerebral function such as memory remains to be seen.

We will not go into the question here of motor versus sensory specificity of responses to stimulation of the pre- and postcentral gyri in man, except to emphasize that at liminal intensity levels the responses were always purely sensory in postcentral gyrus and apparently purely motor in the precentral gyrus.

With respect to the question of which neural components in somatosensory cortex are initially activated at the threshold levels for conscious sensation, some general suggestions come out of this study of stimulus requirements. The analysis of the evidence on depth of responding elements in the motor cortex, as carried out by Hern, Landgren, and Phillips [1962], and Phillips and Porter [1962], encourages one to use a similar approach in sensory cortex. The critical neural components for threshold sensation (*a*) appear to lie in the more superficial layers of the postcentral cortex, and (*b*) are probably orientated vertically (that is, perpendicular to the surface) rather than horizontally. The evidence for (*a*) is, briefly, that unipolar cathodal pulses were found to require only about 70 per cent of the peak current required by anodal ones, in order to achieve threshold levels in each case. Suggestion (*a*) does not exclude the possibility that deeper neural components are also activated directly or transsynaptically by threshold stimuli, but it would indicate that it is the excitation of more superficial components that sets the threshold requirement. If suggestion (*b*) were wrong, that is, if neural components located in superficial layers were oriented horizontally, a bipolar stimulus should prove more effective than a unipolar one. Since, in fact, a unipolar cathodal stimulus was the somewhat more effective one, this supports the suggestion of a vertical orientation for such components. The even greater effectiveness, in terms of current density, of a large (10 mm diameter) unipolar electrode also supports this view.

The unipolar electrode with this large area could achieve threshold (using a 60 per sec pulse frequency) with a current density of less than 0.1 mA per mm^2, as compared with about 1 mA per mm^2 for the usual 1 mm electrode. It is of considerable interest that the threshold sensation with the large electrode was referred roughly to the same size area of the body and had the same quality associated with it as did the one elicited by the smaller electrode. This would indicate that spatial facilitation originating from a relatively large cortical mass can be an important factor in the effective excitation of a small group of neural elements that mediate conscious sensation.

I want to return now to a further consideration of what are probably the most interesting findings in these experiments with cerebral stimulation. These are the observations that, in order to elicit a somatic sensation not only is repetition of liminal stimulus pulses required but also such repetition must go on for about a half a second or so to become effective (parametric region A, above). This is in sharp contrast to peripheral input requirements, in which virtually a single liminal stimulus pulse (or indeed a single nerve impulse) can produce a conscious sensation. Figure 7.1 shows a graph of the minimum intensities required of the cortical stimuli for threshold responses when plotted against the duration of the repetitive train of pulses required at each such intensity. The curves are somewhat idealized, to represent our general experiences with this relationship, but are based upon the actual data found for several subjects. These curves resemble the intensity-duration curves for threshold single pulses that excite nerve fibers, but in the present case we are dealing with train duration, not pulse duration. Lengthening the train duration beyond a certain minimum value produces virtually no change in the minimum intensity required. This level, which we refer to as the liminal intensity, is lower for higher pulse repetition frequencies up to about 100–200 per sec, but it rises again when the pulse frequency goes above this. The mimimum train duration that is required when using a liminal intensity, that is, the point where further shortening of train duration be-

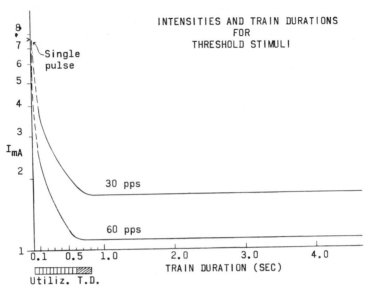

Fig. 7.1. Intensity-train duration combinations for stimuli (to postcentral gyrus) just adequate to elicit a threshold conscious experience of somatic sensation. Curves are presented for two different pulse repetition frequencies, employing rectangular pulses of 0.5 msec duration. "Utilization train duration" is discussed in the text.

gins to require distinctly greater intensities of stimulus, we refer to as the "utilization train duration." This is by analogy with the utilization time of the intensity-duration curve for axons. Most utilization train durations fall into the range of 0.5–1 sec for pulse frequencies from 15–120 per sec, although there have been occasional values as short as 0.2 sec and some as long as 1.5–2 sec. While the mean value of utilization train durations was somewhat lower when higher pulse frequencies were used, the data cannot be assessed for statistical significance of such differences; in any case, there have been subjects in whom there was no reduction of utilization train duration at the greater pulse frequencies (in the 15–60 per sec range).

It should also be noted that we found similar values for utilization train duration with liminal stimulation of the immediate afferent supply to the somatosensory cortex, that is, of its subcortical white matter or of the ventroposterolateral (VPL) nucleus of the thalamus. Such a requirement is not, therefore, something unique to the more abnormal mode of activation of the cortex by direct electrical stimulation.

This relationship of intensity to train duration lends a kind of all-or-nothing aspect to threshold awareness of a sensation. Below the liminal intensity level there is no reportable awareness of a sensation, in contrast to the findings using other criteria of sensory awareness. In addition, for any liminal stimulus with a train shorter than the utilization train duration, the subject reports that he does not feel anything.

One hypothesis to explain the utilization train duration would be that it represents the time required for sufficient summation of excitatory effects up to some critical level. It would also be inferred that the greater liminal intensity required with a lower pulse frequency approximately compensates for the longer pulse interval, in the development of excitatory level during the utilization period. This last could account for the absence of any large effects of change in pulse frequency on the utilization train duration. Another more intriguing hypothesis would be that it is some minimum period of time, *per se*, during which activation of certain neural components must proceed, which is essential for the elaboration of a reportable conscious sensation. This would not require a progressive buildup of excitatory level during the utilization period; rather, the suggestion is that a minimum "activation period" would be necessary even with a constant average level of excitatory actions during the time involved. The evidence we have available thus far appears to favor this second hypothesis, although more definitive types of experiments must still be done in order to settle the issue.

The evidence may be discussed by reference to the diagram in Fig. 7.2. The top line represents the 0.5 msec rectangular pulses at 20 per sec making up a stimulus train at liminal intensity for eliciting conscious sensation. The thresholds for eliciting the direct cortical electrical response (DCR), both its initial negative and the subsequent positive components as recorded from the adjacent cortical surface, were found to be well below those required for eliciting conscious sensory experience. Thus, as seen in line 2, Fig. 7.2, a usually submaximal DCR is already present with the first pulse. This gains in size with the first two or three repetitions of the stimulus pulse. The interesting point with respect to the hypothesis under consideration is that the DCR's remain fairly constant throughout the whole stimulus train, up to and beyond the utilization train duration (except for the rapid initial augmentation, and the decrease in amplitude later in the train in those cases in which a surface-negative shift in steady potential develops). At least for this type of response, then, there is no evidence of a progressive rise in excitatory level throughout the whole period of the utilization train duration.

The third line in Fig. 7.2 indicates that no sensation is elicited until the train has gone on for about 0.5 sec or more. If the train continues beyond the utilization train duration, however, the subjective intensity of the sensation does not increase progressively (except for some uncertainty in a relatively small range of time around the utilization point); the same threshold sensation merely has a longer duration with the longer train.

174 / B. Libet

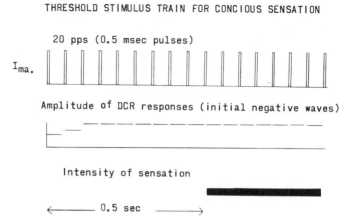

THRESHOLD STIMULUS TRAIN FOR CONCIOUS SENSATION

20 pps (0.5 msec pulses)

$I_{ma.}$

Amplitude of DCR responses (initial negative waves)

Intensity of sensation

←——— 0.5 sec ———→

Fig. 7.2. Diagram of relationships between the train of 0.5 msec pulses at liminal intensity applied to postcentral gyrus, and the amplitudes of the direct cortical responses (DCR) recorded nearby. The third line indicates that no conscious sensory experience is elicited until approximately the initial 0.5 sec of events has elapsed, and that the just detectable sensation appearing after that period remains at the same subjective intensity while the stimulus train continues.

This is remarkable by contrast with the course of the motor response obtained when a similar type of stimulus is applied to the *precentral* gyrus, in the unanesthetized subject. A progressive increase in the motor response during a train of repetitive pulses is often observed even at strengths considerably below that required for a response to a single pulse; once the contraction begins it tends to become progressively more powerful as the train of similar pulses continues. Thus, excitatory processes in the somatosensory cortex, insofar as they are relevant to conscious sensory experience, appear to be maintained at a relatively constant level when the liminal stimulus train continues on beyond the utilization train duration. Such stability in the period following the utilization point does not tell us about the course of development of excitatory processes in the period before this point. It is at least compatible, however, with the suggestion that the relevant excitatory processes have ceased undergoing any further rise in level sometime before the end of the utilization train duration.

Some supporting evidence for the second hypothesis, which suggested a requirement of a minimum "activation period," comes from psychophysical experiments of the type initiated by Crawford [1947] and pursued by others. In these the visual threshold to a brief test flash of light was studied in relation to the timing of a second superthreshold flash [see Wagman and Battersby, 1964]. When the second ("conditioning") flash *followed* the first by as much as 200 msec, the first flash became invisible to the subject unless its intensity was raised considerably. Since the latency of the first evoked potential in the visual cortex is only about 35 msec, it may be presumed that the interaction is a central one. Such psychophysical findings thus indicate that awareness of a near-threshold visual stimulus does not occur for about 200 msec after the initial delivery of impulses to the cortex, and that such awareness can be prevented if there is sufficient interference at any time with the central processes that are going on during this relatively long period following the stimulus [see also Crawford, 1947].

Although the hypothesis of a minimum "activation period" itself has only a tenuous status at present, I will conclude by indulging in some interesting speculative inferences which can be developed from it. The first arises in response to the question of how one may explain the ability of a single peripheral nerve volley to elicit a conscious sensory experience? The answer could lie in the nature of the after-waves which follow the initial evoked potential. Such after-waves have been recorded from the sensory cortex of unanesthetized animals and human subjects by a number of investigators. The after-waves go on for some hundreds of milliseconds, are especially sensitive to conditions which modify the state of consciousness (anesthesia, sleep) and have been reported to change with shifts in attention and learning. They could represent or indicate activation processes which go on normally, in response to peripheral sensory input, during the requisite "activation period." We have not (even with averaging techniques) been able to detect any such after-waves in the DCR which is elicited in the human somatosensory cortex, in response to a stimulus at the liminal strength for eliciting a conscious sensory experience. One may suppose, therefore, that the equivalent of such after-waves must be supplied by the cortical stimulus itself, in the form of repetitive pulses during the activation period.

Secondly, one may speculate that an activation period could be involved in the elaboration or fixation of a memory trace, as we are dealing with a reportable conscious experience. Such a requirement is implicit in the more specific suggestion already proposed by Gerard [1955], that reverberation of activity in neural networks may be involved not only in the fixation of ordinary learned responses, but also in the development of the initial consciousness of an experience. The actual nature of the specific activity that may be critical in this latter connection is, of course, still to be developed, even if the general concept of an activation period is substantiated. It even seems worthwhile to consider the possibility that processes involved in producing memory of an awareness may have some unique differences from those involved in the retention of some types of learned behavioral responses.

Finally, the requirement of a utilization time of 0.5–1 sec indicates that awareness of a sensory experience does not take place immediately after the initial arrival of impulses at the cortex from the periphery. It should be recalled that this requirement was found even for stimuli applied to thalamic VPL nucleus at the liminal intensity for eliciting sensation, that is, when the input to the cortex is delivered via the specific projection afferent fibers. Such a requirement implies then that there is a latency of about 0.5–1 sec before the conscious experience of the sensation begins, at least with threshold levels of input. This inference would seem to hold regardless of what mechanism is postulated for the utilization train duration. Now, as we all know, one can react to a stimulus with a motor response much more quickly than in 0.5–1 sec, even when decisions are involved in making the response. Reaction times as low as 0.05 sec are demonstrable. This then can lead to the further speculative inference that the quick motor reactions which one makes in response to liminal stimuli in everyday life situations may not be mediated by processes at conscious levels, and that they may be confined to unconscious levels. Perhaps only subsequent to the performance of such a quick motor reaction does one become consciously aware of the sensation and response, at least in the sense of awareness having continuity and reportability; or one might remain unaware of it altogether depending upon the circumstances.

ACKNOWLEDGMENTS

The experimental work reported here was carried out in collaboration with a group that included Dr. W. W. Alberts, biophysicist; E. W. Wright, Jr., electronics associate; L. D. Delattre, research assistant in psychology; and the neurosurgeons, Drs. Bertram Feinstein and Grant Levin. The work was done in the Mt. Zion Neurological Institute in San Francisco, and was partially supported by U. S. Public Health Service Grant NB 05061 from the National Institute of Neurological Diseases and Blindness.

DISCUSSION

Chairman: PROFESSOR BREMER

PENFIELD: I have nothing to add to Dr. Libet's very careful, thoughtful analysis.

Our own stimulation of the human brain has been practical; it has always had an ulterior, a therapeutic, purpose of course. Experiment is never a primary purpose. We began in 1928 using the stimulation equipment that

Foerster was using in Breslau. We used a galvanic current for localization and added a faradic current with the greatest caution for fear that the faradic current would produce a major epileptic seizure.

After Dr. Herbert Jasper came to Montreal the apparatus was refined with his guidance. We now use a square wave generator and Dr. Theodore Rasmussen in our clinic has elaborated the parameters of stimulation much more completely than I have but without changing our general conclusions. Our purpose, from the outset, was to try to produce the very beginning of the epileptic seizure that we hoped to cure, without precipitating a major attack. We also used the electrode to establish the functional topography. Thus, as time passed, we stimulated all parts of the human brain. Scars or other lesions may well produce seizures anywhere in the cerebral cortex. In the early days, before we had electroencephalography we had to depend always on the patient to tell us that he felt as though an attack were coming and then we had to use the greatest caution to prevent producing a major convulsive seizure.

As Dr. Libet suggests, we have been impressed by the fact that the findings of Sherrington in cats and then in chimpanzees are borne out during exploration of the human cortex. Facilitation follows stimulation at a cortical point and that applies both to sensory and to motor and to psychical responding areas. There is evidence of fatigue, or inhibition, if one stimulates again too quickly. It is possible also to demonstrate displacement of response, as Sherrington first described it.

LIBET: In reply, I may say that your studies were of course invaluable to us as background in helping us to get into this area of study. Our work is just a beginning into these more quantitative analytical aspects, utilizing one locus. We did not study the sorts of things that you had. For example, we did not study displacement of sensation since we stayed in one place and simply studied the parameters at that point. I might add, however, that the area of projected sensation was not always constant, even though we stayed at one point; that is, even with a threshold stimulus one stimulus might produce a sensation in the tip of an index finger and the very next one with exactly the same parameters, 30 sec or more later, might produce a sensation in a somewhat adjacent area, not precisely the same one.

We did not find facilitation with sensory cortex stimuli lasting beyond the 30-sec interval, although we did find it if we used many stimuli at intensities somewhat above threshold level. So that there may be a difference there; if one stays at the liminal level using train durations of 5 sec or less, then I think you can get by with 30-sec intervals without producing appreciable facilitation on the next threshold point.

PENFIELD: In psychical responses, for example, the elicitation of previous experience, we found a little different kind of facilitation was present. If we produced an experience of one type, or an experience which came from a certain time in the individual's life, one was apt (from the region around within perhaps 3, 4, or 5 cm) to get another experience of the same type and from the same period. There was a certain tendency for the first experience thus to set the type of the later elicited experiences. That is a little different kind of facilitation. When, on the other hand, one jumped quite a long way across the cortex and set the electrode down on interpretive cortex at a distance, the experience summoned came from a different period of life or had different characteristics altogether.

LIBET: This is somewhat analogous to our requirement of a 5-min or so waiting period in order for us to change the modality of the sensation when stimulating at the same point on the sensory cortex; there is some persistence of a subjective quality once you elicit it at a certain point.

PENFIELD: If we went back to the same point with the lapse of a few seconds or a minute or so, we usually had the same experiential response. If, on the other hand, we waited a little longer time and then went back to the same point, another experience would appear.

GRANIT: I wanted to comment on the single fiber elementary sensation experiment. We have had so much information lately on small fibers that we should be very cautious in accepting evidence of that sort, because the small fibers may always contribute to these sensations. I was very impressed by the long time for utilization, but, of course, one can think of so many explanations for it that it is very difficult to put forward anything definitive. The fact in itself is most interesting, namely, that simple sensory developments take such a long time compared with what we know that the brain can do with fast reactions. So I want to compliment you on that finding, which seems to me of great importance.

LIBET: Thank you, Professor Granit. I agree that our experiments have not differentiated conclusively between the various alternative explanations of this long utilization train duration, although the fact is interesting. But we do intend to try to get further evidence on which of the possible hypotheses may be more probable.

MOUNTCASTLE: Dr. Libet, it is the duration in the hypothesis that you discussed at the end of your paper that disturbs me, because I believe that the human experiments which you refer to involve a decision and a discrimination of stimulus that can be made by humans with an intracortical time of 60 msec, as Grey Walter has recently told us. These are conscious reactions. And this does not fit very well with the idea that you need a time of a half second for perception. The difference, of course, may be that the cortex has a very difficult job in weeding out the conscious perception from the abnormal train of events set in motion by the electrical stimulus. I wonder whether one should really translate through to the process of perception what is going on when you pass the current through the cortex, because as Grey Walter showed especially in the learning situation, the human cortex can make a discrimination in a very few milliseconds.

LIBET: I have not seen the reports of the particular experiments you are talking about. One has to watch out for the distinction between making a decision response and then being consciously aware of it. In experiments of the kind you mention that I have looked at in this regard, they have not always been careful to make this distinction.* I am confident that one can

* (Note added later): The experiments reported by W. Grey Walter, referred to by Dr. Mountcastle, were evidently those described in a talk published in the *Ann. N. Y. Acad. Sci., 112*:1, 320–361 [1964]. Subjects could learn to turn off an

make a decision and act very rapidly, but this does not necessarily mean that awareness is involved immediately.

PHILLIPS: Could I ask you to say a little more about the qualities of the sensations that were evoked? I am interested in this partly from the point of view of the last question because, if the sensation is tingling or something abnormal, it may not be recognized as something normally significant in the environment. And the other question in which we are all interested is, how far does electrical stimulation evoke normal function in the cortex? If you ever get normal sensations, then this of course is a very important observation. I think you once told me that generally the sensations are abnormal: pins and needles or tingling or electricity or something of that sort. But if you ever get normal sensations, it is very important to know about those.

LIBET: Yes, that is certainly an important general question. One answer, to the suggestion that some of our findings may be a function of the very abnormal nature of electrical stimulation of the cortex, is that we have substantiated the long utilization train duration with stimuli other than those at the surface of the cortex. We have stimulated in some cases the VPL nucleus, the specific projection nucleus in the thalamus, and got again there at liminal intensity levels the same kind of requirement of a half a second or longer train duration; this, of course, involves stimulating the afferent pathways to the cortex. Stimulating, in one case at least, the subcortical white matter just below the somatosensory cortex gave the same kind of long utilization trains.

Now, as to the qualities of the sensations elicited by cortical stimuli: Although in the majority of cases the response was an abnormal or parasthesia kind of sensation, I would say that in about one third of the individuals a specific kind of quality was reported which was more akin to a natural one.

The most common quality of a more natural kind—this is at the threshold level of stimulation—has been one of a deep pressure sensation, a kind of wave moving about under the skin in the area that is involved. The less common ones have been those of a specific light touch, some reports of what appears to be pure motion without any movement detectable, and also reports of pure heat and pure cold with nothing else involved. So that at the threshold levels, specific qualities certainly do appear, and I am sure that Professor Penfield and others have also obtained reports of specific modalities. The reason for the specific sensations not appearing consistently is another matter, and this gets us into the general question of what is the nature of the activity that has to go on in the somatosensory cortex for the production of a specific kind of quality. I do not think we have time to go into that now, but we do have some evidence along this line to indicate what the reasons may be for our failure to elicit specific qualities consistently.

JASPER: I want to draw Dr. Libet out a little bit on some of these other findings that he did not have time to report. I first thought that perhaps your results might be explained in terms of the threshold required for conduction

unconditional stimulus with an apparent reaction time of 50 msec after its onset, when this stimulus followed a conditional one by a fixed interval (of 1 sec). The question of subjective experience of awareness of the unconditional stimulus, at the moment of response, was apparently not a specific consideration.

out of the cortex. This is known to be much higher when you study the pyramidal tract responses to direct cortical stimulation, where a much higher stimulus
is required to get the impulse to conduct out than to excite the cortex superficially; I think Lord Adrian first showed this with the direct cortical response.
And do you not find the same thing, that it requires many times the threshold
of a direct cortical response to elicit sensation?

LIBET: Not usually. We did have to get above threshold for the direct
cortical response in all cases in order to elicit a sensation. But the threshold
for sensation could be as little as 10 per cent or so greater than that for the
DCR, although it was relatively much greater in some instances. The other
evidence that we have on this point is the fact that a distinctly weaker cathodal
stimulus is required than an anodal one. This indicates that the response is
generated at the superficial end of some neural elements.

JASPER: It does not require conduction out, you think?

LIBET: I do not think so. That is, there may eventually be conduction out,
but I don't think we are directly stimulating efferent elements. The available
evidence indicates that, at the threshold for sensation, we are stimulating something before that point.

PENFIELD: In regard to the response of the sense of movement. I am interested that it appeared so rarely in your liminal stimulation; I think we got
it a little more frequently, probably because we were using just routinely one
volt and perhaps were slightly above liminal strength. From the second sensory area of the cortex, which in man is the downward projection or continuation of the precentral gyrus into the fissure of Sylvius, we more frequently produced a sense of movement and often it was a more elaborate movement; just
as from the supplementary motor area we sometimes got a sense of larger
movements which seemed to include muscles and parts of both sides of the
body.

CHAIRMAN: Before closing this interesting discussion, I want to ask Dr.
Libet a question which may be answered "yes" or "no." Did you in your work
combine a sensory stimulus with electrical stimulus in conditioning experiments,
the sensory being the unconditioned stimulus? Such experiments might be interesting from the point of view of the organization of sensory modalities in the
somatosensory cortex.

LIBET: I agree with you that this might be a very useful approach, and in
fact we have intended to do experiments along such lines, but we have not done
them yet.

REFERENCES

ADRIAN, E. D. What happens when we think, in: *The Physical Basis of Mind*
(ed. by P. Laslett). Oxford: Blackwell [1952].

CRAWFORD, B. H. Visual adaptation in relation to brief conditioning stimuli,
Proc. Roy. Soc. B (London), *134*, 283–302 [1947].

EIJKMAN, E., and A. J. H. VENDRIK. Detection theory applied to the absolute
sensitivity of sensory systems, *Biophys. J.*, *3*, 65–78 [1963].

GERARD, R. W. The biological roots of psychiatry, *Amer. J. Psychiat.*, *112*, 81–90 [1955].

HENSEL, H., and K. K. A. BOMAN. Afferent impulses in cutaneous sensory nerves in human subjects, *J. Neurophysiol.*, *23*, 564–578 [1960].

HERN, J. E. C., S. LANDGREN, and C. S. PHILLIPS. Selective excitation of corticofugal neurons by surface-anodal stimulation of the baboon's motor cortex, *J. Physiol.*, *161*, 73–90 [1962].

LANSING, A. W., E. SCHWARTZ, and D. B. LINDSLEY. Reaction time and EEG activation under alerted and non-alerted conditions, *J. Exp. Psychol.*, *58*, 1–6 [1959].

LIBET, B., W. W. ALBERTS, E. W. WRIGHT, Jr., L. D. DELATTRE, G. LEVIN, and B. FEINSTEIN. Production of threshold levels of conscious sensation by electrical stimulation of human somatosensory cortex, *J. Neurophysiol.*, *27*, 546–578 [1964].

PENFIELD, W., and T. RASMUSSEN. *The Cerebral Cortex of Man. A Clinical Study of Localization of Function.* New York: Macmillan [1950].

PHILLIPS, C. S., and R. PORTER. Unifocal and bifocal stimulation of the motor cortex, *J. Physiol.*, *162*, 532–538 [1962].

WAGMAN, I. H., and W. S. BATTERSBY. Neural limitations of visual excitability. V. Cerebral after-activity evoked by photic stimulation, *Vision Res.*, *4*, 193–208 [1964].

8

Alterations of Perception
After Brain Injury[1]

by H.-L. Teuber

*Massachusetts Institute of Technology,
Cambridge, Massachusetts*

The previous speakers have approached the relation of brain and conscious experience primarily by considering single units; they have surveyed the microstructure of neo- and archicortex, the interplay of inhibitory and excitatory synapses, the possible functional significance in the grouping of neurons into cortical layers and columns, the effects of direct electrical stimulation of the exposed cortex, and the routing of impulses over single fibers in visual and somatic sensory pathways.

It seems evident that such information on structure and function of elements is indispensable, yet it is equally evident that it is far from sufficient. Somehow we must find out, to borrow Lord Adrian's expression, how these myriads of elements interact in the mass; how to define those patterns of neuronal function that enable the structure to mediate conscious experience.

In the absence of this crucial information, we must take care not to lose sight of the question. Professor Mountcastle and Professor Granit have stressed how much can be learned for an understanding of perception by studying activity in single fibers among first-order neurons; I would like to start at the opposite end, so to speak, by considering what else is involved in spatially organized perception beyond the

[1] Acknowledgments: The work reported in this chapter has been aided by the Commonwealth Fund of New York, and by the Rockefeller and Hartford Foundations. Additional support was provided by the National Institute of Mental Health, U. S. Public Health Service, under Program Grant M-5673, and by the National Aeronautics and Space Administration, under Grant NsG-496.

separate and distinct sensory signals. I should like to pose the question as Professor Eccles does in the draft of his second paper, where he says: "How, it may be asked, can my perceptual experience give me such an effective knowledge of the external world that I can find my way around in it and even manipulate it with such success?" To the neuropsychologist, this is the central problem of perception; yet all I can do with it is to describe what normal perception, so considered, seems to entail, and how it breaks down in the presence of various cerebral lesions.

As I look into this room, there is a subjective middle, a to-the-right, a to-the-left, a subjective above and below. This spatial order in its simple form remains a puzzle, even though we know that the retina, and the visual pathways beyond it, are themselves spatially organized. As I move my eyes slowly over the scene, I sense that my eyes are moving, but the visual world stands still. Moreover, as I tilt my head, verticals in the room remain vertical, even though they are now inscribed on a different meridian of my retina. Lastly, I am keenly aware of absent space, of the relation between things now before my senses to those that have been there before—the parts of the room behind my head, the Papal gardens beyond—and while an animal may have such awareness of spatial relations that are not given at that moment to the senses, only man can externalize this awareness in the form of maps or plans.

What I would like to propose is that those three aspects of spatial order are distinct and that we must consider separately (1) the level of immediate *presentation* of visual space; (2) the mechanisms of *compensation* for changes in spatial order, under voluntary change in posture; and (3) the level of *representation* which enables us to deal with spatial relations not immediately given, the ability involved in the finding of routes and in the making of maps. That these three aspects of experienced spatial order are indeed distinct can be shown by considering their selective vulnerability to different cerebral lesions: In the previously normal adult, brain injury implicating the occipital lobes may interfere with presentation, frontal lobe lesions with compensation, and parietal lesions, as is well known, with representation. Such observations on after-effects of injuries fall far short of defining normal function but indicate what separate mechanisms are needed; in this way, these observations help to keep before us those problems which neurophysiology will ultimately have to solve.

A word about the cases on which these observations were based. Over the last twenty years we have dealt primarily with men who had suffered missile wounds penetrating skull, dura, and brain. These studies began during the Second World War in the U. S. Navy and have continued since in New York and Boston. The group of patients in New York numbers 232 men with such brain wounds and 118 control cases with combat injuries of the peripheral nervous system but not of the brain. A more recently assembled group in Boston includes 138 cases of cerebral missile wounds. Most of these men are ambulatory; the majority are gainfully employed. The consequences of their brain injury range from gross and obvious disabilities to minimal changes that would go undetected in routine neurological and psychological examinations. The only principle of selection of these cases is the presence of their lesions rather than any need for clinical attention. They are being seen regardless of whether there have been any complaints or not, and their cooperation is sought by repeated appeals to their altruism. In this way, numerous cases are included which might have been missed in earlier surveys, which have concentrated perforce on those patients who had trouble or thought they did.

In supplemental studies we are trying to compare the effect of brain lesions in man sustained early in life, at birth, or soon afterward, with those incurred through combat injury in the young adult. This work on brain-injured children is accompanied by a number of animal experiments in which early or later lesions are deliberately placed in the brains of rodents, carnivores, or subhuman primates in order to check the observations made on man by repeating them under conditions where site and size of cerebral lesion might be better controlled. The ultimate aim is that set by Lashley a quarter of a century ago—the eventual coalescence of neurology and psychology [Lashley, 1941a].

OCCIPITAL LESIONS AND THE PRESENTATION OF VISUAL SPACE

The effects on vision of direct penetrating wounds in man's optic radiation or visual cortex have been examined in considerable detail [Teuber et al, 1960], yet it is still not clear what a total loss of man's primary visual projection region, defined restrictively as area 17, might entail. The known instances of lesions in man tend to be either too large—overshooting the primary areas—or too small to permit definite conclusions.

In the experimental cat and monkey, some residual vision undoubtedly survives complete removal of striate cortex, although most aspects of spatial patterning can no longer form a basis for the animal's reactions. The now classic work of Kluever [1942] describes the consequence of such radical striate cortex removals in the monkey as permanent change from a normal capacity for perceiving spatially organized visual input to a new and abnormal capacity for reacting to total luminous flux. Such a monkey walks into obstacles and fails to flinch at threatening gestures; in these respects he seems totally blind, yet he can be trained to approach or avoid the dimmer of two targets of equal size, even though he cannot discriminate a triangle from a circle, or horizontal from vertical stripes. Once trained to the dimmer of two equal-sized targets, he will promptly transfer his reaction to the smaller of two targets of equal brightness. Clearly, the animal has lost those invariants which make size or brightness perception possible in the normal state; the intact monkey or man can react to size independently of a wide range of differences in brightness, distance, or angle of the target, or can selectively attend to brightness, taking differences in distance, or area, or angle "into account."

The crucial experiment is one in which a monkey with bilateral striate cortex removal is confronted with two targets, one of which is twice as large but half as bright as the other. Under these stimulus conditions, any discrimination on the part of the operated monkey is impossible, indicating that he does react in such situations to total luminous flux irrespective of the spatial patterning of the input. The full-brained monkey in the same situation can be rapidly trained to select the brighter or the dimmer of the two targets; he can be just as readily trained to pick the larger or the smaller target regardless of their brightness, but he cannot be trained to react to total flux, and even the normal human observer is forced to use a man-made device—an integrating photoelectric meter—to accomplish the same reactions to flux per se.

While these observations on residual vision after total striate cortex removal have held up remarkably well, whenever the experiment has been repeated, there is nevertheless one important addition that needs to be made: Four years ago, during a visit to our laboratories, Dr. Lawrence Weiskrantz noted one further and hitherto unsuspected capacity on the part of monkeys deprived of their primary visual cortex [Weiskrantz, 1963]. During unsuccessful attempts at demonstrating reactions to striped fields, such as the one shown on the left-hand side of the illustration, Fig. 8.1, we ran into a shortage of gray papers. In order to produce a shade of gray equivalent to the black and white

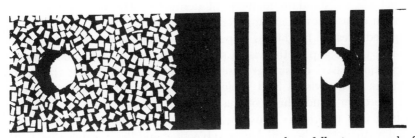

Fig. 8.1. Striped and speckled fields for testing monkeys following removal of striate cortex [after Weiskrantz, 1963].

striped pattern, Mrs. Weiskrantz cut the white stripes into smaller pieces and placed them in irregular distribution over the black background, as shown in the right-hand portion of the illustration. To everyone's considerable surprise, the monkey was capable of discriminating this "speckled" field from any shade of gray. These observations have since been confirmed and extended by Dr. Weiskrantz who believes that at least one further dimension has to be added to the perceptual repertoire of monkeys without striate cortex; in addition to a capacity for distinguishing amounts of luminous flux, these animals can apparently react to "speckledness," or, perhaps, total length of contour.

It would be of great value for our understanding of vision if we could perform the converse experiment, that is, if we could define the visual capacities of an animal which has lost all of its neocortex except for the primary visual area. Because of the paralyzing effect of such extensive cortical removals, it is impractical to inquire in such a direct fashion into the extent of autonomy of the visual cortex. However, one could further exploit the preparation suggested by Professor Sperry [1958] by using cats in which the interhemispheric commissures have been transected and the visual cortex isolated on one side only, by removing most of the neocortex anterior to it. With visual input restricted to that side, visual capacity is drastically reduced. It may turn out to be limited to discrimination of directions of contours, such as vertically versus horizontally striped fields, but extensive tests are necessary to establish the range of residual abilities in such islands of visual cortex.

All of these observations on animals, though obviously incomplete, have considerable bearing on findings in man with partial lesions of optic radiation or visual cortex. In these studies one has the opportunity to ask how visual functions proceed in the presence of a gap in the neural substrate. For instance, in a case such as the one illustrated in Fig. 8.2, an occipital lesion was sustained in combat by a previously normal young adult [Teuber et al, 1960]. This through-and-through wound of the occipital pole resulted in a central island of blindness detectable by standard methods of perimetry. The remarkable feature of such a case lies in an apparent contradiction. On the one hand, the acquired area of brightness appears to correspond in seemingly direct fashion to the gap in the visual system, supporting Sir Gordon Holmes' suggestion based on similar cases from World War I that the central portions of the visual field project to the lips of the calcarine fissure. On the other hand, this scotoma does not seem to enter in any direct fashion into this man's conscious experience. As he looks into a room filled with detail, he still has a subjective middle, a subjective to the left and to the right, an above and below. He is merely aware of some

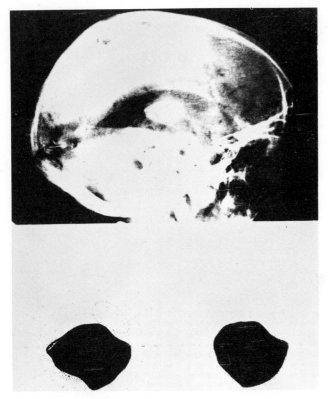

Fig. 8.2. Pneumoencephalogram (above) and visual fields (below) in a case of penetrating missile wound of the occipital lobe.

vague reduction in his visual acuity. When fixating on any given detail in the visual field, he employs a vicarious fovea in the upper margin of the scotoma. Straight lines, plain-colored surfaces, grid patterns, or herringbone patterns are all "completed" across the area of his scotoma. As a result of such completion effects, his functioning visual field seems wider than routine perimetry with isolated targets would seem to indicate.

The apparent direct correspondence between cerebral lesion and perimetric scotoma underscores the puzzling nature of these completion effects, yet it should be stressed that the cerebral lesion may have to exceed a critical size before a permanent scotoma can be demonstrated [Weiskrantz, 1961; see also Teuber et al, 1960]. Moreover, the correspondence may be much less direct in the very young, possibly because much larger lesions are required there for any permanent scotoma. Thus when an occipital lesion is sustained during infancy, as in the

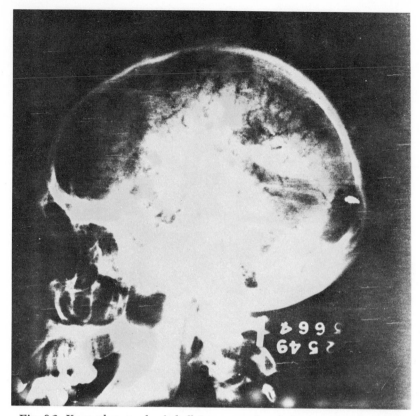

Fig. 8.3. X-ray photograph of skull in a case of early brain injury (at age 1¼) by small-caliber bullet entering posterior parietal region and lodging permanently in the region of the occipital pole. No visual field defect was observed in this case (see text).

instance illustrated in Fig. 8.3, the visual field can escape without demonstrable scotoma. The case illustrated in Fig. 8.3 is that of a middle-aged man who was shot accidentally at the age of 1¼ years, the bullet entering in the parietal region near the midline and lodging permanently in the occipital poles as shown in the X-ray. The location of the lesion would seem to correspond exactly to that which produced the permanent central scotoma illustrated in Fig. 8.2, where the injury was sustained in adulthood. Yet neither ordinary perimetry nor dynamic perimetry after Harms [1965], nor flicker perimetry, nor measurements of regional dark adaptation could detect any consequences of the early lesion in the visual field.

By contrast, in the adult the correspondence between lesions and gaps in the field remains impressive, although these gaps established by perimetric tests are hardly ever represented in the patient's conscious experience. Some of these fields are illustrated in Figs. 8.4 and 8.5, chosen from among the 46 cases of permanent field defects uncovered in the New York group of 232 gunshot wounds of the brain. For instance, our first case of central scotoma surrounded by a seemingly intact periphery can be contrasted with one of central sparing with complete loss of peripheral vision (Fig. 8.4). Here, again, the man's experience of his own defect is limited to some vague awareness of necessity for moving his head in order to gain a full view of peripheral details in his field. Besides that, he performs surprisingly well with his central remnant of vision; earning his living as a mail sorter, he pulls each letter carefully and laboriously across a small area of preserved vision, and then flings it with excellent aim into the appropriate compartment on a shelf provided for this sorting task. He thus has no difficulty in spatial orientation nor any difficulty with the recognition of things seen in the residual field, even though this remnant is surrounded by a ring of complete blindness. Conversely, the man with the central scotoma can promptly

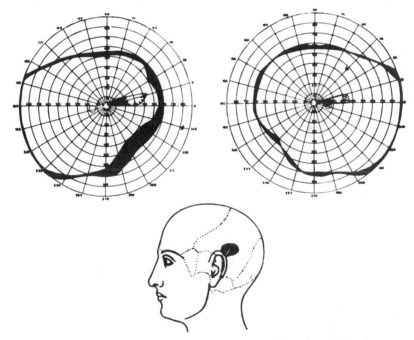

Fig. 8.4. Concentrically contracted fields of vision (above) resulting from penetrating missile wound indicated in diagram (below). Sparing of central area of visual field is probably due to separate vascular supply for the occipital pole [see Teuber et al, 1960].

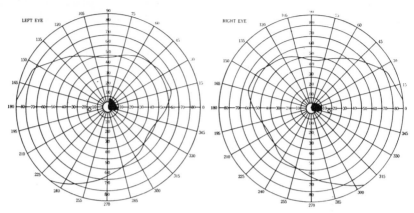

Fig. 8.5. Wedge-shaped scotoma, tapering toward fovea, following penetrating wound of the optic radiation.

discriminate and name any contoured figure that is circumscribed around his scotoma, such as large outlined triangles, squares or circles, thereby invalidating any theory of pattern vision which invokes the role of neural processes within the boundaries of a figure seen.

Even more characteristic of such restricted lesions in the higher visual pathways in man are the small sector scotomata tapering towards the fovea as exemplified in Fig. 8.5. By their very shape, these field defects require certain revisions in our current views on the course and distribution of fibers in man's optic radiation [Teuber et al, 1960]. It must also be noted that nearly all of the field defects we have plotted, while homonymous and geometrically similar in corresponding halves of the monocular visual fields, are rarely congruent, and these departures from strict congruence go beyond the errors involved in current methods of plotting visual fields.

A further feature of defective fields following occipital (or deep temporal, or deep parietal) lesions in man are certain characteristic distortions and displacements of contours in affected portions of the field. Thus, immediately after the wound has been sustained, unless there is transient complete blindness, the patient complains of apparent displacements of objects, in homonymous quadrants or sectors of quadrants. These phenomena, too, have been extensively described [for example, Teuber and Bender, 1949], since they suggest a systematic change in mode of presentation of the sensory input which can persist against the patient's better knowledge during the early stages of recovery from his injury. In some instances, these distortions take the form of reduplication or further multiplication of contours, say, towards the lower left (monocular diplopia or polyopia), as well as perversions in the perception of motion so that a patient might complain that a motorcycle moving past him on the left side is perceived as "a string of motorcycles standing still."

Characteristically, these distortions and perversions in the processing of visual input disappear after the first few weeks or months following the injury. Later on, however, the same or similar disorders may reappear, or appear *de novo*, in the course of *ictal* disturbances, that is, visual fits. These episodic disturbances are associated with abnormal electrographic manifestations over the posterior third of the cerebrum either bilaterally or, by predilection, over the right hemisphere if unilateral. Figure 8.6 shows 15 such cases with recurrent visual fits for whom the center of the bone gap has been circumscribed by a circle indicating the location of their lesions. It is evident that the lesions cluster around the occipital poles or the right posterior temporal and temporoparietal regions. Extreme manifestations of such ictal disorders of contour formation are represented by the paroxysmal polyopia illustrated in Fig. 8.7, and by the rare but important instances of so-called allesthesia for the optic sphere, in which things seen, say, in the left lower quadrant are suddenly and temporarily perceived as if they appeared in the opposite half field, often with 180° reversal.

We are citing these miscarriages of perception not because they are bizarre, but because they underscore the scope of the task involved in the achievement and maintenance of normal spatial organization. Moreover, recent disclosures about the mode of action of single units in the visual cortex and elsewhere suggest the directions which a physiological interpretation of these disorders might take.

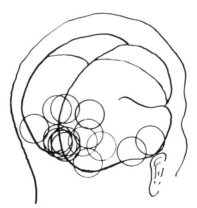

Fig. 8.6. Schematic representation of locations of bone gaps in fifteen cases of penetrating brain wounds followed at varying times by visual fits. Each circle surrounds the center of a cranial defect.

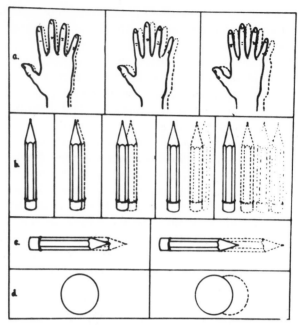

Fig. 8.7. Drawing of typical polyopic images (monocular polyopia) reported by a patient with acute right occipital penetrating trauma [after Teuber and Bender, 1949].

The fundamental discoveries by Hubel and Wiesel about the organization of receptor fields in the visual cortex of cat and monkey [Hubel, 1958; Hubel and Wiesel, 1960, 1965] and the corresponding findings by Lettvin and his coworkers [1959, 1961] on the visual system of frogs and birds make it possible to find at least provisional explanations for some of the most baffling consequences of subtotal destruction of the higher visual pathways. As has already been reviewed elsewhere in this symposium, even the simplest cortical unit in the cat's and monkey's striate area can be influenced by visual input over a rather wide area of the visual field. Schematically speaking, such a unit can be considered as lying at the neck of a funnel opening into the field of view, the funnel being circular in diameter for retinal units [Kuffler, 1953] but elongated and elliptical for cortical units. In a sense, then, each cortical unit looks at far more of the field than lies immediately opposite to it; adjacent neurons have widely overlapping receptor fields so that completion of contours across gaps in the substrate would be quite understandable. The newly disclosed mechanism might also account for the selectivity of such completion which is optimal for color or for single lines, grids, or other internally reduplicative patterns.

Typically, cortical receptor fields of the simplest sort have an excitatory ridge surrounded by inhibitory flanking regions or, conversely, an inhibitory ridge with an excitatory flank or flanks. As a result, the cortical receptor field becomes a detector of visual direction. Thus, a luminous line which is presented within the receptor field at right angles to an excitatory ridge cuts across inhibitory regions as well, and therefore is minimally effective or ineffective in driving the particular cortical neuron. Rotating the luminous line in the frontal plane so as to bring it gradually into alignment with the excitatory ridge will progressively increase the discharges of the unit until alignment with the ridge produces maximal discharge. Different units have systematically different orientational preferences, so that the set of simple receptor fields in the striate cortex can be seen as a system of overlapping direction detectors, extracting information about orientation of contours with considerable redundancy yet great precision. It is noteworthy that in this system, visual direction is represented by the rates of discharges in given units so that one might perhaps conjecture how mistiming of discharges, as by regional distortion of firing rates, could have illusory distortions or displacements of contours as a consequence.

The arrangements we have just reviewed may be equally applicable to the curious phenomena which accompany the transitory scotomata of migraine, particularly those involving the central portion of an otherwise normal visual field. In recording and plotting these episodic disturbances within his own field, Lashley [1941b] noted completion effects for checkerboard and wallpaper patterns whose repetitive lines seemed "filled-in" across the acute functional gaps in his field. Similarly, he related experiences such as the following: While he was traveling by car on a straight Florida highway, a migraine attack set in, with a small paracentral scotoma developing in such a way that appropriate shifting of gaze would make a pursuing highway patrol car disappear, while the road itself, as well as the rest of the landscape, remained subjectively continuous.[2] These completion effects are thus not attributable to a prolonged existence of scotomata, with gradual adaptation to the gap, but are an immediate result of the ways in which the visual field is organized.

Such dissociations of levels can be demonstrated for the completion phenomena seen in chronic cases, in the presence of permanent small scotomata, by employing special techniques. Two test patterns we have used recently are, first, the highly redundant visual patterns studied by

[2] In discussing these and similar completion effects recently in front of a former colleague of Lashley's, Dr. Edward Dempsey, the latter recalled an episode in the Harvard Faculty Club when Lashley suddenly exclaimed, "Dempsey, I have just beheaded you"; and, "but I can still see the wallpaper pattern behind you." (Apparently, a selective completion of the herringbone pattern on the wallpaper across the area where Dr. Dempsey's head had become invisible.)

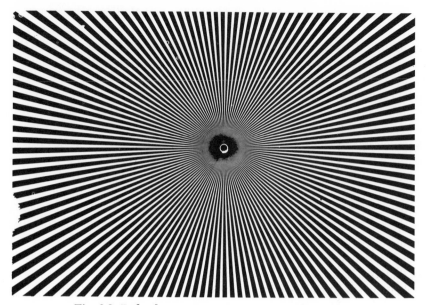

Fig. 8.8. Redundant pattern as used by MacKay [1957].

Professor Donald MacKay [1957], as illustrated in Fig. 8.8, and, second, a display of visual noise such as the random motion of dots obtained from the output of a computer and recorded on an endless loop of film. Patients with small parafoveal scotomata such as the one illustrated in Fig. 8.9 report that they perceive the radiating-line pattern shown on the previous figure without any blank, that is, they "complete" the lines. Correspondingly, they see the random motion of dots in the same fashion as would a normal observer; there thus is completion for visual noise.

Normal observers on inspecting the radiating-line pattern report a subjective streaming or rippling at right angles to the black lines; this illusion can be much enhanced, as has been shown by Professor MacKay, by superimposing this radial line pattern upon the random display. As soon as this is done, one perceives a circular motion of the dots instead of the random bobbing seen without the lines. This induced motion can be clockwise or counterclockwise, with occasional spontaneous reversals in direction. At times, normal subjects will report a complicated swirling motion in both directions, clockwise and counterclockwise simultaneously.

The patient whose visual fields appear in Fig. 8.9 continued to show completion after the line pattern and the noise display had been superimposed. Just as a normal observer, he reported the induced motion effect; specifically he said that the "snow flakes" were swirling in a consistently clockwise motion around the center of the radial line pattern, as soon as that pattern and the noise had been projected together. However, in the parafoveal region corresponding to his scotoma, he did *not* see the induced motion. He delineated this area with his hand, insisting that in that particular region, and there alone, he saw a random bobbing of specks against the background of the continual radial lines. Thus, his scotoma, which had not been within his awareness, had suddenly become entoptically visible under these special conditions of stimulation.

The interpretation of these phenomena remain speculative, but it is quite possible that the completion of these and similar redundant line patterns could be ascribed to the activity of direction detectors in the visual cortex, while the persistent perception of randomly moving dots might be mediated in other structures, at midbrain levels or at cortical levels outside the primary projection system, since the recent animal experiments by Weiskrantz [1963] have indicated a similar persistence of capacity for reaction to "speckled" fields in the absence of primary

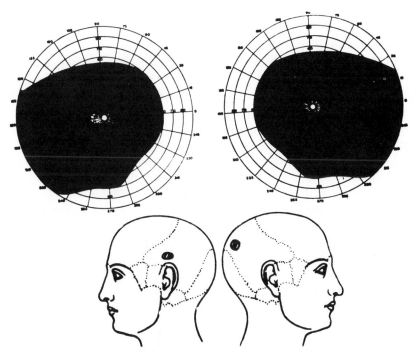

Fig. 8.9. Small paracentral scotoma, the result of a penetrating gunshot wound of right occipital region; this defect was plotted twenty years after the injury.

visual cortex. The induced motion at right angles to the redundant contours in normally functioning parts of the field of vision might possibly be attributed to those hypercomplex cortical units discovered by Hubel and Wiesel [1965] which have two preferential orientations, one at right angles to the other, with selective adaptation for one direction and, hence, spontaneous shifts to the other.

Quite generally, the recent disclosures about cortical receptor fields raise hopes that we might better understand how we manage to see a vertical line as long as our retina is stationary and normally oriented. Paradoxically, however, these major advances in cortical microphysiology make it harder rather than easier to understand why such a vertical line should remain subjectively vertical when our head and eyes are tilted. We believe that a special mechanism needs to be invoked to account for these relative constancies of visual direction, and there is increasing evidence that this compensatory mechanism can be disturbed in cases where visual pathways and visual fields are intact. In fact, maximally effective lesions appear to lie as far from the occipital lobes as possible; they involve the frontal lobes and subjacent basal ganglia.

FRONTAL LOBES AND BASAL GANGLIA: THE COMPENSATION IN PERCEPTION FOR CHANGES IN POSTURE

In discussing the hypothetical mechanisms for compensation it may be well to inquire how an animal far removed from the primates manages to maintain constant orientation in the face of changes in posture. Higher cephalopods, such as the octopus, have image-forming eyes connected with central visual structures capable of detecting and discriminating visual directions, sizes, and certain shapes.

Recent work by Young [1960, 1961] and others [Sutherland, 1957; Wells, 1962] has strongly suggested that the optic lobe of the octopus contains arrays of horizontality and verticality detectors, that is, receptive fields whose preferential orientations are at right angles to each other. It is likely, but not yet proved, that these optic lobes are devoid of obliquely oriented fields. If this is the case, it would be understandable why the octopus can be readily taught to discriminate horizontal from vertical lines but is notoriously incapable of acquiring any discrimination between oblique lines running in opposite directions (such as: / versus \, or \ versus / (see Sutherland [1957] and Fig. 8.10). The question is how the octopus manages to maintain a positive reaction, say, to an objectively vertical line when the animal's eyes are inclined out of their normal primary position.

As it turns out, visual coordinates in the frontal plane are preserved

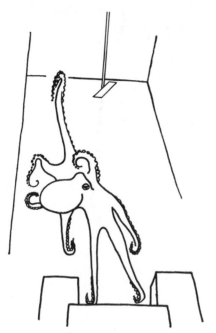

Fig. 8.10. Octopus being trained on discrimination of oblique rectangles (based on Sutherland [1957] and Wells [1960, 1962]).

for this cephalopod by virtue of a peripheral mechanism. The animal's eyes can undergo extensive cyclotorsion and these torsional movements are under control of the statocyst. As the head and eyes are inclined, the eyes counterrotate. Since the animal has a conspicuous horizontal slit pupil, one can readily observe how this slit maintains a constant horizontal orientation so that verticals in the environment continue to fall on the midvertical meridian of the octopus retina, in spite of changes in posture.

If the statocysts are destroyed (as has been done by Wells [1960]), this compensatory control is lost; the eyes roll into various positions unrelated to the gravitation vertical, and visually guided reactions are then determined by the chance position of the eyes. Thus, if the eye is rotated by 45° out of its normal position so that the normally horizontal pupil points 45° downward to the right, the animal will treat a line that is inclined by 45° as if it were a vertical. The coordination remains within the retina, so to speak, in striking contrast to the situation in man, where torsional movements of the eyes are quite limited and the appropriate compensation for head tilts or head movements has to be provided by a central rather than peripheral mechanism [Teuber, 1960].

We have called this postulated mechanism of central compensatory action the "corollary discharge." We assume that each voluntary movement, or change of posture, involves not only the downward discharge to the peripheral effectors, but a simultaneous central discharge from motor to sensory systems preparing the latter for those changes that will occur as a result of the intended movement. A voluntary eye movement which transports contours across the retina would thus leave the spatial order of perception undisturbed, because the impulses to the eye muscles are accompanied by appropriate corollary discharges which preset the visual system for all anticipated shifts in the spatial order of visual inputs. By contrast, when we push against our eyeball, moving it passively, the visual scene jumps, and the same apparent shift of scene is perceived whenever we intend to move our eye but there is inability to move, either by mechanically restricting the globe in the orbit, or by virtue of an acute extraocular palsy.

Such instances of paralysis are particularly revealing, since there is no displacement of contours on the retina; yet any unsuccessful intention to move is experienced as an illusory displacement of the scene in a direction opposite to the intended motion [Kornmueller, 1931]. These illusory motions of contours in the presence of ocular palsy provide the most direct evidence for the continual operation of the compensatory mechanisms which counteract the normally inevitable shifts of input that result from voluntary movement. In paralysis, these counteractive signals turn into illusions, since they are not annulled by the result of the motion. Correspondingly, if one wears spectacles that invert the visual scene, as has been done by Stratton [1897], Kohler [1951], and Held [1961], one will inevitably perceive at first extensive illusory shifts of the scene with every voluntary movement of the eye. This is due to the fact that the compensatory signal is not subtracted from those shifts in contours that result from the eye movements, but is added to these shifts, as a consequence of the optical reversal induced by the spectacles.

All of these considerations go back at least as far as Helmholtz [1867], who included them in an outflow theory about the role of eye movements in perception. He was severely criticized for attributing the compensatory effects to what he called "feelings of innervation"; his critics claimed that they could not discover these feelings among their own introspections. Modern versions of the outflow theory have tried to preserve its essential features while eliminating the postulated feelings of innervation. Such versions were formulated simultaneously and independently by the team of von Holst and Mittelstaedt [1950] and by Sperry [1950] about 15 years ago. We have tried to give these notions the broadest possible meaning; presence or absence of a corollary discharge from motor to sensory systems would determine whether a movement is "voluntary" or "involuntary" [Teuber, 1960, 1961, 1964]. On this view, the corollary discharge would serve as a physiological criterion for self-produced movements in contradistinction to reflexes. However, before developing this proposal further, we would like to summarize the experimental evidence which suggested to us that the integrity of frontal lobes and basal ganglia might play a role in the corollary discharge mechanisms which guarantee that the perceiver sees a vertical line as vertical even though his head and eyes might be tilted.

For the normal observer, vertical and horizontal directions in his field of view depend to some extent on the visual framework, so that the perception of the vertical is better studied under those conditions where the observer faces a single luminous line in the dark. As long as head and body are upright, such a luminous line can be set to the apparent vertical with minimal error, but this task becomes more difficult when the observer's head and eyes are tilted as under the conditions shown schematically in Fig. 8.11. With head and body tilted, say, 30° to the left, the observer will set the luminous line with a slight constant error misplacing it by about 2° to the opposite side, that is, to the right. Conversely, with head and body tilts of 30° to the right, the constant error in setting the vertical will be about 2° to the left. In a sense, then, normal observers not only compensate for their tilts but overcompensate under these conditions to a slight but significant extent. By contrast, men with penetrating brain wounds implicating the anterior third of the cerebrum were found to make significantly larger errors than normals or men with wounds elsewhere in the cerebrum [Teuber and Mishkin, 1954], and similar difficulties with the setting of the visual vertical were encountered more re-

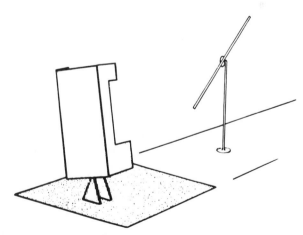

Fig. 8.11. Tilting chair and luminous line, employed in testing human perception of verticality under various conditions of body tilt.

cently in patients with diseases of the basal ganglia, both before and after surgical intervention in the region of the globus pallidus, or of the ventral lateral nucleus of the thalamus [Teuber and Proctor, 1962].

We have suggested elsewhere [Teuber, 1964] that this peculiar symptom of frontal lobe or basal ganglia lesions in man might be analogous to the persistent deficits produced by similar lesions in subhuman forms: the loss of capacity for delayed-response and delayed-alternation tasks, a loss seen in the infrahuman primate and in carnivores after frontal ablations, or equivalently after destructive lesions in the head of the caudate nucleus.[3] Both kinds of symptoms—the trouble on visual-postural tasks in man, and the delayed-response and delayed-alternation deficits in the infrahuman forms, might be interpreted as reflecting a difficulty in maintaining directions in the face of changing posture: In the delayed response task, the monkey cannot recall whether to turn right or left as soon as his own body position has changed in the interval between the presentation of the lure and the moment when he is permitted to make his choice. The visual task likewise seems to involve the problem of maintaining orientation under conditions where posture is abnormal. This deficit, however, should not be described as purely sensory; a number of control experiments have shown that what is involved is an abnormal interaction between vision and posture, in the absence of mere visual or postural deficits. In point of fact, massive frontal lobe damage produces outright changes in the voluntary control of movement, leading to the well-known automatisms of grasping and groping in which visual and tactile inputs gain abnormal control over the motor act [Denny-Brown, 1951]. Conversely, the integrity of frontal lobes and basal ganglia appears to be

---

[3] The vulnerability of delayed-response performance to frontal lesions in the monkey was first noted by Jacobsen nearly thirty years ago [1935]. In its simplest form, the test consists of presenting the animal with two equally appearing food wells, lying side by side; in full view of the animal one of the wells is baited and the lid replaced. An opaque screen is lowered, shielding the food wells for a delay period (usually five seconds) from the animal's view. The screen is raised and the animal permitted to approach the wells. A success is scored, on any given trial, if the animal raises the lid from the baited well, a failure, if he uncovers the unbaited one. The side baited varies in essentially random sequence from trial to trial. Variations of the test include the delayed-alternation task in which the animal has to learn that whichever food well has been baited on the last trial will be empty on the next trial, so that he is forced to shift systematically from trial to trial with intervening delays, during which the opaque screen bars the food wells from view. More recent work has shown that the effective lesions for producing lasting deficits in delayed response and delayed alternation are bilateral removals of the upper and lower banks of the sulcus principalis in the lateral frontal region of the Macaque monkey, and that electrical stimulation of these regions can produce transient failure in performance on the tests during current flow [Stamm, 1961; Weiskrantz et al, 1960]. The same parallelism between behavioral effects of destructive lesions and brief electric stimulation can be shown for the head of the caudate nucleus [Rosvold and Delgado, 1956].

essential for the maintenance of those anticipatory mechanisms which can take the sensory consequences of self-produced movements into account.

The importance of distinguishing active from passive movement and of searching for physiological bases for this distinction is underscored by a further series of experiments which attest to the role of action in perception and coordination. These experiments are being carried out by my colleague in the M.I.T. psychology department, Richard Held, and his co-workers, particularly Alan Hein and Burton White [see Held, 1961; Held and Bossom, 1961; Held and Freedman, 1963; Held and Hein, 1963; White et al, 1964]. In a paradigmatic experiment, normal adults are made to wear prismatic spectacles which displace all visual input by, say, 15° to the left. When these glasses are first worn, consistent misreaching for objects occurs, so that objects are missed by 15° to the right of their true location. However, if such spectacles are worn for one hour, during which the wearer walks actively in an optically structured environment, complete and exact compensation for the visual displacements can be demonstrated. Reaching under visual control has now become accurate again. If the spectacles are then removed, the extent of the adaptation to their use is made evident by the way in which the person now mis-reaches in a direction opposite to that shown during exposure. This post-exposure disturbance, however, is quite transient, lasting a few minutes at most.

On the other hand, if the spectacles are worn for an hour during which the wearer moves passively, for example, while being pushed about in a wheelchair, no compensation to the prismatic spectacles is achieved. This failure to adapt is all the more remarkable since perceived contours sweep over the observer's eyes in the same fashion as under the active conditions of exposure, yet the absence of self-produced movement and, we would say, the absence of the corollary discharge prevent the reorganization of visuomotor function.

In view of the importance of self-produced movement in adapting to perceptual rearrangement, Held and Hein have suggested [1963] that not only maintenance, but also origin of coordination might depend on movements that are self-produced. Accordingly, kittens are raised under special conditions of deprivation; their visual experience is restricted to several hours of daily exercise in the drum shown in Fig. 8.12, where two kittens who are litter mates are given the following contrasting experience: One kitten in each pair walks actively about while carrying the second kitten by means of a harness and pivot arrangement in a gondola, so that the second (the passive kitten) sees the world move past him, while he is being moved. After varying periods of this exposure, covering several weeks from birth up to many months, the visual capacities of active and passive kittens are compared. It then turns out that the active

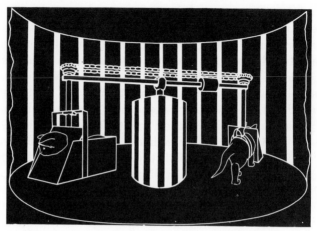

Fig. 8.12. Apparatus used by Richard Held and Alan Hein in studying effects of active and passive exposure of kittens to the visual environment.

kitten has normal form and depth perception as defined by a number of tests, while the passive kitten is merely capable of discriminating luminous flux yet fails to discriminate patterns and depth. This form blindness as a result of passive exposure can apparently be overcome in a few days following release from the passive condition, although it is still possible that further prolongation of the passive exposure might eventually produce irreversible deficits in form and depth perception.

The role of action in the origin of visuospatial order can be defined in yet another way; the kittens are given visual experience as before but in such a way that one eye remains covered. After an hour of contrasting exposure with one kitten active, the other passive, the situations for the two kittens are reversed and the blind patches shifted, so that each kitten in the end has one "active" and one "passive" eye. Under these conditions, the active eye has normal form and depth perception while the passive eye shows the same reduction in visual capacity to mere flux perception which had been found previously when both eyes had been given passive exposure. One of these kittens has been taken by Drs. Held and Hein to the laboratories of Drs. Hubel and Wiesel, who mapped the receptor fields in the animal's visual cortex and compared responses to patterned stimulation evoked through the active and the passive eye. No differences were found, the receptor fields being normal (within the limits of such preliminary mapping), irrespective of whether cortical activity was driven through the active or the passive eye. This finding prompted Dr. Hubel to suggest that the crucial events of interest in sensorimotor coordination must take place at some level higher than the primary visual pathways. We can readily agree with this suggestion, since we are sure that Dr. Hubel would not wish to imply that the correlates of these crucial events would be extracranial!

The role of action in the early stages of perceptual development can also be explored in our own species. One can observe the delays in human sensorimotor development that are produced by the kind of inadvertent deprivation which human infants suffer in certain orphanages and nurseries. A few years ago, Professor Held and his group of coworkers discovered such an orphanage-type nursery in the vicinity of Boston [see White et al, 1964]. In this situation, children were raised from birth with adequate feeding and physical care but without opportunities for playing with adults. Typically, these children lie on their backs in a bland environment, staring at a gray ceiling. Normative studies performed by means of time-sampling techniques and cinematographic records showed conclusively that these children were severely retarded with respect to the appearance of such elementary sensorimotor activities as hand regard, hand clasp, and visually guided reaching for various test objects. Over the first six months of life, the emergence of some of these achievements was found to be delayed by ten weeks or more.

Under these conditions, a regime of "graded enrichment" was instituted with systematic variation of visual stimulation combined with opportunities for increased motor activity. Mobile toys were suspended above the babies' cribs. At various times during the day the infants were placed in prone position, forcing them to elevate their heads. With these or similar maneuvers much of the developmental lag could be overcome, even though a residual delay of about four weeks remained if the attempts at enrichment were instituted only after the second month of life.

Undoubtedly a major task of the organism during the first few months is to make the transition from various automatisms to voluntary movement and to perform a variety of acts under visual control. This in turn requires, in our view, that the spatial order of perception should remain invariant during changes of posture [see also Twitchell, 1965].

We have previously pointed out that integrity of frontal lobes and basal ganglia may be necessary for the proper interaction between vision and posture, since these structures might somehow participate in the compensatory mechanisms needed to maintain or re-establish visuomotor coordination. These views have been strengthened by the results of a recent experiment performed by one of Professor Held's former students, Joseph Bossom, who has extended the rearrangement paradigm to work with monkeys (Fig. 8.13).

Prismatic spectacles mounted on a snugly fitted helmet are worn by the monkey for up to eight hours, during which he actively reaches for

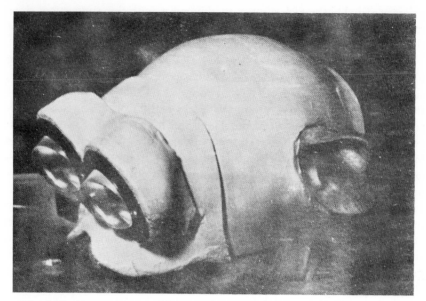

Fig. 8.13. Arrangement used by Joseph Bossom in testing adaptation of visually guided reaching movements in monkeys to displacement of the scene by prismatic spectacles [after Bossom, 1965].

bits of food. At the end of this exposure, normal monkeys have achieved compensation for the prismatic displacement. These experiments were then repeated with more than fifty animals following ablations of various cerebral lobes: occipital, temporal, parietal, or frontal. In line with expectations derived from the earlier studies in man, animals with frontal lobectomy failed to show any adaptation to the prismatic displacement, but all other groups of animals—those with occipital, temporal, or parietal removals—did manage to adapt. The adverse effects of frontal lobectomy on prism adaptation were duplicated by those subcortical lesions which involved the head of the caudate nucleus [Bossom, 1965]. These experiments are thus analogous to our previous results in man where adjustment of the visual vertical under conditions of body tilt was found to be impaired by frontal lesions or, equivalently, by diseases of the basal ganglia.

All of these studies suggest that mechanisms of presentation and of compensation are separable aspects of visual space perception since they are separately disturbable by lesions lying at opposite ends of the forebrain: presentation is vulnerable to posterior lesions, while compensation is impaired by lesions that lie far anterior. Yet there remains at least one further aspect of orientation—the ability to relate ourselves to present *and* absent space, and the capacity of finding routes with or without the aid of maps. This capacity is known to depend quite crucially on the integrity of the parietal lobes.

REPRESENTATION AND THE PARIETAL LOBES

It has long been established that massive and acute lesions of man's parietal lobes can produce severe disorientation in space. In one of the typical cases in our group, a young soldier wandered aimlessly for three days between the opposing lines during the Korean campaign following a penetrating parietal lobe wound which was big enough to admit a fist. For a full year afterwards, he was unable to find his bed in the hospital ward, put his housecoat on backwards, and did not know how to manage his slippers. In spite of these early difficulties, the eventual recovery of this man, injured when he was barely seventeen, was so far-reaching that he managed to achieve and hold an important administrative position requiring frequent trips across the country. At the present stage, his deficits in spatial orientation can be brought out only in especially designed tests, such as the one shown in Fig. 8.14.

This figure depicts the series of fifteen maps which had been employed by Semmes, Weinstein, Ghent, and Teuber [1955] in assessing

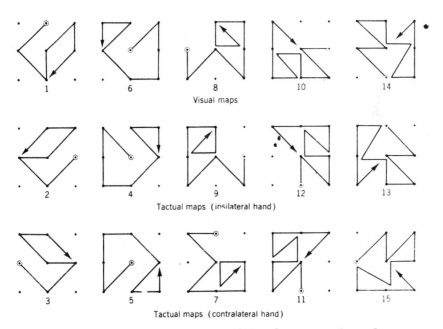

Fig. 8.14. Maps used in tests of route finding [Semmes et al, 1955].

capacity for route finding. The person to be tested is led into a large room where nine dots are marked off on the floor, all equidistant (1.37 m) from each other in a square array. These dots are represented on each of the maps with a line connecting them, indicating where in the room the person tested has to start and which path he is to follow by active locomotion, from dot to dot, until he reaches the goal symbolized by the arrowhead. All maps are carried by the patient, one map at a time; he is not permitted to reorient a map as he looks about. However, one edge of the map, as well as the appropriate wall of the room, have been marked to indicate north. Five of the maps (the top row in Fig. 8.14) are presented visually, being line drawings on a square of cardboard. The remaining maps are made of raised tacks with cords running between them, and these are carried on a tray attached to the patient's chest who palpates them under a black cloth. Five of these "nonvisual" maps are palpated by the patient with the hand contralateral to his major cerebral lesion, and the remaining five with the hand ipsilateral to that lesion. These different modes of presentation of the maps were introduced in order to see whether trouble in route finding after brain injury could be described, as it has often been in the past, as a specifically visual disturbance, that is, a visuospatial agnosia.

As it turned out, trouble in route finding by means of these maps appeared irrespective of the sensory modality through which the maps were presented. Those patients who did have difficulties on this task showed equally inferior performance for the visual and tactual-kinesthetic (or "haptic") modes of presentation. Moreover, this general difficulty in route finding by means of maps was specifically dependent upon the parietal lobes (Fig. 8.15), since only the group with parietal lesions showed a significant deficit. When this group was excluded from the sample of brain-injured patients, the difference between brain-injured and control subjects was reduced to the point where it was no longer significant. This specific deficit consequent upon parietal lesions can be demonstrated for decades following the injury. Thus, spatial representation can be disturbed quite selectively by lesions that are neither occipital nor frontal, but parietal.

Unfortunately, the focal nature of the symptom holds few clues for our understanding of the physiology underlying normal functions involved in this higher-order form of spatial orientation. Representation of absent space involves memory, and there is as yet no physical basis for any form of learning. In fact, Lashley has often suggested that if one took all of the evidence, the old and the new, on neural correlates of memory, learning simply should not occur. Yet it sometimes does, and will eventually have to be explained.

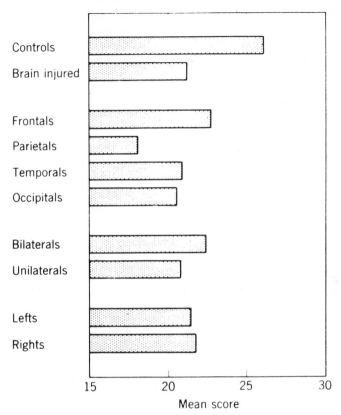

Fig. 8.15. Results of route-finding tests, grouped by location of brain wounds. Scores indicate number of turns correctly made. Only the group with parietal lesions shows significant impairment.

In summary, then, we have tried to show that there are at least three aspects of spatial organization in perception which require the postulation of separate mechanisms. Conscious experience of external space seems to depend first of all, and crucially, on mechanisms of presentation which can be found at various levels of the central pathways. Several effects of focal lesions at these sites are perhaps somewhat more intelligible now than they were only a few years ago. The increase in our understanding is primarily due to recent disclosures on the remarkable extent of "sensory preprocessing of inputs" in occipital receptor fields which can classify their input according to direction and length of lines, edges, color, and movement. These findings on elementary pattern analysis in the visual cortex may account for many of the old observations on "completion" of patterns across scotomata. The new findings may suggest for the first time why completion should be better for certain simple patterns composed of lines than for complex configurations. There might even be a promise of eventual explanation for the sudden subjective tilts and distortions of the presented scene, an explanation which might invoke a transient mistiming of discharges since it appears to be a temporal code that expresses the spatial features of the scene.

Compensation also is somewhat better understood than it was only a few years ago when we elaborated some of these notions on the basis of formulations by von Holst and by Sperry. The corollary discharge mechanism which we have invoked remains a conjecture, but the evidence for quite focal disturbances in such a hypothetical mechanism, after frontal or caudate lesions, has become fairly strong. Neuroanatomical and neurophysiological observations are at least compatible with the view that the cerebral motor systems discharge not only downstream into their peripheral effectors, particularly the musculature, but also, and at the same time, centrally into sensory systems, thus presetting these systems for the consequences of self-produced movements. This motor-to-sensory discharge, or "corollary discharge mechanism," not only provides a vehicle for maintaining spatial order of one's perceptions during movement, but may also allow one to readapt after peripherally imposed distortion, as by displacing or inverting spectacles or pseudophones. The same mechanism might be involved in the original establishment of sensorimotor coordination in the course of early development. The mechanism, in fact, may permit one to distinguish, physiologically, between voluntary and involuntary movement. It may thus provide clues as to how voluntary motor control might arise out of a matrix of compulsory reflex reactions in the neonate [Twitchell, 1965].

Last, we have to account for the amazing accomplishments of spatial orientation in the everyday sense of that term, the ability to find one's way about, to use or to make maps or similar symbolic representations. This aspect of space perception, which is so exquisitely vulnerable to parietal lesions in man, is the hardest to understand since it involves the making and retaining, in memory, of appropriate symbols and their manipulation, and thus indicates a still higher level of conscious experience.

The three aspects of perception here reviewed are not exhaustive; they constitute at best glimpses of neural mechanisms, but are far from providing a theory of human space perception. To attempt such a theory at this time would probably be a hindrance rather than a help in achieving a more complete explanation of human space perception and its neural bases. We are thus making no apology for the absence of a coherent theory, but if an excuse were needed, it could not be put into better terms than those used by Hans Spemann at the end of his Silliman Lectures on embryonic development and induction [1938] where he had this to say:

> It is not my intention to conclude these experimental contributions to a theory . . . with the attempt to construct such a theory myself. . . . Besides, I believe that if the facts are not compiled at random, but gained in a logical proceeding, they will by themselves join together to build up a genuine theory in the original meaning of this word, i.e., a comprehensive view of all the facts afforded by experience.
>
> I should like to work like the archeologist who pieces together the fragments of a lovely thing which are alone left to him. As he proceeds, fragment by fragment, he is guided by the conviction that these fragments are part of a whole which, however, he does not yet know. He must be enough of an artist to recreate, as it were, the work of the master, but he dare not build according to his own ideas. Above all, he must keep holy the broken edges of the fragments (*die Bruchflächen heilig halten*); in that way only may he hope to fit new fragments into their proper place and thus ultimately achieve a true restoration of the master's creation. There may be other ways of proceeding, but this is the one I have chosen for myself.

DISCUSSION

Chairman: PROFESSOR HEYMANS

CHAIRMAN: I would like to ask a question to this top expert in the field of alterations of perception after brain injury.

In cases of arrest of the heart occurring in patients with a carotid sinus syndrome or total heart block, unconsciousness occurs first of all. If the circulation restarts after less than about 5 min of interruption, consciousness is soon restored, but the patient does not memorize the accident.

So I would like to ask whether we have some information concerning alterations in metabolic processes or injuries occurring in some areas of the brain related to this situation of unconsciousness and restoration of consciousness but lack of memory after a period of arrest or marked decrease of blood circulation to the brain.

TEUBER: I believe Professor Penfield can tell us much more about these conditions than I could. Our own experience is essentially limited to cases of transient or persistent amnesia following massive brain injury, concussion, or generalized convulsions. During the recovery period following any of these events, there may be a time when the patient seems to be quite well oriented and capable of responding to what is being said to him, yet he fails to retain any permanent memory of what he or others are saying or doing. In addition to this post-traumatic amnesia, which may reflect interference with the function of basal temporal-lobe structures, there may also be a period of retrograde amnesia, as if memories for events preceding the ictus—memories that would normally have been laid down—had been wiped out. In man, I have never yet seen such retrograde amnesia without some post-traumatic amnesia, although post-traumatic amnesia can be found quite often in the absence of any convincing signs of a retrograde loss. In fact, much of the clinical literature on retrograde amnesia has been questioned, because it is not often clear how much of the trouble in recalling premorbid events might not be a relatively trivial consequence of the memory difficulties for events which follow the trauma.

Because of these ambiguities, a great deal of animal experimentation on retrograde amnesia has been performed. Electroshock-induced convulsions have been the treatment of choice, although more recently cortical spreading depression has also been employed as well as transient arrest of blood flow (in goats), or the topical application of drugs such as puromycin to the rodent hippocampus. These studies do not yet form a coherent picture, but it looks as if even temporary interference with the function of certain rhinencephalic structures might reproduce those features of post-traumatic or post-ictal states in which there is failure in the transfer of memories from their more fragile, short-term state into some more permanent form.

Retrograde amnesia by itself—i.e., without any post-traumatic amnesia—remains almost impossible to obtain. Earlier work with electroshock-induced convulsion in rats suggested that learning based on a series of maze-running trials could be abolished retroactively, by the convulsion, even though the trials preceded the treatment by an hour or more.

More recently, however, Professor Stephan L. Chorover and his colleagues in our department at M.I.T. have shown that effects of so-called one-trial learning in rats are *not* wiped out by a subsequent electroshock-induced convulsion unless the convulsion is induced within seconds of that experience. He believes, therefore, that the so-called consolidation period for memories of this sort is much shorter than has been admitted heretofore,—certainly not more than 10 secs. A comparable result has been obtained in experiments with visual choice reactions in cats by Dr. Helen Mahut in our department. She found that stimulation of the intralaminar nucleus in the cat's thalamus, with current strengths below the thresholds for movement or arrest of movement, interfered with learning, if and only if the stimulation followed a given trial within 10 sec or less. Paradoxically, the same stimulation enhanced learning if it was delivered at the moment of choice. I should add that at this time I am unaware of any crucial electrophysiological or metabolic correlates of these conditions which produce amnesia or possibly hypermnesia, but I hope that Professor Penfield will comment on these issues.

CHAIRMAN: Thank you very much. Don't you think it would be very important to relate to the problem of the location of consciousness some information about basic metabolic processes occurring in these areas?

In a somewhat different context, I would like to tell about my enquiry into the question: what is the derivation of the words "carotid artery" and "carotid sinus"? I had the good luck to find the answer to that question. The name "carotis" was used by Aristotle (300 B.C.), who stated that this name had already been given before him to the arteries in the neck, because a physician observed that compression of the blood vessels in the neck of man induced stupor (sleep), and from this the name carotis from the Greek word *charos* meaning soft, stupor, or sleep. Rufus of Ephesus, however, pointed out that not the compression of the arteries in the neck, but compression of nerve fibers close to those arteries provokes stupor or sleep.

In our opinion, the old physician who compressed the arteries in the neck of man did not compress the blood vessels themselves, but the carotid sinus area, inducing a reflex bradycardia, arterial hypotension, and unconsciousness in a patient with a carotid sinus syndrome.

Vesalius did not use the name "arteria carotidea" in his famous book, the *Fabrica*, but the name "arteria soforotis," thus showing that he knew the meaning of carotis.

THORPE: I would like to make a brief comment which may be relevant. Early in his paper Professor Teuber spoke of the ability to make mental maps as one of the higher achievements of the human brain. I would like to point out that all the evidence points to the fact that the higher insects in their orientation behavior are doing just the same thing—hunting wasp learning the appearance and the surroundings of its nest, using a series of landmarks. It can learn the position and appearance of these landmarks in a matter of a few seconds and remember them for at least 24 or 36 hours. Also it seems worth pointing out that if one is looking for mechanisms in the human brain which are apparently specifically performing this kind of function, one must remember that almost exactly the same thing on a rather smaller scale seems to be done by even the insect's brain served by the insect's compound eye. The compound eye is, of course, totally different in structure from the human eye and the insect brain has hardly any structural resemblance whatever to that of the human being. In fact, considering the nature of the insect sense organs, the insect's achievement in learning, remembering, and utilizing the relative position of landmarks appears little, if at all, inferior to our own.

TEUBER: This is a most illuminating comment. Actually, my main reason for dragging in the octopus was an attempt to illustrate how rather diverse mechanisms in perception might be used to achieve the same end. As I pointed out, the octopus has little difficulty in distinguishing verticals from horizontals as long as we do not interfere with his statocysts. In the octopus, invariance of visual direction is accomplished by an actual reorienting of the eyes, to keep constant relations to gravity. Our own central nervous system, I believe, has to react in a rather different manner to those changes of the visual input which are produced by our changes in posture. I proposed that this is done by means of "corollary discharges" from motor-to-sensory systems. As to the levels on which we can represent external space, including absence of space, here, too, several mechanisms suggest themselves, although the neurological basis of most of them remains obscure. Many lower animals can evidently keep track of their own movements, at least to some extent, and relate these traces to those of past sensory impressions. Still, I would like to think that man's capacity to make more or less permanent records, in the form of maps or other symbolic representations of absent space, is on the same level as his capacity for language.

There may be a foreshadowing of such capacities in lower forms, but I don't believe that these can be identified with a fully evolved mechanism in man.

THORPE: I would like to add two more comments: first, these insects behave as if they had made a map of some kind. Second, the work you refer to by Holst and Mittelstaedt was carried out on insects and fish. So here we are considering three entirely different studies carried out on different types of animal and all of them different from the one we are mainly discussing here.

PENFIELD: I am very much interested in Dr. Heymans' observations and followed his work on the carotid sinus for many years. Turning to the human automaton, it is quite possible to produce this automatic state at operation. It occurs in man spontaneously when a localized epileptic discharge occurs in the critical area. The individual may be quite confused, or he may be able to walk about and perhaps talk in a seemingly reasonable manner. During the whole period, however, the train of his consciousness is not being recorded in the brain. Afterwards he will be completely oblivious of this period. That is what we call an automatic state and it is produced by a localized epileptic discharge in the amygdaloid nucleus which is related to the hippocampus. Electrical stimulation there may also produce it if the stimulus is followed by epileptic afterdischarge.

If the hippocampus is removed in a human being, who has already had an injury to the hippocampus on the other side of the brain (this has happened twice in my experience), you take away his recent memory. The man is completely conscious and adjusted, able to carry on in other ways. I think this is what you are describing.

During old age or with arteriosclerosis, the hippocampus is particularly susceptible to vascular inadequacy. To make a long story short, in elderly people there is a certain loss of recent memory. Associated with this difficulty there is pathological change, sclerosis of the arteries of the cornu ammonis, the hippocampus. That person may have no loss of other mental activities. He may well preserve his keenness of reason.

MAC KAY: I would like to take up this question of "compensation," not to quarrel with what Professor Teuber meant by the term but to draw what seems to be a necessary distinction. I think he used it to mean simply "taking into account the other data," but I wonder whether the most neutral term for this would not rather be *integration*. The trouble is that compensation has been used in the past in connection with a particular theory of the stability of the perceived world, namely, the theory that the changes produced by voluntary movement have to be compensated in the sense of *canceled*. I have indicated in my paper some reasons for dissatisfaction with this theory, so I will not elaborate on these now, but I believe that Professor Teuber was not himself concerned to espouse it.

I am not sure that Held's beautiful experiments support the conclusion that reafference, in the sense of *self-induced* stimulation, is essential for successful readjustment to perceptual arrangement. Howard, for example, in Durham, has shown that if a subject is fitted with prisms, and is not allowed to move, but is repeatedly struck in the teeth by an object which he can see approaching him, this is sufficient to secure readaptation. The conclusion would seem to be that, although obviously error information (in the technical sense) is essential for adaptation, it is not essential that that information be generated by bodily movement. In this case it seems entirely accurate to speak of compensation, since the subject must learn to "aim off," consciously or unconsciously, to offset the action of the prisms. What is compensated here, however, is the motor coordinate system. I cannot see that any safe inferences can be drawn from these experiments in support of the notion that the optical changes produced by voluntary movement have to be removed from the incoming sensory signals. They require to be appropriately *evaluated* but not annulled.

TEUBER: I am almost ready to accept your reclassification of this phenomenon. I still believe, however, that compensation might fit the case discussed in such detail by von Holst, that is, the striking difference between the perceptual consequences of voluntary as against involuntary movements of the eye. A particularly telling instance—to me at least—is the extensive illusory motion of the visual world which results when one wears inverting spectacles. I find these illusory motions easier to understand if I assume that there is a corollary discharge which, after inversion, is added to the reafferent movement instead of being subtracted from it. On the other hand, I am quite ready to grant you that adaptation to distorting or displacing spectacles and similar devices can proceed in more than one way, particularly in the normal adult who has achieved sensorimotor coordination over many years and under very diverse conditions. I would still assume that self-produced output, i.e., voluntary movement, will turn out to be crucial at certain early stages in the origin of normal coordination.

GRANIT: I just wanted to introduce our main theme of consciousness, which Thorpe touched on already, and I point out that we must distinguish clearly between consciousness and comprehension or even integration of the outer world. I would take as an example the vestibular organs which in my opinion do not come to the knowledge of our consciousness at all.

Our unconscious is far more ingenious than our conscious acting. We have, for instance, all these impulses coming from space or, if we analyze them, from vestibular organs, from neck muscles, from the limbs and other postural muscles. You tilt your head and the eyeballs will in no time adjust themselves so as to preserve, as well as possible, the horizontal axis. As I said, there is tremendous ingenuity in the unconscious. I suppose one of the great tasks of future pedagogists will be to learn to get at them.

ECCLES: When passively moved in the absence of visual sensation, I always have a sense of direction of movement and of rotation that gives me a conscious experience which we may call an orientation feeling. I would suggest that we have much more conscious experience from our vestibular mechanism than we are apt to imagine.

TEUBER: My comment on Professor Granit's statement may not be very helpful, but I would like to say that I have often wished that my vestibular system would not intrude upon my consciousness, particularly when I am riding in a plane in turbulent air or when I find myself on a ship in heavy seas.

JASPER: I would like to offer some positive evidence in favor of your hypothesis of effective movement and sensation. We have been studying this question in intact animals, recording from both implanted and macroelectrodes in the visual cortex in conditioning experiments. The striking thing is that changes in responses of even the primary units of the visual cortex with a nonvisual conditioning stimulus occur each time that there is a movement associated with it, affecting the light responsive units of the visual cortex. There was always a change in response of the visual cortex to a light stimulus which had been conditioned to produce a motor response, as compared to identical stimuli which had not been so conditioned.

TEUBER: Undoubtedly, our major task is to find consistent electrophysiological signs of these postulated motor-to-sensory discharges.

REFERENCES

BOSSOM, J. The effect of brain lesions on prism adaptation in monkey, *Psychon. Sci.*, 2, 45–46 [1965].

DENNY-BROWN, D. The frontal lobes and their functions, in: *Modern Trends in Neurology* (ed. by A. Feiling). New York: Paul B. Hoeber, pp. 13–89 [1951].

HARMS, H. Visuelle und pupillomotorische Störungen bei Veränderungen des Okzipitallappens, in: *8th Inter. Congress of Neurology*, Wien [1965].

HELD, R. Exposure history as a factor in maintaining stability of perception and coordination, *J. Nerv. Ment. Dis.*, 132, 26–32 [1961].

———, and J. BOSSOM. Neonatal deprivation and adult rearrangement: Complementary techniques for analyzing plastic-sensory-motor coordinations, *J. Comp. Physiol. Psychol.*, 54, 33–37 [1961].

———, and S. J. FREEDMAN. Plasticity in human sensorimotor control, *Science*, 142, 455–462 [1963].

———, and A. HEIN. Movement-produced stimulation in the development of visually guided behavior, *J. Comp. Physiol. Psychol.*, 56, 872–876 [1963].

HELMHOLTZ, H. VON. *Handbuch der physiologischen Optik.* Leipzig: Leopold Voss, Vol. III [1867].

HOLST, E. VON, and H. MITTELSTAEDT. Das Reafferenzprinzip (Wechselwirkungen zwischen Zentralnervensystem und Peripherie), *Naturwiss.*, 37, 464–476 [1950].

HUBEL, D. H. Cortical unit responses to visual stimuli in nonanesthetized cats, *Amer. J. Ophthalmol.*, 46, 110–122 [1958].

———, and T. N. WIESEL. Receptive fields of single neurons in the cat's striate cortex, *J. Physiol.*, 150, 91–104 [1960].

———. Receptive fields and functional architecture in two non-striate visual areas (18 and 19) of the cat, *J. Neurophysiol.*, 28, 229–289 [1965].

JACOBSEN, C. F. Functions of the frontal association areas in primates, *Arch. Neurol. Psychiat.* (Chicago), 33, 558–569 [1935]

KLUEVER, H. Functional significance of the geniculo-striate system, in: *Biol. Sympos.* (ed. by H. Kluever), 7, 253–299 [1942].

KOHLER, I. Ueber Aufbau und Wandlungen der Wahrnehmungswelt, *Sitzber. Oesterr. Akad. Wiss.*, philohist. Kl., *227*, 1–118 [1951].

KORNMUELLER, A. E. Eine experimentelle Anaesthesie der aeusseren Augenmuskeln am Menschen und ihre Auswirkungen, *J. Psychol. Neurol.*, *41*, 354–366 [1931].

KUFFLER, S. W. Discharge patterns and functional organization of mammalian retina, *J. Neurophysiol.*, *16*, 37–68 [1953].

LASHLEY, K. S. Coalescence of neurology and psychology, *Proc. Amer. Phil. Soc.*, *84*, 461–470 [1941a].

——. Patterns of cerebral integration indicated by the scotomas of migraine, *Arch. Neurol. Psychiat.*, *46*, 331–339 [1941b].

LETTVIN, J. Y., H. R. MATURANA, W. S. McCULLOCH, and W. H. PITTS. What the frog's eye tells the frog's brain, *Proc. Inst. Radio Engr.*, *47*, 1940–1951 [1959].

——, H. R. MATURANA, W. H. PITTS, and W. S. McCULLOCH. Two remarks on the visual system of the frog, in: *Sensory Communication* (ed. by W. A. Rosenblith). New York and Cambridge, Mass.: Wiley and MIT Press, pp. 757–776 [1961].

MACKAY, D. M. Moving visual images produced by regular stationary patterns, *Nature* (London), *180*, 849–850 [1957].

ROSVOLD, H. E., and J. M. R. DELGADO. The effect on delayed-alternation test performance of stimulating or destroying electrically structures within the frontal lobes of the monkey's brain, *J. Comp. Physiol. Psychol.*, *49*, 365–372 [1956].

SEMMES, JOSEPHINE, S. WEINSTEIN, LILA GHENT, and H.-L. TEUBER. Spatial orientation in man after cerebral injury: I. Analysis by locus of lesion, *J. Psychol.*, *39*, 227–244 [1955].

SPEMANN, H. *Embryonic Development and Induction* (Silliman Lectures). New Haven: Yale Univ. Press [1938].

SPERRY, R. W. Neural basis of the spontaneous optokinetic response produced by visual inversion, *J. Comp. Physiol. Psychol.*, *43*, 482–489 [1950].

——. Physiological plasticity and brain circuit theory, in: *Biological and Biochemical Bases of Behavior* (ed. by H. F. Harlow and C. N. Woolsey). Madison: Univ. Wisconsin Press, pp. 401–424 [1958].

STAMM, J. S. Electrical stimulation of frontal cortex in monkeys during learning of an alternation task, *J. Neurophysiol.*, *24*, 414–426 [1961].

STRATTON, G. M. Vision without inversion of the retinal image, *Psychol. Rev.*, *4*, 463–481 [1897].

SUTHERLAND, N. S. Visual discrimination of orientation and shape by the octopus, *Nature* (London), *179*, 11–13 [1957].

TEUBER, H.-L. Perception, in: *Handbook of Physiology: Section 1, Neurophysiology* (ed. by J. Field, H. W. Magoun, and V. E. Hall). Washington, D. C.: Amer. Physiol. Soc., Vol. III, Chapt. LXV, pp. 1595–1668 [1960].

——. Sensory deprivation, sensory suppression and agnosia: Notes for a neurologic theory, *J. Nerv. Ment. Dis.*, *132*, 32–40 [1961].

——. The riddle of frontal lobe function in man, in: *The Frontal Granular*

Cortex and Behavior (ed. by J. M. Warren and K. Akert). New York: McGraw-Hill, Chapt. 20, pp. 410-444 [1964].

TEUBER, H.-L., W. S. BATTERSBY, and M. B. BENDER. *Visual Field Defects after Penetrating Missile Wounds of the Brain.* Cambridge, Mass.: Harvard Univ. Press, pp. vii–142 [1960].

———, and M. B. BENDER. Alterations in pattern vision following trauma of occipital lobes in man, *J. Gen. Psychol., 40,* 37–57 [1949].

———, and M. MISHKIN. Judgment of visual and postural vertical after brain injury, *J. Psychol., 38,* 101–175 [1954].

———, and F. PROCTOR. Some effects of basal ganglia lesions in subhuman primates and man, *Neuropsychologia, 2,* 85–93 [1964].

TWITCHELL, T. E. The automatic grasping responses of infants, *Neuropsychologia, 3,* 247–259 [1965].

WEISKRANTZ, L. Encephalization and the scotoma, in: *Current Problems in Animal Behavior* (ed. by W. H. Thorpe and O. L. Zangwill). Cambridge, Eng.: Cambridge Univ. Press, pp. 30–58 [1961].

———. Contour discrimination in a young monkey with striate cortex ablation, *Neuropsychologia, 1,* 145–165 [1963].

———, C. MIHAILOVIC, and C. G. GROSS. Stimulation of frontal cortex and delayed alternation performance in the monkey, *Science, 131,* 1443–1444 [1960].

WELLS, M. J. Proprioception and visual discrimination of orientation in *octopus, J. Exp. Biol., 37,* 489–499 [1960].

———. *Brain and Behavior in Cephalopods.* London: Heineman [1962].

WHITE, B. L., P. CASTLE, and R. HELD. Observations on the development of visually-directed reaching, *Child Developm., 35,* 349–364 [1964].

YOUNG, J. Z. The visual system of *Octopus:* I. Regularities in the retina and optic lobes of *Octopus* in relation to form discrimination, *Nature* (London), *186,* 836–844 [1960].

———. Learning and discrimination in the *octopus, Biol. Rev., 36,* 32–96 [1961].

9

Speech, Perception and the Uncommitted Cortex[1]

by WILDER PENFIELD

McGill University, Montreal, Canada

William Shakespeare turned to the subject of this symposium when he was writing the play *Richard II.* The imprisoned king emerges from his cell and stands alone upon the stage:

> *I have been studying how I may compare*
> *This prison where I live unto the world:*
> *And for because the world is populous,*
> *And here is not a creature but myself,*
> *I cannot do it; yet I'll hammer it out.*
> *My brain I'll prove the female to my soul;*
> *My soul the father; and these two beget*
> *A generation of still-breeding thoughts,*
> *And these same thoughts people this little world . . .*

During this study week in the Academy of Sciences, as in the little world of Richard's prison, we shall no doubt people the Vatican Gardens with a generation of "still-breeding thoughts." Thoughts, that are of value have their own form of earthly immortality and go on breeding lusty thoughts in other minds.

Pierre Teilhard de Chardin approached the subject of this symposium through his work on the earth's geology and his studies of the skull of Peking Man. "We have seen and admitted," he wrote, "that evolution is

---

[1] Due to the time schedule there was no discussion of this communication as there was following the other papers. However, the general findings of Professor Penfield's paper were extensively discussed at many other times during this conference.

an ascent toward consciousness. That is no longer contested even by the most materialistic, or at all events by most agnostic of humanitarians. Therefore it should culminate forwards in some sort of supreme consciousness."

Père Teilhard, since he was a priest as well as a scientist, felt impelled to face the ultimate problem—that of the supreme consciousness. But it would be unwise for us, meeting here as scientists, to continue the line of his argument toward what he called "the Ego and the All." Like Shakespeare and the common man of today, we must use the terminology of dualism in science, speaking of the brain and the spirit or mind. This does not prejudice eventual judgment as to the nature of things. If we are good scientists, we cannot claim that science has already explained the mind nor that it has thrown any light on man's long continued effort to understand his God. I wonder if it ever will.

Sherrington, once my teacher in physiology, wrote in the second edition of his book, *The Integrative Action of the Nervous System* [1947]: "That our being should consist of two separate elements offers, I suppose, no greater inherent improbability than that it should rest on one only."

It *is* hard for us to conceive of two separate elements. But it is equally incomprehensible that there should be only one element presenting itself as two—the body and the mind. It is a choice, as Sherrington suggests, a choice of two inherent improbabilities. But one of them must be close to the truth, and one of them should be chosen by every responsible man as a faith to live by and to die with.

Meantime, physiologists can only study the two faces of this golden coin, without prejudice, by observation and experiment. It was Hippocrates, in the fifth century before Christ, who urged that authority was to be found in Nature, not in the hypotheses of philosophers.

My own problem is not an easy one because of the nature of the material I have to present. The contempt which intellectuals once had for the barber surgeon lingers on in the minds of men, making it difficult for them to accept the findings of any surgeon on a par with the reports of scientists who study, for example, the virus, the single cell, the earthworm, the guinea pig or the anthropoid ape. I confess that many of us who are surgeons do operate too much and think too little. But we face special problems.

Without stopping to define consciousness, a brain surgeon must act. He must decide when his patient is conscious and when he is unconscious. He must do the best he can to be a good psychologist, a good physiologist, and, above all, a good doctor. He must be a critical observer, a tireless recorder. As an experimenter, he can only be an opportunist. But, on the other hand, disease and accident present to him, from time to time, the most perfect experiments. Then he must be prepared to think as well as act and to do both quickly. When, because he hopes to bring about a cure, he stimulates the brain of a conscious man and perhaps removes a part of the brain, the great opportunity may come and go while the patient is lying hopefully on the operating table.

My purpose in this symposium is to discuss speech, perception, and the mechanisms that seem to condition and to make use of the un-committed cortex. It is my latest study. But it is only a part of the long-continued cooperative effort that began when the Montreal Neurological Institute was founded in 1934. Our work on the brain and our studies of epilepsy opened many approaches to an understanding of conscious-ness, and I am deeply indebted to a brilliant succession of colleagues whose work goes on with ever-increasing excellence, as mine is coming to its close—Rasmussen, Jasper, Boldrey, Hebb, Erickson, McNaughton, Robb, Roberts, Chao, Kristiansen, Milner, Claude Bertrand, Gilles Ber-trand, Feindel, Mullan, Perot, and many others now in Montreal or scattered about the world.

Consciousness is not something to be localized in space. Nevertheless, if we assume that it is a function of the integrated action of the brain, there is placed before us a challenging problem of physiological localiza-tion. This has long been a concern of mine. In 1938, the accumulating evidence that seemed to disprove current beliefs in regard to the organization of function in the cerebral cortex led me to a study entitled, "The Cerebral Cortex and Consciousness," and to the following con-clusion:

"Finally, there is much evidence of a level of integration within the central nervous system that is higher functionally than that to be found in the cerebral cortex, evidence of a regional localization of the neuronal mechanism involved in this integration. I suggest that this region . . . lies below the cortex and above the midbrain. . . . All regions of the brain may well be involved in normal conscious processes, but the indispensable substratum of consciousness lies outside the cerebral cortex, probably in the diencephalon." Final integration, the study continued, may well take place in "those neuronal circuits which are most intimately associated with the initiation of voluntary activity and with the sensory summation prerequisite to it."

Our subsequent experience throws new light on this problem. Man's brain is remarkable among mammals because of the greatly increased volume of cerebral cortex that covers it with deeply folded convolutions. Unlike the cortex of the rat, which is completely motor or sensory except for a small undefined area, most of the human cortex is neither sensory in function nor motor (Fig. 9.1). The temporal and parietal lobes have made their appearance in man as an outbudding from the thalamus

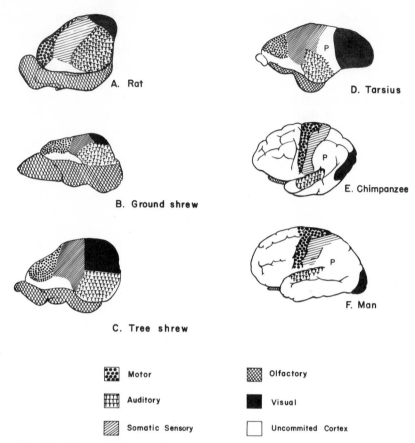

A. Rat

B. Ground shrew

C. Tree shrew

D. Tarsius

E. Chimpanzee

F. Man

▦ Motor   ▨ Olfactory

▦ Auditory   ■ Visual

▨ Somatic Sensory   □ Uncommited Cortex

Fig. 9.1. Mammalian brains from rat to man prepared by Stanley Cobb to illustrate the proportional increase of uncommitted cortex (or undetermined cortex) as compared with sensory and motor cerebral cortex.

which seems to push the visual sensory cortex back and away from the somatic sensory and the auditory sensory.

Because of inborn connections, the sensory and motor areas of man's cortex are committed as to function. Not so the new cortex between the auditory and the visual areas. Its organization and functional connections are finally established gradually during the first decade of life, being devoted to speech on one side and, as I shall show, to perception on the other.

When a patient on the operating table is fully conscious and the hemisphere is exposed on the dominant side (usually left), a gentle electrical current applied to the speech cortex produces immediate interference with his speech mechanism. If, on the other hand, the electrode is applied to the corresponding area on the other side, no aphasia results. But there may be an active response. That is, he may report one of two types of change in his thoughts. Either he is aware of a sudden alteration in· his interpretation of present experience (what he sees and hears seems suddenly familiar, or strange, or frightening, or coming closer or going away, etc.), or, he has a sudden "flashback," an awareness of some previous experience. Although he is still aware of where he is, an earlier experience comes to him and the stream of that former consciousness moves forward again in full detail as it did in some previous period of time. (It may have been a time of listening to music—in a hall hearing an orchestra, or in a café watching an entertainer, or in a church. If asked to do so, the patient can hum an accompaniment to the music. It may be a time of laughing with friends or watching circus wagons as they enter a town long years ago in childhood.)

Similar psychical responses can be induced by stimulation of the temporal cortex that lies farther forward on the nondominant side and on the dominant side as well. Thus, except for the speech area and the audiosensory area, the cortex that covers the superior and lateral surfaces of the temporal lobe on both sides may be taken as a functional unit. We have considered the function of this unit, to be, broadly speaking, interpretive and have called the area from which such responses are obtained the "interpretive cortex" [Penfield, 1959].

The sudden interpretation of the present and the flashback of the past are evidently parts of a scanning mechanism that normally enables an individual to compare present experience with similar past experience automatically.

The Anatomical Record of the Stream of Consciousness

It seems evident that the discovery of an anatomical record of the stream of consciousness may teach us a good deal about the final neuronal integration that constitutes the counterpart of conscious thought. Where the actual record is, we do not know. Certainly it is not in the temporal convolution to which the surgeon's electrode is applied. The stimulating electrode sets up a sequence of neuron activity at a distance by means of axonal conduction from the point of stimulation. In a general study of the *Excitable Cortex in Conscious Man* [Penfield, 1958], I was forced to make a similar conclusion in regard to all the positive responses to electrical stimulation. The mechanism in question is invariably activated in distant gray matter by means of dromic conduction that is similar to the conduction that normally activates the mechanism.

When the stream of consciousness of a previous period of time is caused to flow again, the electrical excitation follows a pathway through a seemingly unending sequence of nerve cells, nerve fibers, and synapses. The path was formed and made permanent by neuronal facilitation. A strip of time seems to run forward again at time's own normal pace, and the individual is aware of the things he selected for his attention then. All of the available sensory information that he had ignored is absent. If he was frightened by the experience, he is frightened again. If he thought the music he is hearing was beautiful, he thinks so again.

Preserved within the anatomical record of the stream of consciousness is all that was once illumined by the searchlight of attention, and only that. The rest has remained in darkness. This is not a summation. It is a selection to which is added the individual's own interpretation which he makes by comparing present with previous similar experience. It is, then, the unaltered record of previous awareness.

SPEECH AND PERCEPTION

This area of human cerebral cortex which, at birth, may be called uncommitted, occupies the superior and lateral portions of the temporal lobe and extends back a little way into the parietal region. While the child is learning to speak and to perceive the meaning of things, something happens in the brain which is startling and unique from the point of view of comparative anatomy. The cortex on one side is devoted to a specific function while in the homologous area on the other side a different function is established: (*a*) the ideational processes of speech, (*b*) the interpretation of present experience by reference to the record of past similar experience.

(*a*) In the left hemisphere (dominant for speech), the major speech area, is that of Wernicke. (The two other ideational speech areas which are in the frontal lobe, Broca's area and the supplementary area, are of secondary importance.) Destruction of the major area results in loss of speech (aphasia). If it occurs before the age of ten or twelve, the homologous area on the nondominant side is made over into a speech area, but it requires a period of a year or more, and during that time the child is aphasic. This transfer does not occur if the accident takes place in adult life.

(*b*) The homologous area of cortex in the nondominant side, which might have been used for the purposes of speech, does not remain "silent." The functional defect produced by a lesion in this area in adult life has been described by many clinicians, as summarized by Critchley. Riddoch called it "visual disorientation" and Brain used the same phrase. Hécaen suggested the term *troubles visuoconstructifs*, or *apractognosia*.

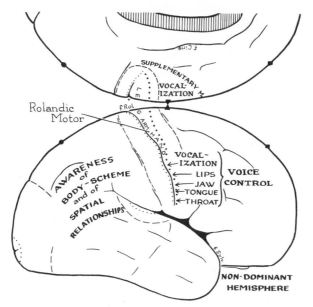

Fig. 9.2. The motor areas related to voice control in the Rolandic area and the supplementary area are the same as those in the other hemisphere. A major lesion in the posterior temporal and parietal region of this non-dominant hemisphere, in adult life, would produce loss of awareness of body scheme and spatial relationships, while the same destruction on the other side would result in complete aphasia.

In the Montreal Neurological Institute, Hécaen made a study of our material [1956]. The conclusion derived from that study may be seen in Fig. 9.2. The critical area for production of this functional defect surrounds the posterior end of the fissure of Sylvius, extending back as far as the interparietal sulcus.

In one patient in our series, a bullet wound (during military service) had scarred this area on the right side, producing epilepsy. The left hemisphere was clearly the dominant one for speech. So I made a complete removal of the area on the right. As hoped, it relieved the man from his seizures but it left him with a severe degree of spatial disorientation. He now lives in a small New Brunswick town. When he leaves his home and turns a corner, where he can no longer see his home, he is lost. But he has solved that problem. He works now quite satisfactorily, he says, in the town's railroad station which is in full view of his home!

What the functional defect would be, if complete removal of the interpretive cortex were carried out in both hemispheres of man, must remain a conjecture. This operation will probably never be done. One may surmise that the defect would be related to other aspects of visual interpretation and to auditory interpretation.

A great deal more is to be learned about the function of the interpretive cortex by stimulation. A complete review of all cases in which electrical stimulation produced experiential responses (or flashbacks) was made by Penfield and Perot [1963], and all cases in which stimulation produced an interpretative response were summarized by Mullan and Penfield [1959].[2] Both types of response are shown in Table 1.

Table 1

Psychical Responses to Electrical Stimulation of Interpretive
Areas of Cortex

A. *Experiential flashback:* Random re-enactment of a conscious sequence from the patient's past.

B. *Interpretive signaling:* Production of sudden interpretations of the present experience, such as *familiar, strange, fearful, coming nearer, going away,* etc.

By summarizing the position of all points where stimulation produced a psychical response, either an interpretive signal or an experiential flashback, it is apparent that the two types of response cover the same general area.

To consider the first group, the location of all points producing signals (illusions) was placed on the map shown in Fig. 9.3. Those that produced a change in interpretation of sounds fell on the first temporal convolution of either side. Production of the signal of familiarity was predominantly from stimulation of the temporal cortex on the non-dominant side and the same was true for alterations of visual interpretation.

Secondly, when all points (from which experiential responses [3] were produced) were summarized on a bilateral map, the result was shown as in Fig. 9.4. There was none in other lobes, none on the hippocampus or in the amygdala, which are not shown, and none on the anterior transverse gyrus of Heschl, which is audiosensory, and none on the occipital cortex, which is visuosensory. Most were on the superior and

---

[2] Stimulation, carefully controlled, does not produce any epileptiform afterdischarge. If recording electrodes show that afterdischarge follows stimulation, the result is not given exact localizing significance. Ordinarily when the current is switched off during deep stimulation, or the electrode is removed following superficial stimulation, the psychical response stops instantly.

[3] Such responses occurred in 40 cases carried out on 40 different patients out of a total series of 1,132 patients who were subjected to craniotomy and exploratory electrical stimulation.

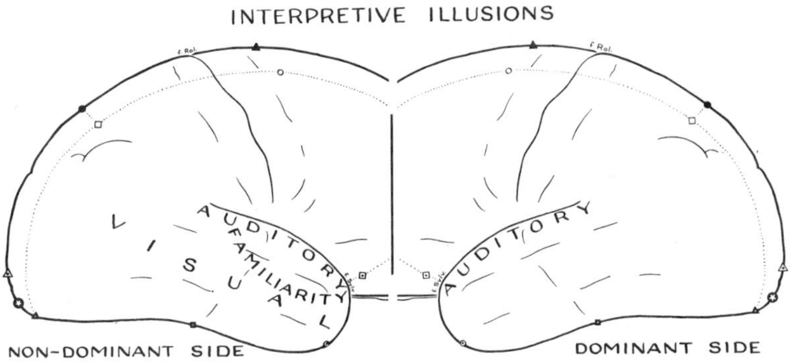

INTERPRETIVE ILLUSIONS

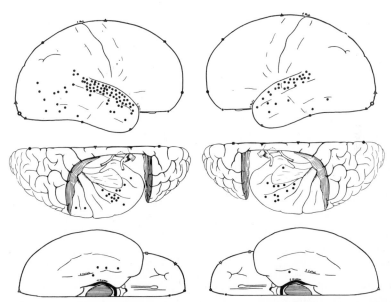

NON-DOMINANT SIDE

DOMINANT SIDE

Fig. 9.3. Summarizing map of areas from which electrical stimulation produced interpretation illusions, or signals. A changed interpretation of things heard (auditory) was produced by stimulation of the first temporal convolution on either side. A change in interpretation of things seen (visual) was produced in the non-dominant side only. The feeling that this had all happened before (*déjà vu,* familiarity) was also produced in the non-dominant side. "Dominant" means side on which speech was localized [from Mullan and Penfield, 1959].

Fig. 9.4. Points of stimulation that produced experiential responses, flashbacks. Hemisphere partly excised to show superior surface of temporal lobe [from Penfield and Perot, 1963].

EXPERIENTIAL RESPONSES

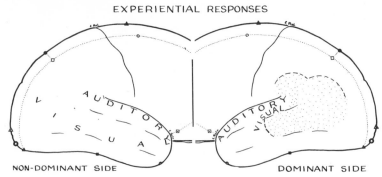

NON-DOMINANT SIDE   DOMINANT SIDE

Fig. 9.5. Summary of experiential responses. The dotted zone indicates ideational speech area [from Penfield and Perot, 1963].

lateral surfaces of the first temporal convolution. They appeared in a scattered distribution on the temporal cortex elsewhere. But they avoided the posterior temporal speech area on the dominant side, although that area was stimulated in a long series of cases.

When the experiential responses were separated into three groups, visual, auditory and combined visual and auditory, the auditory experiences were found to come from points on the first temporal convolutions of both sides (Fig. 9.5). The combined responses came largely from the same convolution. On the other hand, most of the purely visual experiences were produced on the lateral aspect of the temporal lobe of the nondominant hemisphere with a few on the dominant side, just in front of the speech area. This is shown more clearly in Fig. 9.6 where the visual experiences alone are summarized. Compare these figures with the ideational speech map shown in Fig. 9.7.

Let us consider what light this material casts on the nature of perception. When the sudden interpretive signaling is examined, it is clearly no more than the automatic interpretation that comes to all of us when a past experience is repeated. A feeling of "seen before," or "heard before," or in some respect, "experienced before" comes to us even before there is time to think. When true recognition follows, there must have been instantaneous reference to past records.

A selected past is made available—selected by some event in the present. Thus a man apparently forgotten, a place not visited for years, a song familiar in the distant past, is recognized, identified. The recall is so clear that even small changes in the present sensory input coming from eye and ear are recognized, such as the graying of the friend's hair, the windows of a house perhaps altered, in music a new voice or a different musical instrument. These things bring a sense of change as well as the

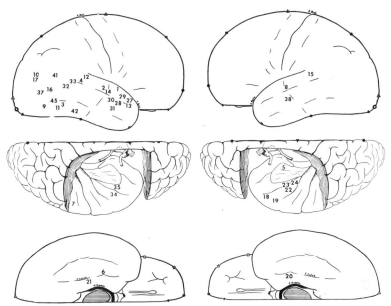

Fig. 9.6. Experiential responses which were purely visual. Figure 9.4 included all such responses, that is, the visual experiences, auditory experiences, and those that were both visual and auditory.

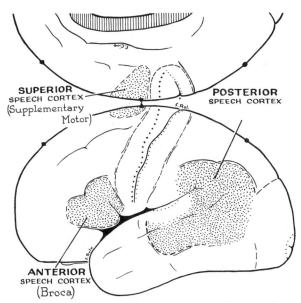

Fig. 9.7. Cortical speech areas of dominant hemisphere as determined by the method of aphasic arrest or electrical interference [from Penfield and Roberts, 1959].

sense of similarity and familiarity. All of this is involved in perception, but it is automatic perception rather than reasoned analysis.

The flashing return of previous similar experience in normal life is very like the flashback produced by electrical stimulation. But the surgeon's electrical recall is completely random while this recall is amazingly selective. After the anterior half of the right temporal lobe had been removed in the case of D.F., she heard a song played by an orchestra each time the stimulating electrode was applied to a specific point on the superior surface of the remaining lobe. The point was stimulated over and over again. Each time, she heard an orchestra playing the same song which began at verse and went on to chorus. When asked to do so, she hummed the air accompanying the music she was made to hear. The tempo of her humming was what would be expected from such an orchestra. She could not remember when she had heard it thus before.

The patient A. Bra., under similar circumstances, was made to hear a certain piece of music by stimulation. She did remember the occasion. It was Christmas Eve in Amsterdam, where she had lived. She seemed to be in a church. It was during the war and there were Canadian soldiers there. (She married a Canadian soldier later and so came to live in Montreal.) The choir sang and she felt again how beautiful it was, even as she lay on the table in the Montreal operating room.

When the temporal cortex of a young South African, J.T., was stimulated, he realized where he was and cried out in astonishment, "Yes, Doctor! Yes, Doctor! Now I hear people laughing—my friends—in South Africa." After I had withdrawn the electrode, he discussed the experience with me. He had seemed to be with two young women, his cousins, on their family's farm. He saw them. They were laughing and he was laughing with them. Still he knew he was really in Montreal and he could still speak to me.

Briefly described, the times that are most often recalled are times during which the individual was paying attention to a scene or to the action of others, a time of predominantly visual experience. Or even more frequently, he was listening to speech or music and the experience was predominantly auditory. Sometimes it was both visual and auditory. The details of all examples of experiential response are included in our final summary [Penfield and Perot, 1963]. Most often the time recalled was neither significant nor important.

For example, stimulation of the superior surface of the anterior part of the first temporal convolution on the right caused the patient, G.F., to say, "I just heard one of my children speaking . . . Frank." She could, she said, "hear the neighboring noises also," by which she meant such things as passing automobiles. She seemed to be in her kitchen and she explained later, "Of course, I have heard Frankie like that many,

many times, thousands of times." She supposed the surgeon had somehow brought all this about—while she was still in the operating room! She thought, too, that she had been able to look into the yard as well, and that she saw the boy there.

A Case Example

We may take the patient, C.H., as a text for discussion. He described his thinking as he lay on the operating table and I mapped out the speech areas. I have often recalled his words. The points where the electrode produced sensory or motor response and those where there was speech interference were marked by numbered tickets placed on the brain (Fig. 9.8). It should be pointed out that the cortex has no means of sensory appreciation and the patient could not know when an electrode was applied to the cortex nor when it was removed. (A square wave generator was used—1 volt, at 2 msec and 60 cycles per sec.) The patient said he felt a tingling sensation in his thumb. This identified the (postcentral) somatosensory gyrus. At 13 there was pulling of the jaw to the right (precentral gyrus).

The stimulating current was stepped up to 2 volts. At point 24, he was called upon to speak but could not do so because of anarthria (interference with motor control of articulation). He knew what he wanted to say. The five small round circles indicate where the electrode was applied without producing any interference with his talking and with no other observable change.

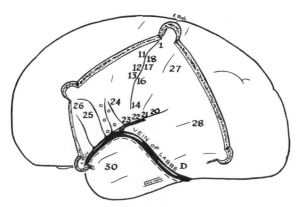

Fig. 9.8. Operative exposure in Case C.H. Electrical interference at points 26, 27, and 28 produced aphasia. The broken line shows the amount of temporal lobe removed as treatment of the focal epilepsy. For complete report see Penfield and Roberts [1959], pp. 113–116.

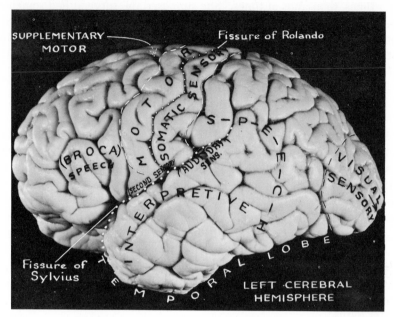

Fig. 9.9. Left cerebral hemisphere (dominant) showing areas devoted to speech, sensation, voluntary movement. The area of cortex from which electrical stimulation produces experiential flashbacks and interpretive signals is labeled "interpretive." There was no overlap between interpretive and speech cortex as judged by stimulation. No experiential or interpretive responses were produced from the speech area as shown in Fig. 9.7 [from Penfield and Roberts, 1959].

After this preliminary exploration I placed the electrode on the posterior speech area at point 28 (3 volts). At the same time an assistant was showing him the picture of a butterfly which he knew he was expected to name. He remained silent although he made a gesture that suggested exasperation. After withdrawal of the electrode, he exclaimed as though with relief: "Now I can talk, butterfly." Then he added, "I couldn't get that word 'butterfly' and then I tried to get the word 'moth.'"

The speech mechanism had failed when called upon. To his surprise, he found himself aphasic. If he had not tried to speak, he would not have known that he was aphasic. This supports the hypothesis that through the central integrating system a particular cortical area can be called into action, while it remains inactive when not so called. In the case of speech, it may well be that the functional arrest is produced by local cortical interference or, very likely, by conduction of current from any one of the three surface speech areas into the underlying pulvinar. Thus the operation of the speech mechanism would be blocked by deep as well as superficial interference.

Seeing the picture, C.H. must have compared it with his own record of past experience and thus perceived the nature of the familiar winged object. Let us assume that action within the brain was as follows: A specific pattern of potentials, which is the electrical equivalent of the *concept* "butterfly," must have moved from a relatively central position in the upper brain stem (diencephalon) to the cortical speech area. Normally the electrical equivalent of the *word* "butterfly" would have flashed back into this central area and he would have been conscious of what the name was.

But, when the name did not appear to him, he tried again, selecting the concept that seemed to him closest to "butterfly." When the appropriately patterned potentials for moth went off, he drew another "blank" and remained silent and frustrated, realizing that he had no words with which to explain. The electrode's current had inactivated the speech mechanism without interfering with the man's capacity to perceive and to reason.

The speech mechanism is clearly a partially separable one. But why, one might ask, should it be assumed that the employment of specialized areas of cortex is made possible by a two-way traffic of electrical potentials between a central integrating area and the cortical area in question? Why should not one cortical area be activated from another such area by means of tangential association fibers?

Surgical experience provides experimental evidence that is a convincing answer. Circumscribed excision of cerebral cortex around the major speech area does not produce aphasia or interfere with speech. Furthermore, similar neighboring removals of cortex about the sensory areas or about the motor area do not impair the accuracy of sensory information or the discriminating control of voluntary movement. These removals, when reconsidered and summarized, form a convincing experiment proving that each of the functional cortical areas carries out its specific function by means of to-and-fro communication with the diencephalon. The initiating demand arriving at the speech area must come from the diencephalon, whether it is an idea calling for a word or a word calling for the idea.[4]

[4] The same is true, as already pointed out, for the cortical motor areas. They are employed for discriminating action by messages arising in the diencephalon. Thus the control of the muscles used in speaking passes through the bilateral area for "voice control" shown in Fig. 9.2. This area can be removed on one side without paralysis of articulation.

Similarly, the conclusion is inescapable that the sensory areas in the cortex are not end stations, as so many physiologists have considered them to be. They are way stations, or interruptions, each on a cortical detour that leads back to a subcortical target. How these way stations make their functional contribution, and just what that contribution may be, remain to be discovered.

When the patient C.H. was shown a picture in the operating room, he evidently referred his visual sensory information to a mechanism for nonverbal perception that had been formed in childhood. In years long past, perhaps during early childhood, he had seen one butterfly and then another. No doubt he focused his attention on the beautiful creature in each experience and heard someone speak its name. Probably he spoke the word for himself as well as he could. When he spoke it a second and a third time, he pronounced it better and eventually he learned to write it. Each time he saw the butterfly he had a clearer conception of form, movement, color. Thus, neuron connections were slowly established that were durable. But he was establishing two neuron mechanisms—one for speech and one for perception.

It may well be that the speech mechanism also has some automatic means of utilizing the neuronal record of the stream of consciousness. There is no way of discovering that. Certainly the interpretive cortex has a means of calling upon it automatically, if the results of electrical stimulation have any meaning.

It is, of course, no more than surmise if I suggest that this scanning mechanism in the interpretive cortex was employed by C.H. when he saw the picture and knew it was that of a butterfly.

There are similarities between the process of verbal perception and nonverbal perception, as one might expect. When a printed word is shown, the speech mechanism is used. When a picture is shown, the other mechanism. But the result is the same. An idea or a concept appears in consciousness. In either case a symbol is translated into an idea. The speech mechanism has a double task. It must work in the opposite direction to translate ideas into words.

SUMMARY

The subdivision of the uncommitted cortex into the speech cortex and the interpretive cortex is well established and fixed by the time a child has entered adult life. When the cortex is mapped out functionally by means of electrical stimulation, the divisions are found to be surprisingly sharp. After hundreds of cases in which stimulation mapping was carried out, there was still no overlap in responses between the speech area and the adjacent areas for visual sensation and for auditory sensation. There is no overlap either between the speech area and the interpretive area immediately anterior to it (see Fig. 9.9; also 9.5 and 9.7).

To summarize briefly: the uncommitted cortex which remains after speech has taken its position may be called, for convenience, the interpretive cortex. Electrical stimulation sometimes produces a sudden change in automatic interpretation of those things of which the individual is at the moment aware. Or, stimulation activates a neuron sequence that constitutes the record of the stream of consciousness. That record is not in the interpretive cortex, but at a distance from the point of stimulation. It is activated by axonal conduction [Penfield, 1958]. The record may be located in the diencephalon, but I suspect that the hippocampus and the amygdaloid nucleus on the two sides may also have something to do with the process of recording experience.

Each patient has told us what the record of consciousness recalled to him. The events are usually so unimportant and the detail so complete that it seems likely the neuronal record may be complete for each individual's waking hours, and yet the strips of time that have been reached by electrical stimulation in the interpretive cortex recall only the times when attention was directed to auditory or visual experiences, or to times in which both were important.

But there are other sorts of human experience which, up to the present, have never been produced thus—times when attention is focused on one's own effort, times of making up one's mind to do this or that, or periods when one was carrying out skilled acts, or speaking and saying this or that, or writing messages and adding up figures. Such things have not been recalled. No one has said, "I am eating and tasting food." No one exclaimed that he was involved in sexual experience, or having a bowel movement, or suffering pain, or weeping, or engaged in athletic competition.

We have had experience with more than 1,000 craniotomies under local anesthesia, about 500 of them in the temporal area. We have stimulated the cerebral cortex of conscious individuals in most areas of the brain, and yet psychical responses have never resulted outside of the area described here as interpretive cortex. From no other area has the neuronal record of consciousness been activated.

Visual and auditory experiences are very important in a man's life and in his individual development. It is apparent that the large area of uncommitted cortex that separates visual-sensory and auditory-sensory areas in man is devoted to the interpretation of the things he sees and hears.

The speech cortex certainly makes a functional contribution to the process of verbal interpretation. The interpretive cortex probably makes a most important functional contribution to nonverbal perception. These are automatic mechanisms which are functionally separable.

There is some degree of functional localization within the interpretive cortex that may be outlined as follows: Interpretation of current visual information is localized usually in the nondominant side in the temporoparietal cortex. Removal of this area (Fig. 9.2) produces, in an adult, loss of awareness of spatial relationships. This is the counterpart of the aphasia produced in an adult by destruction of the speech area. Interpretation of current auditory information is localized largely in the superior and lateral portion of the first temporal convolution of both sides where it surrounds the auditory-sensory cortex (Heschl's transverse gyrus within the fissure of Sylvius).

Finally, the interpretation that "all this has happened before" was a response obtained only from stimulation of the nondominant temporal lobe. Other interpretations, such as fear, are not frequent enough to be localized with certainty.

Discussion

It is easier to say where than it is to explain how. But localization of function in the brain must come first, and because new tools were placed in my hands, I have spent most of my life mapping and localizing. First it was the localization of sensory and motor activity, and later of psychical activity in specific areas of the human cerebral cortex.

Every man has the feeling that he controls his own thinking and directs the searchlight of his own attention, to some extent in any case. And yet, even accompanying this very initiation there must be brain action. At any rate, that is the hypothesis of science. By deciding to prove or disprove that hypothesis, by making up my mind to discover the truth about free will, I am, at the same time, proving the existence of free will. Or so it seems on introspection!

Consciousness continues, regardless of what area of cerebral cortex is removed. On the other hand, consciousness is inevitably lost when the function of the higher brain stem (diencephalon) is interrupted by injury, pressure, disease, or local epileptic discharge. The detailed anatomy and physiology of the diencephalon (which includes the thalamus) are still obscure. Nevertheless, it is clear that within the diencephalon there is a system of nerve fibers and gray matter that communicates directly with the functional units of the two hemispheres.

It is on the action of this system that the existence of consciousness depends. By means of it, the action of cortical mechanisms is started and stopped. Thus it is that the diencephalon and the prosencephalon (or forebrain hemispheres) function together as an integrated unit.

I began to call this hypothetical communication the centrencephalic system after much discussion with my colleagues (especially Stanley Cobb of Boston and Herbert Jasper). It served to call attention to the fact that the so-called cortical association tracts could not account for integration of function in the brain. And it has been and is useful to thoughtful clinicians who understand that the centrencephalic system is only a means of communication, coordination and integration and that it unites the diencephalon with the prosencephalon above, and the mesencephalon below, in functional unity.

Neuronal activity within this system is the indispensable accompaniment of consciousness. On the other hand, to use the misleading word "centrencephalon," or to suggest that such a block of brain exists where consciousness is located, would be to call back Descartes and to offer him a substitute for the pineal gland as a seat for the soul.

It is into the diencephalon that the currents of sensory information come. Patterns of traveling potentials that produce voluntary activity originate here and move out through the motor cortex on either side to the muscles. From here, different areas of cerebral cortex are called into action and carry out their function by means of back-and-forth neuronal activity with the diencephalon. Thus, the differing processes of the mind are made possible through combined functional activity in diencephalon and cerebral cortex, not within diencephalon alone.

Observation of a normal human infant during his waking hours makes it clear that he is conscious. Before long he is evidently making some use of the sensory and motor areas of the cerebral cortex. But he shows little or no superiority over other mammalian sucklings at first. What makes him different, as the years pass, is what he does with his uncommitted cortex. I am ignoring the fateful frontal lobes that contain so much undefined cortex. They have their uses, but that is a matter for later years.

In early childhood, it seems reasonable to suppose that neuronal activity within the diencephalon must have its impact, during the waking hours, upon the uncommitted cortex. That cortex is, after all, an outgrowth from thalamic nuclei (*lateralis posterior et pulvinaris*). This impact must mold and organize the speech cortex on the one hand and the interpretive cortex on the other through the connecting neuron paths. This may be expressed in another way: The child is driven by delighted curiosity to concentrate his attention on what his mother is saying to him and on each new experience that comes to him.

His attention determines the content of each conscious experience and the content of the record of the stream of consciousness. Whatever the mechanism of the control of attention may be, it is safe to predict that its neuronal localization will be discovered in the diencephalon. Here is a subject for future study. The focusing of attention is the final integrative selection that goes along with each successive mental state.

As G. G. Simpson [1958] pointed out, it has generally been assumed "that evolutionary progression in behavior must be accompanied by and cannot proceed either slower or faster than correlated changes in the brain." [5] Simpson quoted Sperry, among others, as authority for such a view. But he added in conclusion "that the point was disputable."

Perhaps, however, without dispute, the facts are capable of changing interpretations. Man is different from lower mammals. He has a language that is spoken and written, and he is therefore part of an evolving society. He has in his brain more extensive areas of undefined and uncommitted cerebral cortex. The connections of the uncommitted cortex that will function are determined only during childhood. To this extent, one might well say that the brain of man is molded by his mind. At any rate, brain organization alters according to the content of the stream of consciousness early in life. The brain is subject to alteration by the teaching that comes to a child and the personal effort that he makes.

Man has no need to wait for a bigger, better brain to come to him by means of the slow process of evolution. How slow the process is, was pointed out by Teilhard de Chardin, when he claimed there had been no measurable change in man's brain since the Ice (Pleistocene) Age, although evolution has "overflowed its anatomical modalities." Evolution of civilized society has been brief, but it is swift and brilliant. This achievement of the mind was made possible when men learned by teaching to mold the human brain. But there is something else that is continuously creative in our society. Men's thoughts live on and go on breeding other thoughts—beliefs, faiths, slogans, propagandas.

Four hundred years after the birth of William Shakespeare we cannot discover how his amazing brain was molded with its vast store of words and its perceptions. Some of the things I have tried to express were prescient shadows in his mind.

"*I cannot do it,*" King Richard said. "*Yet I'll hammer it out.*"

> *My brain I'll prove the female to my soul;*
> *My soul the father; and these two beget*
> *A generation of still-breeding thoughts.*

REFERENCES

Hécaen, H., W. Penfield, C. Bertrand, and R. Malmo, *A.M.A. Arch. Neurol. and Psychiat.*, 75, 400–434 [1956].

Hess, W. *The Biology of the Mind (Bonin).* Chicago: Univ. Chicago Press [1964].

Mullan, S., and W. Penfield. *A.M.A. Arch. Neurol and Psychiat.*, 81, 269–284 [1959].

Penfield, W. *Archiv. Neurol. Psychiatr.*, 40, 417–442 [1938].

[5] W. R. Hess ended his recent book with this conclusion: "Only those contents of consciousness can be developed that correspond to the organization of the brain."

PENFIELD, W. *Res. Publ. Ass. Nerv. Ment. Dis. Proc.*, 30, 513–528 [1950].

———. *Brain*, 81, 231–234 [1958a].

———. *The Excitable Cortex in Conscious Man* (The Sherrington Lectures). Liverpool Univ. Press [1958b].

———. *Science*, 129, 1719–1725 [1959].

PENFIELD, W., and PH. PEROT. *Brain*, 86, 595–696 [1963].

PENFIELD, W., and L. ROBERTS. *Speech and Brain Mechanisms.* Princeton: Princeton Univ. Press [1959].

SHERRINGTON, C. *The Integrative Action of the Nervous System.* Cambridge, Eng.: Cambridge Univ. Press [1947].

SIMPSON, G. G. *Behavior and Evolution.* New Haven: Yale Univ. Press [1958].

TEILHARD DE CHARDIN, P. *The Phenomenon of Man.* New York: Harper [1959].

10

Consciousness

by E. D. ADRIAN

Trinity College, Cambridge, England

One can scarcely come to a meeting of this kind without being reminded of the basic problems that have shaped Western philosophy, the problems of substance and shadow, reality and appearance, mind and matter. They are problems that have been debated since Plato and they have led to all the main developments of philosophic doctrine. As natural scientists I expect most of us prefer to remain uncommitted: our own picture of the universe is clearly not the whole truth but it has been too useful to be far from it and it can always be adapted to include fresh evidence. Yet if we are physiologists it may be difficult to maintain this Olympian detachment. If we are concerned with the sense organs and the central nervous system we are bound to be aware of the difficulties which arise, or have arisen in the past, in relating activities which seem to be shared by the body and the mind.

In his book on *The Analysis of Mind,* Bertrand Russell said this: "Few things are more firmly established in popular philosophy than the distinction between mind and matter. Those who are not professional metaphysicians are willing to confess that they do not know what mind actually is or how matter is constituted, but they remain convinced that there is an impassable gulf between the two and that both belong to what actually exists in the world." It would seem then that the physiologist has that impassable gulf to face as soon as he allows himself to look up from his apparatus.

But Russell wrote that more than forty years ago. I am not at all sure that it is still the popular belief that mind and matter cannot be mixed. There may be a few elderly simple people who are still convinced of the gulf, but the philosophers of our time have all argued so persuasively against it that most of us are prepared to admit that our conviction of it might have been due to some misunderstanding. However much we distrust the metaphysicians, we cannot overlook the fact that the gulf between mental and material can scarcely be called self-evident. It is, or used to be, anathema in the USSR and there must be a large number of the human race who have never suspected its existence.

The change in popular opinion in the twentieth century seems to have been due, in part, to the influence of Mach and William James and the spread of the experimental method into psychology. At all events, by the beginning of the century it was becoming more respectable for psychologists to use some kind of monism as a working hypothesis and even to be whole-hearted behaviorists. McDougall in England kept the flag of dualism flying for a time, but the controversy was becoming a back number by 1914 when the interest had shifted to the more romantic areas revealed by Freud.

Since that time, metaphysicians of all shades have shown a notable unanimity in rejecting the dualist position. They are agreed that the layman's separation of mind and matter will never do and they have given no support to the physiologists who assert that a thought is not the kind of thing which can be expected to depolarize a membrane. They tell us that those who hold such views have no clear conception either of mind or of matter and have been led into error by theological dogma and the ambiguities of language.

Unfortunately their agreement in rejecting dualism has not been coupled with agreement in accepting anything else. Various compromises have been put forward, things or processes which can be viewed as physical or mental according to their context, like Whitehead's *Structures of Activity*, or Russell's *Sensibilia* or Broad's *Sensa*. It is discouraging to find that each of these explanations, which seems so logical when we read it, should fail to satisfy more than the few professional critics whose explanation has been on the same lines; yet it is some encouragement to learn of so many different ways of escape from the mind-body dilemma, and scientists can say, rather patronizingly, that in metaphysics the advance is bound to come by disputation rather than by experimental evidence.

Now physiology and psychology are experimental sciences and they have advanced considerably in their proper spheres during the present century, but have they done any better than metaphysics in bringing mental activity into the same picture as matter, or, alternatively, in showing that it is bound to be excluded? Certainly not much better, but at least it can be said that the gulf has been narrowed, that they have brought mind and matter closer together.

It has never seemed to be necessary to go outside the elastic frame of natural science in describing the action of the sense organs and the signals they send to the brain, but now we can add that there is no need to invoke extraphysical factors to account for any of the public activities of the brain itself. Nowadays a mechanical man could certainly be built to do all, or almost all, that we do ourselves. Someone would have to design and make it, but it could be made to behave as intelligently as we do. The "Universal Turing Machine" can turn its band to any problem. Machinery, in fact, could be constructed to produce most of the facets of human behavior—far more than would have been dreamt of in the period when Condillac imagined the statue coming to life. The comic papers do not exaggerate. Our present-day statue could be designed to speak its thoughts, to answer our questions, to express anger or joy, to recognize friends, form habits and solve problems. It could be made to report introspections and to tell us its hopes and fears.

According to Ross Ashby, and I think we must accept what he says, a machine made on his plan could equal the human brain in the search for knowledge. Naturally there would be differences; unless great pains were taken in its design, we should not expect the robot brain to be so flexibly organized, its different departments might not be so well integrated, and quite apart from such failings we should recognize it as part of a machine and not of a man because it would be made of metals and plastics instead of living cells. We have to admit, however, that to this extent the behaviorist hypothesis seems adequate. As far as our public behavior is concerned, there is nothing that could not be copied by machinery, nothing therefore that could not be brought within the framework of physical science.

Yet for many of us there is still the one thing which does seem to lie outside that tidy and familiar framework. That thing is ourself, our ego, the I who does the perceiving and the thinking and acting, the person who is conscious and aware of his identity and his surroundings. As soon as we let ourselves contemplate our own place in the picture we seem to be stepping outside the boundaries of natural science.

It was William James's rejection of consciousness that made everyone more critical of this particular ghost. He saw no need for separating the thinker and the thoughts and reported that his own search for the "I" revealed only feelings of tension, chiefly in the mouth and throat. At that time, Bergson's philosophy was in the ascendant, and as late as 1911 Bergson maintained that we have a direct and communicable knowledge of our own consciousness. For James, however, consciousness was not an entity but a function, simply the function of knowing.

There are, of course, logical or linguistic difficulties about assigning any meaning to the statement, "I am immediately aware that I am conscious," or even, "I know my own mind." In fact, one has only to read any of the numerous books and papers and reports of symposia in the past ten years to realize the various muddles we are in when we try to give precision to arguments about consciousness or mind. Ryle has made much of these in arguing against the dualist position, the ghost in the machine. But, in general, the psychologists seem to be much more troubled by the grammatical and logical difficulties than are the philosophers. These are on the whole more tolerant and anxious to rescue whatever meaning our statements contain.

How then are we to account for our conviction that we have an immediate awareness of ourselves and that this is the one thing which a machine could not copy?

I used to regard the gulf between mind and matter as an innate belief. I am quite ready now to admit that I may have acquired it at school or later. But I find it more difficult to regard my ego as having such a second-hand basis. I am much more certain that I exist than that mind and matter are different.

Apart from those who are insane, "out of their mind," one does not come across people who do not believe in their individuality, though there are many who do not believe in the separation of mind and matter. Belief in one's existence seems to depend very little on deliberate instruction.

But here we have to rely on evidence which must be derived by introspection. We could construct a machine which would tell us that it was conscious, but we should not believe it. When our fellow men say they are conscious, we believe them because they are much more like ourselves; but we know that many of their ideas and ours have been planted in them and in us by parents or schools fellows; and, for all we know, some of our beliefs about our minds and our awareness may have been acquired in that way. The "I" that I know has been exposed to all the influences of the outside world since my birth. If we wish to reach through to the mind, the individual that has been influenced, we might try to discount all these extraneous factors by comparing the introspections of a great variety of people.

This is easier said than done, for it is usually necessary to elicit introspective reports by direct questioning and it is then more than likely that the report will be unintentionally influenced by the questioner. The horses of Elbefeld were accustomed to giving their master the answer he wanted and the human subject can be equally obliging when the answer will do no one much harm. Questions about the ego need careful framing and impersonal asking if they are to avoid the danger of suggesting the answer which would fit our particular beliefs. It was partly this unreliability of introspective reports which made the behaviorists disregard consciousness in their study of human activity.

Now, in the study of the human ego, introspections are almost all that we have to guide us, but some of the difficulties may not be as serious as we may think. The particular difficulty that the questioner may influence the answer recalls the uncertainty principle in physics, which limits the knowledge we can gain about any individual particle. Observation of that particle is bound to affect its position and velocity, but this does not make it impossible to define the behavior of a system made up of a large number of particles. In a similar way, some kind of statistical treatment might help to compensate for the disturbing effect of the questioner who asks us to report our private data.

Few of us would wish to embark on large-scale statistical comparisons of introspective data, but there are various problems in the psychosomatic field which seem to be badly in need of such treatment. It may be too much to expect that we shall ever find a way of submitting the theories of Freudian psychoanalysis to tests as exacting as those we should use in physics. In our present state of knowledge, it may be more illuminating to express the conflicts of the spirit by parables and myths than by weights and measures—and in any case it would now be very difficult to find people in the Western hemisphere who have not been already biased by popular opinion.

But there is a field of some promise, where the data are less emotionally charged, and it is one more closely related to particular physiological events. This is the field of perception, and I shall mention developments in that field which may be relevant to the problem of our conscious activities, though they might also be used to illustrate the weakness of introspective evidence. There was one, concerned with what is called eidetic imagery, which is in danger of being forgotten nowadays; it dates from the period when German psychology was still under the inspiration of Kraepelin's psychiatric classification and the psychologists then were particularly anxious to divide humanity into different bodily, mental, and temperamental types, the asthenic the pyknic, the schizoid, and so on. Kretschmer's book on *Physique and Character* was published in 1921. Not long after, Jaensch, at Marburg, began to study the perceptual images following optic stimuli and found that they could be used as a guide to the mental and constitutional type. His work on eidetic images roused great interest, for he described them as something between sensations and images. Like physiological after-images, they are always seen in the literal sense, but we do not all see them. They are more often reported by literary or artistic Frenchmen or Spaniards than by scientific Britons or Americans. Sometimes they are little more than sensations and are then seen, like after-images, in the complementary colors; sometimes they are more like memory images, with more detail and variety and appearing in the original colors. Jaensch said that eidetic imagery of this latter kind was rare among average adults, but much commoner in children, and that the eidetic disposition is correlated with nationality, with the particular kind of school teaching, and with certain constitutional factors depending on the thyroid gland.

He found that in schools in certain districts, 85–90 per cent of the children were eidetics. He considered that some of his colleagues had failed to recognize the eidetic type and pointed out that the difference between actually seeing and merely imagining is particularly clear when the eidetic image develops gradually. "Now I see this . . . ," "Now that is beginning to appear," children will say, pointing to a particular spot on the screen. "I know that . . . was also there, but I do not *see* it." In spite of the critics [Allport, *Brit. J. Psychol., XV*, 1924], Jaensch maintained that eidetic phenomena were easily recognizable and reproducible. He was able to develop theories of perception and of education based on their occurrence.

For a time it looked as though Jaensch had discovered something which might be an important bridge between the physiological processes of sensation and the resulting mental experience, but the emphasis was on its value in typology. The general impression seems to have been that, although eidetic imagery exists, Jaensch went too far in thinking that a particular type of response was at all characteristic of the mental and bodily type. The nature of the image seems to depend much more on the situation than on the individual, though it may well be a valuable clue to the way in which visual material is incorporated in the mental organization.

At present, at all events, the study of the body image seems a much more profitable line to follow. It brings together the psychologist, the psychoanalyst, and the clinical neurologist, and it is usually associated with the name of Paul Schilder who was all three. He made observations on eidetic imagery and hypnagogic visions, but was particularly concerned with images dealing with the subject's body and limbs in relation to the outside world, with the boundary between the body and its surroundings, with its relations with space and time and movement. It is to some extent his preoccupation with our ideas of ourselves in relation to the world that distinguishes Schilder's description of the body image from that of earlier workers, Head for instance. The conclusion he reaches is that the body image is constructed gradually, by trial and error. Consciousness is not an independent phenomenon, but consists of the process of trial and error in perception and thought "until the object and the outside world is reached. Consciousness is the attempt to bring experience within a context, we may call this context the ego, from an analytic point of view." The ego, in fact, is a synthesis of our experiences from birth (or before it).

His book *The Image and Appearance of the Human Body* has the sub-title *Studies in the constructive energies of the psyche,* and some of it is hard going for those who are not at home in a Freudian landscape. Some of it also revives our mistrust of introspective reports, particularly when they have been elicited by someone who was clearly a quick-witted and sympathetic examiner with views of his own.

For instance, when Schilder deals with the physiological basis of the body image, he says that "our tactual perception of the skin is felt distinctly below (about 2 cm below) the surface of the optic perception of the body. When we touch an object and gradually diminish the pressure exerted on it, the object and the space between the object and the skin disappear but the sensation in the skin remains. There is at the same time a distinct sensation that the skin is bulging as if reaching for an object."

I have to admit that I do not recognize this description in my own sensations, and there are other passages where, although I can recognize what he describes, I suspect that I should not have done so without his prompting. He quotes, for instance, the reports of six subjects who were asked to imagine a white line, of others asked to describe their sensations in an elevator descending rapidly and then coming to rest. I will not tell you the reports, for you would then be biased for or against them.

Nor shall I try to summarize the more theoretical treatment he undertook, his views on the libidinous structure of the body image and on the difference between his attitude and that of Gestalt psychology. But his views on the physiological basis of the body image include a great many observations made from a more direct physiological and clinical standpoint. He believed that there is no action in which the postural model of the body does not play an important part, and "No sensory experiences that lack spatial qualities." (The term *perception* means that something is going on in space.) Effort or experiment leads to more unified space experience. The body image too is constructed gradually; it can be changed by clothing, by spectacles, or a walking stick. "When people wear enormous masks at the Carnival in Nice they are not merely changing the physiological basis of their body image, but are actually becoming giants themselves."

Schilder does not regard the body image as more than one essential ingredient of the ego, though, like the ego, it is organized by memory and experiment and cannot be maintained without constant effort. I am not convinced that I have understood his description of consciousness as a social act dependent on the resistances of the world, that it consists in "trying to see the context of our experiences by comparing those we find in our outer and inner world." I can only recommend his two books, *Mind, Perception and Thought* and *The Image and Appearance of the Human Body*. Although I cannot follow all the arguments and think some of the evidence is not convincing, at least he makes it clear that our ego and our awareness have many features which are related to bodily events. He makes it very difficult to maintain the belief in an impassable gulf between mind and body.

I am not sure whether more observations on these lines can lead us much further, for what is most needed is corroborative evidence based on data which are not merely reports of introspection but are open to public observation. Fortunately we have evidence of a different kind in the studies of Baldwin, Piaget, and others on the development of intelligent behavior in the child. The picture which Piaget draws is again of a gradual process of establishing the boundary between the self and the external world. He distinguishes first a phase of "absolute realism," where there is no boundary at all, when the child is exclusively concerned with things and confuses himself and the world; then the phase of "immediate realism," where the instruments of thought, names, and words are distinguished from the things but are situated in them. This may last up to eight or nine years, to be followed by the stage of "mediate realism," where they are not in the things but in the body, and finally by the adult phase of "subjectivism," where the thoughts are within ourselves.

Piaget finds that the child's awareness of their own thoughts takes place invariably after the age of seven or eight. It is dependent on social factors through contacts with others. He quotes an interesting passage from Edmund Gosse's account of his own childhood. He had lied to his father and not been found out: he suddenly realized not only that his father was not infallible but that there was a secret belonging to Edmund Gosse and to someone who lived in the same body with him. "There were two of us and we could talk together. It is difficult to define impressions so rudimentary, but it is certain that it was in this dual form that the sense of my individuality now suddenly descended upon me."

Piaget points out that as long as the child believed in his father's omniscience, his own self was nonexistent, in the sense that his thoughts and actions seemed to him common to all. The moment he realized that his parents did not know all, he straightway discovered the existence of his subjective self. It shows how the consciousness of self is not a primitive intuition but results from a dissociation of reality and shows also to what extent this dissociation is due to social factors, to the distinction the child makes between his own point of view and that of others.

There is, of course, a large element of introspection in such evidence, but not in the evidence which shows that it may be seven years or more before the child's ideas of space, size, and direction are organized. Without that organization the distinction between the self and the world can scarcely be as definite as it will be in the adult. That particular ingredient of the ego must be built up by experience. I have to admit that this seems to have little relevance to the question whether a machine could ever become conscious, but it does seem to me to make the question less important.

I will try to sum up the position as I see it now. William James said that his search for the ego revealed only feelings of tension, chiefly in the mouth and throat. No doubt his thoughts took shape to the accompaniment of slight movements of verbalization. Nowadays we should expect to find the whole sensory input from exteroceptors and proprioceptors contributing to the tension, and it is probably better to think of the ego as a summary of the whole structure which has built up the individual since the child began to answer to its name.

But words like "structure," "organization," or "pattern" can often give a false sense of scientific respectability, and they have been used too often as a way of escape from our difficulties. It will be better to avoid them and to end up by giving you the general conclusions reached by the distinguished neurologist Francis Schiller, at a symposium on Brain and Mind in 1951. His paper is called "Consciousness Reconsidered." He is led to conclude that exclusively physiological and exclusively introspective accounts of the subject are incompatible and give rise to artifacts. Although they are complementary, integration of knowledge is hard to achieve because their points of reference and scales of observation are wide apart. "Consciousness" is a logical construction. The ego is a convenient abbreviation, an abstract of a multiplicity of objects from which it is developed. It arises when unconscious processes are integrated; its base line in the individual and in the animal kingdom is arbitrary.

That seems to me to be a reasonable position to have reached. It differs little from Schilder's and Piaget's in essentials. The physiologist is not forced to reject the old fashioned picture of himself as a conscious individual with a will of his own, for the position allows some kind of validity to the introspective as well as to the physiological account.

It admits that the two are incompatible but does not maintain that they must always be so. It would certainly be absurd to suppose that the scientific account will not be altered. Physics has synthesized ideas which once seemed quite incompatible and will probably do so again with great profit; possibly our picture of brain events or of human actions may be changed so radically that in the end they will account for the thinker as well as his thoughts.

DISCUSSION

Chairman: PROFESSOR GRANIT

THORPE: We have heard from Lord Adrian of the prevalent philosophical attitude reflected in the phrase "the ghost in the machine." I shall be referring to this subject myself in a talk to be given at a later session. But I would like in this connection to quote here and now a few sentences illustrating the opposite view from a recent lecture by a distinguished Oxford logician, Professor William Kneale.* Kneale says "We must retain the Platonic notion of mental events which are distinct from anything in the physical world and manifest a special kind of connectedness. The occurrence of such events is part of what we ordinarily intend to assert when we speak of the existence of mind and a presupposition of all the more interesting things we want to say about them."

ADRIAN: That is an example of the swing of the pendulum.

HINSHELWOOD: I have just a very brief question to ask Lord Adrian. I wonder whether he would feel that self-consciousness ceases to be wholly lacking in the public quality that he spoke of when one takes into account the immense degree of coherence that can be achieved in the checking and cross-checking, and in all the variations that can be played upon this checking, in our communications with other people, and in our comparison of our feelings and experiences with theirs. All the elaborate mechanisms of human communication which evolution has produced contribute to this end. It would seem, therefore, that in this way our own consciousness does begin to gain that public quality that Lord Adrian thinks important. I would like to know what he feels about this point of view.

ADRIAN: I think that is quite true, there must be a great deal of corroborative evidences in any verbal reports that we make in that respect and they are public in a sense, but there is a great deal of uncertainty, I think in what we do say, because we are so untruthful, when questioned about our sensations, and when we have no particular certainty about what our sensations are and where or whether we remember something.

ECCLES: I would like to follow up Professor Thorpe's quotation by pointing out that a psychologist, John Beloff, has recently published a book in England entitled *Existence of Mind*, which is a most pointed and effective attack on Rylean philosophy. He there makes the statement that philosophers such as Ryle utilize such a cheap gibe as "the ghost in the machine," when attempting to discredit the brain-mind problem.

ADRIAN: I wish I knew more about the present developments in metaphysics and philosophy in Great Britain and in America. The interest seems to have gone largely into Wittgenstein's ideas and into logical studies, and rather left this question of mind and matter. So that was one reason why I was quoting one of the earlier philosophers who flourished in my young days.

SPERRY: I want to go back to the statement that we can build a mechanical man that can do everything that we can do. I wonder if our engineers are really that far along. There is a view that holds that consciousness may have some operational and causal use and from which it follows that in order to build a machine like the brain one would do well to plan to incorporate consciousness in the design.

ADRIAN: We should do better by incorporating consciousness, but I am merely quoting the people who design theoretical machines.

* Kneale, *On having a mind*, Cambridge [1962].

TEUBER: Unless I misunderstood Lord Adrian, he has specified at least one principal condition in order to make this computer get the first glimpse of consciousness; it would have to tell a lie. Was not that what you said?

ADRIAN: Yes! I would not have said that you could make a machine which would say it was conscious, although it was not: that would be a lie.

TEUBER: I thought of your beautiful citation from Edmund Gosse, Juvenilia.

ECCLES: I would like to invert the present discussion by asking as a neurophysiologist, why do we have to be conscious at all? We can, in principle, explain all our input-output performance in terms of activity of neuronal circuits; and, consequently, consciousness seems to be absolutely unnecessary. I don't believe this story of course; but at the same time I do not know the logical answer to it. In attempting to answer the question, why do we have to be conscious? it surely cannot be claimed as self-evident that consciousness is a necessary requisite for such performances as logical argument or reasoning, or even for initiative and creative activities.

PENFIELD: I had in mind to ask whether the robot could, in any conceivable way, see a joke. I think not. Sense of humor would, I suspect, be the last thing that a machine would have. But I would like to go a little farther and refer to something which I brought out in my own paper this morning: Each man "programs" his own brain by focusing and altering his attention, especially in childhood. In a sense, each individual mind is creating the brain mechanisms, establishing the brain connections that are functional. He does this by the selection of things to which he attends. It is easier to think of it during the earlier years of childhood. The child is establishing the functional pattern of connections. If the brain is tested later by electrical stimulation, it becomes evident that he has done one thing in one part of his cortex and another thing in another. In a sense, the child's mind is stepping in and creating the machinery of the brain.

I throw that concept in hoping for discussion, since there was no time allowed for discussion after my paper.

ADRIAN: That is rather the motion when I think of the consciousness being built up by effort, which children I think first put forward.

CHAIRMAN: I suppose this ends the discussion for the time being, and I suppose that many of us will agree that most of the really important things we perform are quite unconscious.

Developing the Themes of Preceding Papers

DISCUSSION

Chairman: Professor Granit

MAC KAY: I think what baffles us most is the problem of finding an *entity* on the conscious perceptual side to link with a corresponding entity on the physiological side. What I would like to suggest is that in this connection it pays to look for links between *activities* rather than *entities:* instead of talking about consciousness, to talk about conscious-choosing, conscious-perceiving, and the like. By concentrating on activity words we are doing much more than renaming the problem; we are focusing our minds on concepts which can conceivably have direct correlates in the activity that we observe as physiologists. Eddington once made a similar point in connection with atomic physics. *Events* such as electron impact, photon emission, and so on, are good operational concepts; but to try to discuss the electron as an entity, he suggested, was like starting from the phrase "cocking a snook" and ending up by discussing the nature of snooks waiting to be cocked!

SPERRY: I go back just a moment to where Dr. Penfield left off when he spoke of creating the brain connections. I am not questioning the fundamental idea that you are concerned with there, but I would raise the question as to whether any new structures, that is, any new fibers or any new synaptic endings, are created by this learning process. I think it is still an open question as to whether the effects of learning and memory may not be entirely membrane or molecular changes all within an existing network already organized genetically. I don't say this is the case, merely that it is still an open question.

PENFIELD: You mean a new growth of a nerve fiber? I am aware of no evidence to prove this. It is a fine distinction between that and the establishment of pathways through fibers and synapses that are there, associated with the establishment of resistance to passage in other directions. The establishment of persisting patterns is a kind of new creation.

Obviously, the nervous system must be there in the first place. But the point I would make is that, in nonsomatic areas of cortex, early conditioning or programing may take over whole areas. For example, for speech or perception, but not both.

SPERRY: I was not questioning the main concept at all, but for people concerned with the memory problem the distinction becomes critical. Just to assume that new connections are laid down would be going pretty far from their standpoint.

PENFIELD: If the human brain were all of it committed to sensory and motor and other somatic modalities, then we would have to wait for a new lobe to appear. . . . But there is a large area, at least in the human brain, which is flexible and plastic, probably more so than in the brains of lower animals. You agree with that, don't you?

SPERRY: Yes, but the issue is aside from your main point, and I did not want to sidetrack the discussion here.

THORPE: This perhaps ties up with another remark of William James (which I shall be discussing in my talk at a later session) to the effect that consciousness is what you might expect in a nervous system which has become too large to steer itself. I would very much like to know what physiologists think about this. It appeals to me, up to a point, because it seems we have evidence for consciousness at a good many levels in the animal kingdom; and one does need some evolutionary explanation for its having appeared. If James' idea is correct, it suggests that consciousness is to be regarded as a kind of emergent, resulting inevitably from the complexity of design of the brain, considered as an extremely complex piece of neural engineering. But the question for physiologists is whether they think that, in principle, there are a number of important activities which nonconscious brains could not do and which conscious brains can do. This seems to be the crux of the matter.

ECCLES: I am prepared to say that as neurophysiologists we simply have no use for consciousness in our attempts to explain how the nervous system works; that is one side of our problem. But then on the other side, as a person who is a neurophysiologist as I am, the ultimate reality for me is my conscious experiences, which alone are the primary reality. I agree with Eugene Wigner, for example, that there are two levels of reality: there is the primary reality, which is the whole of our conscious experiences, including perceptions, memories, dreams, and there is the secondary or derivative reality of the world, which is a construct from our perceptions. I want to ask people who doubt the existence of consciousness in its own right: what about the world of colors and sounds and smells? Where does that belong except as conscious experiences? It does not exist otherwise.

TEUBER: Since I don't really have an answer to Professor Eccles' question, I want to be historical for a moment. In 1564, three years after this building was erected, Galileo was born; and I think Galileo's greatest contribution to the creation of modern physics was to show to his contemporaries how to extrude pitches and colors and odors from the world. His conception of physics was based on the resolute reduction of the natural world view—the view given to conscious experience; he substituted for the richness of experienced quality of sensations an abstract world composed of matter and matter-in-motion. He cast out pitch and loudness—the subjective dimensions of tones—and introduced instead frequencies and amplitudes of vibrations in a medium. In this fashion, physics was made possible by excluding all of subjective experience except perhaps for feelings of force and resistance, and so the psychology of sensation became a residual problem once physics had become essentially complete.

Thus, physical acoustics set the stage for psychological acoustics, which has to regain, so to speak, the lost qualities of sense. In a corresponding way, the Newtonian reduction of experienced color to vibrations of an ether triggered the modern search for a psychophysics of vision, and, here, too, the physicist created the problems for psychology. With regard to smell—we speak all too easily of chemical sense, but the truth is that we haven't discovered the stimulus yet—the casting-out of subjective qualities of olfaction has been so successful that we have not regained them to this day.

SPERRY: I would question the fact that you do not need consciousness or at least that you know whether you need it or not until one can give a complete explanation of just one simple response that goes through the cortex and involves what we call consciousness. As far as I know, this has never been done yet. We may have some spinal reflexes that are moderately well accounted for, but none where a voluntary response or a perception is involved. We lack any satisfactory picture of the patterning of brain events that go on there, and until we have something better, I doubt you can be sure you don't need a little something extra, something that is a property of that whole central cerebral process that won't come out merely in the activity of the synapses or in the individual cell analysis.

ECCLES: I, of course, in a way agree with that, but neurophysiologists would agree that we have lots of activity that is cortical and that does not reach consciousness. We are all aware, for example, of all these automatic actions that are performed by people in sleep states. We can all do a great many skilled actions without being conscious of them. Then there are pathological conditions, the so-called automatic states, that Professor Penfield and Professor Jasper would know about much more than I. There are all kinds of activities which undoubtedly are cortical and which are highly complicated procedures, yet by testing the patient we can adduce no evidence at all of an associated awareness or conscious experience. The patient will later report no knowledge of what he has done. Isn't that sufficient?

SPERRY: As a simple example I don't think it has ever been shown that you can get a conditioned reflex unless the subject is aware of the stimulus in the sense of consciously experiencing it. Now there is some indication of subconscious learning, but I think it is still controversial; I don't know this literature, but I would be willing to say the majority of the evidence favors the view that the conscious effect is critical, whatever it is.

SCHAEFER: I would then ask Professor Sperry: from where do you know this exactly? And perhaps we should not be bothered so much by your question why we need consciousness; perhaps we could put it the other way round that nature could not make such complicated machines as our brain without this unfortunate by-product of creating some sort of a consciousness, and insofar one should perhaps look at the whole problem only from a methodological point of view.

My opinion is that the first thing we have immediately is consciousness. Eddington put it in one of his books that consciousness is the only thing given us directly and all other things are taken from very far away. This is absolutely true, and I feel that having knowledge of our consciousness is just the very simplest method to have something at all; and everything else comes into play by applying a completely different method, namely, the method of physics and chemistry. It is very difficult to explain and justify how physics has been created by this belief that quantitative data are something which is objective whereas qualitative data are only subjective.

My last point concerns the machine which Lord Adrian mentioned. He does not believe, he says, in a machine which tells us that it has consciousness; and he added the reason, which is, I think, the only reason which really we have not to believe, and that is that all analogs to ourselves are lacking; and we should always consider very carefully how far all our impressions or all our diagnoses of processes going on in the foreign world are based on the logical method of analogizing.

MAC KAY: In the case of a human being, we don't say that his brain is conscious, we say that *he* is conscious; to be conscious is a property of a person, not of his brain. If so, then it is not an empirical question whether a machine can be conscious; it would be a linguistic mistake to say the machine was, just as it would strictly be a linguistic mistake to say that my brain is conscious.

I agree with Professor Schaefer that my own consciousness is a primary datum, which it would be nonsense to doubt because it is the platform on which my doubting is built; but the reality of our own consciousness does not show itself in external behavior that is physically inexplicable—at least we hope as physiologists that it does not! When we come to consider artificial systems, then it is important neither to set tests nor to make claims of a kind that we would not do for the brain. We may properly ask ourselves whether it is possible that an artificial brain and body might "embody" a conscious person in the way that our brain embodies ourselves, but that is very different from asking the nonsense question whether a machine can be conscious.

BREMER: Among the various questions raised by the difficulty of defining consciousness is its relation with memory capacity. There we have clinical evidence which might give an answer to Dr. Thorpe's question. If I understood him well, Dr. Thorpe also raised the question of the operational efficiency brought by consciousness. Well, in epileptic automatisms one might observe subjects who behave quite intelligently, like the best businessman during hours and yet do not have any trace of memory of what they have done during that time. Thus they have behaved like a robot, like a machine. Whether they were conscious or not is for me a matter of convention.

PENFIELD: It seems to me in a sense we are looking at consciousness as though it were a static, stationary thing. Consciousness is a stream. It is a changing phenomenon, continuous except during sleep and coma. It is never twice the same thing; it is a flowing onward of awareness.

Jackson was particularly interested in this phenomenon, which I like to call epileptic automatism. Occasionally when a patient has a localized epileptic discharge in what we now know as the amygdaloid area (Jackson spoke of the temporosphenoidal lobe), the individual becomes automatic. He will have no future recollection of what transpires or what he does. The epileptic discharge interferes with function in the local area in the brain which has something to do with memory recording and conscious control of behavior.

One of the patients that Jackson describes behaved as follows while in such an automatic state. He got up and went to the kitchen and made some chocolate in the dish that was used to feed the cat. In another case, a doctor (who was later shown to have a small tumor in the area of the amygdala) examined a patient during his automatic state. The notes he made during this examination were reasonably accurate. He had no recollection of it, of course. You get different varieties. Sometimes there is no evidence of conscious plan. Evidently in the automatic state the automaton can pay some attention to a purpose, but always he makes no record of his stream of consciousness. That is the one constant feature of the functional deficit. We localize thus a part of the recording mechanism. Of course, all this brings us no nearer to the ultimate nature of consciousness. We can only say that the stream of awareness has a neuronal counterpart and that when this counterpart is activated electrically the stream of consciousness flows again exactly as before.

HEYMANS: I have been listening with very much interest to all those opinions, but I would like to raise a question now as a pharmacologist: whether we ought not to think somewhat more in biochemical terms and not so much in structural, anatomical, and neurological terms while speaking of nervous activities and also of consciousness? We know indeed how easy it is to interfere with many nerve activities and also with activities of the brain and consciousness, by means of some drugs that interfere with the biochemical—mainly the enzymatic processes—in the brain. So-called psychopharmacology is indeed based on biochemical processes.

SCHAEFER: On the last page of my paper you will find attempts to define in a more or less operational way the words "mind," "psyche" (or *Geist, Seele,* in German), and it reads thus: both words are synonyms and are only definable methodologically. The whole of all conscious and subjective phenomena has the quality of "mental" or "psychic" (*geistig, seelisch*). From this definition a hypothetical agent may be deduced which carries these mental (psychic) phenomena in the same formal sense, as previously the agent matter (materia) carries the physical phenomena. This agent, acting as a carrier model, is called mind or psyche. This answers, perhaps, a little of Professor Heymans's question.

GOMES: I want to make a comment to Professor Eccles about his assertion that as a neurophysiologist he cannot see a role for consciousness. Though I am not a neurophysiologist, I feel that his point of view is completely right; neurophysiology is now developed in such a way that one would look in vain, under its light, for a place or for any operational use for consciousness. Is not this obviously aberrant situation due to the fact that neurophysiology is neglecting some basic concepts it should be very specially attentive to from the start? Consciousness is the brand of individuality, that is, of something that exists for itself— clearly self-reflexively or not—and must, consequently, to some extent differentiate itself from the world where it exists. However, neurophysiology studies the nervous processes which underlie conscious life and are necessary for it, completely ignoring the concept of individuality, as if those processes were of the same nature and perfectly continuous with everything else which is going on in the universe.

ECCLES: I am not claiming to have said any final word; all I am claiming to say is that as neurophysiologists we do not take care of consciousness in our concept of the working of the brain, and we go on and on and on showing these beautiful pictures of cortical responses that we have seen, for example, of Andersen's, Creutzfeldt's, Jasper's, and Hubel's, without even considering if these responses are associated with consciousness at all. But the reason for this defect in our approach is, of course, that we are still far too primitive in our outlook as physiologists; we are at the very beginning of this tremendous task of trying to understand brains.

GOMES: I completely agree with Professor Eccles' view again. But I do insist on this point: should not neurophysiologists in general begin to pay some more attention to the concept of individuality as such and to the question of its definition in their field of research, so that questions as important as this one of the meaning of consciousness in connection with the nervous processes should not simply outline a blank? Because, after all, consciousness does exist!

CHAIRMAN: We must close this general discussion for the time being at any rate, and I would like to finish by giving my own declaration— which will be mostly, I suppose, in the nature of an answer to Dr. Thorpe. I belong to the people who were brought up in the Machian philosophy, and to me it has always semed that as physiologists we have, with the aid of consciousness, selected some basic concepts and have created a world in those terms, and that we are still engaged in studying the world in those terms and are making a great number of interesting discoveries, most of them relating to what Dr. Teuber called representation, which is, I suppose, the beginning. But I don't quite agree with Dr. Eccles that we have no use for consciousness; we have no use for it in our actual experiments; but the basis of our concepts, I think, is a conscious isolation of centimeters, grams, seconds as units of operation.

11

Pathophysiological Studies of Brain Mechanisms in Different States of Consciousness [1]

by H. H. JASPER

Université de Montréal, Montreal, Canada

Disturbances in perceptual awareness or states of consciousness due to trauma or disease of the brain in man present many challenging problems to the neurophysiologist interested in brain mechanisms. Such problems are of such enormous variety and complexity that it would be pretentious indeed to propose definitive solutions in the light of the meager neurophysiological knowledge presently at our disposal. This is especially true when one attempts to cross the "no man's land" from brain mechanisms to conscious mental experience. Recent neurophysiological studies have brought to light some new principles which may be brought to bear upon some of these old problems, a few of which I would like to present for the consideration of this conference.

In particular I would like to present for discussion the following problems:

1. In what manner and to what degree is perceptual awareness dependent upon, or independent of, the exact nature of information arriving over the principal sensory pathways?

2. Is there an anatomically distinct neuronal system in some central location, with widespread functional connections with all parts of the brain, involved in the selection of the ever-changing momentary patterns

[1] Based upon work supported by The Committee on Psychobiology of the National Science Foundation of the United States and The Medical Research Council of Canada.

of neuronal activity of perceptual awareness, as opposed to those systems constantly engaged in the unconscious processing of information and in the execution of automatic movements? or,

3. Is that portion or portions of cerebral activity upon which momentary perceptual awareness depends, or upon which it persists for recall in short- or long-term memories, due only to its inherent integrative organization in the brain as a whole whereby a certain pattern out of widely dispersed synaptic circuits may dominate the rest in an ever-changing sequence?

These questions have been discussed at length in several previous symposia and conferences, beginning with the Laurentian Conference in 1953 [Adrian et al, 1954; Jasper et al, 1958; Wolstenholme and O'Connor, 1960; Moruzzi et al, 1963]. However, much new and important neurophysiological data can now be added which should enable us to re-evaluate some previous conceptions and to make possible the formulation of working hypotheses which should lead to some more critical experimental approaches to restricted portions of the age-old problem of the ultimate relationship between brain mechanisms and conscious experience.

It is possible to make a phenomenological distinction between those brain mechanisms which occur with conscious awareness and those occurring under conditions which seem to preclude such awareness (coma, sleep, anesthesia, or inattention) and, in man, those reported as not consciously perceived. Since one is fully aware of the precarious nature of such data, it must be used in as controlled a manner as possible if we are to approach the problem of the distinction between the largely unconscious complex integrative machinery of the brain and those processes peculiarly significant for conscious perceptual awareness.

I do not mean to imply that clinically defined states of consciousness, particularly impaired consciousness, may be considered a homogeneous entity with a common physiological mechanism. There are many different kinds of coma, for example, with a wide variety of neurochemical or pathophysiological causes [Fazekas and Alman, 1962; Perria, 1964]. Our problem is to examine possible common factors in these varied disturbances in brain function which lead to impaired or disturbed perceptual awareness and the associated loss of integrated adaptive responses to environmental stimuli. Bremer [1957a] has expressed it well in describing consciousness as "une qualité particulière du fonctionnement cérébral, caractérisé par une réactivité différentielle et sélective, par l'intégration et l'organisation harmonieuse des actes du comportement, par leur adaptation correcte à la situation du moment." This definition could apply equally well to man and to animals, and would, of necessity, apply to states of unconsciousness in man, or in man deprived of verbal communi-

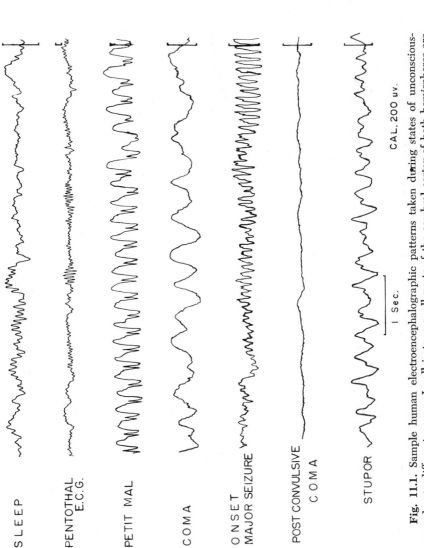

SLEEP

PENTOTHAL
E.C.G.

PETIT MAL

COMA

ONSET
MAJOR SEIZURE

POST CONVULSIVE
COMA

STUPOR

1 Sec.

CAL. 200 uv.

Fig. 11.1. Sample human electroencephalographic patterns taken during states of unconsciousness due to different causes. In all instances, all parts of the cerebral cortex of both hemispheres are involved, with regional differences in the form of abnormality in some instances.

cation. Dependence upon verbal reports of human subjects may be hazardous since such reports also depend upon memory which may be affected independently of other signs of conscious behavior, as will be discussed later.

It was once thought that the EEG might provide a reliable indicator of states of consciousness, but the wide variety of electrical patterns in different forms of unconsciousness (Fig. 11.1), including normal waking patterns in coma [Loeb, 1964] and a pattern similar to that of alertness or arousal in "paradoxical" sleep, has made the relationship between cortical electrical activity and states of consciousness a most complicated one. It seems clear, however, that in all cases of impaired consciousness there are widespread and important changes in the electrical activity of the cerebral cortex, when a fine analysis of this activity is undertaken [Jasper, 1958; Evarts, 1961, 1962, 1963; Verzeano and Negishi, 1961; Hubel, 1959, 1960].

EFFECTS OF LESIONS IN PRIMARY SENSORY SYSTEMS

The remarkable manner by which certain forms of information concerning the outside world, or concerning events within the body itself, are translated into coded messages which proceed to precisely localized specific sensory receiving stations in the brain has been illustrated particularly by Granit and Mountcastle in this symposium. It has been shown by microelectrode recording techniques that certain brain cells are highly specialized for the purpose of receiving or transmitting in a quantitative manner not only the intensity but also the location, the direction of movement, and even the specific pattern of a given stimulus.

We have recently [Jasper and Bertrand, 1964] had the opportunity of confirming the high degree of selectivity and the mechanical precision of the response of single thalamic neurons in conscious man. Although less complete in details, these studies show that even in the human brain, under the conditions existing in an operating room, tactile stimuli or movements of joints elicit regularly reproducible and constant responses in certain thalamic cells, which reflect accurately in coded form the precise location, the intensity, or the direction of change in a given stimulus. In addition, however, we are able to determine whether or not the patient is consciously aware of these stimuli and to study the effects of his attention directed toward them or directed toward something else, so that in one instance he reports a keen awareness of each stimulus and in the other he may not be aware that he has been stimulated. To our surprise, individual cells within the sensory portion of the thalamus (ventrobasal complex) continue to respond faithfully in the same manner to peripheral stimulation, whether the patient is aware of such stimuli or not. However, this is true only for cells confined to sensory nuclei. Mesial and dorsal to these cells, and never intermingled with them, are cells with quite different properties; they do not respond consistently to any form of sensory stimulus. They respond briefly to novel stimuli of many kinds and from almost any part of the body, and rapidly cease responding to repeated stimuli of the same kind. We have called them "novelty" detectors. Their activation does seem to be dependent upon factors important for conscious awareness rather than sensory discrimination, that is, the significance of a given stimulus to the organism.

In physiological experiments in animals, such as the highly discriminative response seen in visual cortical cells described by Hubel and Wiesel (see Chapter 5 by Granit), the animals cannot be aware of such cerebral events, owing to anesthesia. It seems obvious that such data, though giving great insight into how and where the brain receives and processes sensory information, imply that there must be some additional mechanism or neuronal system in the brain which must be activated for conscious perception to take place. There can be no doubt that the brain must depend upon the characteristics of specific sensory systems for the image that is constantly being constructed and projected to form the "reality" of the surrounding world, but one may raise the question as to what degree and in what manner perceptual awareness is necessarily bound to or always controlled by the information arriving over specific sensory pathways. Clinical experience with patients who have an interruption or distortion in sensory transmitting or receiving systems is of interest to this problem, and is considered in further detail by Teuber in Chapter 8.

It is common clinical experience that the brain is able to compensate for loss of major exteroceptive contact with the outside world by creation of a vivid mental life, as in the celebrated case of Helen Keller. In fact, reactions to remaining sources of sensory information and emotional life may be exaggerated in the absence of normal controls from visual and auditory pathways.

A lost limb may be replaced by a phantom limb, often with pain to which the patient exhibits exaggerated emotional reactions. Similarly exaggerated painful emotional reactions occur following a lesion of primary sensory pathways in the thalamus, the well-known *thalamic syndrome*. Loss of normal sensation from the hand due to a lesion of its nerve supply may be replaced by a hand which is excruciatingly painful to the slightest touch, *causalgic pain*. When of long standing, this condition is particularly resistant to surgical treatment. Section of the nerves supplying the painful hand may not bring relief [Livingston, 1943; White and Sweet, 1955]. Such observations suggest that central brain mechanisms upon which conscious sensory experience depends must have the capability of being activated independently of the information arriving over normal sensory input channels. Electrophysiological studies have abundantly confirmed this conclusion by the recording of "spontaneous" neuronal discharge in many cells of all sensory pathways, including the retinae, providing they have not been silenced with anesthesia [Granit, 1955]. For example, the cells of the retinae discharge so actively in total darkness that the total number of impulses in the optic nerve is greater in the non-illuminated eye, the effect of light being, on the average, to reduce the total retinal discharge [Arduini and Pinneo, 1962; Arduini, 1963]. Certainly many central neurons, even in specific sensory systems, show much continuous activity in the absence of deliberate stimulation, and many respond to a stimulus by an arrest or inhibition of their discharge (see Chapter 5 by Granit). Such evidence demands a re-evaluation of the nature of the dependency of the brain upon activation from incoming sensory impulses for perceptual awareness.

In this connection it is pertinent to recall the early experiments of Adrian and Matthews [1934], who showed that the characteristic arrest of the alpha rhythm from the occipital region in man in response to opening the eyes with visual attention occurs in the same manner when the eyes are opened in a completely darkened room, in the absence of visual stimulation, when the subject is attempting to see. It was then demonstrated both in man and in experimental animals that this reaction of the visual cortex could be readily conditioned to nonvisual stimuli ([Jasper and Shagass, 1941a and 1941b], and Fig. 11.2) brought under a degree of "voluntary" control. It is important to note in the example of Fig. 11.2 that the typical changes in the electrical activity from the occipital cortex in man to a visual stimulus (blocking of the alpha rhythm) occurred in the absence of any form of stimulus, owing only to having repeated the visual stimulus at regular 10-sec intervals for 54 consecutive trials. Even before the time for the 55th trial there was an anticipatory blocking of the alpha rhythm, showing a remarkable degree of central control of occipital cortical activity depending upon a conditioned interval of time. It is not known just what neuronal elements in the visual cortex participate in this reaction, but it has been shown that there are many cells in the primary and secondary or paravisual cortical receiving areas in animals which respond to nonvisual stimuli [Jung, 1958; Jung et al, 1963; Jasper, 1963]; and certain cells in the auditory cortex have been shown to respond to auditory stimulation only when the animal appears to be attending to the stimulus, the "attention" units described by Hubel et al [1959]. Such studies show clearly that sensory receiving areas of the cerebral cortex, under conditions compatible with perceptual awareness, are not rigorously stimulus bound, and may be activated independently of the normal influx of specific sensory information. Their

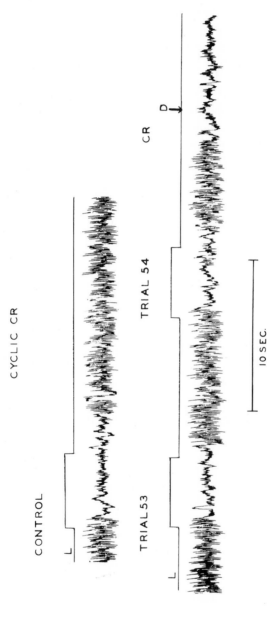

Fig. 11.2. Example of cyclic conditioning of the alpha rhythm from the occipital region in man. Note that after 54 presentations of the light stimulus at regular 15 sec intervals there occurs an anticipatory response (CR) which continues throughout the period when the light would have occurred, even though no stimulus was presented during this time [from Jasper and Shagass, 1941b].

subliminal activation in different states of vigilance alters the nature of their response to specific stimuli [Creutzfeldt and Jung, 1960; Evarts, 1960; Evarts et al, 1962; Fuster, 1961; Fuster and Docter, 1962].

Sensitization and Partial Denervation

It has been demonstrated that nerve centers become hypersensitive to chemical and to electrical excitation after a period of partial denervation [Canon and Rosenblueth, 1949; Stavraky, 1961; Sharpless and Halpern, 1962; Sharpless, 1964]. The presence of the normal flow of sensory influx to these centers appears, therefore, to be necessary to the maintenance of their normal excitability. Compensatory proliferation of remaining synaptic terminals occurs [McCouch et al, 1958], together with chemical alteration in neuronal membranes, causing excessive and abnormal response to minimal excitation and particularly to acetylcholine [Sharpless, 1964]. In partially isolated cortex, for example, after–discharges to electrical stimulation are much prolonged, beginning 5–6 days after denervation [Sharpless and Halpern, 1962], but the increased tendency to after-discharge can be prevented by frequent stimulation, apparently replacing, in effect, the afferent bombardment which the cortex is habitually receiving under normal conditions. This may be one of the mechanisms whereby perceptual awareness may be actually increased and distorted by a decrease in the normal afferent influx. Atrophy and complete functional loss may occur, however, in certain centers permanently and completely deprived of all afferent input [Wiesel and Hubel, 1962, 1963].

It is of particular interest that it is not necessary actually to interrupt the afferent nerve fibers, and to allow them to degenerate for the hypersensitization to occur, although degeneration may be necessary to stimulate proliferation of remaining synaptic terminals. Sensitization occurs even when the nerve fibers or their synaptic or effector junctions are blocked for a sufficient period of time (hours or days) and disappears when these fibers or terminals are allowed to conduct normally again [Thesleff, 1960; Emmelin, 1961; Trendelenberg, 1963]. This may be of considerable significance in explaining some of the effects of sensory deprivation.

Sensory Deprivation and Habituation

Another way to study the nature of the dependency of conscious awareness upon a normal and varied contact with the external environment of the organism is to reduce environmental stimuli to a minimum consistent with life, and to make such remaining stimuli as constant and invariable as possible. The latter results in additional effective sensory deprivation by the process of habituation, that is, decreased responsiveness of the organism to monotonously repeated stimuli without re-enforcement. All experiments on functional sensory deprivation involve a large element of habituation, so that the two processes must be considered together in any attempt to understand the neurophysiological mechanisms underlying the effect of such conditions upon behavior and perceptual awareness.

Habituation is a very general phenomenon in the biological world, being present in lower organisms such as the snail [Holmgren and Frenk, 1961], and probably also in the isolated spinal cord [Kozak, MacFarlane, and Westerman, 1962]. It is to be clearly distinguished from adaptation of sense organs since it occurs under conditions which preclude sensory adaptation and even without reduction in early components of evoked responses in sensory cortex in the cat ([Sharpless and Jasper, 1956] and Fig. 11.3).

In Pavlovian experiments with the conditioned reflex technique, decreased response to monotonously repeated unre-enforced stimuli in a carefully controlled uniform environment produces what has been termed "internal inhibition" and sleep in experimental animals. Sleep can be induced by rhythmic electrical stimulation of a cutaneous nerve in the cat [Pompeiano and Swett, 1962].

The advent of sleep as an escape from monotonous environmental stimuli is a common experience, but of particular importance to individuals engaged in repetitive activities in industry, or in long sustained watches before a radar screen in isolated outposts of the far north, where sustained and accurate observations may be of critical importance. It was because of the danger of false observations under these conditions that experimental studies on human subjects isolated in a soundproof room with a minimal change in environmental stimuli was undertaken in Professor Hebb's laboratories at McGill University [Heron, 1961]. University students were paid to live day and night in as complete isolation as possible, even with greatly restricted movements, virtual absence of external stimuli, and minimal relatively constant stimulation of the body surface. They did sleep excessively in the beginning, but after two or three days they began to be very much disturbed by vivid hallucinations, distorted but active, and sometimes intense conscious experiences which some could or would not stand for long in spite of being paid for doing nothing.

The physiological basis for the tendency of the brain to create its own illusory experiences in compensation for the loss of normal varied

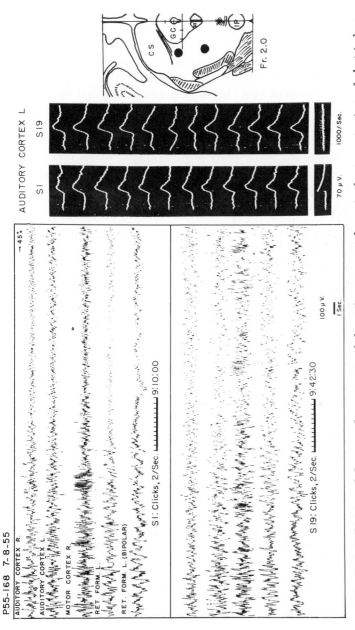

Fig. 11.3. Habituation of the arousal response to clicks at 2 per sec, as shown in the upper tracings of electrical activity from implanted electrodes in the brain of a freely moving unanesthetized cat. The generalized response failed to appear and the animal remained asleep during the 19th presentation of this identical series of clicks. The two columns of oscilloscope tracings on the right were taken of the early responses from the primary auditory cortex before and after habituation. The cross section diagram of the brain stem on the right shows the location of recording electrodes from which the last two tracings of the EEG's were taken [from Sharpless and Jasper, 1956].

influx of sensory information is poorly understood. There can be no doubt, however, of its physiopathological importance in the context of this conference. It provides a dramatic demonstration of the degree to which perceptual awareness may be dissociated from its dependence upon peripheral sensory processes and become largely centrally determined or grossly distorted, though not diminished in intensity, when the controls of a constant and varied contact with the outside world are reduced over a sufficiently long period of time. It has been postulated that the process of denervation sensitization may also play a role in such phenomena, but far more complex mechanisms may be also involved. Unfortunately, neurophysiologists have very little to offer when challenged with the task of attempting to explain the many gross disturbances in perceptual awareness in mental diseases, though the possibility of reproducing some of them by hallucinogenic drugs (such as lysergic acid diethylamide, LSD) has opened up avenues of experimental study which show great promise for the future [Evarts, 1957, 1962].

On the Significance of the So-called "Nonspecific" Neuronal Systems: The Centrencephalic Integrating System, or the Reticular Activating System

In spite of the weight of clinical and experimental evidence which has been reviewed in numerous symposia and conferences since the Laurentian Conference in 1953 concerning the anatomical identification and functional importance of a separate "centrencephalic" or "reticular" neuronal system whose activation is required for neuronal activity in the brain to be translated into conscious awareness, thorough proof of this hypothesis is still lacking. Dr. Perria has summed up the present situation very well in his introduction to a recent conference in Genoa on The Physiopathology of States of Consciousness [Perria, 1964] as follows: "Nevertheless, there are still perplexities and zones of shadow on the wide problem of the neural mechanisms underlying consciousness, both in the field of research and in that of clinical pathology." Brodal, reviewing the anatomical evidence, concludes that "Anatomically the RF of the brain stem has no entity" which is in agreement with the conclusion of the late Dr. Olszewski ten years before at the Laurentian Conference. Brodal asks "whether it is not timely to deprive the RF of some of its supremacy as concerns consciousness, and to consider this, like so many other functions, as being more or less dependent on the whole brain." A similar point of view was expressed by other participants in this conference based upon clinical as well as experimental evidence for the importance of states of activation of the cortex as a whole, and of other brain structures which seem of critical importance in the determination of states of consciousness.

Kristiansen recalls Penfield's statement [1957] that

> . . . it would be absurd to suppose that central integration could take place without implication and employment of cortical areas selected appropriately to the needs of the organization that faces the brain mechanism. To suppose that centrencephalic integration is possible without utilization of the cortex would be to return to the thinking of Descartes and to enthrone again a spiritual homunculus in some area such as the nearby pineal gland. It would be equally absurd to consider that the reticular formation is functionally separable from the cortex.

Penfield states the problem well when he emphasizes functional interaction rather than localization, and selection of only certain cortical processes by some as yet unknown process to be dominantly involved in perceptual awareness. He might have added that it is also absurd to assume that all of the multitudinous activities of the brain as a whole can be simultaneously involved in the perceptual awareness of a given moment. The more refined our anatomical and electrophysiological techniques become, the more highly specialized do we find the individual neurons and local assemblies in different parts of the brain. Even the more complex functions appear to have their regional localization, not necessarily involving "the brain as a whole." It seems more consistent with such facts to assume that each "bit" of perceptual awareness (in the sense of information theory) is restricted to a highly specific and limited assembly of neurons. What then constitutes the neurophysiological basis for a distinction between conscious and unconscious levels of neuronal integration? To reverse the question, by what mechanism are myriads of actively integrating and transmitting neuronal networks excluded from the unified perceptual awareness of a given moment? Is it not possible that there are also neuronal systems of most highly complex innervation, which are specialized for conscious perceptual awareness rather than to attempt to attribute this function to the "brain as a whole"? It may be analogous to the fact that relatively few cells in the visual cortex respond to diffuse illumination of the retina as a whole [Hubel and Wiesel, 1962], but require highly specific patterns in the visual field for their excitation. It is true that more careful analytic physiological studies have proved that the reticular system is far from homogeneous in function as well as in structure, that the activating system is composed of both inhibitory and excitatory components, and that it may possess a more specialized internal organization than was originally supposed. But does the fact that the functional and structural properties of the retina, the lateral geniculate body, and the visual cortex are different, and that highly integrative processes take place in all, prevent one from speaking of "the visual system" as a unit of specialized function? Is it not possible, therefore, to conceive of an interconnected neuronal network composed of heteromorphous neuronal elements extending throughout the brain stem and into the diencephalon, with widespread to-and-fro connections to the cerebral cortex (possibly including specialized cortical interneurons, but excluding direct participation of the major sensory and motor transmitting systems), which may have, among other functions, a peculiar specialized significance in neuronal transactions or interactions of critical importance to conscious awareness?

CHEMICAL CORRELATES OF CORTICAL ACTIVATION

Recent studies of Shute and Lewis [1963] have shown that there may be a chemical specificity to certain neurons belonging to the physiologically determined diffuse projection system of upper midbrain and thalamus, and significantly also to cells of the hippocampus. These cells were shown to contain high concentrations of intracellular cholinesterase, in contradistinction to thalamic cells of the specific sensory relay nucleus. This was considered to provide support for the suggestion made by Bremer [1957] and others [Desmedt and La Grutta, 1957; Smirnov and Ilyuchenok, 1962; Hernandez-Peon, 1964] that desynchronizing activation or "arousal" of the cortex of brain stem origin may be mediated by acetylcholine or a related cholinergic substance. Support for this conclusion has been recently provided by the demonstration that the rate of release of ACH from the cortex is definitely increased during arousal of brain stem origin, and is apparently absent in undercut cortex, deprived of its afferent supply [MacIntosh and Oborin, 1953; Mitchell, 1963; Sie, Jasper, and Wolfe, 1965; Kanai and Szerb, 1965].

In experiments on rate of liberation we have found that unilateral destruction of the mesial brain stem at the mesodiencephalic junction, sparing the lemniscal sensory pathways, caused a marked reduction in ACH output from the cortex of the hemisphere showing constant sleep spindles, as compared with the intact side when samples from the two sides were taken simultaneously (3.6 to 1.4 ng per min per cm², see Table 1). This would be consistent with the proposal of Shute and Lewis and also with the conclusion that the diffuse projection system may be cholinergic as distinct from the (unknown) mediator for specific sensory synapses. These results are consistent with the conclusions of Pepeu and Mantegazzini [1964; also Mantegazzini and Pepeu, 1964], who found that the ACH content of cortical tissue was much higher in the synchronized "sleeping" hemisphere on the side of a hemisection of the

Table 1

The Effect on Cortical ACH Release of Left Hemisection at Mesodiencephalic Level, Followed by Complete Section in an Atropinized Preparation

ACH Release (ng per min; 15 min samples)

Neuraxially Intact		Hemisection, Left		Complete Section	
Left	Right	Left	Right	Left	Right
(pooled)		(sectioned)		(pooled)	
3.33		1.60	3.44	0.74	
3.70		1.54	3.45	0.77	
4.30		1.18	3.85	0.83	
3.10		1.43	3.57	0.74	
3.61 ± 0.32					
		1.43 ± 0.19	3.57 ± 0.19	0.77 ± 0.04	
Mean % of control mean 100		38.6	98.9	21.3	

brain stem, with a lower content in cortex of the opposite hemisphere which had shown a waking EEG pattern prior to extraction. This implies increased rate of liberation in aroused cortex, as we found independently. This was recently confirmed by Kanai and Szerb [1965], who believed that specific sensory cortical areas may be also partially cholinergic, but separation of the two systems was not effectively carried out in their experiments. A possible neurohumoral function of ACH should also be considered [Koelle, 1962; Desmedt and La Grutta, 1957].

The microelectrophoretic studies of Krnjević and Phillis [1963] clearly demonstrated that certain cortical cells can be activated by ACH, the activation being blocked by atropine. The slow onset and prolonged effect was consistent with a muscarinic type of cholinergic receptor. Of considerable interest was the fact that ACH release was blocked by chloralose in spite of the marked enhancement of specific sensory-evoked potentials which characterize the action of this drug. It was concluded by these authors that ACH was not the mediator for specific sensory terminals in the cortex, but must be related to other synaptic sites controlling the spontaneous activity or after-discharge to specific afferent volleys.

ACH has long been known to have a remarkable facilitating action upon cortical after-discharge and spontaneous rhythms. It may be noted also that Bremer has pointed out that one of the most characteristic features of the "aroused" cortex, as compared with that in "sleep" due to a brain stem section or to light barbiturate anesthesia, is a change in the character of the after-discharge to a specific afferent volley [Bremer and Bonnet, 1950; Bremer, 1959, 1961].

Recently, in continuing experiments with Celesia with an improved superperfusion technique, we have found higher rates of ACH liberation (3–4 ng per min per cm^2) in the intact cat without general anesthesia, showing largely an aroused EEG pattern, with a reduction to about 2 ng per min per cm^2 during normal sleep without brain stem section.

These studies prove that the marked changes in the state of activation of the cortex of nonspecific brain stem or diencephalic origin produce important changes in cortical reactivity which may have a specific chemical basis, affecting particularly spontaneous activity and late sensory responses or after-discharge. That other chemical changes may occur in activated cortex, including a decrease in "inhibitory" substances, is shown by the work of Jasper, Khan, and Elliott [1965, Table 2].

Table 2

Release of GABA
from the Surface of the Cerebral Cortex

Preparation	ECoG Pattern	No. of Samples	GABA Released μg/hr/cm^2 Average S.D.	
Neuraxially intact	Aroused	4	0.60 ± 0.20	
Cervical section "Encéphale isolé"	Aroused	6	0.66 ± 0.26	
Midbrain section "Cerveau isolé"	Sleep	17	2.09 ± 0.60	
Left midcollicular hemi-section				
Right hemisphere	Aroused	2	0.80	1.01
Left hemisphere	Sleep	2	2.12	2.60

ON THE SIGNIFICANCE OF THE PROLONGATION AND ENHANCEMENT OF RESPONSE IN CORTICAL SENSORY SYSTEMS

There is considerable evidence to suggest that diminished awareness due to anesthesia or even natural sleep affects principally the later com-

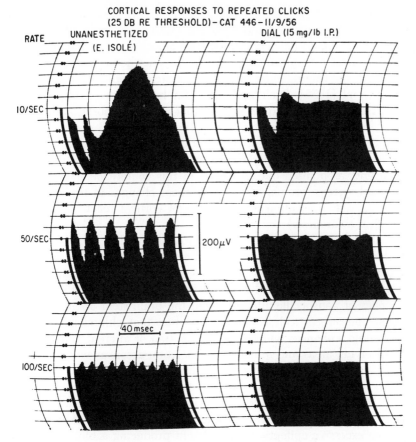

CORTICAL RESPONSES TO REPEATED CLICKS
(25 DB RE THRESHOLD) – CAT 446 – 11/9/56

Fig. 11.4. Average auditory cortical responses to repeated clicks in the cat before and after the administration of Dial anesthesia (15 mg per kg i.p.). Number of responses averaged: 600 at 10 per sec, 3,000 at 50 per sec, 6,000 at 100 per sec [from Goldstein et al, 1959].

ponents of evoked responses to afferent volleys. This is particularly clear in computer-averaged responses, as illustrated in Fig. 11.4 [from Goldstein et al, 1959], for the auditory cortex. For example, Evarts [1963] was able to show a facilitation only in the late responses of single cells in the visual cortex of the cat during waking as compared to natural sleep, there being no significant change in the early unit responses. Such evidence suggests that, even though initial primary activation of cortical sensory cells may be little affected in conditions which preclude conscious awareness, the elaboration of sensory information to involve additional neurons even in sensory cortex itself, and the prolongation of response in time, may be of critical importance [Fleming and Evarts,

1959; Brazier, 1957, 1958; Andersson, 1965]. This is consistent with the observation of Yamamoto and Schaeppi [1961], who showed that it was principally the long latency units in both cortex and brain stem reticular formation which were primarily affected by anesthesia, rather than a special effect on the reticular activating system alone, as suggested by French et al [1953]. Such studies should be extended into even much longer times with techniques such as that used by Robertson and Evans [1964], who showed acceleration in visual cortical cell discharge lasting 20 to 40 minutes following a single brief flash of light. Such prolonged effects are of obvious importance also to theories of neural mechanisms of learning, as pointed out by Eccles in this conference. (Of course, in the visual system, prolonged photochemical changes in the retina must be considered in addition to conditions of cortical reactivity as related to level of awareness.)

It has been postulated that conduction of impulses from cortical sensory receiving areas to a centrencephalic system of neurons may be critical for conscious awareness. This may well be true, but perhaps only following extensive cortical elaboration, re-enforced by the activating influences of nonspecific afferents from the brain stem upon widespread cortical and subcortical structures. The fact that chloralose anesthesia, for example, enhances widespread conduction of afferent volleys in sensory receiving areas and in cortical association areas, as well as in "nonspecific" portions of thalamus and brain stem, even though the animal appears to be unconscious, shows that simple conduction of afferent volleys to the "centrencephalic system" is not sufficient for conscious awareness to occur. This is probably analogous to the unconscious state resulting from excessive epileptic bombardment producing a blockade of integrative functions of the systems critical to conscious awareness. This implies that a certain level of integration, rather than simple activation of certain neuronal systems, is critical to the existence of conscious awareness. The fact that chloralose also blocks the release of ACH in the cortex suggests that critical chemical reactions in only certain classes of cortical neurons may be a necessary accompaniment of the type of activation necessary to translate information processing into conscious awareness. It seems clear, at any rate, that marked changes do occur in cortical activity in conscious as opposed to unconscious states of the brain, and that the importance of the centrencephalic or reticular system of the brain stem probably lies not in its importance as a localization of conscious processes, but in its remarkable and widespread interactions with more specialized neuronal systems, somehow determining which of these functional systems is to gain momentary predominance in the on-going sequence of conscious awareness. It would seem wrong to call this a nonspecific function in the broad sense of the word, for in neuronal systems what could be more specific than the complex reactions which provide that increment of integrated activation necessary for conscious awareness.

The importance of critical interactions between subcortical and cortical mechanisms in the determination of states of consciousness is shown also in recent analyses of the mechanism of the spike and wave of experimental "petit mal" epileptic attacks, a most fascinating physiopathological process capable of reversibly turning off and on the mechanisms of conscious awareness. Although reproduced experimentally by electrical stimulation of the brain stem and mesial thalamus, the slow wave of the complex has been recently shown to be associated with a prolonged hyperpolarizing inhibition when recorded from intracellular microelectrodes in the cerebral cortex [Pollen, 1964]. Thus the neuronal systems which serve to project such a disturbance over wide areas of the cerebral cortex may be concentrated in a "centrencephalic" system of brain stem and thalamus. Profound alterations in cortical function itself must be associated with the impaired state of conscious awareness which characterizes the petit mal seizure, even though certain relatively automatic cortical functions seem to be preserved to some degree in some cases [Penfield and Jasper, 1954].

LESIONS OF THE BRAIN AFFECTING MEMORY RECORDING MECHANISMS
INDEPENDENT OF CONSCIOUS AWARENESS AND SHORT-TERM RECALL
OF PRESENT EXPERIENCE

In man, bilateral lesions of the hippocampal formation or the mesial portion of the diencephalon [Scoville and Milner, 1957; Penfield and Milner, 1958; Milner, 1958; Stepien et al, 1960; Stepien and Sierpinski, 1960, 1964], without involvement of specific sensory pathways, result in the inability to preserve long-term memories. Such individuals appear quite alert and intelligent, substituting old memories for the absence of memory for present experiences, except for a few minutes time, sometimes prolonged by deliberate repetition. I do not intend to present such evidence in detail, but only to point out that the problem of the neurophysiology or neurochemistry of memory recording may be dissociated from that of conscious awareness. We are just as ignorant of the intimate mechanisms of one as of the other, though we may be better guided as to where to look.

Sperry has shown quite clearly, as have others, that certain specific memories seem to be laid down in different regions of the cerebral cortex and of one hemisphere after section of the corpus callosum. Why then are long-term memories not laid down in man in the absence of certain critical subcortical structures? It would seem that the problem is similar to that of conscious awareness, in which regions of the brain stem and diencephalon also seem to be of critical importance [Lindsley et al, 1950; Cairns, 1952; French, 1952; Kristiansen, 1964]. Interaction between cortical and subcortical projection systems may be necessary, possibly involving specific re-enforcing or "fixing" processes, somehow linking those widespread neuronal circuits or "assemblies" [Hebb, 1949] into a dynamic pattern whose code must be engraved in a remarkably permanent manner on the brain. Certainly the changes in synaptic function consequent upon repetitive activity alone will never explain such long-term memories, for they are as selective as are the processes of conscious awareness. But one cannot "locate" memories in the subcortical structures so essential to their establishment since the importance of these systems seems related to their interaction with other parts of the brain, particularly with neuronal processes of the cerebral cortex [Cobb, 1952; Jasper, 1960, 1964].

Summary

In this paper the attempt has been made to bring to the attention of this conference certain clinical physiopathological conditions involving disturbances or loss of perceptual awareness and memory in relation to experimental neurophysiological studies on the brain of man and animals. It is apparent that attempts to explain the more complex clinical conditions on the basis of present neurophysiological knowledge is most unsatisfactory and fraught with the hazards of premature speculation. Without pretending to be able to reach definitive conclusions, certain working hypotheses may be formulated as a guide to future research.

It seems clear that perceptual awareness is not rigorously stimulus bound, nor is it dependent solely upon the transducer properties of peripheral receptors and the manner in which the impulses they generate are conducted and transformed to reach specific receiving stations of thalamus and cerebral cortex. Compensatory hypersensitivity may develop in central sensory systems of the brain following decreased afferent influx, and decreased sensitivity of alerting mechanisms may result from monotonous insignificant stimuli resulting in decrease in level of awareness. Central sensory systems may be activated in the absence of immediate sensory influx by "nonspecific" control mechanisms which also regulate their reactivity to incoming sensory information.

Evidence from the effect of acute local lesions of the brain in man which cause loss of perceptual awareness, as well as comparable lesions in experimental animals, suggests that neuronal systems in the central core of brain stem and diencephalon are either directly or indirectly involved in brain mechanisms critical to perceptual awareness, when indirect effects upon the circulatory or metabolic state of the brain as a whole can be satisfactorily ruled out. This hypothetical "centrencephalic" system of neurons is in constant interaction with the cerebral cortex as well as with subcortical synaptic stations. It seems to be this special form of interaction, involving widespread neuronal elements in cortical and subcortical structures, which determines the nature of the highly selective and specialized form of integration necessary for conscious awareness. Evidence is brought forward which suggests that this involves particularly the later elaboration of sensory influx, with a prolongation of response duration, and that it may depend upon synaptic mechanisms which are anatomically and chemically distinct from those involved in the transmission of sensory information, cholinergic synapses being probably of particular importance in the cortical component of this process.

Local brain lesions affecting the hippocampal system bilaterally and related portions of the brain stem and mesial thalamus in man may prevent the storage of long-term memories without affecting immediate perceptual awareness and short-term recall. This does not imply a localization of memory traces in these structures, since recall of already established memories is preserved. It seems to depend upon an interaction between these structures and selective on-going neuronal processes in cerebral cortex where essential components of the permanent memory trace are laid down. It may be of importance that cholinergic synapses are also particularly prominent in the hippocampus, though the nature of this critical interaction is completely obscure. As for conscious awareness, the prolongation in time of activity in special integrative neuronal networks may be most important for their preservation in memory.

Perceptual awareness as well as memory recording can also be prevented by excessive synchronous rhythmic discharge involving the same neuronal systems upon which they normally depend, as in certain forms of epileptic attack, and with chloralose anesthesia. This implies that a certain level of integration, as well as specific activation, is necessary for perceptual awareness as well as for memory recording to take place.

DISCUSSION

Chairman: PROFESSOR GRANIT

BREMER: I fully agree with the conclusion of Dr. Jasper's report concerning the great importance of the late events in cortical sensory potentials for perceptual integration and for the laying down of memory traces. Already in my early work I insisted on that notion. I had been struck by the fact that, in barbiturate narcosis, the primary-evoked potential was increased at a time when what I called the fast after-discharge of the response, a local phenomenon, had disappeared. Apparently, conscious perception requires a prolongation of cortical activation already in the sensory receptive area itself and also, as you suggest, in association areas connected intimately with the last one.

Another point on which I wish to comment concerns your humoral and pharmacological observations. They seem to me very interesting and important, indeed, especially the data concerning the concentrations of acetylcholine and gamma-aminobutyric acid in various areas and in various functional conditions of the brain. Yet, the importance of these changes does not necessarily mean, I think that you would agree, that they do relate to mediation processes. Even for acetylcholine the question can be raised. One may ask if it could not sometimes represent a local hormone in the brain in the sense given to that term by Burn and Feldberg.

A curious and certainly important fact which struck me again in hearing you is that your method, which recalls MacIntosh and Oborin's work, required, as in their experiments, the application of atropine in order to obtain detectable amounts of acetylcholine at the pial surface of the brain cortex.

JASPER: Though the illustration I gave happened to be of an animal with atropine, atropine is not necessary at all.

BREMER: Anyhow, there is evidence, based on microphysiological recordings and electrophoretic application of acetylcholine, that there are in the brain cortex cholinoceptive cells. In one of these papers the significant fact was mentioned that the cholinoceptive cortical cells were the ones which, when activated physiologically, gave long repetitive discharges.

JASPER: I did not have time to elaborate on the atropine effects, which are certainly very critical here for understanding. The rate of liberation without atropine is of the order of 2–4 ng per min cm^{-2}, and in the atropinized preparation this may be as high as 12 ng per min cm^{-2}. While increasing the liberation of acetylcholine, atropine prevents the activity of acetylcholine on the cortex, and at the same time the activated picture is changed to a sleeping picture, even though there is far more acetylcholine being liberated than before. Eserine or prostigmine also changes the EEG picture; the correlation between the acetylcholine and the EEG is altered by the presence of eserine.

I should also refer again to the finding of Pepeu and Mantegazzini, who explained their results by postulating that with less liberation there is more storage, and hence the higher ACH content of the sleeping cortex. So we have very complex relations where atropine will block the use of acetylcholine by blocking the receptive sites, thus allowing more to accumulate; and it allows more to accumulate if the ACH is not liberated in the sleeping cortex.

CHAGAS: A part of the question I wanted to ask Dr. Jasper was now just answered in the extremely interesting considerations which he forwarded in reply to Professor Bremer. But I would still like to ask him whether he thinks that the data we have already gathered on nervous unit analysis is sufficient for the explanation of increased conduction during chloralose anesthesia, or how, at any cost, he would actually explain the phenomenon.

JASPER: I have to assume chemically specific cells and that chloralose blocks the cholinoceptive units, which has been shown by Krnjević and Phillis in their microelectrode studies; and at the same time, chloralose enhances the noncholinergic primary sensory pathway, and so the responses in nonsensory areas as well. However, it blocks the elaboration of this volley within the cortex as well as the fine elaboration in other areas. So that there must be this integrative or elaborative concept of impulse transmission in specialized neuronal networks, which has to go into the picture of the physiology of consciousness as well as simple conduction.

ANDERSEN: You showed very beautifully how the intracellularly recorded hyperpolarizing potentials occurred simultaneously with the slow waves in the petit mal electrocorticogram. I wondered if, by your thalamic stimulation in the petit mal situation, you have an increased barrage of thalamocortical volleys, so that you produce large inhibitory potentials in a great number of cells, and reduce the number of active cells in the cortex. The petit mal unconsciousness could thus be related to the number of active cortical cells. Is that possible?

JASPER: I would agree with you only to the extent that the cortex participates in this petit mal process, but not to the extent that it is only the activation of more cortical cells that does it. Any other pattern of activation and even activation in different ways will not produce this pattern, so that there must be a specificity both to the type of afferent activation and to the timing as well.

REFERENCES

ADAMS, R. D., G. H. COLLINS, and M. VICTOR. Troubles de la mémoire et de l'apprentissage chez l'homme. Leurs relations avec des lésions de lobes temporaux et du diencéphale. *Physiologie de l'Hippocampe.* Paris: Colloque du Centre National de la Recherche Scientifique, pp. 273–295 [1962].

ADRIAN, E. D., and B. H. C. MATTHEWS. The Berger rhythm: Potential changes from the occipital lobes in man, *Brain,* 57, 355–384 [1934].

———, F. BREMER, and H. JASPER, eds. *Brain Mechanisms and Consciousness.* Oxford: Blackwell, 556 pp. [1954].

ANDERSSON, S. H. Intracellular postsynaptic potentials in somatosensory cortex of the cat, *Nature,* 205, 297–298 [1965].

ARDUINI, A. The tonic discharge of the retina and its central effects, in: *Brain Mechanisms, Progress in Brain Research.* Amsterdam: Elsevier, Vol. 1, pp. 184–206 [1963].

———, and L. PINNEO. Properties of the retina in response to steady illumination, *Arch. Ital. Biol.,* 100, 425–448 [1962].

BRAZIER, M. A. B. A study of the late response to flash in the cortex of the cat, *Acta Physiol. Pharm. Néerl.,* 6, 692–714 [1957].

———. Studies of evoked responses by flash in man and cat, in: *Reticular Formation of the Brain* (ed. by H. H. Jasper, L. D. Proctor, R. S. Knighton,

W. C. Noshay, and R. T. Costello). Boston: Little, Brown, pp. 151–168 [1958].

BREMER, F. Altération caractéristique et semblable des réponses sensorielles des zones de projection de l'écorce cérébrale dans le sommeil spontané et dans le sommeil barbiturique. Comparaison avec l'action de la narcose éthérique, *Boll. Soc. Ital. Biologia Sperimentale, 13*, 96–102 [1938].

————. De quelques problèmes posés par la physiopathologie des altérations de la conscience. Premier Congr. Internat. Soc. Neurol. Seconde Journée Commune. Rapports et discussions. *Acta Med. Belg.* (Brussels), p. 237 [1957a].

————. Médiateurs chimiques et activités nerveuses centrales chez les vertèbres, *Actualités Pharmacologiques, 10*, 1–45 [1957b].

————. Neurophysiological mechanisms in cerebral arousal, in: *The Nature of Sleep* (ed. by G. E. W. Wolstenholme and M. O'Connor), Ciba Foundation Symposium. London: Churchill, pp. 30–50 [1961].

————, and V. BONNET. Interprétation des réactions rhythmiques prolongées des aires sensorielles de l'écorce cérébrale, *Electroenceph. Clin. Neurophysiol., 2*, 389–400 [1950].

CAIRNS, H. Disturbances of consciousness with lesions of the brain stem and diencephalon, *Brain, 75*, 109–146 [1952].

CANON, W. B., and A. ROSENBLUETH. *The Supersensitivity of Denervated Structures.* New York: Macmillan, p. 245 [1949].

COBB, S. On the nature and locus of mind, *Amer. Med. Ass. Arch. Neurol. Psychiatr., 67*, 172–177 [1952].

CREUTZFELDT, O. D., and R. JUNG. Neuronal discharge in the cat's motor cortex during sleep and arousal, in: *The Nature of Sleep* (ed. by G. E. W. Wolstenholme and M. O'Connor), Ciba Foundation Symposium. London: Churchill, pp. 131–170 [1960].

DESMEDT, J. E., and G. LA GRUTTA. The effect of selective inhibition of pseudocholinesterase on the spontaneous and evoked activity of the cat's cerebral cortex, *J. Physiol., 136*, 20–40 [1957].

EMMELIN, N. Supersensitivity following "pharmacological denervation," *Pharmacol. Revs., 13*, 17–37 [1961].

EVARTS, E. V. A review of the neurophysiological effects of lysergic acid diethylamide (LSD) and other psychotomimetic agents, *Ann. N. Y. Acad. Sci., 66*, 479–495 [1957].

————. Effects of sleep and waking on activity of single units in the unrestrained cat, in: *The Nature of Sleep* (ed. by G. E. W. Wolstenholme and M. O'Connor), Ciba Foundation Symposium. London: Churchill, pp. 171–187 [1961].

————. A neurophysiological theory of hallucinations, in: *Hallucinations* (ed. by L. J. West). New York: Grune and Stratton, pp. 1–14 [1962a].

————. Activity of neurones in visual cortex of cat during sleep with low voltage fast EEG activity, *J. Neurophysiol., 25*, 812–816 [1962b].

————. Photically evoked responses in visual cortex units during sleep and waking, *J. Neurophysiol., 26*, 229–248 [1963].

EVARTS, E. V., E. BENTAL, B. BIHARI, and P. R. HUTTENLOCHER. Spontaneous discharge of single neurons during sleep and waking, *Science, 135,* 726–728 [1962].

FAZEKAS, J. H., and R. M. ALMAN. *Coma: Biochemistry, Physiology and Therapeutic Principles.* Springfield, Ill.: C. C Thomas, 114 pp. [1962].

FLEMING, T. C., and E. V. EVARTS. Multiple response to photic stimulation in cats, *Amer. J. Physiol., 197,* 1233–1236 [1959].

FRENCH, J. D. Brain lesions associated with prolonged unconsciousness, *Arch. Neurol. Psychiatr., 69,* 727–740 [1952].

———, and H. W. MAGOUN. Effects of chronic lesions in central cephalic brain stem of monkeys, *AMA Arch. Neurol. Psychiatr., 68,* 591–608 [1952].

———, M. VERZEANO, and H. W. MAGOUN. A neutral basis of the anesthetic state, *AMA Arch. Neurol. Psychiatr., 69,* 519 [1953].

FUSTER, J. M. Excitation and inhibition of neuronal firing in visual cortex by reticular stimulation, *Science, 133,* 2011–2012 [1961].

———, and R. F. DOCTER. Variations of optic evoked potential as a function of reticular activity in rabbits with chronically implanted electrodes, *J. Neurophysiol., 25,* 324–336 [1962].

GOLDSTEIN, M. H., Jr., N. Y.-S. KIANG, and R. M. BROWN. Responses of the auditory cortex to repetitive acoustic stimuli, *J. Acoust. Soc. Am., 31,* 356–364 [1959].

GRANIT, R. *Receptors and Sensory Perception.* New Haven: Yale Univ. Press, Vol. 12, p. 369 [1955].

HEBB, D. O. *The Organization of Behaviour: A Neuropsychological Theory.* New York: Wiley [1949].

HERNANDEZ-PEON, R. A cholinergic limbic forebrain-midbrain hypnogenic circuit, *Electroenceph. Clin. Neurophysiol., 17,* 444–445 [1964].

HERON, W. Cognitive and physiological effects of perceptual isolation, in: *Sensory Deprivation.* Cambridge, Mass.: Harvard Univ. Press, pp. 6–33 [1961].

HOLMGREN, B., and S. FRENK. Inhibitory phenomena and "Habituation" at the neuronal level, *Nature, 192,* 1294–1295 [1961].

HUBEL, D. H. Single unit activity in striate cortex of unrestrained cats, *J. Physiol., 147,* 266–283 [1959].

———. Electrocorticograms in cats during natural sleep, *Arch. Ital. Biol., 98,* 171–181 [1960].

———, C. O. HENSON, A. RUPERT, and R. GALAMBOS. Attention units in the auditory cortex, *Science, 129,* 1279–1280 [1959].

———, and T. N. WIESEL. Receptive fields of single neurones in the cat's striate cortex, *J. Physiol., 148,* 574–591 [1959].

———. Receptive fields of cells in striate cortex of very young, visually inexperienced kittens, *J. Neurophysiol, 26,* 994–1002 [1962].

JASPER, H. H. Recent advances in our understanding of ascending activities of the reticular system, in: *Reticular Formation of the Brain* (ed. by H. H. Jasper, L. D. Proctor, R. S. Knighton, W. C. Noshay, and R. T. Costello). Boston: Little, Brown, pp. 319–331 [1958].

JASPER, H. H. Evolution of conceptions of cerebral localization since Hughlings Jackson, *World Neurology, 1,* 97–112 [1960].

———. Studies of non-specific effects upon electrical responses in sensory systems, in: *Brain Mechanisms, Progress in Brain Research.* Amsterdam: Elsevier, Vol. 1, pp. 272–293 [1963].

———. Some physiological mechanisms involved in epileptic automatisms, *Epilepsia, 5,* 1–20 [1964].

———, and G. BERTRAND. Exploration of the human thalamus with microelectrodes, *The Physiologist, 7,* 167 [1964a].

———. Stereotaxic microelectrode studies of single thalamic cells and fibres in patients with dyskinesia, *Am. Neurol. Assoc. Trans., 89,* 79–82 [1964b].

———, R. T. KHAN, and K. A. C. ELLIOTT. Amino acids released from the cerebral cortex in relation to its state of activation, *Science, 147,* 1448–1449 [1965].

———, L. D. PROCTOR, R. S. KNIGHTON, W. C. NOSHAY, and R. T. COSTELLO. *Reticular Formation of the Brain.* Boston: Little, Brown, 766 pp. [1958].

———, and C. SHAGASS. Conditioning the occipital alpha rhythm in man, *J. Exp. Psychol., 28,* 373–388 [1941a].

———. Conscious time judgments related to conditioned time intervals and voluntary control of the alpha rhythm, *J. Exp. Psychol., 28,* 503–508 [1941b].

JUNG, R. Coordination of specific and nonspecific afferent impulses at single neurones of the visual cortex, in: *Reticular Formation of the Brain* (ed. by H. H. Jasper, L. D. Proctor, R. S. Knighton, W. C. Noshay, and R. T. Costello). Boston: Little, Brown, pp. 423–434 [1958].

———, H. H. KORNHUBER, and J. S. FONSECA. Multisensory convergence on cortical neurones, in: *Brain Mechanisms, Progress in Brain Research.* Amsterdam: Elsevier, Vol. 1, pp. 207–240 [1963].

KANAI, T., and J. C. SZERB. Mesencephalic reticular activating system and cortical acetylcholine output, *Nature, 205,* 81–88 [1965].

KOELLE, G. B. A new general concept of neurohumoral functions of acetylcholine and acetylcholinesterase, *J. Pharm. Pharmacol., 14,* 65–90 [1962].

KOZAK, W., W. V. MACFARLANE, and R. WESTERMAN. Long-lasting reversible changes in the reflex responses of chronic spinal cats to touch, heat and cold, *Nature, 193,* 171–173 [1962].

KRISTIANSEN, K. Neurological considerations on the brain mechanisms of consciousness, *Acta Neurochirurgica, 21,* 289–314 [1964].

KRNJEVIĆ, K., and J. W. PHILLIS. Acetylcholine-sensitive cells in the cerebral cortex, *J. Physiol.* (London), *166,* 296–327 [1963].

LINDSLEY, D. B., L. H. SHREINER, W. B. KNOWLES, and H. W. MAGOUN. Behavioral and EEG changes following chronic brain stem lesions in the cat, *Electroencephalogr., 2,* 483–498 [1950].

LIVINGSTON, W. K. *Pain Mechanisms. Physiologic Interpretation of Causalgia and Its Related States.* New York: Macmillan, 253 pp. [1943].

LOEB, C. Electroencephalograms during coma, *Acta Neurochirurgica, 12,* 270–281 [1964].

MacIntosh, F. C., and P. E. Oborin. Release of acetylcholine from intact cerebral cortex, *Abst. XIX Int. Physiol. Congr.*, 580–581 [1953].

McCouch, G. P., G. M. Austin, C.-N. Liu, and C.-Y. Liu. Sprouting as a cause of spasticity, *J. Neurophysiol.*, 21, 205–216 [1958].

Mantegazzini, P., and G. Pepeu. Increase of cortical acetylcholine induced by midbrain hemisection in the cat, *J. Physiol.*, 173, 20–21 [1964].

Mitchell, J. F. The spontaneous and evoked release of acetylcholine from the cerebral cortex, *J. Physiol.*, 165, 98–116 [1963].

Moruzzi, G., A. Fessard, and H. H. Jasper, eds. *Brain Mechanisms, Progress in Brain Research.* Amsterdam: Elsevier, Vol. 1, 493 pp. [1963].

Penfield, W. Consciousness and centrencephalic organization. *Premier Congr. Inter. Sci. Neurol.*, Bruxelles, 21–28 juillet, 1957 (2e journée commune, pp. 7–18) [1957].

———, and H. H. Jasper, *Epilepsy and the Functional Anatomy of the Human Brain.* Boston: Little, Brown, 896 pp. [1954].

———, and B. Milner. Memory deficit produced by bilateral lesions in the hippocampal zone, *AMA Arch. Neurol. Psychiatr.*, 79, 475–498 [1958].

Pepeu, G., and P. Mantegazzini. Midbrain hemisection: Effect on cortical acetylcholine in the cat, *Science*, 145, 1069–1070 [1964].

Perria, L. Introductory remarks to the International Symposium on the physiopathology of the states of consciousness, *Acta Neurochirurgica*, 12, 161–165 [1964].

Pollen, D. A. Intracellular studies of cortical neurones during thalamic induced wave and spike, *Electroenceph. Clin. Neurophysiol.*, 17, 398–404 [1964].

Pompeiano, O., and J. E. Swett. E.E.G. and behavioural manifestations of sleep induced by cutaneous nerve stimulation in normal cats, *Arch. Ital. Biol.*, 100, 311–342 [1962].

Robertson, A. D. J., and C. R. Evans. Single-unit activity in the cat's visual cortex: Modification after an intense light flash, *Science*, 147, 303–304 [1965].

Scoville, W. B., and B. Milner. Loss of recent memory after bilateral hippocampal lesions, *J. Neurol. Neurosurg. Psychiat.*, 20, 11–22 [1957].

Sharpless, S. K. Reorganization of function in the nervous system—use and disuse, *Ann. Rev. of Physiol.*, 26, 357–388 [1964].

———, and H. H. Jasper. Habituation of the arousal reaction, *Brain*, 79, 655–680 [1956].

———, and L. Halpern. The electrical excitability of chronically isolated cortex studied by means of permanently implanted electrodes, *Electroencephal. Clin. Neurophysiol.*, 14, 244–255 [1962].

Shute, C. C., and P. R. Lewis. Cholinesterase-containing systems of the brain of the rat, *Nature*, 199, 1160–1164 [1963].

Sie, G., H. H. Jasper, and L. Wolfe. Rate of ACH release from cortical surface in encephale and cerveau isolé cat preparations in relation to arousal and epileptic activation of the E.C.G., *Electroenceph. Clin. Neurophysiol.*, 18, 206 [1965].

Smirnov, G. D., and R. Y. Ilyuchenor. Cholinergic mechanism of cortical activation, *Fiziol. Zh.* (Leningrad), 48, 1441–1445 [1962].

STAVRAKY, G. M. *Supersensitivity Following Lesions of the Nervous System.* Toronto: Univ. Toronto Press, 210 pp. [1961].

STEPIEN, L. S., J. P. CORDEAU, and T. RASMUSSEN. The effect of temporal lobe and hippocampal lesions on auditory and visual recent memory in monkeys, *Brain, 83,* 470–489 [1960].

————, and S. SIERPINSKI. The effect of focal lesions of the brain upon auditory and visual recent memory in man, *J. Neurol. Neurosurg. Psychiat., 23,* 334–341 [1960].

————. Impairment of recent memory after temporal lesions in man, *Neuropsychologia, 2,* 291–303 [1964].

THESLEFF, S. Effects of motor innervation on the chemical sensitivity of skeletal muscle, *Physiol. Revs., 40,* 734–752 [1960].

TRENDELENBURG, U. Supersensitivity and subsensitivity to sympathomimetic amines, *Pharmacol. Revs., 15,* 225–276 [1963].

VERZEANO, M., and K. NEGISHI. Neuronal activity in wakefulness and sleep, in: *The Nature of Sleep* (ed. by G. E. W. Wolstenholme and M. O'Connor), Ciba Foundation Symposium. London: Churchill, pp. 108–130 [1961].

WHITE, J. C., and W. H. SWEET. *Pain, Its Mechanisms and Neurosurgical Control.* Springfield, Ill.: C. C Thomas, 736 pp. [1955].

WIESEL, T. N., and D. H. HUBEL. Single-cell responses in striate cortex of kittens deprived of vision in one eye, *J. Neurophysiol., 26,* 1003–1007 [1962].

————. Effects of visual deprivation on morphology and physiology of cells in the cat's lateral geniculate body, *J. Neurophysiol., 26,* 978–993 [1963].

WOLSTENHOLME, G. E. W., and M. O'CONNOR, eds. *The Nature of Sleep,* Ciba Foundation Symposium. London: Churchill [1960].

YAMATOTO, S., and U. SCHAEPPI. Effects of pentothal on neural activity in somato-sensory cortex and brain stem in cat, *Electroenceph. Clin. Neurophysiol., 13,* 248–256 [1961].

12

Neurophysiological Correlates of Mental Unity

by F. Bremer

Faculté de Médicine, Brussels, Belgium

Situation of the Problem

The neurophysiological problem raised by the behavioral singleness of all goal-seeking creatures had until recently attracted little attention from the studies of nervous mechanisms. The reason for this apparent lack of interest is perhaps to be found in the fact that behavioral singleness becomes mental unity in man and that physiologists feared to incur the reproach of adhering to a unifying concept recalling the Cartesian description of "la petite glande qui se trouve environ le milieu des concavités du cerveau et est proprement le siège du sens commun." The body-mind relationship remained as a metaphysical problem, not as a scientific one [Pirenne, 1950]. Yet, one may wonder whether it is not time for abandoning this attitude of resignation.

Behavioral cohesion is, in all higher metazoa, the outcome of the progressive integration of multifarious sensory messages correlated with internal informations stored as innate patterns and as individual memory traces. At each step of the integration process, the bilateral symmetry of the sensitive teguments and of the muscle machinery requires the maintenance of a dynamic equilibrium between the paired halves of a chain of interconnected nervous ganglia headed by a brain ganglion, itself structurally paired, which collects the messages of distance receptors and is the seat of "decision units" [Bullock, 1961] of shifting location. In the human brain the left cerebral hemisphere of the right-handed takes presumably the initiative of most motor decisions because it elaborates the symbolic integrations of language and praxis. However, as we shall see from the report of our colleague Sperry, the right hemisphere, when freed from the dominance of the left one, reveals its praxis autonomy. Besides, the comparative clinical study of the neurological effects of left and right retrorolandic lesions has demonstrated the fact that nonverbal achievements depend more markedly upon the right than the left hemisphere. This is specially the case for spatial and somatic gnostic integrations [Hécaen, 1962; Teuber, 1962; Elithorn, 1964]. The interpretation of this particular dominance of the right hemisphere is still a matter of debate.

Notable advances in the knowledge of the neurophysiological correlates of behavioral and mental singleness in higher mammals have been made in the last fifteen years. Three mechanisms of cerebral synergy have been demonstrated and analyzed experimentally: (*a*) the interhemispheric exchange of sensory informations and the transmission of motor decisions by way of the cerebral commissures, among which the corpus callosum is by far the most important: (*b*) the unifying influence produced on the brain activities by the energizing impulses emitted by brain stem and thalamic reticular structures; (*c*) the neuronal convergence and interaction in the visual area of impulses issued from corresponding receptive fields of the two retinas.

THE COMMISSURAL LINK

The psychophysiological characteristics of the commissural synergy mechanism have been admirably described and analyzed by Myers [1955, 1956, 1959, 1962] and by Sperry and his associates [1958, 1962, 1964]. In the cat and monkey, this mechanism seems to represent essentially an operation of interhemispheric transfer and the resultant duplication of gnostic and praxic memory traces. The patterned structure of the mnesic material communicated—its information content—has apparently more importance for the process of transfer than the particular commissural fibers involved in the interhemispheric transfer. This would account for the large functional equipotentiality found by Myers [1959, 1962] between the subdivisions of the posterior segment of the cat's callosum in the transfer of simple visual discriminations.

In the interhemispheric transmission which can be demonstrated electrophysiologically in acute experiments on the unanesthetized cat's brain for a volley of impulses in a thalamo-cortico-cortical circuit [Bremer and Terzuolo, 1955], the principle of homotopy of callosal connections apparently applies. Indeed, the spatial distribution and the voltage differences of the contralateral-evoked potentials correspond well, in

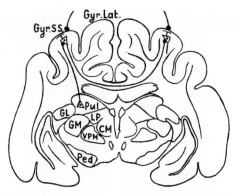

Fig. 12.1. Anatomical schema of the experiment demonstrating interhemispheric transfer, via corpus callosum, of the receiving area response. In this drawing the bipolar electrodes stimulating the thalamic specific nucleus are inserted into N. pulvinar (cf. Fig. 12.3).

general, to the ones of the cortical responses evoked directly by the thalamic stimulus within the homolateral receiving area (Figs. 12.1 and 12.2). This apparent contradiction between the psychophysiological data and the electrophysiological ones should be attributed to the complexity of the intermediary processes normally involved in interhemispheric transactions, a complexity which has its expression in the phenomena of sensory and motor equivalencies, perceptual generalization and abstraction.

The electrophysiological experiments have revealed that the callosal impulses exert a long-lasting facilitatory effect on the reactivity of the area which receive them (Fig. 12.3). The regularity with which this facilitatory process is observed and its long duration are an indication of the propensity of callosal impulses to the laying down of memory traces.

The duplication of cortical engrams mediated by the corpus callosum, and also by the anterior commissure, which by connecting the two temporal poles contributes apparently to the transfer of visual discrimination habits in the monkey [Downer, 1962], should at first sight oppose rather than favor behavioral singleness. But in man the commissural system functions also as a mechanism allowing the immediate transcortical communication of information by a hemisphere at the request of the other one, as well as the utilization by the receiving half brain of patterns of skilled actions stored in the dominant hemisphere, including the engrams of language [Trescher and Ford, 1937; Maspes, 1948; Gazzaniga, Bogen, and Sperry, 1962, 1963; Sperry, 1964; Geschwind, 1962]. This functioning principle does not yet hold for learned

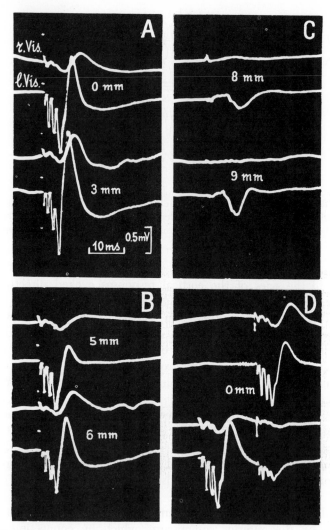

Fig. 12.2. Callosal interhemispheric transfer of the response of the visual area to a thalamocortical volley of impulses. Cat, *encéphale isolé*. In A to C the lower traces show the response of left cortical areas to a stimulus (0.3 msec; 1.5 V) applied on the left geniculate body; the upper ones, the transferred response recorded from symmetrical regions of the right hemisphere; in each pair of traces, the distance of the left and right monopolar recording electrodes from the mesial border of the visual area is indicated in mm. Notice: (1) in A to C the parallelism of the changes of the homolateral and contralateral potentials resulting from the symmetrical displacement of the recording electrodes along the stereotaxic coordinate, and (2) in D, the parallel reduction of the homolateral and transferred responses to a second thalamic shock applied 20 msec after the first one of the pair.

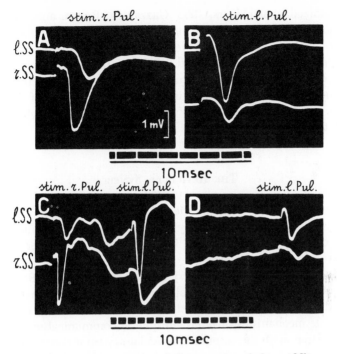

Fig. 12.3. Interhemispheric transfer of the response of the middle suprasylvian gyrus to a pulvinar stimulus. Callosal facilitation. Cat, *encéphale isolé*. Recordings from symmetrical points of the right (lower traces) and left (upper traces) suprasylvian gyrus. (A) Stimulus on right pulvinar. (B) Stimulus on left pulvinar. Notice the latency of the transcortical responses and the reciprocity of the interhemispheric transfer. (C) Succession of the responses to right and left pulvinar stimuli (recorded at a lower speed). (D) Left pulvinar stimulus applied alone. Notice in C (by comparison with the response to the same stimulus in D) the marked facilitation of the response to the left (direct) pulvinar stimulus, resulting from the precession of the right pulvinar stimulus. The relayed callosal response to this left pulvinar stimulus is also increased, as a consequence of the facilitation of the direct one [Bremer, 1958].

pattern discriminations in the rat [Bures and Buresova, 1960; Russell and Ochs, 1963]. But it is already discernable in the cat [Myers, 1962] and it is certainly valid for subhuman primates: in the monkey, the callosum would allow the use, by the untrained side, of visual patterned memory traces laid down in the trained hemisphere only [Downer, 1962].

In the chiasma-split cat and monkey, the functional conflict between the two hemispheres when they are asked to achieve two opposite visual discriminations, a conflict which disappears after the section of the callosum, is a clear indication of the importance of the great cerebral commissure for mental unity. The split-brain animal and also the callosotomized man [Myers, 1962; Gazzaniga, Bogen, and Sperry, 1962, 1963; Sperry, 1964] behave in many experimental situations as if each of their cerebral hemispheres were unaware of what is happening in the opposite one, as if they had in these circumstances two separate brains, each one endowed virtually with a power of decision and command. Yet, very little betrays in the ordinary behavior of the operated subjects the disruption of mental unity, the disclosure of which requires special psychophysiological tests.

THE RETICULAR SYNERGY

This situation raises the question of the existence of interhemispheric mechanisms of cerebral synergy, functionally less specific than the callosal one, yet able to maintain behavioral singleness after the callosal commissurotomy.

Since the experiments of Sperry and his group [1962, 1964] have excluded other potential commissural structures, such as the thalamic massa intermedia, the roof of the brain stem, and the cerebellum, at least as indispensable mechanisms of interhemispheric communication, the floor of the brain stem, with the ascending reticular system it contains, remains as the possible candidate for the supposed compensation. Experimental arguments, in agreement with anatomical ones, may be quoted in support of this hypothesis: (a) dispensability of the forebrain commissures for the interhemispheric transfer of simple visual and other crude learned discriminations [Myers, 1962; Sperry, 1962, 1964]; (b) bilateral cerebral extension of the various manifestations of electrocortical arousal produced by a unilateral brief stimulation of the mesencephalic tegmentum [Moruzzi and Magoun, 1949], including, as shown by Fig. 12.4, the most sensitive of these arousal effects which is the reticular potentiation of the visual area response to an optic nerve shock [Dumont and Dell, 1960; Bremer and Stoupel, 1959]; (c) similar bilaterality of cerebral arousal effects resulting from a unilateral stimulation of various neocortical areas after a complete section of the callosum [Bremer and Terzuolo, 1954]; (d) the fact that brain stem structures contribute with the callosal system to the maintenance of the bilateral synchronism which characterizes the electrogenesis of the resting brain [Bremer, 1958].

The strong homolateral predominance of the tonic influence exerted by synchronizing impulses ascending from the pontine tegmentum [Cordeau and Mancia, 1959] should not be considered as an objection against this body of physiological data indicating that the reticular formation, with the thalamic nonspecific system [Jasper, 1949; Enomoto, 1959], may act as a long loop commissural link and a synergy mechanism

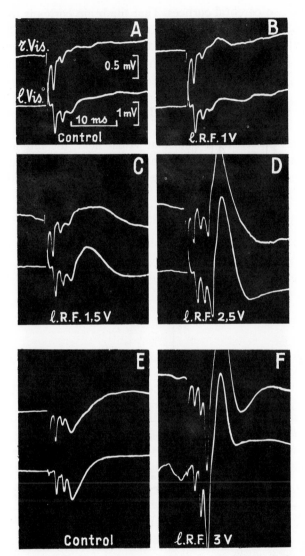

Fig. 12.4. Bilateral facilitatory effect exerted on a cortical-evoked potential by a unilateral reticular midbrain stimulation. Cat, *encéphale isolé*. Simultaneous recording of the responses of the right (upper traces) and the left (lower traces) visual areas to a stimulus (0.3 msec pulse) applied on the right optic nerve. (A) Control traces. (B, C, D) Facilitatory effect exerted by the precession (at 60 msec) of a brief tetanus (five shocks at 200 per sec) applied at increasing voltages on the left tegmentum at 5 mm from the midline. E and F control and facilitated responses recorded 90 min after D. Notice the practically equal facilitatory effects of the left reticular stimulation on the evoked potentials of both visual areas.

between the two cerebral cortices. That the brain cortex is indispensable for the interhemispheric transfer of memory traces, even in the rat, has been proved by experiments using the spreading depression technique [Bures and Buresova, 1960; Russell and Ochs, 1963].

BINOCULAR INTERACTION

In animals possessing a binocular visual field, the interaction in the visual cortex of impulses issued from corresponding right and left retinal areas and converging on the same cortical neurons should constitute

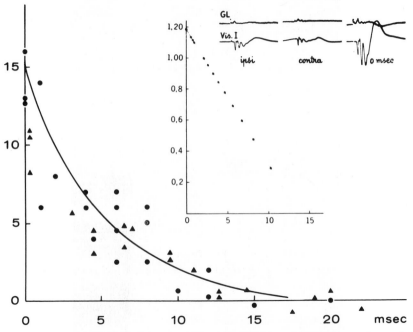

Fig. 12.5. Facilitatory interaction of binocular optic nerve shocks on the evoked potential of visual area. Cat, *encéphale isolé*. Ordinates: percentage of facilitation (given in hundreds per cent) of the response of the striate area to a contralateral optic nerve shock, produced by the precession of a homolateral stimulus at the intervals given in abscissa. The two stimuli were juxtaliminal for the cortex when applied alone (see inset). The graph is constructed from the results of two experiments. Notice: (1) that at the zero interval the potentiation of the visual area response reaches 1,500 per cent and that the facilitatory effect decays along an exponential curve; (2) that the lateral geniculate potential and the radiation potential in the visual area response (traces in the inset) do not participate to the facilitatory process: they show simple algebraic summation at the zero interval [Bremer, 1964].

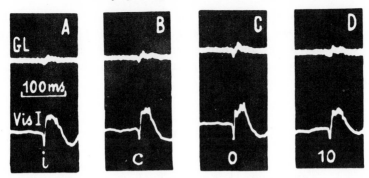

Fig. 12.6. Occlusive effect of the interaction of binocular flashes on the evoked potential of visual area. Cat, *encéphale isolé*. A and B responses of the lateral geniculate body (upper traces) and visual area (lower traces) to ipsilateral and contralateral glow tube flashes. (C) Responses to the two flashes applied simultaneously. (D) Responses to the two flashes at 10 msec interval. Notice: in C, the almost complete occlusion effect on the cortical-evoked potential and the algebraic summation of the geniculate focal potentials; in D, the complete absence of cortical response to the contralateral flash applied after the homolateral one, contrasting with the distinct response of the geniculate to the same stimulus [Bremer, 1964].

a contributory mechanism for perceptual and behavioral singleness. Already in the cat this convergence, demonstrated electrophysiologically by reciprocal facilitation (Fig. 12.5) and occlusion effects (Fig. 12.6), is of such an extent that the great majority of the sensory neurons of the visual area can be described as being binocular [Hubel and Wiesel, 1962; Bremer, 1964; cf. Grüsser-Cornehls and Grüsser, 1961]. The fact that the visual association cortex adjacent to the visual area is the origin of corticifugal oculomotor impulses increases the qualification of this binocular interaction of optic impulses as a contributory mechanism to behavioral cohesion. The interaction of the crossed and uncrossed visual systems within the same hemisphere has been demonstrated by psychophysiological observations [Myers, 1956, 1962; Muntz and Sutherland, 1964]. It represents the long-term manifestation of the neuronal heterosynaptic convergence whose short-term aspects are the summation or occlusion of paired binocular stimuli.

It is interesting to mention in this context the absence of binocular post-tetanic potentiation of the visual area response to a testing optic nerve stimulus [Hughes, Evarts, and Marshall, 1956; Bremer, 1964]. This lack of binocular postactivation potentiation, which is accounted for by the heterosynaptic character of the neuronal convergence in the receiving area, suggests that the pathways from the geniculate layers to the visual cortex are monosynaptic ones, allowing no convergence before the cortical neurons responsible for the evoked potential.

The contour of the monocular visual fields seems to be unmodified in man after section of the callosum [Akelaitis, 1941] and in the case of its agenesis [Jeeves and Rajalakshmi, 1964]. The fusion of the two halves of the visual field does apparently not involve a commissural mechanism [cf., however, Whitteridge, 1964].

UNDEFECTIBLE MENTAL UNITY

With the reservation of the uncertainty concerning the possible effect of a median splitting of the brain stem tegmentum completing the cerebral commissurotomies, the fact is that none of the surgeries aiming at the disruption of the hemispheric synergy has been found capable of altering seriously, "in the common activities of daily life," the behavioral singleness of the cat or monkey and the mental unity of man [Sperry, 1964]. The restrictions which this unity suffered as a consequence of these aggressions were essentially of a perceptual nature in the animal, perceptual, phasic and praxic in man. In both, they were without any overt influence on their volitional conducts.

Mental unity remains intact in man after large lesions of the dominant hemisphere, destroying in it the areas where the symbolic integrations of language are elaborated. Sleep does not affect it seriously. In dreams, the threads of the self remain tied together in spite of the most chaotic space and time disorientations. Besides, behavioral singleness does not depend on the complete functioning of mnemonic mechanisms. In epileptic automatisms, extremely elaborated conducts, having sometimes all the appearances of adequate and intelligent voluntary acts, may leave no memory trace [see Jasper, 1964]. The same amnesia follows apparently the well-coordinated and goal-seeking automatisms evoked, with their accompaniment of affective manifestations, by the electric stimulation of hypothalamic or amygdaloid structures in the free-moving cat [Hess, 1954; Hunsperger, 1963]. Such facts suggest the existence of hierarchical differences between otherwise similar behaviors, corresponding to levels or degrees of neuronal integration.

Again, in focal cortical irritations, should they be pathological or created, as in Penfield's observations [1952], by an electric current stimulating topically a temporal gyrus, the revival of audio-visual memories may evoke a hallucinatory scenery, impressed on the woof of the familiar reality, without revealing the impairment to the coherence of the self which one should expect from this mental diplopia [Jasper, 1964]. The same comment may apply to the visual hallucinations of the self (*heautoscopie* of the French authors). This illusion of a "double" does not affect mental singleness more than the normal perception of a mirror image, which in fact it often looks like.

These difficulties should not obliterate the light which experimental work has begun to project on one of the fundamental aspects of the mind-brain problem. Yet, until the principles of perceptual integration will be understood, the integration mechanisms revealed by the neurophysiological data represent little more than a gross framework in a neuronal communication system of a formidable structural and dynamic complexity.

DISCUSSION

Chairman: LORD ADRIAN

GRANIT: I would like to raise a point here which I would not have been able to raise a year ago, and this is that these experiments of Professor Bremer would have been theoretically difficult to understand because they only demonstrate facilitations. Why is there no elaboration in terms of both inhibition and excitation? The visual image, as we know, is a very complex pattern of excitation and inhibition spread out in cortical space, and if there is a point to point representation of that visual image in the other hemisphere, a pure facilitation would miss these essential features. With the intracellular recording of the effects of stretch receptors on the motoneurons, we saw that it is immaterial for the process of depolarization whether the synaptic message produces an excitation or inhibition. No sooner do you facilitate the cell by depolarizing it from the inside by current than inhibitions come out with their right sign and the excitations come out with their right sign. So I think that I have now a new understanding of Professor Bremer's experiments. I think that a general facilitation by the commissural path could be of importance for the elaboration of a specific image in terms of both inhibition and excitation.

BREMER: I would certainly agree that commissural impulses do not exert only facilitatory effects on the brain cortex. There are good reasons to believe that inhibitory actions are produced as well. Yet, to my knowledge, the clearest demonstration of such inhibitory effects produced by a callosal volley has been brought by the study of animals in which the callosum had been previously cut in order to eliminate the orthodromic impulses and only leave the antidromic ones, acting probably by inhibitory recurrent collaterals [Asanuma and Okamoto, *Jap. J. Physiol.*, 9, 473, 1959]. That does not exclude the possibility that orthodromic influences should involve inhibitory processes as well. In the complicated commissural transfer process disclosed by psychophysiological experiments, excitation and inhibition should be closely associated in elaborate patterns.

But the fact is there that the facilitatory effect of callosal conditioning impulses is of such a regularity and amplitude in electrophysiological experiments on the non-narcotized brain that it must have an important significance in the dynamics of interhemispheric exchanges.

GRANIT: Possibly I did not explain my idea well. I suspect that you misunderstood me. What I meant to say was that it would be quite sufficient to have depolarization alone and yet to have both inhibitory and excitatory patterns come out with their respective signs. This point was elaborated at the end of my paper.

GOMES: I am particularly interested in the problem of the definition and the preservation of individuality, which, of course, is closely dependent on the singleness of behavior; hence I ask Professor Bremer what will happen if the structure which he calls vicarious in the transference of information between the two hemispheres—the ascending reticular system—is also sectioned?

BREMER: The destruction, in the brain-stem core, of the central structures belonging to the so-called activating reticular system results in such a deep lowering of all transactional activities of the creature that all traces of what the French call *vie de relation* disappears. The sagittal splitting of the brain-stem floor produces a similar, although less severe and less enduring syndrome, complicated, however, by the motor disturbances resulting from the section of tract decussations and by unexplained visual disturbances [see Sperry, 1962, 1964]. Its study after recovery from the initial syndrome might sometime afford an answer to your question and give a direct demonstration—or refutation—of the postulated compensation which corticosubcortical circuits provide after the loss of all commissural interhemispheric links. For the present, the preservation of the behavioral singleness of the split-brain mammal by means of a long-loop reticular link remains a working hypothesis.

ECCLES: That is a very interesting idea. I would like to ask how long is the transmission time? It must be about double what you get from stimulating the lateral reticular formation and recording from the cortex; but what is the total transmission time down to the reticular function and back again on the long loop?

BREMER: The question you raise is a difficult one. Terzuolo and I [1954] could regularly record, in the *encéphale isolé* cat, focal potentials of the mesencephalic reticular formation in response to single shocks applied on various neocortical areas. The latency of these responses varied from 10 to 12 msec. But ascending reticular volleys, in the animal not anesthetized with chloralose, gave very little evidence of evoked potentials at the cortical level, in spite of the fact that they powerfully potentiated sensory responses. Therefore it is difficult to measure the total transmission time taken in a cortico-reticulo-cortical circuit. I understand the bearing of your question. Your concern is that the loop would require time. But, when one considers that all our nervous machinery works with repetitive impulses, it does not seem it would matter much if there was a delay of a few milliseconds for these purposes.

MAC KAY: I wonder whether a "long loop" between the two cortices of a split brain is what we need in order to preserve "unity." Might it not be that the unity shown in the behavior of such cases, like that of certain political movements spread over different countries, is attributable not to long loops of direct communication between them, but to effective communication between each and a normative central organization in the unsplit remainder?

BREMER: I think that the mechanism of interhemispheric integration you suggest for the preservation of behavioral unity of the split-brain animal can easily be incorporated into the concept of a cortico-subcortical long loop, compensating for the lost cerebral commissures. Your idea underlines the autonomy of the central compensatory and supplementary organization and the normative control it exerts on the higher functions of the brain. But the long loop hypothesis does not imply that a centrencephalic organization, for example the ascending reticular system, acts as a mere passive relay between the two dissociated cortices.

REFERENCES

AKELAITIS, A. J. Studies on the corpus callosum. II. The higher visual functions in each homonymous field following complete section of the corpus callosum, *Arch. Neurol. Psychiat.*, 45, 788–796 [1941].

BREMER, F. Physiology of the corpus callosum, in: *The Brain and Human Behavior*, Proceedings of the Association for Research in Nervous and Mental Disease. Baltimore: Williams & Wilkins, Vol. 36, pp. 424–448 [1958].

———. Etude électrophysiologique de la convergence binoculaire dans l'aire visuelle corticale du chat, *Arch. Ital. Biol.*, 102, 333–371 [1964].

BREMER, F., and C. TERZUOLO. Contribution à l'étude des mécanismes physiologiques du maintien de l'activité vigile. Interaction de la formation réticulée et de l'écorce cérébrale dans le processus du réveil, *Arch. Int. Physiol.*, 62, 157–178 [1954].

———. Transfert interhémisphérique d'information sensorielles par le corps calleux, *J. Physiol.* (Paris), 47, 105–107 [1955].

BREMER, F., and N. STOUPEL. Facilitation et inhibition des potentiels évoqués cérébraux dans l'éveil cérébral, *Arch. Int. Physiol.*, 67, 240–274 [1959].

BULLOCK, T. H. The problem of recognition in an analyzer made of neurons, in: *Sensory Communication.* Cambridge, Mass. and New York: MIT Press and Wiley, pp. 717–724 [1961].

BURES, J., and O. BURESOVA. The use of Leao's spreading cortical depression in research on conditioned reflexes, in: *The Moscow Colloquium on electroencephalography of higher nervous activity 1959, EEG and Clin. Neurophysiol.*, Suppl. 13 of the *EEG Journal*, pp. 359–376 [1960].

CORDEAU, J. P., and M. MANCIA. Evidence for the existence of an electroencephalographic synchronization mechanism originating in the lower brain stem, *EEG Clin. Neurophysiol.*, 11, 551–564 [1959].

DOWNER, J. L. Interhemispheric integration in the visual system, in: *Interhemispheric Relations and Cerebral Dominance.* Baltimore: Johns Hopkins Press, pp. 87–100 [1962].

DUMONT, S., and P. DELL. Facilitation réticulaire des mécanismes visuels corticaux, *EEG Clin. Neurophysiol., 12,* 769–796 [1960].

ELITHORN, A. Intelligence, perceptual integration and the minor hemisphere syndrome, *Neuropsychologia, 2,* 327–332 [1964].

ENOMOTO, T. F. Unilateral activation of the non-specific thalamic system and bilateral cortical responses, *EEG Clin. Neurophysiol., 11,* 219–232 [1959].

GAZZANIGA, M. S., J. E. BOGEN, and R. W. SPERRY. Some functional effects of sectioning the cerebral commissures in man, *Proc. Natl. Acad. Sci., 48,* 1765–1769 [1962].

———. Laterality effects in somesthesis following cerebral commissurotomy in man, *Neuropsychologia, 1,* 209–215 [1963].

GESCHWIND, N. A human deconnection syndrome, *Neurology, 12,* 675–685 [1962].

GRÜSSER-CORNHELS, U., and O. J. GRÜSSER. Reaktionmuster im zentralen visuellen System von Fischen, Kaninchen und Katzen auf monocular und binocular Lichtreize, in: *Neurophysiologie u. Psychophysik des visuellen Systems. Symposion Freiburg–Br. 1960.* Berlin: Springer, pp. 275–287 [1961].

HÉCAEN, H. Clinical symptomatology in right and left hemispheric lesions, in: *Interhemispheric Relations and Cerebral Dominance.* Baltimore: Johns Hopkins Press, pp. 215–243 [1962].

HESS, W. R. *Das Zwischenhirn, Bâle: Benno Schwabe* [1954].

HUBEL, D. H., and T. N. WIESEL. Receptive fields, binocular interaction and functional architecture in the cat's visual cortex, *J. Physiol., 160,* 106–154 [1962].

HUGHES, J. R., E. V. EVARTS, and W. H. MARSHALL. Post-tetanic potentiation in the visual system of cats, *Amer. J. Physiol., 186,* 483–487 [1956].

HUNSPERGER, R. W. Comportements affectifs provoqués par la stimulation électrique du tronc cérébral et du cerveau antérieur, *J. Physiol.* (Paris), *55,* 45–98 [1963].

JASPER, H. H. Diffuse projection systems: The integrative action of the thalamic reticular system, *Electroencephal. Clin. Neurophysiol., 1,* 405–19 [1949].

———. Some physiological mechanisms involved in epileptic automatisms, *Epilepsia, 5,* 1–20 [1964].

JEEVES, M. A., and R. RAJALAKSHMI. Psychological studies of a case of congenital agenesis of the corpus callosum, *Neuropsychologia, 2,* 247–252 [1964].

MASPES, P. E. Le syndrome expérimental chez l'homme de la section du splenium du corps calleux: Alexie visuelle pure hémianopsique, *Rev. Neurologique, 80,* 100–13 [1948].

MORUZZI, G., and H. W. MAGOUN. Brain stem reticular formation and activation of the EEG, *EEG Clin. Neurophysiol., 1,* 455–473 [1949].

MUNTZ, W. R. A., and N. S. SUTHERLAND. The role of crossed and uncrossed optic nerve fibers in the visual discrimination of shape by rats, *J. Comp. Neurol., 122,* 69–77 [1964].

MYERS, R. E. Interocular transfer of pattern discrimination in cats following section of crossed optic fibers, *J. Comp. Physiol. Psychol., 48,* 470–473 [1955].

MYERS, R. E. Function of corpus callosum in interocular transfer, *Brain, 79,* 358–363 [1956].

————. Localization of function in the corpus callosum, *Arch. Neurol., 1,* 74–77 [1959].

————. Transmission of visual information within and between the hemispheres: A behavioral study, in: *Interhemispheric Relations and Cerebral Dominance.* Baltimore: Johns Hopkins Press, pp. 51–73 [1962].

PENFIELD, W. Memory mechanisms, *Arch. Neurol. Psych., 67,* 178 [1952].

PIRENNE, M. H. Descartes and the body-mind problem in physiology, *Brit. J. for the Philosophy of Sci., 1,* 43–59 [1950].

RUSSELL, I. S., and S. OCHS. Localization of a memory trace in one cortical hemisphere and transfer to the other hemispheres, *Brain, 86,* 37–54 [1963].

SPERRY, R. W. Physiological plasticity and brain circuit theory, in: *Biological and Biochemical Bases of Behavior.* Madison: Univ. Wisconsin Press, pp. 401–424 [1958].

————. Some general aspects of interhemispheric integration, in: *Interhemispheric Relations and Cerebral Dominance.* Baltimore: Johns Hopkins Press, pp. 43–49 [1962].

————. The great cerebral commissure, *Scient. American, 211,* 42 [1964].

————, R. E. MYERS, and A. M. SCHRIER. Perceptual capacity of the isolated visual cortex in the cat, *Quart. J. Exper. Psychol., 12,* 65–71 [1960].

TEUBER, H. L. Effects of brain wounds implicating right or left hemisphere in man: Hemisphere differences and hemisphere interaction in vision, audition, and somesthesis, in: *Interhemispheric Relations and Cerebral Dominance.* Baltimore: Johns Hopkins Press, pp. 131–157 [1962].

TRESCHER, J. H., and F. B. FORD. Colloid cyst of the third ventricle. Report of a case; operative removal with section of the posterior half of corpus callosum, *Arch. Neurol. Psychiat., 37,* 959–973 [1937].

WHITTERIDGE, D. Visual pathways and visual centres. Meeting in honour of Lord Adrian, March 1964. *IBRO Bull., 3,* 75 [1964].

13

Brain Bisection and Mechanisms of Consciousness

by R. W. Sperry

*California Institute of Technology,
Pasadena, California*

During the past decade we have been engaged in studies in which the brain is surgically divided down the middle into right and left halves. The behavioral performances of cats and monkeys following brain bisection have led to the conclusion that each of the surgically separated hemispheres must sense, perceive, learn, and remember quite independently of the other hemisphere [Sperry, 1961a, 1961b; 1964a, 1964b].

The past two years these studies have included two human patients in whom similar disconnection of the hemispheres had been performed in an effort to help control severe epileptic seizures [Bogen and Vogel, 1962; Gazzaniga, Bogen, and Sperry, 1962, 1963, 1965]. The findings most relevant and interesting to the subject of the conference are best illustrated in the latter subjects and I will therefore focus on the human material. The surgery in these patients included complete section of the corpus callosum and the anterior and hippocampal commissures plus the massa intermedia in one case. In the other case the massa intermedia was judged to be absent in the course of the operation [Bogen and Vogel, 1962].

It was hoped that this surgical disconnection of the hemispheres as indicated above might help prevent the spread of epileptic seizures from one to the other hemisphere in these patients, that it might help to retain consciousness in one hemisphere during the onset of the attack at least, and that it might further reduce the severity of the attack by eliminating a powerful avenue for mutual bilateral reinforcement, particularly in the generalized phase. Postsurgical epileptic-like seizures in our colony of split-brain monkeys that have had the same surgery tend to be confined to one side and centered in the distal joints of the arm and leg on the one side. That the surgery would, in addition, reduce the incidence of the attacks to practically zero and permit reduction in the amount of medication, as has been the case in both patients, was something of a surprise bonus, and our fingers are still crossed on this latter point.

These studies represent a team effort: The surgical treatment was initially recommended by Joseph Bogen after extensive consultations. The surgery was performed by Philip Vogel at the White Memorial Hospital in Los Angeles. Most of the psychological testing has been administered by Michael Gazzaniga in our laboratory, with the writer collaborating and aiding in a general consultant and advisory capacity.

Everything we have seen so far indicates that the surgery has left these people with two separate minds, that is, two separate spheres of consciousness. What is experienced in the right hemisphere seems to be entirely outside the realm of awareness of the left hemisphere. This mental division has been demonstrated in regard to perception, cognition, volition, learning, and memory. One of the hemispheres, the left, dominant or major hemisphere, has speech and is normally talkative and conversant. The other, the minor hemisphere, however, is mute or dumb, being able to express itself only through nonverbal reactions. (Hence: "mental duplicity" from this surgery but no "double talk.")

Fortunately, from the patient's standpoint, the functional separation of the two hemispheres is counteracted by a large number of unifying factors that tend to keep the disconnected hemispheres doing pretty much the same thing from one part of the day to the next. Ordinarily there would appear to be a large common denominator of similar activity going in each most of the time. When we deliberately induce different activities in the right and left hemispheres by means of various testing procedures, however, it then becomes evident that each hemisphere is oblivious to the cognitive experience of the other.

This is illustrated in many ways. For example: the subject may be blindfolded and some familiar object such as a pencil, a cigarette, a comb, or a coin placed in the left hand. Under these conditions, the mute hemisphere connected to the left hand feeling the object perceives and appears to know quite well what the object is. Though it cannot express this knowledge in speech or in writing, it can manipulate the object correctly, it can demonstrate how the object is supposed to be used, and it can remember the object and go out and retrieve it with the same hand from among an array of other objects either by touch or by sight. While all this is going on, the other hemisphere meanwhile has no conception of what the object is and, if asked, says so. If pressed for an answer, the speech hemisphere can only resort to pure guesswork. This remains the case just so long as the blindfold is kept in place and all other avenues of sensory input from the object to the talking hemisphere are blocked. But let the right hand cross over and touch the test object in the left hand; or let the object itself touch the face or head as in demonstrating the use of a comb, a cigarette, or glasses; or let the object make some give-away sound, like the jingle of a key case, then immediately the speech hemisphere also comes across with the correct answer.

The same kind of right-left mental separation is seen in tests involving vision. Recall that the right half of the visual field, along with the right hand, is represented together in the left hemisphere, and vice versa. Visual stimuli such as pictures, words, numbers, and geometric forms flashed on a screen directly in front of the subject and to the right side of a central fixation point, so that they are projected to the dominant speech hemispheres, are all described and reported correctly with no special difficulty. On the other hand, similar material flashed to the left half of the visual field and hence into the minor hemisphere are completely lost to the talking hemisphere. Stimuli flashed to one half field seem to have no influence whatever, in tests to date, on the perception and interpretation of stimuli presented to the other half field.

The subjects fail on such simple tasks, for example, as that involved in discriminating whether red and green half fields presented together are the same or different in color where the response involves only a simple nodding or shaking of the head "yes" or "no"—in other words, with everything favoring any cross integration that might be present. The same task caused no difficulty to either hemisphere when the two colors or other stimuli were presented within the same half retinal field and hence projected to the same hemisphere.

Comparison of the directional tilt of broad straight lines running across the visual field and interrupted in the center of the screen went easily, again, when both parts of the bar fell in one field; but when the two parts fell in right and left fields separately, the subjects were unable to indicate whether the two bars were lined up straight across the midline or at an angle. When the response in this test involved manual copying of the perceived lines, the initial result was for each hand to record and draw only the part of the line within its own half of the visual field, the other half being omitted. When both hands had a pencil and worked simultaneously, both parts of the line were drawn correctly, indicating double simultaneous perception and response. With further practice, Case II has learned gradually to reproduce the lines from both half fields with either hand. Meantime, the verbal response has remained firmly lateralized, indicating that the change reflects an improvement in the bilaterality of motor control rather than in the sensory or perceptual sphere. The dominant hemisphere, in particular, has good motor control over both hands, even to the point where the left hand, at one year after surgery, can be used again for simple writing. Testing shows this left-hand writing is controlled from the left hemisphere.

Note in passing that the observed disconnection effects, as in the foregoing examples, do not show up readily in ordinary behavior. They have to be demonstrated by flashing the visual material fast enough so that eye movements cannot be used to sneak the answers into the wrong hemisphere. In the testing of tactile perception in right and left hands, vision has to be excluded with a blindfold, auditory cues must be eliminated, and the hands must be kept from crossing, and so on. The overall condition is amazingly normal considering the state of the brain. The second patient, less handicapped by other medical complications than the first case, has been able since surgery to run her house and to do the family cooking. She also goes out to the market, watches television, and attends full three-hour shows at the drive-in theater, all without complaining about any particular splitting or doubling in her perceptual experience. Her family believes that she still does not have as much initiative as previously in her house cleaning, in which she used to be meticulous, and that her general spatial orientation is not as good as before—for example, she does not find her way back to the car at the drive-in theater as readily as she used to. In the early months after surgery there were complaints about difficulty with short-term memory. By now, some eight months later, there seems to be much improvement in this regard, though not complete recovery. Involvement of the hippocampal fornix would have to be ruled out before effects such as the latter can be ascribed to the commissurotomy per se. Lack of coordination in activities that require close cooperation between the hands was also an early complaint that has become much less bothersome as the months go by.

Functional independence of the hemispheres is more readily apparent in Case I than in Case II. In the first case, the left hand and left half visual field and left half of the cutaneous field of the torso all function together without trouble. This left side experience, however, cannot be integrated with stimuli coming in from across the midline. The same was true for the right hand, right half of the torso and right half visual field. Construction of spatial relations and perspective in drawing went better with the left side and the minor hemisphere, whereas language functions were decidedly better on the right side and in the dominant left hemisphere. In the second case, the functional right-left separation is no longer so clear-cut and simple, although it was very similar during the first months after surgery while trophic shock, from the commissural sections, was still strong. Voluntary motor control of the left arm and hand was much more severely affected than that of the right in the early weeks after surgery. By the seventh month, either hand was being controlled from either hemisphere, which made it much more difficult to determine which hemisphere was involved in a given activity.

One finds plenty of evidence, especially in Case II, that the minor, dumb, or mute hemisphere really does perceive and comprehend, even though it cannot express verbally what it sees and thinks. It can point out with the left hand a matching picture from among many others that have been flashed to the left field, or it can point to a corresponding object a picture of which had been flashed in the left field screen. It can also pick out the correct written name of an object it has seen flashed on the screen, or even vice versa, that is, it can read a name and retrieve the designated object. In other words, the dumb right hemisphere in the second patient is not entirely stupid or illiterate; it reads a word like *cup, fork,* or *apple* flashed to the left field and then picks out the corresponding object with the left hand. While the left hand and its hemisphere are thus performing correctly, however, the opposite hemisphere, again, has no idea at all which object or which picture or which name is the correct one, and makes this clear through its verbal as well as other responses. In such tests you frequently have to convince the talking hemisphere to keep quiet and to let the left hand go ahead on its own, in which case it will usually pick out the correct answer.

These minor differences of opinion between the right and the left hemisphere are seen rather commonly in testing situations. For example, the left hand is allowed to feel and to manipulate, say, a toothbrush under the table or out of sight behind a screen. Then a series of five to ten cards is laid out with names on them like *ring, key, fork,* and so on. When asked what the test object was, the subject may tell you that the toothbrush in the left hand is a *ring* or some other irrelevant object that happens to come to mind. However, when instructed to point with the left hand, the speechless hemisphere deliberately ignores the erroneous verbal opinions of its better half and goes ahead independently to point out the correct answer, in this case the card bearing the word *toothbrush.*

As far as we can see, about the only avenue remaining for direct communication between the two cognitive entities, *mind-right* and *mind-left,* is that of extrasensory perception. If any two minds should be able to tune in on each other, one might expect these two to be able to do so. Thus far, however, there is no evidence that such effects have any appreciable influence in the test performances.

The stimulation of a point on the face in these people with separated hemispheres is doubly perceived, the stimulus being projected bilaterally into each hemisphere. In this situation there are presumably two separate systems perceiving, that is, conscious of the same thing, in the same way that two separate brains in two separate people look at and perceive the same event straight in front of them. In a normal person, also, it would appear that there must be much the same sort of double sensing by the left and also by the right hemisphere—at least there is no way to rule it out. Normally each hemisphere perceives on its own, but the one influences the other, inhibiting or facilitating particular features to keep the effect harmonious and consistent. It would seem to follow that normally there are in a sense two competent perceivers in each cranium; one, for example, that sees the right and another that perceives the left half of the visual field. One can further fractionate normal consciousness on temporal as well as spatial dimensions as in fatigue states, for example, all with implications of questionable significance so far as scientific analysis is concerned.

The presence of conscious comprehension in a hemisphere is hardly demonstrable in the absence of some mode of expression. If speech and writing are excluded as they are in the minor hemisphere or in other kinds of brain damage, more devious testing procedures are required. One is impressed with the ease with which a patient's intellect and conscious capacity, in general, may be misjudged as a result of defects or losses that may be confined mainly or entirely to the mechanisms of expression.

The conscious awareness of the minor hemisphere produced by this vertical splitting of the brain often seems so remote to the conversant hemisphere as to be comparable in effect perhaps to the situation produced by a spinal transection. It makes one wonder if we can really rule out, as I have implied earlier [Sperry, 1964b], the alternative contention of those who maintain that spinal cords, loaves of bread, and even single molecules have a kind of consciousness. Either way, the inferences to be drawn regarding the evolution and elaboration of consciousness in its various states and the valuation that we can put on its respective manifestations remain, for most practical purposes, much the same.

We are often asked if the disconnected hemispheres must not also have each a will of its own and if the two do not then get into conflict with each other. During the first half year after surgery, particularly with the first patient, we got reports suggesting something of the kind. For example, while the patient was dressing and trying to pull on his trousers, the left hand might start to work against the right to pull the trousers down on that side. Or, the left hand, after just helping to tie the belt of the patient's robe, might go ahead on its own to untie the completed knot, whereupon the right hand would have to supervene again to retie it. The patient and his wife used to refer to the "sinister left hand" that sometimes tried to push the wife away aggressively at the same time that the hemisphere of the right hand was trying to get her to come and help him with something. Such antagonistic movements were much less a bother in Case II, though they were present in minor degree during the early months after surgery. These conflicting and dissociated movements of right and left hands are pretty well restricted to situations where the reactions of left and right hand are easily made from the same common supporting posture of body and shoulders. Generally speaking, there are so many unifying factors of this kind and others in the situation, and functional harmony is so strongly built into the undivided brain stem and spinal networks by express design, that one does not see much overt expression, or motor overflow into action, at least, of such conflicts between will power-right and will power-left.

This matter of having two free wills packed together inside the same cranial vault in these patients reminds us that free will is one of the most treasured features of the conscious process and also one of its most controversial properties from the scientific and philosophic stand-points.

(This and the following as well as much of the foregoing is taken from an earlier communication [Sperry, 1964b] of the writer, mainly for reason of expediency in the face of a difficult deadline. Use of the earlier discussion has the advantage, however, of showing that the opinions and implications included are not slanted for the present occasion, but represent the ordinary give and take in scientific thinking.)

Unlike *mind, consciousness,* and *instinct, free will* has not made any notable comeback in behavioral science in recent years. Most behavioral scientists will refuse to recognize the presence of free will in brain function. Every advance in the science of behavior, whether it has come from the psychiatrist's couch, from microelectrode recording, from brain splitting, from the use of psychomimetic drugs, or from the running of cannibalistic flatworms, seems only to reinforce that old suspicion that free will is just an illusion like the rise and setting of the sun. The more we study and learn about the brain and behavior, the more deterministic, lawful, and causal it appears.

In other words, behavioral science tells us that there is no reason to think that any of us here today had any real choice to be anywhere else, nor even to believe in principle that our presence here was not already in the cards, so to speak, five, ten or fifteen years ago. I do not like or feel comfortable about this kind of thinking any more than you do, but so far I have not found any satisfactory way around it. Alternatives to the rule of causal determinism in behavior that I have seen proposed so far, as, for example, the inferred unlawfulness in the dance of subatomic particles, seem decidedly more to be deplored as a solution than desired.

This is not to say that in the practice of behavioral science we have to regard the brain as just a pawn of the physical and chemical forces that play in and around it. Far from it. Recall that a molecule in many respects is the master of its inner atoms and electrons. The latter are hauled and forced about in chemical interactions by the overall configurational properties of the whole molecule. At the same time, if our given molecule is itself part of a single-celled organism like paramecium, it in turn is obliged, with all its parts and its partners, to follow along a trail of events in time and space determined largely by the extrinsic overall dynamics of *Paramecium caudatum.* And similarly, when it comes to brains, remember always that the simpler electric, atomic, molecular, and cellular forces and laws, though still present and operating, have all been superseded in brain dynamics by the configurational forces of higher-level mechanisms. At the top, in the human brain, these include the powers of perception, cognition, memory, reason, judgment, and the like, the operational, causal effects and forces of which are equally or more potent in brain dynamics than are the outclassed inner chemical forces.

You sense the underlying rationalization we are leading to here: "If you can't lick 'em, join 'em." If we cannot avoid determinism, accept and work with it. There may be worse "fates" than causal determinism. Maybe after all it is better to be properly imbedded in the causal flow of cosmic forces, as an integral part thereof, than to be on the loose and out of contact, free-floating, as it were, with behavioral possibilities that have no antecedent cause and hence no reason or any reliability for future plans or predictions.

In line with this, just one more point: If one were assigned the task of trying to design and build the perfect free will model—let us say the perfect all-wise decision-making machine to top all competitor's decision-making machines—consider the possibility that instead of trying to *free* the machinery from causal contact, it might be better perhaps to aim at the opposite: that is, to try to incorporate into the model the potential value of *universal causal contact;* in other words, contact with all related information in proper proportion—past, present and future.

It is clear that the human brain has come a long way in evolution in exactly this direction when you consider what goes on between its input and output in the process of making a decisive response. Consider just the amount and the kind of information and causal factors that our multidimensional intracranial vortex draws into itself, scans, and may then bring to bear on the process of turning out one of its "preordained decisions." Potentially included, thanks to memory, are the events and the collected wisdom of most of a human lifetime. We can add to this, given a trip to the library, the accumulated knowledge of all recorded history. And to all the foregoing information we can further add, thanks to reason and logic, much of the future forecast and predictive value extractable from all this data, not to mention the creative insights that evolve from the interplay of new constellations of all the foregoing. Maybe the total here falls considerably short of universal causal contact, and maybe it is not even quite up to the kind of thing that evolution has going for itself over on Galaxy Nine, and maybe we must grant, in spite of all, that any decision that does eventually come out is still causally determined. Nevertheless, this kind of thing is, in a sense, a very long jump in the direction of freedom from the original slime mold, the Jurassic or Cretaceous sand dollar, or even the 1964 model orangutan.

Following are some further heterogenous excerpts added from earlier communications [Sperry, 1952, 1964b] and included, here out of context, for their bearing on issues in the problem of consciousness:

Prior to the first appearance of conscious awareness in evolution, the entire cosmic process, science tells us, was only, as someone has phrased it, "A play before empty benches," colorless and silent at that because, according to our present physics, prior to the advent of brains there was no *color* and no *sound* in the universe, nor was there any flavor or aroma and probably rather little sense and no feeling or emotion. Before brains the universe was also free of pain and anxiety.

All of these conscious phenomena can now be generated by the surgeon's electrode tip applied to the proper regions of the exposed conscious brain. These conscious effects can be triggered also of course by the proper external stimuli, but, more interestingly, by centrally initiated dream states, illusion-ogenic and hallucinogenic agents. That is, they don't depend on the outside world, but may be generated centrally. But always and only, within and by a brain. There is no more important quest in the whole of science probably than the attempt to understand those very particular events in evolution by which brains worked out that special trick that has enabled them to add to the cosmic scheme of things: color, sound, pain, pleasure, and all the other facets of mental experience.

In searching brains for clues to the critical features that might be responsible for consciousness, I have never myself been inclined to focus on the electrons, protons, or the neutrons of the brain; nor either on its atoms; and with all due respect to biochemistry and the N.R.P., I have not been inclined to look particularly at the little molecules of the brain nor even at its big macromolecules in this connection. It has always seemed rather improbable that even a whole brain cell has got what it takes to sense, to perceive, to feel or to think, on its own. The "search for psyche" in my own case at least has been directed mainly at higher level configurations of the brain like specialized circuit systems—and not just any juicy central nerve network that happens to be complex and teeming with electrical excitation. I have been inclined to look rather at circuits specifically designed for the express job of producing effects like pain, or high C, or blue-yellow, circuits of the kind that one finds above a high transection of the spinal cord, but not below —circuits with something that may well be present in the tiny pinhead dimensions of the midbrain of the color-perceiving goldfish, but lacking in the massive spinal cord tissue of the ox, circuits that are profoundly affected by certain lesions of the midbrain and thalamus, but remarkably little altered by complete absence of the entire human cerebellum. And if it actually came to laying money on the line, I would probably bet first choice on still larger cerebral configurations, configurations that include the combined effects of both (*a*) the specialized circuit systems like the foregoing, plus (*b*) a background of cerebral activity of the alert waking type. Take away the specific circuit, or the background, or the orderly activity from either one, and the conscious effect is gone.

It is common observation that destruction of a brain part through disease, trauma, anoxia, etc., commonly leads to an irreversible permanent loss of the corresponding facet of mental awareness with consequent reduction and crippling of the cognitive self. In this and in the many other evidences that consciousness is directly tied to the properly functioning brain mechanism, the student of brain function finds little to encourage the almost universal hope of the human brain for perseveration of something of its perceiving self following cerebral arrest. This is in line with the prevailing view that consciousness is an emergent property of certain specialized cerebral circuits in action, that is, circuits that are living and unanesthetized and engaged in a normally alert form of activity.

For scientists and engineers involved in computer design it has become a not entirely impractical question to ask whether consciousness is necessarily and inevitably tied to *living* hardware. In this connection, I do not see anything in the above view that excludes the possibility that consciousness might be present in a machine or electronic device, provided it could carry out the kinds of objective functions and processes that the brain handles. This is very different, however, from saying that there is an inner conscious aspect to everything.

In fact, I have often thought that a computer with a sense of pain and pleasure, not to mention color perception, hearing, and other feelings in the conscious introspective sense might well be a much more proficient computer than a similar machine without the conscious properties. For adaptive and complex reactions, consciousness may not be necessary, but when it comes to learning that involves memory, conscious centers become a tremendous asset. This reasoning favors the view that consciousness may have real operational value, that it is more than merely an overtone, a by-product, epiphenomenon, or a metaphysical parallel of the objective process.

If we continue to ask what variables in brain function are correlated with what variables in conscious experiences [Sperry, 1952], and enough of us concentrate our brain research in this direction, the nature of consciousness and its relation to brain process is bound to become increasingly clear. In this day of information explosion it would not be too surprising if some of us present may live to know the full answer.

DISCUSSION

Chairman: LORD ADRIAN

PENFIELD: I think this has been a most startling presentation of these two cases, and it helps to answer certain questions that we have in mind. It is clear that in perception one hemisphere can work with the record of consciousness that is within that same hemisphere, and it is clear, too, that the record of the stream of consciousness is laid down in duplicate in the two sides. This is something that we have always suspected, but as far as I know it has never been proved before; and if I could make a little sketch on the board I can show how this applies to our thinking with regard to the record of the stream of consciousness.

You see here the undersurface of the brain with the midbrain cut across and the cerebellum and pons removed. You see on either side of the midbrain the undersurface of the hippocampus. Now this area is often injured at birth by herniation of the brain through the opening of the incisura of the tentorium. It is squeezed through, and so you have one hippocampus injured, or both, at the time of birth; and we are quite clear that in some of our patients who suffer from temporal lobe epilepsy the cause of the attacks is the scarring of the hippocampus (and often the temporal lobe) produced by the pressure while the baby's head passes through the birth canal. In one distressing case I removed the anterior part of the temporal lobe on the left hoping to cure the attacks, but leaving the hippocampus in place. Then after more than three years, as the patient was not cured, I removed the left hippocampus. He improved as far as attacks were concerned but his memory for recent years was lost [Milner and Penfield, 1955]. Further study led to the conclusion that the right hippocampus had been destroyed at birth. We were forced to conclude that bilateral absence of the hippocampus meant loss of the memory record. With the hippocampus intact on one side, his memory had been normal. He retains his skill as a draftsman and earns his living, but he cannot recall such things as what he had for breakfast today. It is apparent that the memory record in one side is normally the duplicate of that in the other hemisphere under normal conditions. It is located in the hippocampus, together with its connections in the diencephalon. This would explain the findings in these two cases reported by Professor Sperry.

SPERRY: Attempts to produce similar effects in monkeys and other animals have been rather disappointing, suggesting probably that there have been some rapid changes in the course of primate evolution to make the hippocampal structures so critical in man for recent memory. I assume you do not imply that all memory, including that for language, is laid down on both sides. In this connection, language comprehension, I suppose, must be distinguished from speech; it is the motor expression especially, speech and writing, that is most lateralized. But there seems to be much individual variation in these higher-level functions, that is, in the organization of speech, for example, and the functional organization of the corpus callosum in general, so that what applies to one person may not apply to the next. In a small percentage of the population, you recall, Milner found speech to be bilateralized.

MOUNTCASTLE: I would very much like to know, Dr. Sperry, something about the performance of these patients using auditory input, which you did not say anything about. It would be especially interesting to know what happens when the verbalizing hemisphere provides erroneous information to the other hemisphere which can itself respond correctly to somesthetical or visual input.

SPERRY: We have not run any specific tests on auditory functions—except incidentally where speech is involved. The minor hemisphere will use the speech emanating from the major hemisphere, and this is sometimes a means of effecting a kind of cross-integration; for example, if a familiar sample object is placed in the right hand while the subject is blindfolded, the left hand is unable to pick out by palpation the same or a matching object from among others. However, if the subject is allowed to name out loud the sample object in the right hand, then the left hand does find the correct object. Similarly, the left hand can be used to retrieve an object named aloud by the experimenter. At the same time, remember that if the given object is placed in the left hand or retrieved by the left hand without auditory or other cues accessible to the major hemisphere, then the speech hemisphere is unable to name or otherwise indicate any perception of such an object, which is perceived only by the minor hemisphere.

TEUBER: I would just like to ask a question to clarify my understanding of the description you gave of the second of the two cases. Was there a return of capacity not only to write with the left hand, but also to read simple words in the left half field, or did I misunderstand your presentation?

SPERRY: No, you state it correctly.

TEUBER: I would find that most remarkable in view of the repeated trend to interpret difficulties in object recognition, or rather, object naming, by the left hand to an interruption of the callosal commissure.

SPERRY: You first asked about writing and about visual comprehension and now you are speaking of tactile recognition and naming?

TEUBER: As I understood it, it was the left visual half-field that could recognize the word written and the left hand that could identify the appropriate object.

SPERRY: Let us go through that again slowly, you say that the left hand feels an object or the left field looks at a word?

TEUBER: A word is presented to the left visual field; the left hand feels for the appropriate object and finds it. This is how I understood your statement.

SPERRY: The left half-field can read the name of a familiar object, or the object may be placed in the left hand. Either way, the left hand can then retrieve the corresponding object, using either tactile or visual guidance. That is, we have intermodal transfer here within the minor hemisphere as well as comprehension of the printed word.

BREMER: Did I understand that the alexia in the left half-field, which was a consequence of the callosotomy, disappeared after a short time?

SPERRY: It did in the second patient.

BREMER: It did disappear! That is the reason of Dr. Teuber's surprise and my surprise too.

SPERRY: Yes, but remember that a small percentage of people have rather full bilateralization of speech, and also remember that it is only comprehension we are demonstrating here, not motor expression. This same person cannot speak and cannot write with the minor hemisphere, but she can draw simple pictures. She can write with the left hand, but by testing this with lateralized visual or tactile input, we infer this to be governed through the major hemisphere which, as I mentioned, now has considerable control over the left as well as the right hand. With a pen, for example, placed in the left hand out of sight, she can pick out the correct printed name of the test object and can retrieve it and show how it is used, but cannot write any answer. Only after she is told it is a pen, or after the information otherwise reaches the major hemisphere, can she write the answer.

ANDERSEN: Are the two brain halves asleep and alert and awake at the same time?

SPERRY: As far as we know, yes. We have never seen any lateralization of sleep-waking states.

GRANIT: Did you make the minor hemisphere do any mathematical calculations?

SPERRY: We tried, but unsuccessfully. Apparently the minor hemisphere cannot calculate, even to the extent of doubling the numbers 1 to 4.

SCHAEFER: May I ask if the person had awareness on her dominant side —the feeling of something strange happening—because only such a feeling could indicate to us that something besides that system is still acting and that a second ego was somewhere acting besides that in the dominant hemisphere. And then, in respect of free will, I would strongly suggest that, in this case, we adopt a purely methodological point of view because free will is something that comes out of the introspective judgment of man on his own nature. At the same time you can have a feeling of free will and yet there is a complete determination as judged from the outside. That is the common experience of psychiatrists, so I feel that we should tell philosophers that free will is a completely subjective thing, which is, I believe, in complete agreement with what you stated before.

SPERRY: Occasionally, in the case of the first patient, especially, there was reference to numbness or tingling in the left arm. This could be explained in terms of slight positive sensory effects from the left side being projected to the major hemisphere, that is, uncrossed projection in the somesthetic pathways. In the visual sphere and in the somesthetic system more generally, the absence of distinct complaints about abnormalities in left-sided sensation or perception is the striking thing. I have been inclined to compare this to the absence of complaints about scotomata from occipital lobe damage.

Yes, I believe your relegation of "free will" to the subjective realm while keeping behavior completely determined from the standpoint of objective study, psychiatric treatment, etc., seems consistent; but, of course, it still obliges one to acknowledge that everything he has done, he had to do and could not have done otherwise in the circumstances.

PHILLIPS: May I try to focus this discussion by referring to a sentence in the printed summary? "Each of the separate hemispheres seems to have its own conscious awareness." Now, as I understand, in the second patient the nondominant hemisphere could be regarded as a computer which can read the word "cup" and then select a cup from a miscellany of objects. Now, was the individual conscious of that? What were the subjective statements of the patient about her ability to perform that act?

SPERRY: I can only go back to the statement that someone made here yesterday—namely, that we tend to infer consciousness by analogy; in people, we accept it and in objects we don't.

PHILLIPS: This individual human subject was able to speak to you, but was not able to make any statement that implied consciousness in her computer, which could read the word and select a cup from a collection of objects.

SPERRY: The minor hemisphere may be likened to an aphasic brain in which the centers for speech and writing have been damaged. When an aphasia is reversible, the subject's account of his memory of the aphasic period suggests he had been conscious even though he had been unable to express himself. That the minor hemisphere in these adult cases will ever be able to recount any of the current experiences seems doubtful.

Consider the effect of a stimulus applied to the forehead of our subject which will then be projected to both hemispheres because of the bilateral cortical representation of head and face. The sensation in each hemisphere is presumably identical with respect to its localization, timing, and its general quality. In other words, there are two similar but separate conscious experiences, one in each hemisphere, and I am not sure but what the same is true under normal conditions with the corpus callosum intact. There is nothing particularly disturbing about such a lack of unity in consciousness if one does not try to make consciousness some kind of entity in itself, instead of a functional property of the brain in action.

GOMES: Your communication of facts is most challenging for me. When the two hemispheres of the brain of an individual are separated, some very significant disturbance in the system of control of actions of the individual must occur. It is even amazing that the individual is able to perform usual actions with the ordinary degree of coordination which you have observed in your patients. I ask you, therefore, what do you observe in purposely contrived cases in which there is a conflict between the two hemispheres? Could not such defects be attributed in principle to the difficulty of control of motor action which the individual with a split brain has? But this is not an alternative to your interpretation of the existence of two separate minds, and sometimes even of two separate wills. I ask you whether this conflict is not apparent and the result rather of this interruption of the normal system of control of motor reactions in connection with visual and other kinds of perception.

SPERRY: I don't at the moment see how this would account for all the results, that is, all the evidence indicating independence of perception, learning, and memory. In regard to motor control, there was in the first few months a strong apraxia of the left hand, indicating, as Professor Bremer pointed out, that the mediation of voluntary activity of the left hand is normally dependent on the callosum, especially where language and language-dependent thinking is involved.

MAC KAY: I am following up Dr. Phillips' question. I am intrigued by the apparent resemblances between the automatisms which Dr. Penfield reported, and the sorts of behavior of which people are unaware when they are concentrating (I mean these split-brain people) on data coming in through one hemispheric system. What I am asking is whether this evidence really justifies us in saying that there are really two minds here. Aren't we all conscious of executing minor automatisms, for instance, raising eyebrows, and so forth, when our mind is concentrating on something else? I remember once talking to someone in my bedroom when intending to change my shirt and finding myself putting on my pajamas in the course of the discussion, because we had gone on talking and I had automatically carried out a routine which I might have done consciously if I had intended. Under those circumstances, we might say whimsically that I had another mind that was trying to make me go to bed or something, but the common-sense description is that I had left some of my learned routines to run because I was attending to something else. Now why should we say that there are two minds in these individuals? Why shouldn't we say rather that they are capable in a way that we are not, because of the corpus callosum, they are capable of attending to part of their hemispheric activity at a time?

SPERRY: Everything indicates that the minor hemisphere has its own sensations, perceptions, and memories and that it is capable of at least a little comprehension and thinking. Also the fact that it can learn would seem important here. In monkey experiments we have found that this learning can proceed concurrently and simultaneously in the disconnected hemispheres, one hemisphere learning the opposite of the other. We have seen a few indications of emotional feeling generated in the minor hemisphere, like a broad smile following the completion of a test task with the left hand, a smile which the subject was unable to explain verbally; or the reverse, frowning at an incorrect verbal response or an inept performance by the right hand when only the minor hemisphere knew the correct answer!

MAC KAY: Yes, but the kind of model which I will be talking about tomorrow would also show this behavior.

SPERRY: Is there anything then that would not apply just as well to the dominant hemisphere?

MAC KAY: I don't think that either hemisphere is conscious. I don't think that it makes sense to attribute consciousness to cerebral hemispheres. What I am saying is that the person is conscious and there is only one person that is conscious, but he has a split control system, and that he is, therefore, able to pay attention to one half at a time in a way we cannot because of the commissural coupling.

SPERRY: Perhaps this depends on one's definition of consciousness. If you think of it in terms of its simplest elements, the raw sensations like the color red, for example, the colors, sounds, taste, touch, smell, and the like, as I have done, then wouldn't it appear most reasonable to assume the presence of conscious sensation in the minor hemisphere when that hemisphere is selecting correctly one of two colors? Dr. Thorpe has to use similar reasoning when it comes to consciousness in various animal species.

CHAIRMAN: I expect that we are all bursting with questions, but I think it will do us good to keep them in store for a bit and think over the results of this extraordinarily interesting communication.

REFERENCES

BOGEN, J. E., and P. J. VOGEL. Cerebral commissurotomy in man, *Bull. Los Angeles Neurol. Soc.*, 27, 169–172 [1962].

GAZZANIGA, M. S., J. E. BOGEN, and R. W. SPERRY. Some functional effects of sectioning the cerebral commissures in man, *Proc. Natl. Acad. Sci.*, 48, Part 2, 1765–1769 [1962].

———. Laterality effects in somesthesis following cerebral commissurotomy in man, *Neuropsychologia*, 1, 209–215 [1963].

———. Observations on visual perception after disconnection of the cerebral hemispheres in man, *Brain*, 88, 221–236 [1965].

SPERRY, R. W. Neurology and the mind-brain problem, *Amer. Scientist*, 40, 291–312 [1952].

———. Cerebral organization and behavior, *Science*, 133, 1749–1757 [1961a].

———. Some developments in brain lesion studies of learning, *Fed. Proc.*, 20, Part I, 609–616 [1961b].

———. The great cerebral commissure, *Scient. American*, 210, 42 [1964a].

———. *Problems Outstanding in the Evolution of Brain Function*, 1964 James Arthur Lecture on the Evolution of the Human Brain. New York: Amer. Mus. Natl. Hist. [1964b].

14

Conscious Experience and Memory

by J. C. Eccles

Institute for Biomedical Research, Education and Research Foundation, American Medical Association, Chicago, Illinois; formerly Professor of Physiology, Australian National University, Canberra, Australia

Conscious Experience

Introduction

I have chosen the expression "conscious experience" in preference to the simple term *consciousness* in order to stress the experienced character of consciousness in all its aspects. I prefer this expression to the term *experienced integration* or EI that was employed by Fessard [1954] in his distinguished contribution to the symposium *Brain Mechanisms and Consciousness*. Nevertheless, "experienced integration" has the advantage of stressing the integrative character of brain action in the synthesis of conscious experiences from the most diverse sensory inputs. Fessard builds his contribution around the answers to three fundamental questions: "What neuronal activity is most likely to correspond to the existence of EI? How can we conceive of the integrative process that transforms an assembly of separately active neurone pools in the brain into a unified pattern? Where are all these processes likely to take place?" And much of our discussion at this symposium will relate to these three questions.

In recent decades the word "mind" or the term *concept of mind* has been philosophically unfashionable. Philosophers of great influence, such as Ryle and Ayer, have claimed that the problem of brain and mind is illusory and due to verbal confusions or category mistakes. Nevertheless neurophysiologists and neurologists have continued to wrestle with the

problem of brain and mind, regarding it as the most difficult and fundamental problem confronting man; and now we can be encouraged by a
recent book *The Existence of Mind* [Beloff, 1962] that certainly reestab-
lishes the philosophical status of the brain-mind problem. In addition,
I give two quotations from a recent lecture "Two Kinds of Reality" by
Eugen Wigner, Nobel laureate in physics, in order to illustrate how important and urgent the problem of consciousness is to a theoretical
physicist.

> . . . There are two kinds of reality or existence: the existence of my
> consciousness and the reality or existence of everything else. This latter reality
> is not absolute but only relative. . . . Excepting immediate sensations, the
> content of my consciousness, everything is a construct, . . . but some con-
> structs are closer, some farther, from the direct sensations. [These constructs
> are, of course, the physical world.]
> . . . As I said, our inability to describe our consciousness adequately,
> to give a satisfactory picture of it, is the greatest obstacle to our acquiring a
> rounded picture of the world.

Because conscious experience is the immediate and absolute reality,
it is necessary that I base my account of it on my own experience, adopt-
ing a purely personal or egocentric method of presentation, which may
be called methodological solipsism. My conscious experience is all that
is given to me in my task of trying to understand myself; and it is only
because of and through my experience that I come to know of a world
of things and events and so to embark on the attempt to understand it.
Furthermore, I have to consider the totality of my conscious experiences,
not only here and now, but of all my past. Because of the experiences
that can be recalled in memory, and so re-experienced, I recognize my
unity and identity through all past vicissitudes; it is memory that gives
me that continuity of inner experience which belongs to me as a self; and
this inner experience comprises not only my memories, but all the sequences of imagery, ideas, desires, volitions, and emotional feelings that
characterize my waking life, and, in addition, it includes my dreams and
hallucinations. Sherrington [1940], in his book (*Man on His Nature*),
has written most movingly on the self, as may be illustrated by the following quotation:

> This "I," this self, which can so vividly propose to "do," what attributes
> as regards "doing" does it appear to itself to have? It counts itself as a
> "cause." Do we not each think of our "I" as a "cause" within our body?
> "Within" inasmuch as it is at the core of the spatial world, which our percep-
> tion seems to look out at from our body. The body seems a zone immediately
> about that central core. This "I" belongs more immediately to our awareness
> than does even the spatial world about us, for it is directly experienced. It *is*
> the "self."

In contrast to this inner experience I have experiences or perceptions that are derived from activation of my sensory receptors. It is solely from such perceptual experiences that I derive the concept of an external world of things and events, which is a world other than the world of my inner experience and which even includes my body, the "body image" of neurology. I would agree with Wigner that this external world has the status of a second-order or derivative reality. How, it may be asked, can my perceptual experiences give me such an effective knowledge of the external world that I can find my way round in it and even manipulate it with such success? So effective is this practical operation that I am not conscious of this problem in my whole experience of practical living; my body and its environment appear to be directly known to me. This attitude towards perceptual experiences can be termed naive or direct realism, which has of course been rendered untenable by modern neurophysiology.

Neurophysiological Events Relating to Perception

We can now be sure of the initial stages in the process whereby stimulation of receptor organs gives rise to a perceptual experience. We owe our understanding of the coding of such stimulation into trains of nerve impulses to the pioneer contributions of Adrian and his school; and the processes of transmission through the serial synapses on the pathway to the cerebral cortex have already been illuminated by the contributions to this symposium by Mountcastle [1965], Granit [1965] and Creutzfeldt [1965]. In this pathway there has been much integration in the coded information, but this can be but a prelude to the unimaginably complex integrational procedures in the cerebral cortex that have been so effectively discussed by Fessard [1961].

Indubitable evidence of the convergence of sensory information in the cortex is provided by those experiments in which a single cortical neuron is shown to be activated from several different sensory inputs. Multisensory convergence onto cortical neurons has been studied very intensively by Jung and his collaborators [Jung, 1961; Jung, Kornhuber, and da Fonseca, 1963; Kornhuber and Aschoff, 1964]; and also by Dubner and Rutledge [1964]. For example, in Fig. 14.1 a neuron in the para-auditory cortex was excited both by light and by vestibular stimulation. Similar convergence of two or three sensory modalities was observed in all cortical areas investigated, both in the primary receiving areas and in the associative areas of the cortex. Buser and Imbert [1961] have obtained comparable results in an extensive study on multisensory neurons. For example, in Fig. 14.2 a neuron in the perisigmoid cortex was excited not only by somatosensory impulses from each limb (Al, Ar, Pl, Pr), but also by a light flash (V), a click (A) and by V + A in close succession.

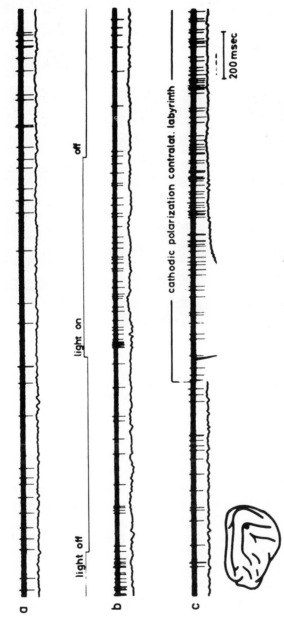

Fig. 14.1. Extracellular responses of neuron in an association area of the neocortex (the para-auditory cortex). (a) Gives spontaneous activity in darkness; (b) shows that it responds to light and is transiently depressed by the onset of darkness; (c) shows that it is strongly excited from the contralateral labyrinth [Jung, Kornhuber, and da Fonseca, 1963].

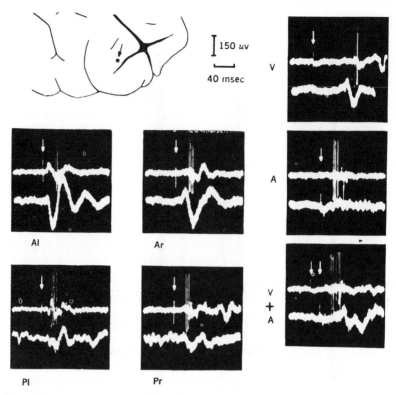

Fig. 14.2. Extracellular responses of a neuron in the perisigmoid cortex of a cat in deep chloralose anesthesia. Arrows signal stimuli to each limb; anterior, A; posterior, B; l, left; r, right. All evoked responses of the unit that was otherwise silent. V is flash, A is click, and V + A is combined flash plus click [Buser and Imbert, 1961].

I should also refer to the recent very comprehensive report of sensory integration in the cortex as signaled by evoked potentials and their interaction [Albe-Fessard and Fessard, 1963]. Provisional attempts have been made to discover the physiological significance of these convergence patterns, but for our present purpose it is sufficient to document this evidence that there are now hundreds of examples of multisensory convergence on single cortical neurons in all parts of the cerebral cortex, as well as in all the subcortical centers.

It is difficult to conceive the complexity actually obtaining in propagation over neuronal chains, where each neuron is linked to hundreds of other neurons and where the convergence of many impulses within a few milliseconds is necessary in order to evoke a discharge from any one neuron. It is therefore desirable to study the properties of simple models of networks as has been done by Burns [1951] and by Fessard [1954, 1961]. For example, Fig. 14.3 is such a model formed by the synaptic connections between 16 cells. Simplification has also been achieved by neglecting inhibitory action and by reducing the number of excitatory synapses made by each axon to no more than three; and, correspondingly, it has been assumed that any cell is made to discharge by the activation of two or more synapses on its surface. The synaptic connections of Fig. 14.3 have been designed to illustrate one remarkable and important property of a neuronal network, namely, that two completely different inputs at A (A_1A_2 in the upper picture or A_3A_4 in the lower picture) can be transmitted through the same pattern of cell connections (A to B to C to D), crossing each other and emerging as completely different outputs at D (D_3D_4 in the upper picture and D_1D_2 in the lower). An interval of some milliseconds between the two wave fronts would eliminate interference by neuronal refractoriness or by summation of synaptic excitations. It will be noted that along the fringe of the advancing wave front in Fig. 14.3 there are subliminally excited neurons (C_1, D_1, D_2 in the upper picture). Such "fringe neurons" give opportunity for growth of a wave if other influences should also subliminally activate them.

Thus we are introduced to the concept of lability of a wave front. It may be diminished by inhibitory or depressant influences, and so ultimately be extinguished, or it may be enhanced by factors aiding in the activation of "fringe neurons." It will also be appreciated that, if a wave front moves into neuronal pathways having interconnections of suitable configuration, it may bifurcate into two waves propagating independently; while, conversely, two wave fronts propagating at the same time into the same pool of neurons would coalesce and give an onwardly propagating wave having features derived from both waves, with additional features due to the summation.

It will be realized that in the neuronal network of the cerebral cortex the factors involved in transmission of a wave front are vastly more complicated than in the simplified model of Fig. 14.3. In the first place, each neuron would make very many synaptic contacts with other neurons, and also receive from many more—probably from hundreds. Perhaps as many as one hundred neurons would be involved in each stage of an effectively advancing wave front and not 2 or 3 as in Fig. 14.3, so this wave would sweep over 100,000 neurons in one second. An advancing wave would also be branching at intervals, often abortively, and coalescing with other waves to give a complex spatiotemporal pattern.

Figure 14.4 is a diagrammatic illustration by Fessard [1961] to show the manner in which three neuronal assemblages could process repetitive trains of impulses reaching them at various frequencies as indicated.

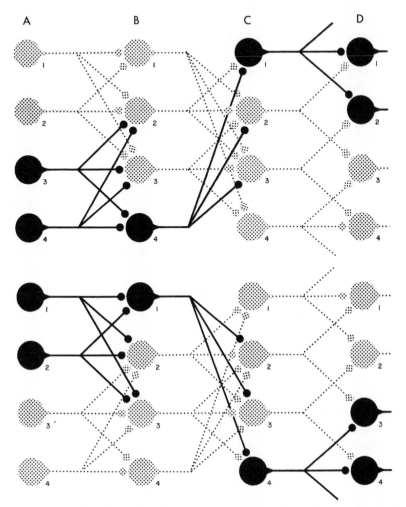

Fig. 14.3. Model of a highly schematic neuronal network to illustrate the simplest case of propagation along a multilane pathway. There is exactly the same anatomical network in the upper and lower diagrams. The synaptic connections of the twelve cells in columns A, B, and C are drawn, cells with impulses being shown light grey, while the silent cells are black. The assumption is that a cell fires an impulse if it is excited by two or more synapses (also light grey). Thus an input A_1A_2 results in an output discharge of D_3D_4 (upper diagram), whereas an input of A_3A_4 gives an output of D_1D_2 (lower diagram). Neurons B_2B_3 and C_2C_3 are activated in the crossing zone for both these inputs. This diagram suffers from the serious defect that it ignores inhibition.

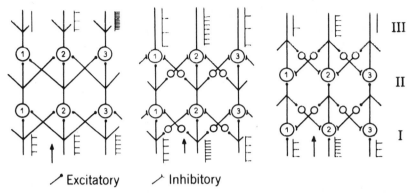

/ Excitatory   / Inhibitory

Fig. 14.4. Three diagrams illustrating possible modes of action of neuronal networks. In each the input is shown in three channels below, the frequencies being indicated by the assumed impulse discharges on vertical lines. The outputs are shown above with similar indications of the discharge frequencies. The identification of excitatory and inhibitory synapses is shown below. Thus the first diagram shows purely excitatory synapses and illustrates how an increasing selectivity of response may be produced. The other two diagrams illustrate the action of feed-forward and feed-back inhibition in increasing the specificity of the output [Fessard, 1961].

The first is a purely excitatory network in which an input at stage I is transformed into a much more selective output at stage III. In the second, afferent collateral inhibition serves likewise to heighten the contrast between input (stage I) and the output (stage III) frequencies. In the third, recurrent collateral inhibition acts similarly, but more effectively, so that lines 1 and 3 are virtually silenced at stage III. In Chapter 2 I gave illustrations of both these types of inhibitory action on cortical neurons. The role of inhibition in sharpening zones of neuronal activation has been very thoroughly studied in the visual cortex by Hubel and Wiesel [1962] and by Jung [1961] and his collaborators. Undoubtedly cortical inhibition is of great importance in suppressing the incessant background neuronal discharges of the awake brain, and so heightening the signal to noise ratio.

Despite the obscurity of the integrated neuronal events that subserve the elaboration of the perceptual process, it is a general postulate [cf. Fessard, 1961; Mountcastle, 1965] that for every perception there is a specific spatiotemporal pattern of neuronal activity in the neuronal networks of the cerebral cortex and the related subcortical ganglia. The transmission from sense organ to cerebral cortex is by a coded pattern of nerve impulses that is quite unlike the original stimulus to that organ, and the spatiotemporal pattern of neuronal activity that is evoked in the cerebral cortex would be again different and would contain synthetic elements deriving from afferent inputs from other sense organs. Yet, as a

consequence of these cerebral patterns of activity, I experience perceptions which in my private perceptual world are "projected" to the external world; it may be to the surface of the body or even within it; or,
as with sight, hearing, or smell, to the outside world.

The Relationship of the Perceptual World to the External World

In response to sensory stimulation, I experience a private perceptual
world which must be regarded, neurophysiologically, as an interpretation
of specific events in my brain. Hence I am confronted by the problem:
how can these diverse cerebral patterns of activity give me valid pictures
of the external world? Usually this problem is discussed in relation to
visual perception. There seems to be an extraordinary problem in explaining how impulses from the retina when relayed to the cerebral cortex
give a picture of the external world with all its various objects in three-
dimensional array and endowed with brightness and color. This epistemological problem has led to much philosophical confusion when it has
been discussed on the assumption that fully patterned visual perception
is an inborn property of the nervous system. On the contrary, visual perception is an interpretation of retinal data that has been learned through
association with sensory information provided by receptors in muscles,
joints, skin, and the vestibular apparatus. The prime importance of active
movement in this development of visual perception has been demonstrated in elegant experiments by Held and Hein [1953]. The three-
dimensional world pictures which result from my visual experience are
primarily based on perceptual data derived from active movements and
touch, and are the end product of a long effort of progressive learning
by trial and error. As a well-trained adult, it is difficult for me to realize
that my earliest learning occurred in a cot with movement of limbs under
visual observation; and thereafter the field of visual education was extended by crawling, walking, and still other modes of locomotion so that
my sphere of observation was progressively further extended. I judge
distance and space as distance and direction that could be traveled, if I
so wish; and so I orientate the world around myself. Thus my three-
dimensional perceptual world is essentially a "kinesthetic world"; it is
initially bounded by the cot, but has thereafter been enormously extended in range and subtlety.

The learning processes of early childhood are largely unremembered,
but I can remember many early efforts to evaluate distance and size, as
well as the errors of judgment that I made when confronted by strange
environments where familiar clues were lacking. Fortunately, I do not
have to rely on memories from infancy, for there are well-documented
accounts by von Senden [1962] of adults who were given patterned vision
for the first time by the removal of congenital cataracts from their eyes.

They reported that their initial visual experiences were meaningless and quite unrelated to the spatial world that had been built up from touch and movement. It took many weeks and even months of continual effort to derive from visual information a perceptual world that was congruent with their "kinesthetic world" and in which as a consequence they could move with assurance. Similar evidence is provided by Riesen's [1947, 1958] experiments on chimpanzees that were reared in darkness and then transferred to an illuminated world. It took many months of training before they could skillfully use visual experience in guiding movement. A further illustration of the way in which learning can transform the interpretation of visual information is provided by Stratton's [1897] experiences when a system of lenses was placed in front of one of his eyes (the other being covered) so that the image on the retina was inverted with respect to its usual orientation. For several days the visual world was hopelessly disordered. Since it was inverted, it gave an impression of unreality and was useless for the purpose of apprehending or manipulating objects. But as a result of eight days of continual effort, the visual world could be sensed correctly and then became a reliable guide for manipulation and movement. There have been many recent confirmations of these early experiments with many additional observations of most intriguing variety [Köhler, 1951; Held and Bosson, 1961; Mikaelian and Held, 1964].

These experiments establish that, as a consequence of trial-and-error learning, the brain events evoked by sensory information from the retina are interpreted so that they give a valid picture of the external world that is sensed by touch and movement, that is, the world of visual perception becomes a world in which I can effectively move. Actually, this perceptual world is much more synthetic than we imagine; for example, it normally remains fixed and stable when the images on the retina are moved in the most diverse ways by naturally occurring body, head, or eye movements, but not, for example, when the eye is moved by an applied pressure. The kinesthetic information from all these natural movements as well as the sensory information from the vestibular apparatus is synthesized with the retinal information. The action of this automatic correcting device for visual perception is best appreciated when there are disturbances of vestibular function; under such conditions there is gross movement of the visually perceived world, which gives rise to the sensation of vertigo.

Further problems are involved in attempting to understand how the brain events derived from the various sensory inputs can give me not only my own private perceptual world, but also experiences that are shared by other observers and which as a consequence I have come to regard as manifestations of an external world. Communication between observers serves to establish the existence of a world that is virtually identical to many observers. Its manner of operation is best illustrated by giving instances where there are differences between observers. For example, when observers differ in their perception of colors, as revealed by tests in color mixing and matching, we resolve this discrepancy not by rejecting color as an attribute of an external world common to all observers, but by classifying some observers as defective in color perception. Again, a subject under the influence of a hallucinogenic drug, such as mescaline, experiences a wealth of imagery that is not shared by other observers close by. It is readily appreciated that such a discrepancy does not cast doubt on the validity of the external world that is derived from the shared perceptual world of these observers; instead, the exceptional experiences that occur under the influence of mescaline or in other disordered cerebral functions are classified as hallucinations. It will be realized that, when observers report one or other of these exceptional features of their perceptual worlds, the situation is customarily handled in a "common sense" way so that the status of a real external world independent of observers is not impugned.

The Objective-subjective Dichotomy

It would seem that the status of the external world is assured, for it has a reality that apparently transcends all the imperfections in the perceptual equipments of the observers. In this way there has arisen the contrast between the reality of the external or objective world on the one hand and, on the other, the subjectivity of our perceptual experiences with all their personal bias and distortion. It is generally believed that the former alone provide a sound basis for scientific investigation. However, this objective-subjective distinction is illusory, being derived from a misinterpretation and a misunderstanding, as has been convincingly argued by Schrödinger [1958]; for example, he says:

> Without being aware of it and without being rigorously systematic about it, we exclude the Subject of Cognizance from the domain of nature that we endeavour to understand. We step with our own person back into the part of an onlooker who does not belong to the world, which by this very procedure becomes an objective world. This situation is the same for every mind and its world, in spite of the unfathomable abundance of "cross-references" between them. The world is given to me only once, not one existing and one perceived. Subject and object are only one. The barrier between them cannot be said to have broken down as a result of recent experience in the physical sciences, for this barrier does not exist.

The illusory nature of the objective-subjective dichotomy of experience is further illustrated by what might be called a spectrum of perceptual experiences. (*A*) Vision of an object that can be confirmed by touching it, so giving it form, and which can in this same manner be sensed by and reported upon by their other observers with addition of color, the perception of the object thus achieving public status. (*B*) Pin prick of a finger can be witnessed by an observer as well as by the subject, but the pain is private to the subject; however, each observer can perform a similar experiment on himself and report his observation of pain, which in this way is shared and so achieves a public status. (*C*) The dull pain or ache of visceral origin cannot be readily duplicated in another observer, yet clinical investigators have provided a wealth of evidence on the pains characteristic of the visceral diseases, and even of referred pains, so that reports of visceral pain achieve indirectly a kind of public status. Similar considerations apply to such sensations as thirst or hunger. (*D*) Unlike the preceding three examples, mental pain or anguish is not a consequence of stimulation of receptor organs; yet again a kind of public status can be given to such purely private experiences, for there is a measure of agreement in the reports of subjects so afflicted. Similar considerations apply to other emotional experiences: anger, joy, delight in beauty, awe, fear. (*E*) The experiences of dreams or of memories are even more uniquely private, belonging as they do still more exclusively to the realm of inner experience; yet again a kind of public status is established by the wealth of communication that there is between observers.

It can be claimed that all transitions exist between any two successive examples of this spectrum, which conforms very well with the postulate that every one of the various experiences is associated with specific patterns of neuronal activity in the brain. Apparently such specific patterns can sometimes be evoked by electrical stimulation of the brains of epileptic patients. Penfield and Jasper [1954] have given fascinating accounts of the way in which electrical stimulation of the temporal lobe of the cerebrum will evoke vivid and detailed memories of long-forgotten incidents (cf. Chapter 9).

The conclusion is that every observation of the so-called objective world depends in the first instance on an experience which is just as private as the so-called subjective experiences. The public status of an observation is given by symbolic communication between observers, in particular through the medium of language. By means of this same method of communication, our inner or subjective experiences can likewise achieve a public status. We report such experiences to others and discover that they have like experiences to report to us. A large proportion of our literature is concerned with such verbal communications of inner experiences, either of the author himself or of the characters that he so creates.

The Representative Theory of Perception

When I re-examine the nature of my sensory perceptions, it is evident that these give me the so-called facts of immediate experience and that the so-called external world or "objective world" is a derivative or representation of certain types of this private and direct experience. But this "representative theory of perception" [Beloff, 1962] must not be confused with idealist monism, for the implication is that my perceptual world is my symbolic picture of the "objective world" and thus resembles a map. This map or symbolic picture is essential so that I can act appropriately within this "objective world"; and, as we have seen, it is synthesized from sensory data so as to be effective for this very purpose. It is built upon spatial relations, but is also given symbolic information in terms of secondary qualities. For example, colors, sounds, smells, heat, and cold, as such, belong only to the perceptual world. Furthermore, it is part of my interpretation of my perceptual experience that my "self" is associated with a body that is in the "objective world"; and I find innumerable other bodies that appear to be of like nature. I can exchange communications with them by bodily movements that give rise to perceptual changes in the observer, for example, by gestures or at the more sophisticated level of language, and thus discover by reciprocal communication that they too have conscious experiences resembling mine. Solipsism becomes for me no longer a tenable belief. There is a world of selves, each with the experience of being associated with a body that is in an "objective world" comprising innumerable bodies of like nature and a tremendous variety of other living forms and an immensity of apparently nonliving matter.

Cerebral Events and Conscious Experience

I now return to the key problem in perception which can be expressed in the question: How can some specific spatiotemporal pattern of neuronal activity in the cerebral cortex evoke a particular sensory experience? We can dimly perceive a relationship between brain states and consciousness when we consider the neuronal activity of the cortex in states of unconsciousness, that is, when stimulation of sense organs fails to evoke a sensory experience. The electroencephalogram reveals that in such states there may be either a very low level of neuronal activity, as in coma, concussion, anesthesia, and deep sleep, or a very high level of stereotyped and driven activity, as in convulsions. On the contrary, the electrical activity of the awake brain indicates that a large proportion of the neurons is occupied in an intense dynamic activity of great variety [cf. Fessard, 1961]. Under such conditions it has been postulated that at any instant a considerable proportion of the neurons would be passing through levels of excitation at which the discharge of an impulse would be problematical, such neurons being "critically poised" with respect to the generation of impulses [Eccles, 1953]. Diagrams of activated neuronal networks as in Figs. 14.3, 14.4 can form the basis of imaginative constructs of spatiotemporal patterns that would develop if such inputs were superimposed on high levels of background activity. It has further been postulated that consciousness is dependent on the existence of a sufficient number of such critically poised neurons, and, consequently, only in such conditions are willing and perceiving possible. However, it is not necessary for the whole cortex to be in this special dynamic state. There is clinical evidence that excision of a large part of the cerebral cortex does not interrupt consciousness; and in convulsions, unconsciousness does not supervene until the convulsive activity has invaded a large part of the cortex. Furthermore, I would suggest that the transcendent performance of the central nervous system is a consequence of its amazing complexity, not only structural, but also dynamic, which is of a much higher order than any other organized system in the universe.

On the basis of this concept we can face up anew to the extraordinary problems inherent in a strong dualism. Interaction of brain and conscious mind, brain receiving from conscious mind in a willed action and in turn transmitting to mind in a conscious experience. But let us be quite clear that for each of us the primary reality is our consciousness—everything else is derivative and has a second-order reality. We have tremendous intellectual tasks in our efforts to understand baffling problems that lie right at the center of our being; but as Eugene Wigner [1964] asks: "Have we any right to expect a solution to such fundamental problems when the efforts made have been trivial relative to the extreme nature of the problem?"

MEMORY

Introduction

The word "memory" is a term now being used for a very wide range of phenomena that involve the storage of information and the retrieval or read-out of this information. Hence we have genetic memory, as, for example, may be illustrated by the bald statement of Eigen's [1964] that "DNA for instance has memory." Also the term is used in relationship to immunology (immunological memory). Such diversity of usage means that the term *memory* becomes practically valueless. I shall adhere to the original restricted sense, and associate memory with that property of the central nervous system whereby it is effective both in the storage and retrieval of information. This property has been termed *psychic memory,* and may be considered to have two components, learning and remembering.

It is generally recognized that there are two varieties of psychic memory. First of all there are brief memories for seconds or at most minutes, many examples of which have recently been considered by Brown [1964]. One example is the ability to repeat sequences of numbers that have been read out. After a few seconds or minutes this memory is lost beyond all recall. Following Hebb [1949], Gerard [1949], and Burns [1958], one can postulate that such a memory is subserved by a spatiotemporal pattern of propagated impulses. So long as this specific pattern is preserved in dynamic operation, retrieval is possible. The spatiotemporal pattern forms a dynamic engram such as Lashley would have envisaged. The second kind of memory is distinguished by its enduring character, even for a lifetime, and has been shown in many experiments to survive, even when the central nervous system is reduced to a quiescent state, as by deep anesthesia, coma, or extreme cooling. Such memories must therefore have as a basis some enduring change that is built into the fine structure of the nervous system, and that is often referred to as a "memory trace," so that we have what is called the "trace theory of memory" [Gomulicki, 1953]. There is an immense literature on what we may term the *learning process*, which includes the phenomena of conditioned reflexes. It is impossible here to review it, but reference can be made to Morrell [1961b] for a recent comprehensive survey. I will confine my treatment to the possible synaptic mechanisms concerned in learning and recall.

As a neurologist, I would assume that in long-term memory a structural change is essentially synaptic, but before considering this postulate in detail, I should refer to some recent alternative suggestions that are built upon a supposed analogy between psychic memory and either genetic memory [Hydén, 1959] or immunological memory [Szilard, 1964]. I do not propose to consider Szilard's theory of memory and recall because it is based on several unacceptable assumptions in regard to the mode of operation of synapses.

Molecular Memory

No doubt everybody is familiar with the great popularity that has been achieved by Hydén's theory, so-called "molecular memory." The claim is repeatedly made by exponents of molecular memory, or in the more extensive field now called molecular neurology [Schmitt, 1964], that the theories of conventional neurology have been most unfruitful and that they neither have sufficient precision in formulation nor sufficient experimental basis. In view of this criticism it is surprising to find that theories of molecular memory are remarkable for extreme extrapolation beyond the experimental evidence. By very elegant techniques, Hydén [1959, 1964] has actually shown that nerve cells involved in a variety of learning situations have an increased RNA content, and they also often show an increase in the ratio of purine to pyrimidine bases (actually of adenine to uracil). One can readily agree that activity of nerve cells is likely to be associated with an increased protein production, which, of course, is dependent on the increased RNA content; but this is very inadequate evidence for the elaborate theory that has been developed by Hydén and which involves assumptions that are contrary to a great deal of neurophysiological evidence and for which there is no experimental support whatsoever. These deficiencies of the theory of molecular memory have recently been pointed out by Dignam and Sporn [1964], and the review of Hechter and Halkerston [1964] should also be consulted.

The theory of molecular memory makes a series of postulates which may be listed in serial order. (1) In an acute learning situation there are specific time patterns of frequency responses set up in neurons. (2) In some way, not stated, any particular specific frequency pattern (also called a modulated frequency) causes DNA to produce uniquely specific RNA. (3) This RNA in turn synthesizes specific proteins in the soma of the neuron. (4) These proteins in turn give rise to the production of the transmitter substance. Essentially it is postulated that a particular modulated frequency of activation by these four sequential operations results in a chemical specification of neurons, so that (5) a similar temporal pattern at some later stage evokes by a resonance-like reaction an increased transmitter production. Hydén [1964] further develops this postulate: "A chemical specification of neurons in learning, involving synthesis of chromosomal RNA and specified proteins, reacting on modulated frequencies in millions of neurons in different parts of the brain, stronger in some, weaker in others, would also fit the conception that a complicated task is learned and remembered, not as a series of bits, but in whole contexts. More easily specified areas of the brain, for example, the hippocampus in mammals, would get a more dominant position in learning."

It is evident to neurophysiologists that this speculation derives from the postulate that the frequencies of impulse discharge by nerve cells carry an extraordinary specificity of coded information. The intensive study of many varieties of neurons in the central nervous system certainly shows wide varieties in their temporal patterns of impulse discharge, but it does not show sharp specificity either in the patterns or in the frequency of discharge. In particular, the frequencies of discharge vary over wide ranges dependent upon the intensity of activation. One must reject the postulate that specificity is carried by some frequency modulation in the manner required by Hydén's theory. The immense wealth of neuro-anatomical and neurophysiological data provides the framework for all the specificity that is required from the brain, and there is no necessity whatever for the speculative suggestions of additional specificity dependent upon frequency modulation. There is the further unacceptable postulate in Hydén's theory of molecular memory (No. 5 above) that there is a kind of resonance phenomenon involved in the recall by a subsequent frequency modulation resembling that responsible for the initial chemical specification. Furthermore, the evidence for the immense number of differently specified RNA molecules, one for each memory, is merely a significant change in the ratio of purine to pyrimidine bases, which could signify only two RNA's, yet thousands of millions are assumed to be specified. Later we shall see that Hydén's elegant demonstration of RNA increase in a learning situation can be built into the classical growth theory of learning; and, in fact, must be a necessary postulate of this theory, though of course there is no requirement of such a high order of chemical specification of this RNA.

Synaptic Properties and Memory

There have been in the past many attempts to attribute learning to the development and growth of synapses [Ramón y Cajal, 1911; Hebb, 1949; Tönnies, 1949; Eccles, 1953, 1961; Young, 1951]; and I would suggest that we can now develop this postulate further, or at least that it is justifiable to speculate about the way in which synapses could be changed by activity, and so in this way develop further the original growth theory of learning. Common to all these synaptic explanations of learning is the general concept that a given sensory input results in a uniquely patterned activation of central neurons; and, according to this explanation, a subsequent re-presentation of this input would tend to be channeled along the same pathways because of the increased efficacy of the synaptic actions exerted by all those neurons that were activated by the initial presentation. There would thus be a further reinforcement of the synapses responsible for the unique pattern of activation and response, with consequently a more effective channeling; and so on, cumulatively, for each successive application of that sensory input. Necessarily, the postulated changes in synaptic efficacy must be of very long duration—days or weeks. There is no way in which relatively brief durations of synaptic change for each synapse of a serial arrangement can sum to give a more prolonged change.

Unfortunately, it has not yet been possible to demonstrate experimentally that excess use produces prolonged changes in synaptic efficacy. The experiments have been performed on the spinal cord in order to take advantage of the precise experimental procedures that can there be applied in the quantitative evaluation of synaptic action [Eccles and MacIntyre, 1953; Eccles, Krnjević and Miledi, 1958; Beránek, Hník, Vyklický and Zelená, 1961; R. M. Eccles, Kozak and Westerman, 1962]. The failure to demonstrate a synaptic basis of learning at the spinal cord level [cf. Eccles, 1964] certainly confirms the general belief that it is a stereo-typed structure, poorly endowed with plastic properties that may be presumed to be very well developed with synaptic connections at the higher levels of the nervous system. I would like now to consider four distinctive properties of cerebral neurons and synapses, relative to their counterparts in the spinal cord, and, furthermore, to discuss their possible significance in relation to the learning process.

Frequency Potentiation

In Fig. 14.5 the same motoneuron in the cervical enlargement of a baboon spinal cord is subjected to a brief repetitive monosynaptic bombardment from two different sources, by afferents from the large stretch receptors of forelimb muscles (A), and by impulses descending the pyramidal tract (B) [Phillips and Porter, 1964]. There is a great contrast in the two responses: the six afferent volleys from the muscle receptors typically evoke a maintained level in the sizes of the successive EPSP's at 200 per sec; the first EPSP generated by the pyramidal tract volley is about the same size as with the first muscle afferent volley, but suc-

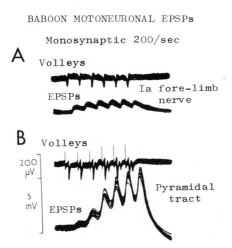

Fig. 14.5. Effect of repetitive activation on the sizes of excitatory postsynaptic potentials. Lower traces of A and B are intracellular records from a motoneuron in the cervical enlargement of a baboon spinal cord, while downward deflections in the upper traces of A and B give the sizes of the presynaptic volleys produced by stimulating a forelimb muscle nerve (A) and the pyramidal tract (B). All records formed by superposition of several faint traces. Note potential scales for presynaptic and intracellular records [Phillips and Porter, 1964].

cessively there is an enormous increase in size, the last EPSP being increased about ten times. This shows that synapses made by pyramidal cells have an extraordinarily efficient mechanism for greatly increasing their effectiveness when they are stressed by high frequency of stimulation. I would suggest that in synapses showing this remarkable plasticity, some residual potency is likely to remain, and this could be the synaptic basis for a trace theory of memory.

It could be objected that, though these synapses are formed by cerebral pyramidal cells, they actually exist in the spinal cord and hence are not a convincing illustration of a high level of plasticity in the cerebral neurons. As yet there seems to be no equivalent experiment on synapses in the cerebral cortex, but there is a considerable potentiation of the successive EPSP's produced by repetitive pyramidal tract stimulation and recorded intracellularly from a pyramidal neuron not invaded antidromically [Eccles, 1966, Fig. 2.1D; Phillips, 1961, Fig. 5]. The latency of these EPSP's and their ability to follow frequencies as high as 200 per sec [Armstrong, 1965] suggest that they are produced by monosynaptic action of the axon collaterals of pyramidal cells. The frequency potentiation of cerebral synapses should be further investigated.

Inhibitory Postsynaptic Potentials

Intracellular recording from a variety of cerebral neurons reveals that their postsynaptic inhibitory potentials are much longer and larger than with spinal neurons. For example, with pyramidal cells of the hippocampus, the IPSP's may be as large as 20 mV and have a duration of 200 to 500 msec [Kandel, Spencer, and Brinley, 1961; Andersen, Eccles, and Løyning, 1963, 1964], which contrast with spinal neurons where the IPSP's are no more than one tenth the size and have a duration of 20 msec at most, as illustrated in Fig. 14.6. IPSP's of neocortical pyramidal cells and of Purkinje cells of the cerebellum are also much larger and longer than spinal IPSP's. Another distinctive feature of the postsynaptic inhibition of cerebral neurons is that it is very largely produced by a concentration of inhibitory synapses on the soma and the axonal origin therefrom, which gives it a great strategic advantage in the suppression of impulse discharge [Andersen, Eccles, and Løyning, 1963, 1964; Andersen, Eccles, and Voorhoeve, 1963, 1964].

These unique features of cerebral IPSP's may not be directly concerned in the synaptic mechanism of learning, but at least they indicate that in the brain some of the synapses have highly developed properties that are not matched in the spinal cord. The original assumption was that synapses at all levels of the nervous system did not differ greatly in properties; consequently the plastic properties responsible for learning were sought experimentally in the spinal cord where more rigorous testing was

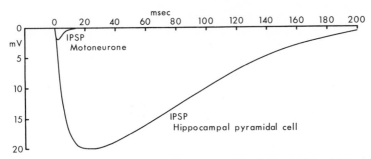

Fig. 14.6. Superimposed traces on the same potential time sides of intracellular recordings to illustrate the very large difference between the maximal IPSP's produced by a group Ia volley in a motoneuron and by the recurrent inhibitory pathway to a hippocampal pyramidal cell.

possible [Eccles and McIntyre, 1953; Eccles, Krnjević and Miledi, 1958; R. M. Eccles, Kozak and Westerman, 1962]. It is now clear that this was mistaken strategy and the postulated plasticity must be sought for experimentally in cerebral synapses.

Neuronal Complexity

Another special feature of the most prominent cerebral neurons, such as pyramidal cells and Purkinje cells, is the extraordinary wealth of dendrites and the synaptic receptive surfaces thereon. For example, it has been calculated that a Purkinje cell has as many as 60,000 dendritic spines, each with a synapse [Fox and Barnard, 1957], while with large cortical pyramidal cells the number is probably in excess of 10,000. Evidence is accumulating that all these spine synapses are excitatory. In many of these large neurons, excitatory synapses can generate local responses or even propagating impulses in the dendrites. For example, with hippocampal [Spencer and Kandel, 1961; Andersen, 1960a, 1960b] and neocortical [Purpura and Shofer, 1964] pyramidal cells and Purkinje cells [Eccles, Llinás, and Sasaki, 1966], integration of synaptic activity is not simply a consequence of the electrotonic convergence of excitatory and inhibitory synaptic activity onto the initial segment of the axon. Probably the initiation of impulses is not here uniquely determined, as is usually the case with the motoneuron [Coombs, Curtis and Eccles, 1957; Eccles, 1957, 1964]. The diagram of the diverse synaptic contacts on a hippocampal pyramidal cell (Fig. 14.7; and Hamlyn [1963]) certainly suggests that much of the integration is effected peripherally in the dendrites. Consequently, these cerebral neurons have a complexity of operation that contrasts with the simplicity that seems to characterize spinal neurons. Again, it is not suggested that this complexity is directly involved in the synaptic changes

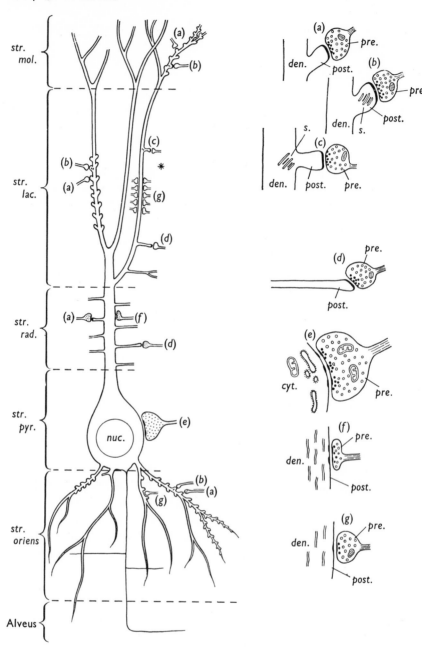

Fig. 14.7. Drawing of a hippocampal pyramidal cell to illustrate the diversity of synaptic endings on the different zones of the apical and basal dendrites, and the inhibitory synaptic endings on the soma. The various types of synapses marked by the letters *a–g* are shown in detail to the right [Hamlyn, 1962].

responsible for learning; nevertheless, it should not be overlooked in the general conceptual development of a theory of learning.

Dendritic Spine Synapses

Ever since the first synaptic theory of learning was proposed, it has been a general postulate that activity tended to cause a growth of synapses. The detailed observation of synapses by electron microscopy now allows more specific postulates to be developed in relation to this synaptic growth. For example, Hamlyn [1962] noted that a special structure, the spine apparatus, was often located postsynaptically in dendritic spines of neocortical and hippocampal pyramidal cells, but was not present with spine synapses at lower levels of the nervous system; hence he suggested that it might be concerned with learning. More directly apposite are the small secondary spines that Hámori and Szentágothai [1964] observed to be budded off from the main dendritic spines of Purkinje cells and to form, as it were, secondary synapses (Fig. 14.8). Since the number of these secondary spines was extremely variable from preparation to preparation, it was suggested that their frequency might depend on previous activity. Such a postulated development of microstructure with activity certainly would accord well with the general postulates of a growth theory of learning. Hebb [1949] and Konorski [1950] have suggested that synaptic multiplication may be the structural basis of learning. Moreover, it has now been demonstrated that the development of secondary spines is a feature of the dendritic spines of the cerebrum as well as of the cerebellum [Van der Loos, 1964].

It is of interest to recall that the dendritic spines were recognized in the early investigations with light microscopy, being called gemmules (Fig. 14.9), but usually [cf. Ramón y Cajal, 1911, 1934], they were not regarded as synaptic. It was further recognized by Ramón y Cajal [1934] that the gemmules developed late, and, in fact, gemmule development was employed as a sign of functional maturation of cortical neurons. The possible synaptic function of gemmules was suggested by Chang [1952], who quoted earlier work on the extreme susceptibility of gemmules to toxins, which had suggested a synaptic function for gemmules. It would be of great interest to have a rigorous study of the postnatal development in number, size, and complexity of dendritic spines (or gemmules).

Discussion

It is pertinent now to recall the evidence of Hydén and Morrell that there is an increase in the RNA content of neurons subjected to excess stimulation. Presumably in the synaptic growth theory of learning it must be postulated that RNA is responsible for the protein synthesis required for growth. However, this postulated growth would not be the

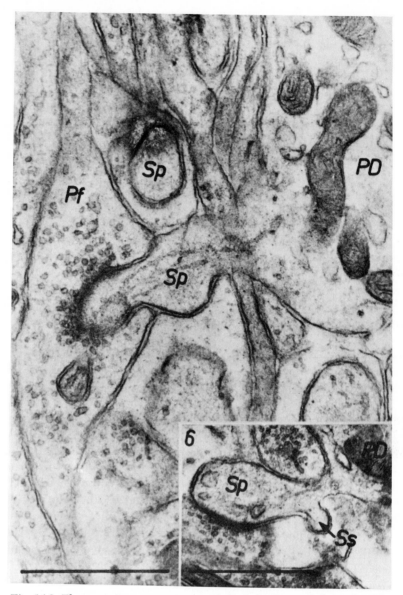

Fig. 14.8. Electron microscopic pictures of the molecular layer of the cerebellum showing parallel fibers, some being swollen with synaptic vehicles, and making synapses with the dendritic spines (Sp) of Purkinje cells. Secondary spines (Ss) are shown budding from spines and in the inset entering into synaptic contact with a parallel fiber [Hámori and Szentágothai, 1964].

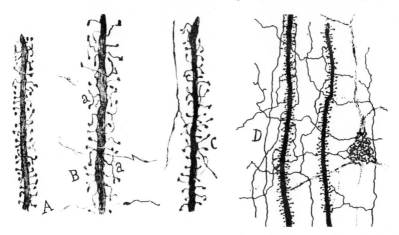

Fig. 14.9. Dendritic spines on neocortical pyramidal cells. (A) rabbit; (B) child of two months; (C) month old cat, visual region [Ramón y Cajal, 1934]; (D) adult rat, showing two dendrites and also the pericellular nest on a pyramidal cell [Chang, 1952].

highly specific chemical phenomenon postulated in Hydén's molecular theory of learning. The specificities are encoded in the structure and in the synaptic connections of the nerve cells, which are arranged in the unimaginably complex patterns that have already been formed in development. From then on, all that seems to be required for the functional development that we call learning is merely the microgrowth of synaptic connections already in existence. The flow of specific information from receptor organs into the nervous system will result in the activation of specific spatiotemporal patterns of impulse discharges. The synapses so activated will grow to an increased effectiveness; hence the more a particular spatiotemporal pattern of impulses is replayed in the cortex, the more effective become its synapses relative to others. And, by virtue of this synaptic efficacy, later similar sensory inputs will tend to traverse these same neuronal pathways and so evoke the same responses, both overt and psychic, as the original input.

Dingman and Sporn [1964] have reviewed several experiments that indicate a relationship between the RNA content of the nervous system and learning ability. First, Morrell [1961a] finds an increase in the RNA of nerve cells forming an epileptogenetic mirror focus in the cerebral cortex, which may be regarded as a neurophysiological model of memory. Second, Dingman and Sporn [1961] find that a decrease of functional RNA depresses the rat's ability to learn a new maze, and Gerard and colleagues [1963] report that under the same conditions, "fixation of experience" requires a longer time, whereas an increased RNA concentration shortens the time for fixation. Finally, there have been several reports that long-term administration of yeast RNA improves memory function. These experimental observations need further testing and control, but it can provisionally be recognized that they are readily assimilable into the growth theory of learning.

SUMMARY

We may summarize this discussion of the structural basis of memory by stating that memory of any particular event is dependent on a specific reorganization of neuronal associations (the engram) in a vast system of neurons widely spread over the cerebral cortex. Lashley [1950] has convincingly argued that "the activity of literally millions of neurons" is involved in the recall of any memory. His experimental study of the effects of cortical lesions on memory indicates that any particular memory trace or engram has multiple representation in the cortex. Furthermore, Lashley concludes that any cortical neuron does not exclusively belong to one engram, but on the contrary, each neuron and even each synaptic junction would be built into many engrams. We have already seen that the systematic study of the responses of individual neurons in the cortex and in the subcortical nuclei is providing many examples of this multiple operation.

DISCUSSION

Chairman: LORD ADRIAN

GOMES: I would ask Professor Eccles how can he reconcile his views about a synaptic mechanism of memory with the ablation experiments conducted by Lashley. One cannot suppose that the recording of a so-called memory trace is effected upon a group of neighboring neurons, because, according to the results of Lashley's experiments, no particular cortical area can be identified as being essential for the retention of habits acquired previously to an ablation. On the other hand, the hypothesis that each single engram is diffused throughout different regions of the brain would seem even more inadequate; and the more so, the greater the diffusion is, because in this case the destruction of any small area would entail the disruption of all the traces having some component in this area.

ECCLES: Lashley did not think that his theory was contrary to his experimental results. He interpreted his experiments as indicating multiple representation of the engrams. The engram is not just some particular fixed wiring diagram, but it is a tremendous complex of pathways, so that any one memory is actually laid down in many places. I am sure Dr. Sperry would agree that before the brain was split the engrams subserving a particular memory were laid down in both hemispheres, with the corpus callosum helping in the transfer to an enormous degree.

MAC KAY: The question I would like to raise is not intended in any way to depreciate the importance of synaptic changes, but to draw attention to a further possible way of storing information, particularly suitable in a communication net where propagation time is significant, as it is not in a normal electrical net. What I have in mind is the possibility of adaptive modification, not only to the spatial but also to the temporal structure of neural networks. Consider, for example, a railway network. If you want to make it impossible for people to travel across country from A to B, you may of course simply withdraw one link in the chain of connections; but a more refined method (not unknown in our country) is to speed up the service on one line, so that the would-be traveler arrives at a junction to find his train gone. So a change in either the spatial or temporal structure of such a time-sensitive network can have equally drastic effects on its dynamics.

What I want to suggest is that in the nervous system, particularly in its dendritic ramifications, the potential information storage capacity of adaptive modifications in the time domain would seem to be at least as great as in the space domain*; and, since the physical change required (in fiber diameter, for example) can be spread over the whole length of each fiber, rather than concentrated in the minute region of a synapse at its end, it might in principle be capable of proportionately greater long-term stability. Such changes in fiber diameter with use are not unknown. A mechanism on this principle would show itself to best effect in richly interconnected networks of the kind described by Professor Eccles, where specific sensitivities to highly complex temporal rhythms and relationships could be evolved and stored in great numbers. Do we have any reason to believe that the nervous system does not use it?

ECCLES: I don't know how such a factor could be utilized in the nervous system. You would have to formulate this question with due respect to the fact that all neuronal networks would be repetitively activated. There is not a single volley coming up from receptors, but there is a repetitive discharge from each receptor, as Lord Adrian has shown. Hence, I think, for the purpose of information storage we cannot utilize variations in the propagation times of the individual axons.

ANDERSEN: It is, of course, very tempting to look for morphological changes that could be related to plasticity in the nervous system. I think really that the evidence at hand is very scarce indeed, and a few of the ideas that Professor Eccles proposed really have evidence against them. For example, the spine apparatus is not restricted to cortical neurons. Furthermore, in the dendrites the synapses are on the stems as well as on the spines. Then, with

---

* D. M. MacKay. Operational aspects of some fundamental concepts of human communication, *Synthèse*, 9, 182–198 [1954]; Self-organization in the time domain (in) *Self-Organizing Systems 1962* (ed. by Yovits, Jacobi, and Goldstein). Spartan Books, pp. 37–48 [1962]; D. M. MacKay and W. S. McCulloch. The limiting information capacity of a neuronal link, *Bull. Math. Biophys.*, 14, 127–135; 15, 107 [1952].

regard to the postulated budding of the dendritic spines, a very strange fact is that if you follow the development of mouse cortex for a few days, you find that these extended spines shrink, and in the adult animal you find fewer of them than at birth. Maybe these animals remember less as they grow! What we should look for, I think, are more subtle changes than just the surface area of synaptic contact.

CHAGAS: I would completely agree with Professor Eccles' criticism of Szilard's hypothesis, but I am less skeptic than he about Hydén's theory. I really suppose that one has to consider very marked molecular changes in long-termed memory. It should also be noticed in relation to this, that some recent work on denervation of a very highly synaptic organ has produced a change on the pattern of molecular weights of some proteins, which seems to indicate that modifications in synaptic activity may have some very significant effects on the molecular patterns of postsynaptic structures.

ECCLES: I am grateful for any suggestions about the way in which synaptic action can be enhanced by usage. In my verbal report I did leave out the comment that undoubtedly Hydén's work is important, and that there is evidence that RNA is concerned in learning; but not in the specific manner that Hydén postulated.

BREMER: Among the various factors from which memory retention depends, it may be useful to mention the input by which the cerebral machinery has been put in action. Behavioral conducts involving apparently the same patterns of efferent impulses may differ radically in regard to the laying down of memory traces. As I have already mentioned in my report, the stimulation of hypothalamic or adjacent regions, in the free-moving cat, induces a spectacular display of rage and aggressiveness unaccompanied by any manifestation of immediate memory. The same emotional outburst, when evoked by a natural stimulation, would have been followed by a long-lasting behavior disturbance.

REFERENCES

ALBE-FESSARD, D., and A. FESSARD. Thalamic integrations and their consequences at the telencephalic level, in: *Progress in Brain Research*, Vol. I. *Brain Mechanisms* (ed. by G. Moruzzi, A. Fessard, and H. H. Jasper), pp. 115–154 [1963].

ANDERSEN, P. Interhippocampal impulses. II. Apical dendritic activation of CAI neurons, *Acta Physiol. Scand.*, 48, 178–208 [1960a].

———. Interhippocampal impulses. III. Basal dendritic activation of CA3 neurons, *Acta Physiol. Scand.*, 48, 209–230 [1960b].

———, J. C. ECCLES, and Y. LØYNING. Recurrent inhibition in the hippocampus with identification of the inhibitory cell and its synapses, *Nature* (London), 198, 540–542 [1963].

———. Location of postsynaptic inhibitory synapses on hippocampal pyramids, *J. Neurophysiol.*, 27, 592–607 [1964].

———, J. C. ECCLES, and P. E. VOORHOEVE. Inhibitory synapses on somas of Purkinje cells in the cerebellum, *Nature* (London), 199, 655–656 [1963].

ANDERSEN, P., J. C. ECCLES, and P. E. VOORHOEVE. Postsynaptic inhibition of cerebellar Purkinje cells, *J. Neurophysiol.*, 27, 1138–1153 [1964].

ARMSTRONG, D. M. Synaptic excitation and inhibition of Betz cells by antidromic pyramidal volleys, *J. Physiol.*, 178, 37P–38P [1965].

BELOFF, J. *The Existence of Mind.* London: Macgibbon & Kee [1962].

BERÁNEK, R., P. HNÍK, L. VYKLICKÝ, and J. ZELENÁ. Facilitation of the monosynaptic reflex due to long-term tenotomy, *Physiologia Bohemoslovenica*, 10, 543–552 [1961].

BROWN, J. Short-term memory, *Brit. Med. Bull.*, 20, 8–11 [1964].

BURNS, B. D. Some properties of the isolated cerebral cortex of the unanaesthetized cat, *J. Physiol.*, 112, 156–175 [1951].

———. *The Mammalian Cerebral Cortex.* London: Arnold, 119 pp. [1958].

BUSER, P., and M. IMBERT. Sensory projections to the motor cortex in cats: A microelectrode study, in: *Sensory Communication* (ed. by W. A. Rosenblith), Symposium on Principles of Sensory Communication. New York: Wiley, pp. 607–626 [1961].

CHAMBERLAIN, T. J., P. HALICK, and R. W. GERARD. Fixation of experience in the rat spinal cord, *J. Neurophysiol.*, 26, 662–673 [1963].

CHANG, H. T. Dendritic potential of cortical neurons produced by direct electrical stimulation of the cerebral cortex, *J. Neurophysiol.*, 14, 1–21 [1951].

———. Cortical and spinal neurons. Cortical neurons with particular reference to the apical dendrites, *Cold Spr. Harb. Symp. Quant. Biol.*, 17, 189–202 [1952].

COOMBS, J. S., D. R. CURTIS, and J. C. ECCLES. The generation of impulses in motoneurones, *J. Physiol.*, 139, 232–249 [1957].

CREUTZFELDT, O. D. Information transmission in the visual system, in: *Brain and Conscious Experience* (ed. by J. C. Eccles). Berlin: Springer [1966].

DINGMAN, W., and M. B. SPORN. Molecular theories of memory, *Science*, 144, 26–29 [1964].

DUBNER, R., and L. T. RUTLEDGE. Recording and analysis of converging input upon neurons in cat association cortex, *J. Neurophysiol.*, 27, 620–634 [1964].

ECCLES, J. C. *The Neurophysiological Basis of Mind: The Principles of Neurophysiology.* Oxford: Clarendon Press, 314 pp. [1953].

———. *The Physiology of Nerve Cells.* Baltimore: Johns Hopkins Press, 270 pp. [1957].

———. The effects of use and disuse on synaptic function, in: *Brain Mechanisms and Learning* (ed. by J. F. Delafresnaye). Oxford: Blackwell, pp. 335–352 [1961].

———. *The Physiology of Synapses.* Berlin: Springer, 316 pp. [1964].

———. Cerebral synaptic mechanisms, in: *Brain and Conscious Experience.* Berlin: Springer [1966].

———, K. KRNJEVIĆ, and R. MILEDI. Delayed effects of peripheral severance of afferent nerve fibres on the efficacy of their central synapses, *J. Physiol.*, 145, 204–220 [1959].

ECCLES, J. C., R. LLINAS, and K. SASAKI. Intracellularly recorded responses of the cerebellar Purkinje cells, *Exp. Brain Res., 1,* 161–183 [1966].

——, and A. K. McINTYRE. The effects of disuse and of activity on mammalian spinal reflexes, *J. Physiol., 121,* 492–516 [1953].

ECCLES, R. M., W. KOZAK, and R. A. WESTERMAN. Enhancement of spinal monosynaptic reflex responses after denervation of synergic hind-limb muscles, *Exp. Neurol., 6,* 451–464 [1962].

EIGEN, M. Chemical means of information storage, and readout in biological systems, *Neurosciences Research Program Bull.,* May–June 1964, pp. 11–22 [1964].

FESSARD, A. Mechanisms of nervous integration and conscious experience, in: *Brain Mechanisms and Consciousness* (ed. by J. F. Delafresnaye). Oxford: Blackwell, pp. 200–236 [1954].

——. The role of neuronal networks in sensory communications within the brain, in: *Sensory Communication* (ed. by W. A. Rosenblith), Symposium on Principles of Sensory Communication. New York: Wiley, pp. 585–606 [1961].

FOX, C. A., and J. W. BARNARD. A quantitative study of the Purkinje cell dendritic branchlets and their relationship to afferent fibres, *J. Anat.* (London), *91,* 299–313 [1957].

GERARD, R. W. Physiology and psychiatry, *Amer. J. Psychiat., 106,* 161–173 [1949].

GOMULICKI, B. R. *The Development and Present States of the Trace Theory of Memory.* Cambridge, Eng.: Cambridge Univ. Press [1953].

GRANIT, R. Sensory mechanisms in perception, in: *Brain and Conscious Experience* (ed. by J. C. Eccles). Berlin: Springer [1966].

HAMLYN, L. H. An electron microscope study of pyramidal neurons in the Ammon's horn of the rabbit, *J. Anat.* (London), 97, 189–201 [1963].

HÁMORI, J., and J. SZENTÁGOTHAI. The "crossing over" synapse. An electron microscopy study of the molecular layer in the cerebellar cortex, *Acta Biol. Hung., 15,* 95–117 [1964].

HEBB, D. O. *The Organization of Behaviour.* New York: Wiley [1949].

HECHTER, O., and I. D. K. HALKERSTON. On the nature of macromolecular coding in neuronal memory, *Perspect. Biol. Med., 7,* 183–198 [1964].

HELD, H., and J. BOSSOM. Neonatal deprivation and adult rearrangement: complementary techniques for analyzing plastic sensory-motor coordinations, *J. Comp. Physiol. Psychol., 54,* 33–37 [1961].

——, and A. HEIN. Movement-produced stimulation in the development of visually guided behavior, *J. Comp. Physiol. Psychol., 56,* 872–876 [1963].

HUBEL, D. H., and T. N. WIESEL. Receptive fields, binocular interaction and functional architecture in the cat's visual cortex, *J. Physiol., 160,* 106–154 [1962].

HYDÉN, H. Biochemical changes in glial cells and nerve cells at varying activity, *Proc. Fourth Inter. Congr. Biochemistry* (ed. by Hoffmann-Ostenhof). London: Pergamon, Vol. 3, 64–89 [1959].

——. Introductory remarks to the session on memory processes, *Neurosciences Res. Program Bull.,* May–June, pp. 23–38 [1964].

JUNG, R. Neuronal integration in the visual cortex and its significance for visual information, in: *Sensory Communication* (ed. by W. A. Rosenblith), Symposium on Principles of Sensory Communication. New York: Wiley, pp. 627–674 [1961].

———, H. H. KORNHUBER, and J. S. DA FONSECA. Multisensory convergence on cortical neurons. Neuronal effects of visual, acoustic and vestibular stimuli in the superior convolutions of the cat's cortex, in: *Progress in Brain Research*, Vol. 1, *Brain Mechanisms* (ed. by G. Moruzzi, A. Fessard, and H. H. Jasper), pp. 207–240. Amsterdam: Elsevier [1963].

KANDEL, E. R., W. A. SPENCER, and F. J. BRINLEY. Electrophysiology of hippo-campal neurons. I. Sequential invasion and synaptic organization, *J. Neurophysiol.*, 24, 225–242 [1961].

KÖHLER, I. Über Aufbau und Wandlungen der Wahrnehmungswelt, *SB Öst. Akad. Wiss.*, 227, 1–118 [1951].

KONORSKI, J. The mechanisms of learning, *Symp. Soc. Exp. Biol.*, 4, 409–431 [1950].

KORNHUBER, H. H., and J. C. ASCHOFF. Somatisch-vestibuläre Integration an Neuronen des motorischen Cortex, *Naturwissenschaften*, 51, 62–63 [1964].

LASHLEY, K. S. In search of the engram, *Symp. Soc. Exp. Biol.*, 4, 454–482 [1950].

MIKAELIAN, H., and R. HELD. Two types of adaptation to an optically-rotated visual field, *Amer. J. Psychol.*, 77, 257–263 [1964].

MORRELL, F. Lasting changes in synaptic organization produced by continuous neuronal bombardment, in: *Brain Mechanisms and Learning* (ed. by J. F. Delafresnaye). Oxford: Blackwell, pp. 375–392 [1961a].

———. Electrophysiological contributions to the neural basis of learning, *Physiol. Rev.*, 41, 443–494 [1961b].

MOUNTCASTLE, V. B. The neural replication of sensory events in the somatic afferent system, in: *Brain and Conscious Experience* (ed. by J. C. Eccles). Berlin: Springer [1966].

PENFIELD, W., and H. H. JASPER. *Epilepsy and the Functional Anatomy of the Human Brain*. Boston: Little, Brown, pp. 1–896 [1954].

PHILLIPS, C. G. Some properties of pyramidal neurones of the motor cortex, in: *The Nature of Sleep* (ed. by G. E. W. Wolstenholme and M. O'Connor), Ciba Foundation Symposium. London: Churchill, pp. 4–24 [1961].

———, and R. PORTER. The pyramidal projection to motoneurones of some muscle groups of the Baboon's forelimb, in: *Progress in Brain Research*, Vol. 12, *Physiology of Spinal Neurons* (ed. by J. C. Eccles and J. P. Schadé), pp. 222–245. Amsterdam: Elsevier [1964].

PURPURA, D. P., and R. J. SHOFER. Cortical intracellular potentials during augmenting and recruiting responses. I. Effects of injected hyperpolarizing currents on evoked membrane potential changes, *J. Neurophysiol.*, 27, 117–132 [1964].

RAMÓN y CAJAL, S. *Histologie du Système Nerveux de l'Homme et des Vertébrés*. Paris: Maloine, Vol. II, 993 pp. [1911].

———. Les preuves objectives de l'unité anatomique des cellules nerveuses, *Trab. Lab. Invest. Biol. Univ. Madr.*, 29, 1–137 [1934].

RIESEN, A. H. The development of visual perception in man and chimpanzee, *Science, 106,* 107–108 [1947].

———. Plasticity of behavior: Psychological aspects, in: *Biological and Biochemical Bases of Behavior* (ed. by H. F. Harlow and C. N. Woolsey). Madison: Univ. Wisconsin Press, pp. 425–450 [1958].

SCHMITT, F. O. Molecular and ultrastructural correlates of function in neurons, neuronal mets, and the brain, *Neurosciences Research Program Bull.,* May–June, pp. 43–66 [1964].

SCHRÖDINGER, E. *Mind and Matter.* London: Cambridge Univ. Press, 104 pp. [1958].

SENDEN, M. VON. *Space and Sight* (tr. by P. Heath). London: Methuen [1960].

SHERRINGTON, C. S. *Man on His Nature.* Cambridge, Eng.: Cambridge Univ. Press, 413 pp. [1940].

SPENCER, W. A., and E. R. KANDEL. Electrophysiology of hippocampal neurones. IV. Fast prepotentials, *J. Neurophysiol., 24,* 272–285 [1961].

STRATTON, G. M. Vision without inversion of retinal image, *Psychol. Rev., 4,* 463–481 [1897].

SZILARD, L. On memory and recall, *Proc. Nat. Acad. Sci., 51,* 1092–1099 [1964].

TÖNNIES, J. F. Die Erregungssteuerung im Zentralnervensystem, *Arch. Psychiat. Nervenkr., 182,* 478–535 [1949].

VAN DER LOOS, H. Personal communication [1964].

WIGNER, E. Two kinds of reality. Unpublished lecture [1964].

YOUNG, J. Z. Growth and plasticity in the nervous system, *Proc. Roy. Soc. B, 139,* 18–37 [1951].

15

The Functional Significance of Sleep with Particular Regard to the Brain Mechanisms Underlying Consciousness[1]

by G. MORUZZI

Istituto di Fisiologia dell' Università, Pisa, Italy

INTRODUCTION

The physiology of sleep is an appropriate subject in a symposium devoted to conscious experience. This theme was discussed in several reports at the Ste. Marguerite Symposium on Brain Mechanisms and Consciousness, whose proceedings were published just ten years ago [Delafresnaye, 1954].

Kleitman [1963] has pointed out that the level of consciousness is determined by "the degree of one's ability to utilize the past and contribute to the future" (l.c. p. 5). Consciousness is usually defined by the ability: (1) to appreciate sensory information; (2) to react critically to it with thoughts or movements; (3) to permit the accumulation of memory traces. If one accepts these definitions and these criteria, there is little doubt that during sleep there is either no consciousness at all or (during

[1] The original work carried out at Pisa and quoted in the present report was made with the support of the Office of Scientific Research, OAR, through the European Office, U.S.A.F. [Arduini et al, 1963; Moruzzi, 1960, 1963a], and of the National Institute of Neurological Diseases and Blindness, N.I.H., P.H.S., U.S.A. [Baust and Berlucchi, 1964; Baust, Berlucchi, and Moruzzi, 1964; Bizzi et al, 1964; Gassel et al, 1964, 1965a, 1965b; Giaquinto et al, 1963a, 1963b, 1964a, 1964b; Marchiafava and Pompeiano, 1964].

345

dreaming) a very low level of consciousness. This statement obviously does not imply that wakefulness is synonymous with consciousness or that bodily manifestations of sleep must be absent when consciousness is absent or very low, as is certainly the case of several new-born mammals or in the adult animal after decerebration. We sleep with our brain as well as with our body, as von Economo [1929] pointed out several years ago, and there is ample evidence that the two aspects of sleep may be dissociated with experimental procedures. In this report we shall be concerned only with the sleep of the brain in the adult, normal mammal.

Although our information on the brain stem mechanisms involved in drowsiness, sleep, and arousal have greatly developed during the last years, we are still unable to explain why we must spend nearly one third of our life in a state of unconsciousness. Whether one likes it or not, what Professor Eccles called at the Ciba Symposium on sleep [Wolstenholme and O'Connor, 1961, p. 1] a period of "abject mental annihilation" is necessary for our life. Experiments of sleep deprivation show that sleep may be only postponed for some days. The ability to sleep is a matter of life or death.

Sleep and death. The verses of the poets, from Lucretius [2] to Shakespeare, the sculptures on the tombs in our cathedrals remind us of what seemed to be the obvious, straightforward explanation of sleep: a period of recovery, which is made possible by a kind of reversible death, involving the almost total inactivation of the brain and of most of the functions in the somatic sphere. It is the nervous system which needs this period of recovery, as shown by the fact that the refreshing experience of sleep is lacking altogether when we lie for several hours in bed, immobile but sleepless. Since the recovery of the skeletal muscles occurs at its best when they are fully relaxed, reasoning by analogy led to the conclusion that a prolonged period of inactivity was also required for the recovery of the brain neurons, of those at least which are not concerned with the regulation of visceral functions essential for life.

That the inactivity was far from being complete was immediately recognized when the classical investigations of Berger, Adrian, and Bremer appeared. The idea which had been accepted since Bremer's classical experiment on the *cerveau isolé* was that whenever the tonic activity which is going on within the cerebrum, the *tonus central,* fell below a critical level, wakefulness and awareness were no longer possible, and sleep occurred [Bremer, 1938]. Thus sleep would simply be due to the inability to remain awake [see Kleitman, 1963 for reference]. Experiments carried out in the late forties [Moruzzi and Magoun, 1949; see Rossi and Zanchetti, 1958; Magoun, 1959; Moruzzi, 1960, 1963a, 1963b

---

[2] *De Rerum Natura,* III, 917–918.

for references] suggested that the slackening of brain activity was due to the reduction of a diffuse facilitatory influence exerted on the cerebrum by the ascending reticular system, while total inactivation of this system was regarded as the cause of the coma.

MAIN LINES OF PROGRESS IN SLEEP PHYSIOLOGY SINCE THE STE. MARGUERITE SYMPOSIUM

This was the situation in 1953, when the theme of the present symposium was the subject of the Ste. Marguerite Colloquium. The next step of the present report will be to review the progress made during the last decade.

The main results obtained during the last ten years may be summarized as follows:

1. Behavioral sleep is not necessarily associated with synchronization of the activity of brain neurons. There are episodes of desynchronized sleep, associated with rapid eye movements, twitching of the limbs and atonia of the antigravity muscles. These episodes have been observed in several mammals, including man, where they seem to be associated with dreams. They are correlated with the appearance of spike-like potential oscillations in the nucleus reticularis pontis caudalis and in the lateral geniculate body.

2. Several lines of evidence suggest the existence, within the medulla and the lower pons, of EEG synchronizing structures, antagonistically oriented with regard to the activating reticular system and probably related with the onset of sleep.

I have dealt at length with these recent results in a Harvey Lecture [Moruzzi, 1963a] and I refer to it for a detailed account on the literature and for the bibliography. I shall devote the time that remains available not to the positive achievements of the last decade, but rather to those aspects of sleep physiology where the results of recent investigations have led to a disquieting crisis in our conceptions.

Whether the physiologists thought that sleep was due to an active inhibitory process or to passive deafferentation [Moruzzi, 1963a], they tacitly agreed upon the concept that the ultimate result was a striking reduction of the overall activity of the body and of the brain, a period lasting several hours during which unknown processes of recovery took place. There is little doubt that the activity of the body is strikingly reduced with respect to active wakefulness, although this is certainly not the critical phenomenon in sleep; but our difficulties arise from the fact that recent physiological evidence has failed to confirm the hypothesis that the overall activity of the brain abates during sleep.

I am not disturbed by the fact that oxygen consumption of the cerebrum does not appear to be appreciably decreased during sleep [Kety, 1961]. We know that in striated muscle physiological rest, as shown by the absence of action potentials, is not associated with a decrease of metabolic activity, at least until full recovery has been completed. Although the ability of the central nervous system to contract oxygen debt is indeed very limited, we are so ignorant about the slow processes of recovery which occur in the neurons or in the glia cells, that it would be unwise to speculate on determinations of oxygen consumption. They concern, moreover, the entire brain.

The microelectrode investigations carried out by Evarts [1962, 1964] on the neocortex of normal, unanesthetized mammals confront us, however, with a problem that can no longer be ignored. Although the pyramidal tract neurons of monkey's motor cortex showed a reduction in the average frequency of discharge from wakefulness to synchronized sleep, the majority of nerve cells not giving rise to pyramidal fibers actually discharged more rapidly during synchronized sleep than during relaxed wakefulness [Evarts, 1964]; nor was a decrease in impulse frequency observed during synchronized sleep in the units of the cat's visual cortex as compared with the waking state, of course in the absence of retinal stimulation [Evarts, 1962].

Finally, the rate of discharge of neurons of the visual cortex was always significantly greater during the desynchronized than during the synchronized phase of sleep [Evarts, 1962]. An enhancement of the integrated pyramidal activity had been found by Arduini, Berlucchi, and Strata [1963] during the desynchronized phase of sleep in the unrestrained, unanesthetized cat, an effect which Marchiafava and Pompeiano [1964] showed later to be mainly associated with the outbursts of rapid eye movements. Evarts [1964] came to a similar conclusion by recording from single pyramidal tract neurons of the monkey's motor cortex.

Significant progress along the same lines has been recently reported by Evarts [1965a, 1965b]. He has been able to identify in the unrestrained, unanesthetized monkey pyramidal tract neurons with large and small cell bodies on the basis of the latencies of their antidromic response to pyramidal stimulation. Units with short latencies of response tended to be phasically active during contralateral movements, became almost inactive during relaxed wakefulness, and showed an increase in discharge frequencies during synchronized sleep. Units responding with long antidromic latencies, on the other hand, tended to be tonically active during wakefulness and their frequency slowed down from wakefulness to synchronized sleep. Nevertheless, even during synchronized sleep their mean discharge frequency remained always greater than that of the large cells, in the same experimental situation.

Summing up, even during the less active phase of sleep the neurons of the motor and visual cortices never rest; indeed, some of them seem to be, paradoxically, more active during synchronized sleep than during relaxed wakefulness. A further phasic enhancement of their activity occurs during the desynchronized phase.

SLEEP AS RECOVERY FROM PLASTIC ACTIVITY

Apparently the neuronal populations which have been studied so far in projection areas of the neocortex never "sleep." To express this concept more rigorously, there is nothing, in their behavior during sleep, which may be regarded as the counterpart of the state of almost complete inactivity that characterizes a fully relaxed skeletal muscle. This may not appear entirely surprising after all. We know that there is no need for a long-lasting state of inactivity in the large populations of neurons of the respiratory or vasomotor centers or in the inhibitory areas of the cerebellar cortex. Apparently there is plenty of time for their recovery during the intervals between the discharges of impulses, disregarding the additional possibilities represented by rotation of activity. Evarts' investigations have led to the unexpected conclusion that this is true also for the large neocortical neurons which have been investigated so far.

There are other neural functions, however, which cannot go on indefinitely. They must be interrupted for long periods of time. The neural activities related to consciousness are the typical examples of these labile functions. The usual fast processes of recovery, lasting a few milliseconds, are apparently unable to cancel altogether the effects of past neuronal activity, when higher nerve functions are concerned. Some chemical changes slowly accumulate, either in the neurons or in the glia cells, or at some synapses. A full recovery can then be achieved only after a very slow process, one that requires the interruption of the neural activities underlying consciousness for long periods of time: several hours in animals with monophasic sleep patterns. There would be probably no need to sleep if recovery were concerned only with fast processes, such as those related to sodium or potassium pumps or the activity of enzymes, such as cholinesterase and cholinacetylase.

It is extremely unlikely that the cells related to these higher nervous functions are among those investigated so far in the microelectrode studies on sleep. Maybe we are not even concerned with nerve cells, but only with specialized synapses lying upon them, such as those located at the level of the spines of the dendrites. I leave out every reference, since the problem of the synaptic changes underlying enduring psychic memory has been extensively reviewed at this symposium by Professor

Eccles [1966b; also 1964, pp. 255–260]. According to our hypothesis it is for the sake of these nerve cells, or these highly specialized synapses, that we do sleep.

There are, of course, many other events which occur during sleep in widespread regions of the central nervous system and in the body. The activity of the Betz cells, that of the preganglionic parasympathetic neurons of the Edinger-Westphal nucleus or of the vagal cardioinhibitory center are undoubtedly greatly affected by sleep. These changes have a physiological significance, which in the majority of cases is now easily understood. However, we should try to separate quite clearly from its epiphenomena, at least conceptually, the hard core of the problem of sleep.

Some of these epiphenomena, both in the autonomic (myosis, brady-cardia) and in the somatic spheres (closure of the eyes, relaxation of the antigravity muscles, inability to stand), had impressed men a long time before the beginning of the experimental era. Actually, bodily manifesta-tions of sleep gave rise to most of the old hypotheses, and inspired master-pieces of art, such as Michelangelo's "Night." They are epiphenomena, nevertheless, as shown by the fact that birds sleep while perching and that the typical lying position of sleep is lacking in ruminants, which during most of the night keep the thorax upright and the eyes open [see Balch, 1955]. There are reports of physiological lagophthalmos also in man [see Kleitman, 1963]. After all, there would be no need to remain unconscious several hours in order to relax one's musculature or to reduce the amount of the sensory barrage.

The old hypothesis that, during learning, enduring changes occur in the fine structures of some synapses has been revived by electron micros-copy, and is supported by the observation that enduring psychic memory persists after complete blackout of the brain produced by extreme cooling [see Eccles, 1964; pp. 255–260]. These plastic changes are likely to require their own processes of recovery, which are quite different from those related with membrane polarization and synaptic transmission. After all, the so-called "fatigue" produced by several hours of learning also requires a very slow process of recovery. *Sleep appears, therefore, to play a major role in the recovery from plastic activities.* It is perhaps not without sig-nificance that so much time is spent in sleep by young infants when so many new synapses are being formed; and when one learns so much, incidentally, by trial and error through association of sensory information. Professor Eccles [1966b] has devoted in this symposium a section of his report to the problem of how the interpretation of retinal data is being learned during the earliest period of life through association with sensory information from muscle, joint, and skin. His analysis leads to the conclu-sion that during the few hours of wakefulness of the young infant the effort devoted to learning is likely to be by far greater than during any other period of the adult life. As we grow old, our ability to learn, and to become conditioned, decreases; we require less and less sleep. Plastic changes are reduced and our need of the slow processes of recovery is also reduced.

I have considered here only the development of sleep in man. Perhaps more attention should be devoted, also from the point of view of comparative physiology, to the relationships between patterns of sleep and ability to learn and to be conditioned, with particular regard to the effort which is actually spent in voluntary or involuntary learning during the different periods of life. The striking difference in the EEG and behavioral patterns of sleep between the ruminants and other domesticated animals like the cat, dog, or the horse [Bell, 1960], or between new-born lambs and adult sheep [Ruckebusch, 1963] might perhaps be studied also with regard to this aspect of the problem.

If our hypothesis is correct it would be the very reason of sleep, not a mere accident, that we spend such a great portion of our life unconscious. To know what is the ultimate result of sleep is a problem of macromolecular biology, a problem about which our ignorance is complete; one, however, that is closely related to the theme of this symposium: brain and consciousness.

NEURAL STRUCTURES INVOLVED IN THE SLOW RECOVERY FROM PLASTIC ACTIVITY

During the last thirty years, electrophysiology has been instrumental in the tremendous progress of our knowledge on the neural mechanisms underlying the onset of sleep and the phenomenon of arousal. The contrast with our complete ignorance on the functional significance of sleep is therefore particularly surprising. Is there a way to help the neurochemist to join the neurophysiologist in an attack along new lines of endeavor? I see at the present two possibilities of attack: (1) at the level of the cerebral cortex, and (2) at the level of the brain stem.

Plastic changes may occur everywhere throughout adult life, but for some neurons, and possibly for some areas of the cerebral cortex, they are likely to have overwhelming importance. Fast processes of recovery may dominate, for example, at the level of the large Golgi I cells of the neocortex. There would be little need of sleep for these nerve cells, as well as for the neurons controlling circulation and respiration. Technical improvements might well permit one to record also from smaller nerve cells, and I have already reported that this attempt has recently been made, quite successfully, by Evarts [1965a, 1965b]. A careful exploration of the association areas of the cortex might well lead to the discovery of units whose discharge constantly abates or even disappears during sleep. Such a discovery would open new fields of investigation to the physiologist and to the biochemist, since all structures related in one way or the other to these units—glia cells, specialized synapses—would be important for the physiology of sleep, as well as for the general problem of the interrelations between brain and consciousness.

The second approach is still represented by the study of the brain stem structures involved in the regulation of sleep. The integrative function of the central nervous system is certainly disrupted during sleep, as far as the higher neural activities are concerned. An animal asleep may still present some fragments of the responses to the environment that occur during wakefulness, but certainly its reaction is no longer the integrated response of an individual. The relation between several hypnagogic phenomena and schizophrenia has been repeatedly stressed. This loss of the animal's ability to react as a unit to the environment is, however, produced and controlled by some structures, which are mainly localized within the brain stem. Without this control, neurons would sleep at random and we might spend most of our life in a *dormiveglia*. We are unconscious one third of our time in order to be really awake and fully conscious the other two thirds.

It is obvious that these regulating structures of the brain stem must be informed in some way about the needs of plastic recovery of the cerebrum. Very little can be said at the present time in support of the old hypotheses of humoral information. Neural messages from the cerebrum to the brain stem are more likely to be important. They are not essential, however, as shown by the fact that fragments of sleep behavior (I would hesitate to call "sleep" these postural and ocular manifestations) are clearly present in anencephalous children and in the decerebrate cat [see Jouvet, 1962], when no information is transmitted by the cerebrum. Hence we are led to the hypothesis that the brain structures related to sleep are particularly sensitive, for some unknown reasons, to the needs of recovery which are related to the plastic activity carried out during wakefulness. Similarly, the cells of the carotid body are particularly sensitive to the metabolic changes produced by a fall of arterial pO_2, and the functional significance of the chemoceptors is to protect all cells from the dangers of anoxia.

What one needs, therefore, is to find a signal of the beginning and of the end of the process of the inactivation of the ascending reticular system which is responsible for the appearance of sleep, or a signal of an increase of activity in the antagonistically oriented synchronizing system. To obtain *direct* evidence of the changes in the *overall* activity of the brain stem regulating system is a very difficult task. The physiologist may be easily informed on the activity of the carotid chemoreceptors by recording the impulses from the Hering nerve. Such a direct approach is by far more difficult to utilize in the brain stem, since the efferent pathways of the activating reticular system, of the synchronizing system, as well as of the pontine structures related to desynchronized sleep, cannot be studied in isolation. Neither do we know the exact origin of the spike discharges we record with our extracellular microelectrodes in the intact animals, nor whether these discharges represent the cause, or the consequences, of the state of sleep. It is mainly because of these tremendous difficulties that physiologists have been obliged to rely on indirect evidence, such as EEG synchronization, or behavioral phenomena. Great progress has been made in this way, but we still do not know how changes in brain stem activity influence the cerebral cortex or the thalamus in such a way as to produce a condition which is clearly incompatible with the maintenance of consciousness.

SLEEP AND INHIBITION

In the previous section we have been concerned with two problems: (1) *where* are the neurons located which are mainly involved in plastic activities? and (2) *how* brain stem regulation permits concentration in a given period of the nychthemeron, usually during the night, all processes of slow recovery involving loss of consciousness.

If one starts from the hypothesis [see Eccles, 1966b] that the structural changes involved in all kinds of plastic activities are essentially synaptic, a distinction should be made between those synapses which "learn" and those which are concerned in the routine task of transmitting impulses along stereotyped, inborn pathways. If our assumption is correct, there would be no need of sleep for these synapses, or for those neurons for which this type of synaptic activity has overwhelming importance. The neurons of the spinal cord and of the respiratory and vasomotor centers of the medulla belong to this category. If our assumption is correct, we sleep merely (or mainly) in order to permit recovery of those synapses which are able to "learn," and of those neurons which are mainly concerned with their activity.

The synaptic changes underlying plastic activity are seldom stable, occasionally they may be indeed extremely labile, as can be inferred from the study of memory and of conditioned reflexes. During alertness, memory traces are intensively built and intensively destroyed. Were we able to "see" the macromolecular picture at the level of the "learned synapses," at the end of a prolonged period of wakefulness we should be probably more impressed by the ruins than by the new constructions.

Fit quasi paulatim nobis per membra ruina.[3]

The verse of Lucretius might still be chosen to epitomize what happens at the end of a prolonged period of wakefulness, but the "ruins" which accumulate little by little until we succumb to sleep are likely to be mainly present at the level of the "learned synapses," not throughout the central nervous system, and still less (as it was taught in the Epicurean doctrine) throughout our limbs [see Moruzzi, 1964].

Again, Sherrington's [1946, p. 252] definition of sleep, "a phase to be thought of less as quietude than restorative activity *in what has suffered wear and tear,*" [4] probably applies mainly to the learned structures. The recuperation of the routine synapses, which are involved in all kinds of inborn stereotyped activities, occurs during wakefulness, in the short intervals between all-or-none discharges. Thus "learned synapses" might be compared to the center of a modern metropolis, where new building cannot occur without tearing down the old constructions, while the "routine" synapses might be compared to the streets of those old little cities where little changes can be observed from year to year.

These considerations may permit us to examine from an entirely new point of view—the recuperation of the learned synapses—the old problem of sleep and inhibition. It is difficult to conceive how the hypnic recovery from previous plastic activity that occurs at the level of a synapse lying, for example, on one spine of a cortical dendrite may coexist with synaptic transmission at the level of that spine. I would even say that the sheer arrival of impulses to the presynaptic endings may not be easily reconciled with such a kind of slow recovery. A total arrest of the bombardment of impulses is more likely to contribute to the slow processes of restoration. This arrest might well be produced by localized inhibitory processes, although this is not necessarily the only explanation, as we shall see later.

The term *inhibition* has frequently been used in a rather loose way in the history of sleep physiology. Let us first of all stress the obvious point that a decrease of firing is not necessarily due to inhibition. It may be brought about by defacilitation. Professor Granit [1966] has shown in this symposium that, without some biasing organization of interneurons depolarizing the cell membrane of the motoneuron, the afferent barrage is dissipated as synaptic activation noise. This principle is likely to have wide validity and may be utilized for explaining phenomenon such as spinal shock or the patterns of coma produced by mesencephalic transection. A fall of the tonic activity of the ascending reticular system may produce sleep by a process of deactivation; and there is no place for inhibition in the classical formulation of the deafferentation theory of sleep. Nothing, of course, will prevent us from thinking that inhibitory

---

[3] *De Rerum Natura,* VI: 942.
[4] Italics are ours.

processes are involved in the chain of events leading to sleep, even if we accept the reticular hypothesis. We have first to prove, however, that presynaptic or postsynaptic inhibition occurs in the cerebrum, in the brain stem, or in the spinal cord during sleep, and that these phenomena are causally related to sleep.

It is an attractive hypothesis that the synchronizing structures of the lower brain stem inhibit the activating reticular system at the onset of sleep, that during sleep the brain is partially isolated from the sensory receptors through centrifugal inhibition, or, finally, that the recovery of a given synapse is protected by presynaptic inhibition. There is no direct proof, however, that these hypotheses are true. Direct evidence might be provided only by intracellular recording, which has never been carried out in this kind of experiment.

A critical review may be centered around two questions:

Are there active processes of inhibition during sleep? And if a positive reply is given:

Is inhibition causally related to the slow processes of recovery occurring during sleep, or is it simply related to epiphenomena of sleep, such as the control of movements or of the sensory inflow?

The next three sections will be devoted to an analysis of recent results which clearly demonstrate, in our opinion, that active inhibition is indeed present during sleep at the level of the spinal cord. We shall see, however, that no clear-cut proof has yet been obtained that inhibitory processes are involved in the control of the sensory inflow or in the sleep behavior of cortical neurons. Available evidence simply suggests that the inhibitory hypothesis is a likely one. It may be regarded as an assumption that deserves to be tested with appropriate experiments.

DESCENDING INHIBITORY INFLUENCES ON THE SPINAL CORD DURING THE DESYNCHRONIZED PHASE OF SLEEP

Both tendon and cutaneous reflexes are strongly depressed during human sleep [see Kleitman, 1963], but this well-known clinical observation does not necessarily imply that during sleep descending inhibitory volleys impinge upon the spinal cord. Partial withdrawal of the tonic facilitatory influence exerted by the descending reticular system, or by the Deiters nuclei, might also produce hyporeflexia. Actually, this event would be likely to occur as a consequence of the process of brain stem deactivation, which has been postulated as the cause of sleep.

The inhibitory hypothesis had been put forward by Tarchanoff in 1894, but the proof that during sleep inhibitory volleys descend from suprasegmental centers to the spinal cord has been obtained only recently by

Pompeiano and his collaborators. They have shown that during the desynchronized phase of sleep two kinds of inhibitory influences—one, tonic and another one, phasic in nature—arise in the brain stem. For the sake of simplicity only the inhibition of monosynaptic reflexes will be examined. However, polysynaptic reflexes [Giaquinto, Pompeiano, and Somogyi, 1963a, 1963b] and pyramidal movements have also been shown to be strikingly inhibited during desynchronized sleep [Marchiafava and Pompeiano, 1964]. The last phenomenon might provide an explanation of one of the most terrifying experiences during nightmares, the inability to move.

Tonic Inhibition of the Heteronymous Monosynaptic Reflex

Giaquinto, Pompeiano, and Somogyi [1963a, 1963b; 1964a, 1964b] have studied in the intact, unanesthetized cat the monosynaptic response of the *lateral* gastrocnemius motoneurons to stimulation of Group Ia proprioceptive fibers of the *medial* gastrocnemius nerve. This weak, heteronymous monosynaptic reflex can be obtained with a single electrical shock, only after post-tetanic potentiation (Fig. 15.1), and is entirely blocked throughout the duration of the desynchronized phase of sleep (Fig. 15.1F,G). The response to tetanic stimulation of the same Group Ia muscle afferents is only slightly depressed, with respect to arousal, during the synchronous phase (Fig. 15.2), but is strikingly and constantly inhibited during desynchronized episodes of sleep (Fig. 15.3).

Since the heteronymous monosynaptic reflex can no longer be obtained in the hindlimb soon after thoracic transection of the spinal cord, one might maintain that withdrawal of a descending facilitatory influence would give rise, during desynchronized sleep, to a kind of reversible, functional spinal shock. This mechanism of defacilitation is not conflicting with the inhibitory hypothesis, but would simply make it unnecessary.

Experiments of multistage chordotomy, carried out at thoracic levels, have demonstrated the existence of a descending inhibitory influence which actually appears to be quite striking during the desynchronized phase of sleep. After dorsal chordotomy (Fig. 15.4A,B), there was no spinal shock, and the hypnic modulation of the reflex response to tetanic stimulation of Group Ia muscle afferents was present. Spinal shock occurred when dorsal and ventral chordotomy were combined together (Fig. 15.4G).

Two hours and ten minutes after this combined chordotomy the reflex was again present, and, as before, it disappeared during desynchronized sleep. Two days later the lesion was extended dorsally to the ventral part of one lateral column (Fig. 15.4H). After recovery, the reflex was again present ipsilaterally, and again it disappeared during

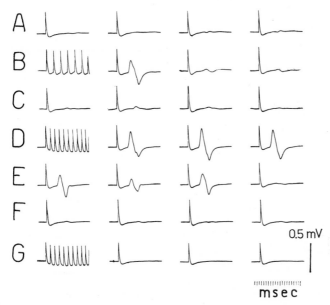

0.5 mV

msec

Fig. 15.1. Post-tetanic potentiation of the heteronymous monosynaptic extensor reflex. Unrestrained, unanesthetized cat. Experiment made five days after implantation of the electrodes. The extensor monosynaptic reflex was recorded electromyographically (CRO) from the left *lateral* gastrocnemius muscle, following stimulation of the central stump of the left *medial* gastrocnemius nerve at 0.05 msec pulse duration. The stimulus intensity was suprathreshold for the group Ia muscular afferents and remained the same for all the records.

(A) Single shock stimulation of the medial nerve, repeated once every 5 sec, does not produce any detectable reflex response of the lateral gastrocnemius muscle, on a background of relaxed wakefulness.

(B,C) Following a volley of electrical pulses at 320 per sec, 4 sec in duration, applied on the same background of wakefulness, single shock stimulation of the same medial nerve produces a reflex response, whose amplitude decreases in the following sweeps. C is the direct continuation of B.

(D,E) Following a tetanus at 500 per sec, 4 sec in duration, applied on the same background, single shock stimulation produces a reflex response of larger amplitude, which declines more slowly (compare C and D); E is the direct continuation of D.

(F,G) Complete abolition of the potentiating effect of a tetanic stimulation at 500 per sec, 4 sec in duration (G), when the experiment is carried out on a background of desynchronized sleep. For latency measurements see original paper [from Giaquinto, Pompeiano, and Somogyi, 1964a, Fig. 1].

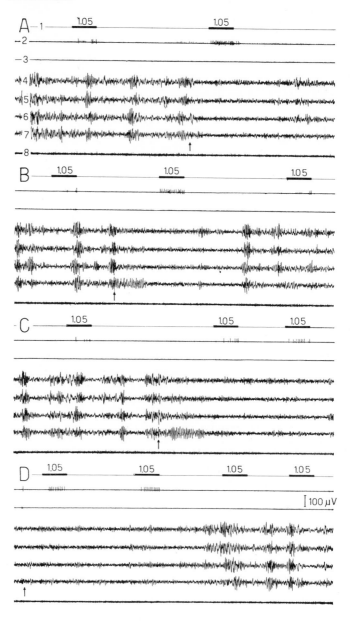

Fig. 15.2. Facilitation of the reflex response to stimulation of Group Ia muscle afferents by arousing stimuli. Unrestrained, unanesthetized cat. Stimulation of the central end of left medial gastrocnemius nerve at 100 per sec, 0.05 msec pulse duration at stimulus intensities slightly above (1.05 T) the threshold (T) for eliciting

desynchronized sleep (Fig. 15.5). This time, however, the tonic facilitation of suprasegmental structures was no longer required, as shown by the fact that the reflex was present soon after complete thoracic transection. Hence the sleep modulation that occurred immediately before this final, complete transection could only be due to descending inhibitory volleys. This experiment is made possible by the fast recovery from spinal shock in the cat, and by the presence of only a partial overlapping, within the lateral columns, of the descending inhibitory and facilitatory paths. Apparently the descending inhibitory pathways are located dorsally to those (for example, the Deiters spinal tract) which are responsible for the tonic supraspinal facilitation. Bizzi, Pompeiano, and Somogyi [1964] have come to the same conclusion, through an entirely different approach, by recording with microelectrodes from the Deiters nucleus of the unanesthetized, unrestrained cat. No decrease of firing was observed when the symptoms of desynchronized sleep (atonia, depression of spinal reflexes) appeared on the record.

Phasic Inhibition of the Homonymous Monosynaptic Reflex

The homonymous monosynaptic reflex has been recently studied by Gassel, Marchiafava, and Pompeiano [1964] in the intact, unanesthetized cat. They recorded the electromyographic response of a muscle to single shock stimulation of its motor nerve. Following a technique usually adopted in man for eliciting the H-reflex, the intensity of stimulation was subliminal or just liminal for motor fibers. In this way, antidromic contamination was largely avoided, although stimulation turned out to be supraliminal for Group Ia muscle afferents.

The homonymous monosynaptic response is a much stronger reflex, and the tonic inhibitory influence occurring in the desynchronized phase of sleep is apparently too weak to suppress it. However, whenever the

---

the reflex by stimulating Group Ia muscle afferents. In this and in Figs. 15.3 and 15.5 all values are expressed in multiples of this threshold (T). Bipolar records. (1): Stimulus marker. (2, 3): EMG of the left *lateral* gastrocnemius muscle (2) and of the left tibialis anterior muscle (3). (4, 5, 6, 7): EEG record from left (4) and right (6) parietotemporal, and from left (5) and right (7) temporo-occipital. (8): EMG from posterior cervical muscles.

Potentiation of the reflex after A, trigeminal stimulation (slight movement of the vibrissae); (B) photic stimulation (flash of light); and (C,D) acoustic stimulation (short lasting whistle). All these maneuvers, indicated by arrows, produced EEG arousal. D is the direct continuation of C. The arousing effect of a first acoustic stimulus applied in C is potentiated in D by a second whistle. The reflex is particularly evident during the background of induced EEG desynchronization, but it is greatly reduced or disappears on the EEG pattern of synchronization [from Giaquinto, Pompeiano, and Somogyi, 1964a, Fig. 4].

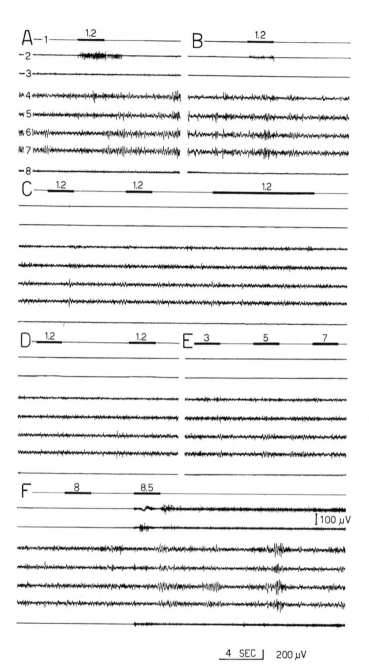

Fig. 15.3. Spinal reflexes produced by stimulation of Group Ia muscle afferents and of flexor afferents abolished during desynchronized sleep. Unrestrained, unanesthetized cat. Experiment made 48 hours after implantation of the electrodes, and

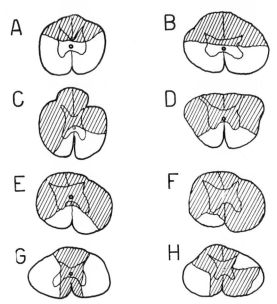

Fig. 15.4. Schemes of spinal cord lesions. (A,B) Spinal cord lesions at T_{12} in two different cats. (C,D,E,F) Spinal cord lesions performed in rostrocaudal direction at different levels between T_{10} and L_1 in the same cat. (G,H) Spinal cord lesions performed at T_{11} (G) and T_{12} (H) in another cat [from Giaquinto, Pompeiano, and Somogyi, 1964b, Fig. 1].

outbursts of rapid eye movements appear, the reflex response may be abolished altogether (Figs. 15.6, 15.7, 15.8). Since during acute spinal shock the reflex is only temporarily depressed, but never abolished, the conclusion is drawn that the descending barrage of inhibitory impulses is phasically enhanced whenever the rapid ocular movements occur.

---

16 hours after partial cordotomy performed under ether at T_{12} (see Fig. 15.4, B). Records as in Fig. 15.2.

(A) Response to stimulation of Group Ia muscle afferents at 100 per sec, 0.05 msec pulse duration (1.20 T) on a background of EEG synchronization. (B) 77 sec after A: great reduction of the reflex during the initial stage of desynchronized sleep (see cervical atonia). (C) 70 sec after B: complete abolition, during desynchronized sleep, of the same reflex even when (right), the duration of the stimulus train is increased from 2.3 to 9.3 sec. (D) (Immediately after C): no effect obtained by increasing the rate of stimulation up to 400 per sec (left side) and 500 per sec (right side). (E) (40 sec after D): stimulation of the nerve at 100 per sec at progressively increasing stimulus intensities, recruiting also the flexor reflex afferents (3, 5 and 7 T). (F) Immediately after E. Arousal of the animal occurs (and reflex responses) only at 8.5 T [from Giaquinto, Pompeiano, and Somogyi, 1964b, Fig. 7].

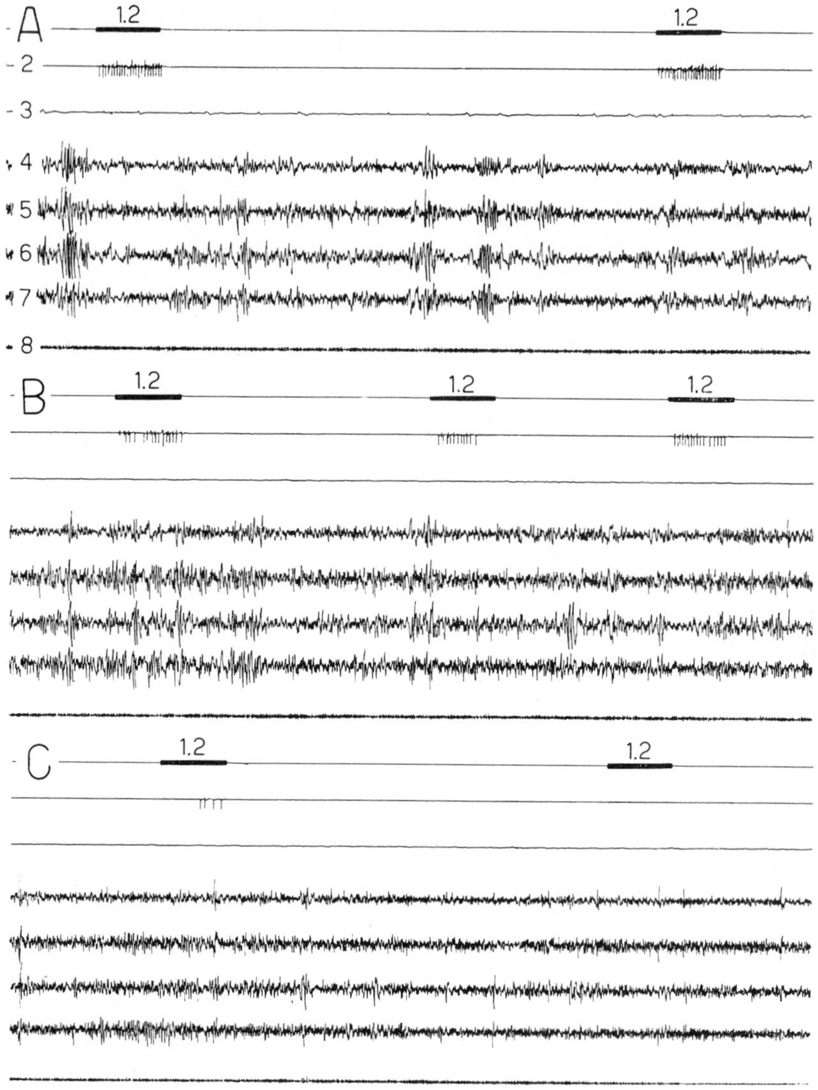

Fig. 15.5. Demonstration of the inhibition of spinal reflexes during desynchronized sleep. Unrestrained, unanesthetized animal; stimulation and records as in Fig. 15.2. One day after the chronic implantation of the electrodes, the animals were submitted to bilateral section of the dorsal and ventral funiculi at T_{11} (Fig. 15.4G). Soon after the section, a condition of spinal shock appeared which was over after 2 hr and 10 min. When an episode of desynchronized sleep occurred, a complete abolition of the reflex could be observed. Two days after the implantation of the electrodes the lesion was enlarged at T_{12} to affect also the medial part of the left ventrolateral funiculus (Fig. 15.4H). The recovery of the reflex after this section occurred quickly. All records were taken one day after this last cordotomy.

(A) Reflex on a background of EEG synchronization. (B) Five min after A. Slight reduction of the reflex. (C) (Soon after B): striking reduction (left) and abolition (right) of the reflex during the initial stage of desynchronized sleep (see cervical EMG). (D) (Soon after C): complete silence in the cervical EMG, total abolition of the reflexes. (E) The episodes of desynchronized sleep continue, the rate of stimulation is raised to 500 per sec, and reflex responses appear only at 1.3 T and 1.5 T. (F) (65 sec after E): back to synchronized sleep, reflex present as in A [from Giaquinto, Pompeiano, and Somogyi, 1964b, Figs. 9, 10].

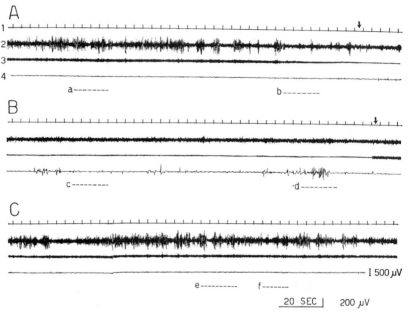

Fig. 15.6. Episodes of desynchronized sleep during which homonymous mono-synaptic reflexes were recorded. Unrestrained, unanesthetized cat. (1) Signal of single shock stimulation of left tibialis nerve: one every 4 sec, 0.05 msec pulse dura-tion, intensity 1.06 times threshold (T) for motor fibers; (2) occipito-occipital EEG; (3) EMG of posterior neck muscles; (4) record of the outbursts of rapid eye movements (REM). Calibration at 500 μV applies only to channel 4. The arrows indicate the beginning and the end of the episode of desynchronized sleep. See legends of Figs. 15.7 and 15.8 (same experiment) for explanation of horizontal bars a to f [from Gassel, Marchiafava, and Pompeiano, 1964, Fig. 4].

Presynaptic versus Postsynaptic Inhibition: The Recurrent Discharge of the Alpha Motoneurons During Sleep

The demonstration by Giaquinto, Pompeiano, and Somogyi [1963a, 1964] of a tonic depression of spinal reflexes coincident with the desyn-chronized phase of sleep was soon confirmed, in almost the same experi-mental situation, by Kubota, Iwamura, and Nimi [1964] and by Bal-dissera, Broggi, and Mancia [1964]; while the observations of Gassel, Marchiafava, and Pompeiano [1964] on phasic enhancement in the inhibition of the homonymous monosynaptic reflex, in correspondence with the outbursts of rapid eye movements, have just been reproduced by Hodes and Dement [1964] in a study on the sleep modulation of the human H-reflex. To summarize the present situation, the *tonic* inhibition of spinal activities, which goes on throughout the desynchronized phase

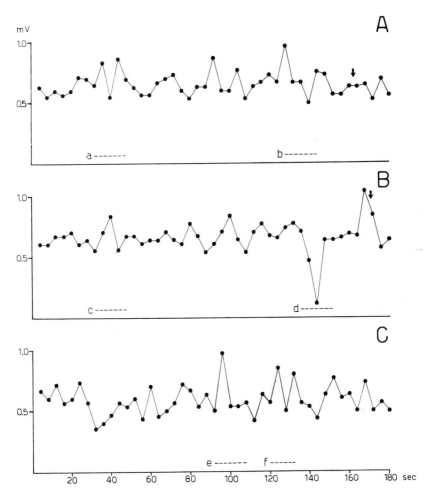

Fig. 15.7. Phasic depression of the homonymous monosynaptic reflex during the rapid ocular movement period of desynchronized sleep. Diagram showing changes in amplitude of the EMG response of flexor digitorum brevis (CRO) to stimulation of left tibial nerve in the experimental situation of Fig. 15.6. The two arrows and the horizontal bars a to f correspond to those of Fig. 15.6. Note that the reflex response was not altered by the change from synchronized to desynchronized sleep, but that a dramatic depression occurred when the response was recorded during the rapid eye movements (d). See also Fig. 15.8d [from Gassel, Marchiafava, and Pompeiano, 1964, Fig. 5].

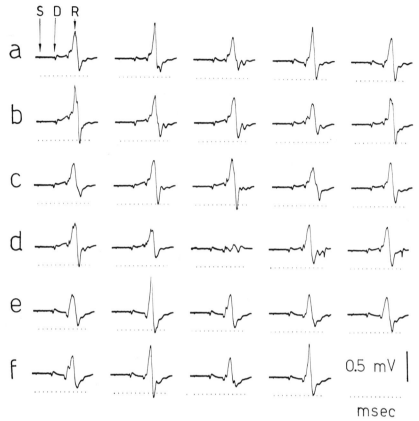

Fig. 15.8. Modulation of the homonymous monosynaptic reflex during sleep. CRO records a to f correspond to the horizontal bars a to f of Figs. 15.6 and 15.7. S is shock artefact; D, direct motor action potential; R is the reflex. (a,b) Variability of the reflex on background of EEG synchronization. (c) No significant change in amplitude during desynchronized sleep in the absence of rapid eye movements. (d) Phasic depression of the monosynaptic reflex during a burst of REM. (e,f) Controls taken on a background of EEG synchronization. Note the small amplitude as well as the stability of the direct motor action potentials (D), indicating that the intensity of the shocks applied to the nerve, which was slightly supraliminar for the motor fibers, remained unmodified throughout the experiment [from Gassel, Marchiafava, and Pompeiano, 1964, Fig. 6].

of sleep, appears to be *phasically* enhanced when outbursts of rapid eye movements occur.

Recent experiments by Gassel, Marchiafava, and Pompeiano [1965a, 1965b] have shown that the recurrent response of the alpha motoneurons to their antidromic activation can be easily detected on the unrestrained, unanesthetized cat. It is markedly reduced throughout the desynchronized phase of sleep, that is, during the tonic depression of the spinal reflexes. Several reasons discussed in the full papers (l.c.) lead to the conclusion that this effect is due to postsynaptic inhibition of the alpha motoneurons. It can be reproduced by stimulating the medial bulboreticular formation, after decerebration. Since the phasic enhancement of the inhibition of the homonymous monosynaptic reflex that occurs in correspondence with the bursts of rapid eye movements can never be observed on a background of recurrent discharge, Gassel, Marchiafava, and Pompeiano have put forward the hypothesis that the phasic inhibition of the monosynaptic reflexes is presynaptic in nature.

The Problem of the Inhibitory Control of Sensory Inflow During the Desynchronized Phase of Sleep

The episodes of low voltage fast sleep are usually associated, both in man [Williams et al, 1964] and cats [see Jouvet, 1962], with an increase in the threshold of auditory arousal.[5] We are not concerned here with the central mechanism of the phenomenon. The auditory system represents, however, an ideal subject for the study of the problem of the centrifugal control of the sensory receptors. The existence of Rasmussen's olivo-cochlear tract is well documented anatomically [Rasmussen, 1946, 1953, 1960], and its electrical stimulation is known to inhibit the click-evoked neural responses of the round window [Galambos, 1957; see Desmedt, 1962, for literature], an effect abolished by strychnine [Desmedt and Monaco, 1960].

Baust, Berlucchi, and Moruzzi [1964] have made an attempt to see whether the click-evoked round window responses are inhibited by Rasmussen's system during the desynchronized episodes of sleep, that is, when the spinal cord is submitted to the barrage of descending inhibitory volleys.

If one disregards the experiments in which the click-evoked responses were led from the cochlear nucleus, in consideration of the fact that the effects might also be due to a central mechanism, there are in the literature only the unpublished results of Galambos, Rupert, and Simmons (quoted by Galambos [1960]) which are related to this theme. They reported that changes in the neural cochlear responses occurred as a consequence of sleep in the intact, unanesthetized cat, and stated that this effect disappeared after tenotomy of the middle ear muscles. However, no data on the correlations of these changes with the usual electrophysiological manifestations of sleep were reported in the short account

[5] For older literature see Kleitman [1963].

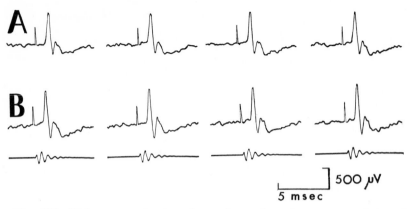

Fig. 15.9. Slight tonic reduction of neural round window response during desynchronized sleep. Unrestrained, unanesthetized cat, with intact middle ear muscles. During a lull between outbursts of rapid eye movements, in the phase of desynchronized sleep (A), the amplitude of round window neural responses to clicks is slightly reduced with respect to an immediately following period of sleep synchronization (B). The shape of the click monoaurally applied through a microphone is shown in the lower trace (under B) [from Baust, Berlucchi, and Moruzzi, 1964, Fig. 2].

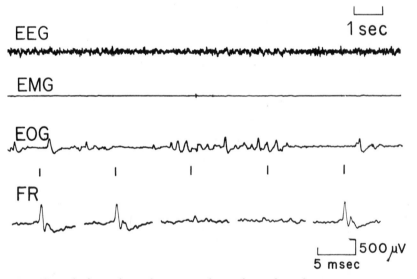

Fig. 15.10. Striking phasic depression of neural round window response occurring synchronously with an outburst of rapid eye movements, during desynchronized sleep. Unrestrained, unanesthetized cat, with middle ear muscles intact. Upper three tracings: cortical EEG, EMG of neck muscles, and electronystagmographic (EOG) record of outbursts of rapid eye movements, recorded during an episode of desynchronized sleep. Vertical marks below the EOG indicate the time of click stimulation, while the corresponding strips of the CRO records of round window responses have been placed below (FR). In association with a prolonged outburst of REM, the third neural response is strikingly reduced and the fourth is abolished [from Baust, Berlucchi, and Moruzzi, 1964, Fig. 3].

368

given by Galambos [1960], so that it would be impossible to draw from their results the conclusion that Rasmussen's control of the cochlea is not involved during the desynchronized phase of sleep.

Baust, Berlucchi, and Moruzzi [1964] recorded simultaneously—in the free moving, unanesthetized cat—the EEG, the cervical EMG, the electronystagmogram, and the round window neural responses to clicks. They found a slight tonic decrease of the amplitude of the N_1 responses during desynchronized sleep (Fig. 15.9), and reported that further striking reduction occurred in coincidence with the rapid eye movements (Fig. 15.10). This effect, however, was abolished by tenotomy of the middle ear muscles, and the electromyogram of M. tensor tympani and stapedius showed a powerful contraction in coincidence with the rapid eye movements (Fig. 15.11). Baust and Berlucchi [1964] also investigated the effect of sleep on the auditory reflexes of the middle ear muscles.

The phasic blockade of the neural response is not due, therefore, to an

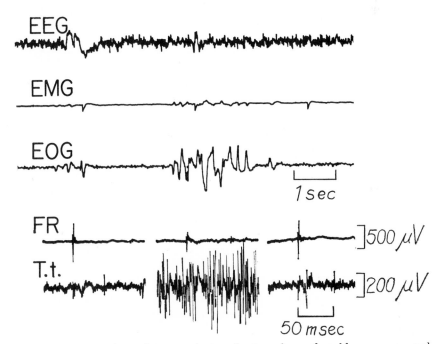

Fig. 15.11. Correlation between phasic reduction of neural cochlear response and twitches of intraaural muscles. Unrestrained, unanesthetized cat, with middle ear muscles intact. The first three tracings are ink-writer recordings arranged as in Fig. 15.10. The lower two tracings are the corresponding strips of CRO records from round window (FR) and tensor tympani (T.t.). Note striking phasic reduction of round window response to click, associated with outburst of REM and contraction of M. tensor tympani [from Baust, Berlucchi, and Moruzzi, 1964, Fig. 7].

outburst of inhibitory impulses descending along Rasmussen's fibers. The intensity of stimulation of the hair cells, not their excitability, is decreased in coincidence with the outbursts of rapid eye movements occurring during the desynchronized phase of sleep.

Summing up, there is no evidence of the existence of a centrifugal inhibitory influence on the auditory receptors during the phases of sleep which are characterized by strong spinal inhibition. This conclusion is not necessarily true for other sensory systems, and investigations on this aspect of the problem are now in progress in our laboratory.

Data and Hypotheses on Sleep and Inhibition in the Cerebral Cortex

The problem of the inhibitory mechanisms of the cerebral cortex has been dealt with extensively at this symposium by Professors Eccles [1966a] and Jasper [1966]. We shall be concerned only with recurrent inhibition in the pyramidal tract neurons of the motor cortex, since this theme has been intensively investigated during the last years. The existence of inhibitory interneurons driven by collaterals of the pyramidal fibers seems well established [Phillips, 1959; Crawford et al, 1963; Stefanis and Jasper, 1964; Asanuma and Brooks, 1965; Brooks and Asanuma, 1965]. Recurrent spinal cortical inhibition has been regarded very much on the lines of the present interpretation of the functional significance of the Renshaw system in the spinal cord, that is: (i) as a safety device to dampen excessive discharge; and (ii) as a mechanism for sharpening focal responses of cortical neurons to localized sensory stimuli [see Brooks and Asanuma, 1965a]. Some authors believe that intracortical recurrent inhibition is blocked by strychnine or tetanus toxin, as in the spinal cord [see Brooks and Asanuma, 1965b; Jasper, 1966], while negative results have been reported by other investigators [Crawford et al, 1963].

Evarts devoted three important papers [1964, 1965a, 1965b] to a microelectrode analysis of the pyramidal tract neurons during sleep in the monkey. He compared his results with those obtained by Adrian and Moruzzi [1939] by recording, under different kinds of anesthesia, from fibers of the cat's pyramidal tract. Although the experimental situation is markedly different, an examination of the two groups of records leads to some interesting considerations.

During wakefulness the monkey's pyramidal discharge is continual and rather regular (Fig. 15.12). It is surprisingly similar to that observed in the cat when $MgSO_4$ anesthesia is so light that pinching of the foot evokes slow withdrawal of the limb (Fig. 15.13).

During synchronized sleep, one observes, again in the unanesthetized monkey, short bursts of impulses interspersed with periods of inactivity

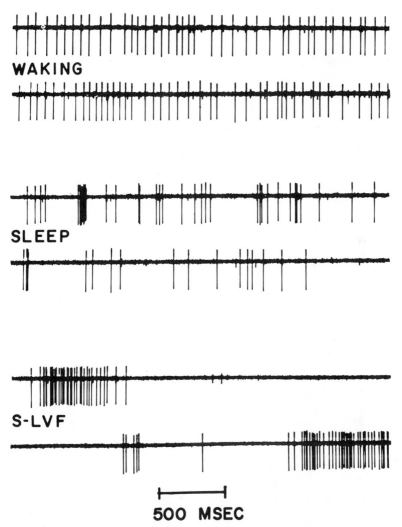

500 MSEC

Fig. 15.12. Patterns of discharge of pyramidal tract neurons during wakefulness and the two stages of sleep. Intact, unanesthetized monkey. During wakefulness the discharge is regular, without any tendency to clustered firing (top). During synchronized sleep there are bursts interspersed with periods of relative inactivity (middle). During low voltage fast activity (S-LVF), burst duration increases, intervening periods of inactivity become longer, and discharge frequency rises (bottom) [from Evarts, 1964, Fig. 1].

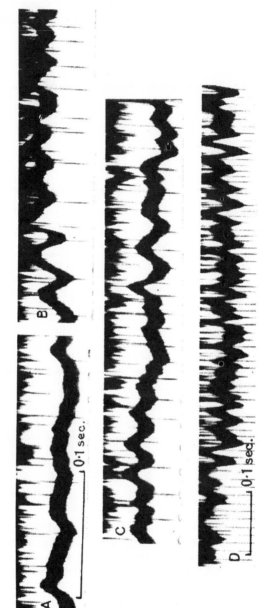

Fig. 15.13. Patterns of pyramidal discharge during activation of the motor cortex. Cat during light MgSO$_4$ anesthesia, permitting slow withdrawal of the limb when the foot is pinched. Single unit discharge from pyramidal decussation (top trace) and potentials from motor cortex (bottom trace) A, before, B, C, D, after pinching the foot, producing a gradual increase in frequency of the cortical waves. The rate of pyramidal discharge is 25 per sec in A, 50, 80, 90 per sec in B, C, D. D is a slower record [from Adrian and Moruzzi, 1939, Fig. 17].

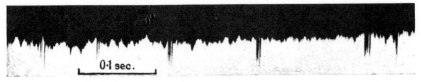

Fig. 15.14. Tendency to clustered firing of pyramidal tract neurons during barbiturate anesthesia. Cat anesthetized with dial. Single unit pyramidal discharges showing multiple outbursts (2–3 impulses each). The groups of impulses correspond with the groups of slow potential waves of the motor cortex [from Adrian and Moruzzi, 1939, Fig. 9].

(Fig. 15.12). Incidentally, a tendency to clustered firing has also been found, again during synchronous sleep, in the lateral geniculate body [Hubel, 1960], in the striate cortex [Hubel, 1959], and in the suprasylvian association cortex [Evarts et al, 1962]. It is interesting to note that during barbiturate anesthesia—a condition admittedly quite different from this stage of sleep, but characterized as well by cortical synchronization—the pyramidal tract neurons present short high frequency outbursts, composed of only two or three impulses, which occur synchronously with the slow 10 per sec cortical waves (Fig. 15.14). Adrian and Moruzzi [1939] pointed out that double or triple impulse groups were constantly absent under conditions of light $MgSO_4$ anesthesia, while Creutzfeldt and Jung [1961] reported that the clustered firing of the cortical motor units disappeared during arousal in the *encéphale isolé* cat. It is tempting to think that the mechanisms which prevent clustered firing during arousal are depressed during synchronized sleep, and blocked by barbiturate anesthesia.

Evarts [1964] has shown that during desynchronized sleep the duration of each burst, as well as that of the intervals of silence, greatly increases in the pyramidal tract neurons of the unanesthetized monkey's cortex (Fig. 15.12). Marchiafava and Pompeiano [1964], by recording the integrated pyramidal discharge, have shown that these phasic enhancements of the corticofugal activity occur synchronously with the bursts of rapid eye movements. The patterns of unit discharge during these outbursts are surprisingly similar, although the frequency is much lower, to that which one observes when convulsive outbursts are recorded from pyramidal units of the anesthesized cat after local strychninization of the motor cortex (Figs. 15.15, 15.16).

If local strychnine acts by abolishing the recurrent inhibition which usually damps the excessive discharge of Betz's cells, Evarts' hypothesis [1964] that during sleep the inhibitory intracortical neurons are depressed would be a challenging one. Such a depression would start during synchronized sleep, and might reach its highest intensities during the

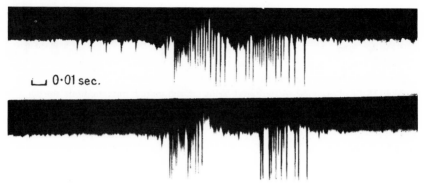

⌐_⌐ 0·01 sec.

Fig. 15.15. High-frequency pyramidal outbursts separated by intervals of silence after local strychninization of motor cortex. Cat anesthetized with dial. After local application of one per cent strychnine on the motor cortex. Although rate of unit firing is higher, the patterns of discharge resemble that of desynchronized sleep [from Adrian and Moruzzi, 1939, Fig. 29].

desynchronized phase. Even then the inhibitory interneurons might still be put into action by the recurrent collaterals, whenever a critical level of temporal summation is reached. Evarts [1964] has pointed out that the well-known tendency of epileptic seizures to occur during sleep might perhaps be explained along these lines.

It should be pointed out, however, that we have so far no evidence that recurrent intracortical inhibition is depressed during sleep, although this theme might be approached experimentally. The similarity between strychnine outbursts and those occurring in cortical neurons during desynchronized sleep provides only suggestive evidence. This evidence is

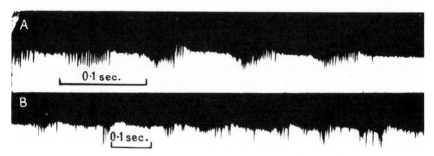

A

⌐___ 0·1 sec. ___⌐

B

⌐0·1 sec.⌐

Fig. 15.16. End of the effect of local strychninization of the motor cortex. Cat anesthetized with dial. Towards the final stage of local strychninization the high-frequency pyramidal outbursts occur in groups at 10 per sec, as before strychnine (A). A few minutes later the number of impulses in each outburst has greatly decreased, and the patterns are similar to those produced by dial anesthesia alone (B) [from Adrian and Moruzzi, 1939, Fig. 33].

weakened, moreover, by the fact that the mechanism of action of local strychnine on the cerebral cortex is still in doubt. As we have recalled above, negative [Crawford et al, 1963] or weak [Brooks and Asanuma, 1965b] results on recurrent inhibition have been obtained after intravenous injections of the drug, whereas positive results were reported after local injection of tetanus toxin [Brooks and Asanuma, 1965b].

It is interesting, nevertheless, to examine Evarts' hypothesis from the angle of our considerations on the slow recovery of the "learned" synapses. Actually, the function of cortical interneurons in the regulation of the rate of firing is one which is likely to involve mainly routine synapses. However, it would not be unthinkable that a lot of learning occurs in all kinds of functions concerned with the sharpening of the response of the individual cortical cells to different patterns of highly localized sensory stimulation. The depression of the inhibitory interneurons would then be specifically related to the slow process of recovery from plastic activity. Whether this depression is due to withdrawal of reticular facilitation, to localized processes of inhibition, or to both mechanisms, remains a matter for speculation.

CONCLUSIONS

There is little doubt that active inhibitory processes are at work during sleep, at least during its desynchronized phase. This has been clearly proved, in my opinion, by the investigations of Pompeiano and his colleagues as far as the mechanism of the hypnic depression of spinal reflexes is concerned. Plastic changes, however, are likely to be of minor importance in the history of spinal synapses, although their presence at segmental levels can be inferred from the old observations of Di Giorgio [1929; for literature see Dow and Moruzzi, 1958]. Anyway, there is little doubt that slow processes of recovery are unlikely to be extensively needed within the spinal cord. On the whole, spinal inhibition during desynchronized sleep seems to be an aspect of the regulation of the sleep of the body. It is undoubtedly an important aspect, since the ability to maintain a posture or to carry out movements would be useless, and might become occasionally dangerous, when the animal is unconscious. It is an aspect, nevertheless, which is clearly unrelated with what appears to be the hard core of sleep physiology, the slow recovery of the "learned" synapses.

We have seen that it is only likely, but by no means proved, that active inhibitory processes are involved in the slow reintegration of the synapses occurring in the neocortex. Actually, there was no place for inhibition in the original formulation of the reticular hypothesis. An attempt to see how far the reticular explanation of sleep may be reconciled with the mechanisms considered in the present review may well close this article. This last section may also be used as a summary of the main considerations presented in the previous sections.

A doctrine on sleep should take into account not only the neurophysiological mechanism of the phenomenon, but also its functional significance. The latter aspect has been rather neglected so far, notwithstanding the sweeping progress made during the last thirty years by the electrophysiological investigation of sleep. It is very important, nevertheless, even from a strictly neurophysiological standpoint. If we were able to express, in physiological and biochemical terms, what the aims of sleep are, it would become at once easier to understand the functional significance of the multifarious neural events which have been observed during the different stages of sleep.

Saying that sleep is concerned with the recovery of the neurons is tantamount to expressing a self-evident truth, and such a statement is, moreover, so vague as to become almost meaningless. An attempt should be made, first of all, to circumscribe the field of our interest. One may start by saying that there are at least two kinds of recovery in the nervous system.

Fast recovery processes are related with conduction and synaptic transmission of nerve impulses, that is, essentially with changes of membrane permeability. Ion pumps, enzymatic activities related with breakdown, and resynthesis of the chemical mediators belong to these fast recovery processes, which are completed in a few milliseconds and do not require any interruption in the activity of large populations of neurons. Sleep is not required for these fast recovery processes, which probably predominate in what we have called the "routine" synapses, the overwhelming majority in the lower nervous structures involved in inborn, stereotyped activities.

There are, moreover, *slow recovery processes,* which can occur only when the activity of other neuronal populations is interrupted or severely disorganized for long periods of time. The hypothesis is made that slow recovery is related to the plastic activities, which are probably present everywhere, but predominate in the neural structures associated with the higher nerve functions, and above all with consciousness. Hence, sleep should not be regarded as a period of recovery for the entire cerebrum, but only (or mainly) as a period of recuperation for these synapses where plastic (macromolecular) changes occurred during wakefulness, as a consequence of higher nervous activities such as those involved in learning or conditioning. Following Eccles [1966b], we assume that these plastic changes occur at the level of these learned synapses, but of course the biochemical processes related to the recuperation may take place also in the postsynaptic soma or in the neighboring glia cells. A further working hypothesis might be that small interneurons are more strongly affected than the large neurons of the neocortical projection areas by these slow recovery processes. Some or most of these interneurons might be inhibitory in nature and would be closely related to the ascending reticular system, as suggested by the blockade of the discharge of large cortical cells of the projection areas that occurs at the moment of arousal [Whitlock, Arduini, and Moruzzi, 1953].

If all these slow recovery processes were not concentrated in a given period of time, we should spend our life in a kind of *dormiveglia*. We should never be really awake or completely asleep. What rightly seems to us to be a disorder in the higher nervous activities, sleep, must be produced in an orderly manner. This is the meaning of the sleep-controlling structures of the brain stem. Sleep of the body is simply a consequence of the existence of a period of blackout in our higher nervous activities. It is simply a consequence of the state of sleep. The aim of sleep, however, is not to provide a period of recuperation for our body nor even for several structures of the central nervous system. This recovery could perfectly well be achieved without sleep.

According to the reticular hypothesis, a critical level of the tonic facilitatory influence exerted by the ascending flow of reticular impulses is required in order to maintain wakefulness. We may add that as wakefulness progresses—up to the unphysiological condition of sleep deprivation—more and more support is required by the brain stem, probably because the efficiency of the learned synapses involved in the processes of plastic activity gradually decreases. The fight against an overpowering tendency to sleep is usually carried out by performing voluntary movements, or simply by standing and by increasing the isometric contraction of the muscles of the jaw. Strong cutaneous stimulations and mental effort are also usually effective. These efforts may be regarded as attempts to increase the activity of the ascending reticular system by intensifying the barrage of sensory and cortico-reticular impulses impinging upon it. This energizing influence of the ascending reticular system is not needed by, or appears to be by far less important for, the large projection neurons of the neocortex, which are likely to be mainly devoted to routine tasks.

We have followed so far the main lines of the deafferentation hypotheses, with only two limitations, namely: (1) that sleep concerns *primarily* not the whole cerebrum, nor even the entire neocortex, but only those neurons or synapses which are the seat, during wakefulness, of particularly intense plastic activities; (2) that sleep results not merely from withdrawal of brain stem facilitation—the usual explanation of spinal shock—but that a gradual fall in the excitability of the cerebral structures, requiring slow processes of recovery, is also essential for the onset of sleep.

This simplified scheme does not require that an active process of inhibition be exerted upon the structures undergoing the process of slow recovery. The mass inhibition of cortical neurons which Pavlov had postulated certainly does not exist, but it would be impossible to deny that strategically placed interneurons or synapses may be inhibited during sleep, either presynaptically or postsynaptically. There is certainly no need to invoke the presence of such an inhibition to explain our falling asleep after a prolonged and exacting period of wakefulness. We are purposely refraining, moreover, from taking into account the position of the diffuse projection nuclei of the thalamus or of the subcortical mechanisms of synchronization. We would only like to state that one may explain the onset of sleep simply by postulating that some neurons of the ascending reticular system share the same properties of the interneurons of the cerebrum with regard to the need of prolonged periods of rest.

Obviously, the need of a slow process of recovery will be different in the different parts of the cerebrum. It will be related to metabolic processes and to the amount of plastic activity which went on during the period of wakefulness. What matters is that the blackout of the cerebrum occurs simultaneously, or almost simultaneously, in all its different districts. We certainly oversleep with regard to the needs of multitudes of neurons, but any integrated behavior—and the concentration of sleep in a given period of time is certainly the expression of an integrated behavior—requires a situation of privilege for those neurons that are called to take, or to influence, the main decisions. When arousal is not purposely or fortuitously produced by sensory stimulation, one might think that the regions of the brain which are the first to recover will increase the activity of the ascending reticular system through cortico-reticular and thalamo-reticular paths. There are certainly several kinds of interrelations between cerebrum and brain stem which may explain the gradual deepening of sleep, its maintenance for several hours and its disappearance at the moment of a spontaneous arousal.

We have stated above that there is no need to postulate inhibitory processes for explaining our inability to remain awake after a prolonged wakefulness—still more so after sleep deprivation. But it would be more difficult to explain, without the existence of brain stem structures antagonistically oriented with regard to the ascending reticular system, the sleep produced by conditioning or by monotonous sensory stimulations [Moruzzi, 1960], or that represented by a daytime nap, or the obvious tendency to oversleep of the domestic cat. Even the clinical cases of narcolepsy cannot be easily explained with the deafferentation hypotheses. A detailed review of the literature on the synchronizing structures of the lower brain stem has been given elsewhere [Moruzzi, 1960, 1963a]. They may act by inhibiting the activating reticular system or by antagonizing its influence at thalamic levels. Both antagonistic systems of the brain stem appear to be tonically active.

The classical experiment of Hess is probably correlatable with the activity of these synchronizing structures, and the work of Schlag and Chaillet [1963] on the descending influence exerted by the midline nuclei of the thalamus on the brain stem reticular formation appears to be particularly important in this respect. Even Jouvet's views on neocortical sleep [1962, 1965b, 1965c] might be easily reconciled with the existence of synchronizing structures within the brain stem [see Moruzzi, 1965].

This is only an attempt to draw the main lines of a doctrine on sleep. We have purposely refrained from taking into account the contingent aspects of the phenomenon. Atonia and absence of the righting reflexes, eye closure and myosis, EEG synchronization or low voltage fast activity —in short, most of the multifarious behavioral and electrophysiological signs of sleep—are contingent phenomena, since sleep may occur without them. They are related with important neurophysiological mechanisms, which deserve to be fully investigated. However, it is unlikely that their study will lead us to reach the hard core of hypnic physiology.

Also the episodes of low voltage fast sleep, and the dreams which have been shown in humans to be associated with them, are closely related to the process of slow recovery. The experiments carried out in man by Dement [1960] and in the cat by Jouvet et al [1964] clearly show that there is a specific need for desynchronized sleep. After deprivation of desynchronized sleep, the percentage of it rises from about 20 per cent to 60 per cent of the total duration of the recovery sleep. Apparently part of the process of slow recovery may be accomplished only during the episodes of desynchronized sleep, but the relationship between them and synchronized sleep is yet completely unknown. The work of Jouvet [1962, 1965a] and his colleagues [Jouvet, Jouvet and Valatx, 1963] clearly suggests, anyway, that the pontile structures involved in the production of these episodes of sleep may still become periodically active after chronic decerebration.

Desynchronized sleep is characterized by an eruption of phasic phenomena, some excitatory (clonic twitches) and some inhibitory in nature, as reported in the previous sections of this report. Several observations [see Jouvet, 1962] suggest that pontine structures are at the origin of these outbursts of brain stem activity. It is extremely likely, moreover, that the excitatory and the inhibitory phenomena are closely related, since they are so clearly associated in their occurrence. This chapter of sleep physiology appears to be a promising field for future investigation.

DISCUSSION

Chairman: PROFESSOR MOUNTCASTLE

BREMER: I should like to raise two questions in relation with Professor Moruzzi's topics.

The first one concerns what one could name the teleological aspect of sleep. It seems at first sight unescapable to admit that the "purpose" of sleep, in the higher mammals at least, is to give the nerve cells and their synapses the due rest they deserve. But I wish to point out a difficulty which results from the great varieties of sleep among mammals, and I am glad that we have among us a zoologist who may confirm and enlarge my information and its bearing. It concerns the sleep of the seals. I have been told that, when lying on the shore, they sleep during two minute spells, then they awake, raise the head, apparently to be sure that a polar bear is not in view, and then go to their precarious sleep again. This succession of brief sleep-and-waking spells is said to be regularly repeated during the whole resting time of the animals, as if they had an internal clock in their brain. With such brief periods of sleep, would a real neuronal recovery be possible?

My second remark is related to the search for inhibitory processes, at the cortical level, in sleep. It is certainly an important finding that, during activated sleep, there is a strong inhibition going down to the spinal cord. But this fact concerns the physiology of the sleep syndrome, not the sleep mechanism itself. And I must again conclude that in spite of the efforts to find true inhibitory processes at the cortical level during sleep, we may say that, up to now, it has been a failure. I do not deny the possibility of such direct suppressive processes. But, if one neglects that other unknown represented by the so-called activated or paradoxical sleep—in the light of Moruzzi and Magoun's and my own work—the depression aspects of the brain cortex functioning in sleep can be satisfactorily explained by the interruption of ascending energizing impulses; hence the absence of clear evidence of direct inhibitory processes at the cortical level does not disturb me too much!

MORUZZI: Concerning the first part of Professor Bremer's remark, I agree that a comparative approach would be quite stimulating, particularly in view of the fact that the neural activities involved in learning, conditioning, etc., are extremely variable in the different animals. A study of sleep in the invertebrates might be rewarding. The honeybees, for example, are certainly able to learn, as von Frisch beautifully showed, but there is little doubt that the main effort of their central nervous system is devoted to the routine tasks of their instinctive life. The main difficulty, of course, is to find criteria of the presence of true sleep, or even of a lower level of wakefulness, in low animals. It would be dangerous to extrapolate from the bodily manifestations of sleep in mammals and birds. Periods characterized by absence of movements do not necessarily mean presence of sleep, at least in the sense this term is generally used.

Concerning the second question of Professor Bremer, I agree that the demonstration of an inhibitory modulation of the spinal cord during desynchronized sleep, which has been given by Pompeiano and his colleagues, is related to neural control of the body during sleep. Its functional significance is probably to prevent or to reduce movements when the animal is unconscious, an event which is more likely to occur during sleep. The feeling of being unable to move, an agonizing experience of nightmares, is probably dependent on the inhibition of the motoneuronal response to pyramidal volleys, which has been shown by Marchiafava and Pompeiano.

THORPE: I am glad that Professor Bremer has raised this point of the comparative approach to the study of sleep because it does present a great many interesting problems. Perhaps the most outstanding thing to me is the apparently great difference between quite closely related animals in their sleep requirements. A great many birds, for instance, sleep apparently normally during the hours of darkness, and their time of going to rest is very closely correlated with the fading of the light. Thus they show preparations for going to rest during a solar eclipse. On the other hand, many birds in the northern regions appear to sleep little, if at all, during the summer, remaining active during the whole 24-hour period. Still more extraordinary is the fact that—as had long been suspected—(a proof has now been provided by Dr. David Lack) the common swift (*Apus apus*) frequently spends whole nights in the air. In the coastal regions of eastern England the careful observer can see parties of swifts going high into the air at dusk and then, while flying in wide circles in an excited manner, drifting slowly out over the North Sea until they disappear. Their presence far out over the sea has been confirmed by pilots, and in the morning the coastal watcher may see them returning landwards to continue their aerial feeding. The swift, therefore, seems to be a bird in which, at any rate for certain periods, sleep can be completely dispensed with—unless one supposes, which seems highly improbable, that the birds take what we might call cat naps between wing beats!

Coming to the fish, we find that a great many species apparently remain actively swimming all night, although they do not maintain shoal formation. This shoal formation is primarily a visual matter and so the group tends to disrupt at night when the light fails and be reformed in the morning. However, fish which live on reefs, and particularly tropical reef fishes, apparently do go to sleep. I myself have been fortunate enough to see a striking demonstration of this at the Marine Biological Laboratory at Bimini in the Bahamas. The research station there is provided with areas of the shallow sea which have been fenced in, the wire of the fencing going down to the sea bottom. In these enclosures, marine creatures varying in size from quite small fish on the one hand, to large turtles and even porpoises on the other, can be retained. Some of these pens contain large numbers of tropical reef fishes, and one can go out at night along the catwalks around the edge of the pen and with a lighted torch observe the nocturnal behavior of the reef fishes. Such fish are mostly laterally flattened; that is, they are deep and very narrow, and one can see them lying down night after night as if sleeping. It was very noticeable that one or two of the larger fish which had been in the pens for a long time were always to be seen in the same places at night, as if they had first choice of the best spots while the others which were either smaller or had been put in more recently had to make do with the second best. So in quite closely related fishes you may have some species which apparently remain in normal swimming activity all night and others which go to sleep. Presumably, under natural conditions these reef fishes have small holes and crannies in the reef where they can rest with impunity more or less safe from predators. I suggest that a physiological study of two closely related species of fish, one of which lives in reefs and one which is pelagic, would be of very great interest.

As Professor Bremer has said, the same kind of thing apparently applies to seals and to many mammals. When we come to the insects the evidence is much more difficult to interpret because in this group we have not the obvious signs of sleep which are to be found in vertebrate animals. Nevertheless, in some insects there are what appear to be specific "sleep attitudes"; and there is also a change in the arrangement of the pigment in the eyes during such periods of apparent sleep. Beyond this, however, one can say very little about sleep in the invertebrates. It is true that one gets the impression that bees inside the hive are active all through the night, but this, of course, is only a statistical affair. It may well be that individual bees take regular periods of sleep, even though the whole hive is never quiescent at any one time. It would, I think, nevertheless, be very well worthwhile to investigate the night activities of a population of marked bees. As far as I am aware this has not been done.

CHAIRMAN: I would like to make one or two comments; I think that in relation to the problem of the need for cerebral versus somatic sleep, the situation in the porpoise is of interest. The porpoise has been shown, I think fairly clearly, to sleep, one hemisphere at a time, so that his bodily movements maintaining his up-down swimming movements in the water and breathing are maintained. Apparently he closes one eye and synchronizes one hemisphere at a time, which is a rather interesting variant of sleep.

The second point is that you have put in the introduction to your talk what is at least to me a completely new idea that the requirement of sleep is due to some accumulation of a slow process going on in the cerebral cortex; and I presume you mean this in relation to the metabolism of large molecules in some way associated with the continued growth of axons. The question I would like to ask you is, what sort of a signal can be obtained which is the influence affecting the brain stem mechanism controlling forebrain excitability that is derived from this accumulated need in the cerebral cortex? We need some transmission of information here.

MORUZZI: The reply to the important question of Professor Mountcastle should be introduced by a definition of the plastic activities. Some of them are related to the formation of new synapses, an event which is of course more likely to occur in the young animals, particularly among those which are born immature. In this period of life the central nervous system is concerned with a task which is both anatomical and biochemical in character.

In the adult animal, most of the plastic changes are unlikely to be related to the formation of new synapses. The study of the plastic activities would mainly concern, therefore, the macromolecular biology rather than synaptology. These considerations might explain why so much time is spent asleep in the young mammals. However, this may not be the only reason, since, when the cerebral cortex is still immature, the corticoreticular mechanisms producing arousal are of course absent.

There is little doubt, as Professor Mountcastle has pointed out, that the accumulated need of slow recovery occurring, say, in the cerebral cortex should influence in some way the action exerted on the cerebrum by the brain stem mechanisms controlling wakefulness and sleep. The simplest explanation is that because of the growing accumulation of a need of slow recovery the brain neurons involved in the plastic activities would require more and more the facilitating support of the ascending reticular system. At a critical moment the ascending facilitation would be unable to support the critical level of cortical tone which is required for the maintenance of wakefulness. This explanation is in line with the reticular version of the passive doctrine of sleep. However, the tonic activity of the ascending reticular system may also gradually decrease during wakefulness, either because of intrinsic properties of the reticular system (whose tasks are, of course, particularly heavy during alertness) or as a consequence of inhibitory signals arriving from the cerebrum. The synchronizing structures of the lower brain stem might be involved in this cerebral control of reticular activity.

JASPER: First, regarding your difficulty with inhibition and strychnine, I don't know whether Canadian cats are different from Australian cats, but we have now 26 confirmed pyramidal tract cells with intracellular recording in which the antidromic type of inhibition was abolished with strychnine, and even reversed to a depolarizing potential. But there is another kind of inhibition: the inhibition that results from orthodromic stimulation of the thalamus, and we showed many years ago that this occurred without evidence of change in intracellular membrane potential in the pyramidal tract neurons. This kind of inhibition is not affected by strychnine, and I think we have pretty clear evidence now that you cannot make a generalization about inhibition in the cortex with regard to strychnine.

I would like to draw you out a little bit, Professor Moruzzi, if I could. You decided not to include your work on the effect of rhythmic repetitive stimulation because of the lack of time. This is related not only to your considerations, but to some of Professor Eccles' assumptions regarding the facilitation of neuronal pathways with activity. It is well known that repeated activity, if continued in a rhythmic manner in a fixed system of neurons, does not facilitate conduction, but it blocks reaction. I suppose it is a phenomenon that Pavlov described in his inhibitory theory of sleep, which was based upon the observation that repeated presentation of stimuli in the learning situation without reinforcement regularly induced sleep in the animal, which he described hypothetically as spreading inhibition. This remarkable development of a failure of responsiveness with identically repeated monotonous stimuli is, I think, a very fundamental part of this whole question, and is a method of inducing sleep in all of us!

MORUZZI: Monotonous sensory stimulation leads to sleep, an effect that has been intensively investigated by Pavlov. I have made the hypothesis, at the Moscow Symposium [Moruzzi, 1960], that Pavlovian sleep is mediated by the synchronizing structures of the lower brain stem. This technique of gradually producing sleep is a very useful one, and might be utilized in an attempt to study how the antidromic inhibition of pyramidal neurons, which was the subject of the fascinating group of experiments just reported by Professor Jasper, is affected by sleep and wakefulness.

CHAGAS: In his brilliant paper, Professor Moruzzi referred to the recovery of tired, overworked neurons as the primary cause of sleep, or of the need of it. This would lead us to the consideration of sleep in a molecular level, as Dr. Mountcastle might say.

I would suppose that for small molecules in living animals, the turnover time parameters would possibly give us significant indications; however, for macromolecules the problem becomes much more complex, and the time elements involved are completely out of rhythm with sleep. It may, in fact, become extremely difficult to know exactly the significance of pools and transfers of molecules. In any event, the extrapolation from one case to the other seems rather doubtful.

ECCLES: I am fascinated by the suggestion of Professor Moruzzi that the plastic properties of the nerve cells may be those that require this period of inactivity or rest during sleep. This is a very valuable and original suggestion which seems to give us new conceptual possibilities. I can appreciate that after the immense barrage of impulses or information that has been poured into the nervous system during the day, these microgrowth and regression processes would be required in order to reconstitute the nervous system for the next day. In regard to Dr. Jasper's comment about strychnine, I have not investigated strychnine action on the neocortex. But certainly with the hippocampus, with the thalamus, and with the Purkinje cells of the cerebellum, the hyperpolarizing IPSP's are not significantly changed by quite large intravenous doses of strychnine; nor are, of course, the inhibitory phenomena produced by these potentials.

ANDERSEN: I worked quite a lot with Dr. Curtis who performed the experiments on the neocortex; and I think there is, so it seems, a difference between Australian and Canadian cats! Dr. Curtis ejected glutamic acid electrophoretically from an extracellular microelectrode and so he was able to maintain the cells at a given firing rate. On this background, he fired an antidromic volley up the pyramidal tract. In a large number of cells, after the intravenous injection of strychnine, there was no change in the duration of the recurrent inhibitory period.

REFERENCES

ADRIAN, E. D., and G. MORUZZI. Impulses in the pyramidal tract, *J. Physiol.*, 97, 153–199 [1939].

ARDUINI, A., G. BERLUCCHI, and P. STRATA. Pyramidal activity during sleep and wakefulness, *Arch. Ital. Biol.*, *101*, 530–544 [1963].

ASANUMA, H., and V. B. BROOKS. Recurrent cortical effects following stimulation of internal capsule, *Arch. Ital. Biol.*, *103*, 220–246 [1965].

BALCH, C. C. Sleep in ruminants, *Nature*, *175*, 940–941 [1955].

BALDISSERA, F., G. BROGGI, and M. MANCIA. Modificazioni del riflesso spinale monosinaptico e polisinaptico nel gatto normale non anestetizzato durante le varie fasi del sonno e della veglia, *Rend. Accad. Naz. Lincei, Cl. Sc. Fis. Mat. e Nat.*, Ser. VIII, *36*, 539–542 [1964].

BAUST, W., and G. BERLUCCHI. Reflex response to clicks of cat's tensor tympani during sleep and wakefulness and the influence thereon of the auditory cortex, *Arch. Ital. Biol.*, *102*, 686–712 [1964].

———, and G. MORUZZI. Changes in the auditory input in wakefulness and during the synchronized and desynchronized stages of sleep, *Arch. Ital. Biol.*, *102*, 657–674 [1964].

BELL, F. R. The electroencephalogram of goats during somnolence and rumination, *Animal Behaviour*, *8*, 39–42 [1960].

BIZZI, E., O. POMPEIANO, and I. SOMOGYI. Spontaneous activity of single vestibular neurons of unrestrained cats during sleep and wakefulness, *Arch. Ital. Biol.*, *102*, 308–330 [1964].

BREMER, F., L'activité électrique de l'écorce cérébrale et le problème physiologique du sommeil, *Boll. Soc. Ital. Biol. Sper.*, *13*, 271–290 [1938].

BROOKS, V. B., and H. ASANUMA. Recurrent cortical effects following stimulation of medullary pyramids, *Arch. Ital. Biol.*, *103*, 247–278 [1965a].

———. Pharmacological studies of recurrent cortical inhibition and facilitation, *Amer. J. Physiol.*, *208*, 671–681 [1965b].

CRAWFORD, J. M., D. R. CURTIS, P. E. VOORHOEVE, and V. J. WILSON. Strychnine and cortical inhibition, *Nature*, *200*, 845–846 [1963].

CREUTZFELDT, O. D., and R. JUNG. Neuronal discharge in cat's motor cortex during sleep and arousal, *The Nature of Sleep*, in: Ciba Foundation Symposium. London: Churchill, pp. 131–170 [1961].

DELAFRESNAYE, J. F., ed. *Brain Mechanism and Consciousness*. Springfield, Ill.: C. C Thomas, xv + 556 pp. [1954].

DEMENT, W. The effect of dream deprivation, *Science*, *131*, 1705–1707 [1960].

DESMEDT, J. E. Auditory-evoked potentials from cochlea to cortex as influenced by activation of the efferent olivo-cochlear bundle, *J. Acoust. Soc. Am.*, *34*, 1478–1496 [1962].

———, and P. MONACO. Suppression par la strychnine de l'effet inhibiteur centrifuge exercé par le faisceau olivo-cochéaire, *Arch. Int. Pharmacodyn.*, *129*, 244–248 [1960].

DI GIORGIO, A. M. Persistenza, nell' animale spinale, di asimmetrie posturali e motorie di origine cerebellare, *Arch. Fisiol.*, *27*, 519–542 [1929].

DOW, R. S., and G. MORUZZI. *The Physiology and Pathology of the Cerebellum.* Minneapolis: Univ. Minnesota Press, xvi + 675 pp. [1958].

ECCLES, J. C. *The Physiology of Synapses.* Berlin: Springer, 316 pp. [1964].

———. Cerebral synaptic mechanisms, in: *Brain and Conscious Experience* (ed. by J. C. Eccles). New York, Springer-Verlag [1966a].

ECCLES, J. C. Conscious experience and memory, in: *Brain and Conscious Experience* (ed. by J. C. Eccles). New York, Springer-Verlag [1966b].

ECONOMO, C. VON. Schlaftheorie, *Ergebn. Physiol.*, 28, 312–339 [1929].

EVARTS, E. V. Activity of neurons in visual cortex of the cat during sleep with low voltage fast EEG activity, *J. Neurophysiol.*, 25, 812–816 [1962].

———. Temporal patterns of discharge of pyramidal tract neurons during sleep and waking in the monkey, *J. Neurophysiol.*, 27, 152–171 [1964].

———. Relation of discharge frequency to conduction velocity in pyramidal tract neurons, *J. Neurophysiol.*, 28, 216–228 [1965a].

———. Relation of cell size to effect of sleep in pyramidal tract neurons, in: *Sleep Mechanisms* (eds. K. Akert, C. Bally, and J. P. Schadé), *Progress in Brain Research*, Vol. 18:91, Amsterdam: Elsevier Publishing Co. [1965b].

———, E. BENTAL, B. BIHARI, and P. R. HUTTENLOCHER. Spontaneous discharge of single neurons during sleep and waking, *Science*, 135, 726–728 [1962].

GALAMBOS, R. Suppression of auditory nerve activity by stimulation of efferent fibers to cochlea, *J. Neurophysiol*, 19, 424–437 [1956].

———. Studies of the auditory system with implanted electrodes, in: *Neural Mechanisms of the Auditory and Vestibular Systems* (eds. G. L. Rasmussen and W. F. Windle). Springfield, Ill.: C. C Thomas, pp. 137–151 [1960].

———, A. RUPERT, and F. B. SIMMONS. Unpublished observations quoted in Galambos [1960].

GASSEL, M. M., P. L. MARCHIAFAVA, and O. POMPEIANO. Tonic and phasic inhibition of spinal reflexes during deep, desynchronized sleep in unrestrained cats, *Arch. Ital. Biol.*, 102, 471–499 [1964].

———. An analysis of the supraspinal influences acting on motoneurons during sleep in the unrestrained cat. Modification of the recurrent discharge of the alpha motoneurons during sleep, *Arch. Ital. Biol.*, 103, 25–44 [1965a].

———. Modulation of the recurrent discharge of alpha motoneurons in decerebrate and spinal cats, *Arch. Ital. Biol.*, 103, 1–24 [1965b].

GIAQUINTO, S., O. POMPEIANO, and I. SOMOGYI. Reflex activity of extensor and flexor muscles following muscular afferent excitation during sleep and wakefulness, *Experientia*, 19, 481–482 [1963a].

———. Supraspinal inhibitory control of spinal reflexes during natural sleep, *Experientia*, 19, 652–653 [1963b].

———. Supraspinal modulation of heteronymous monosynaptic and of polysynaptic reflexes during natural sleep and wakefulness, *Arch. Ital. Biol.*, 102, 245–281 [1964a].

———. Descending inhibitory influences on spinal reflexes during natural sleep, *Arch. Ital. Biol.*, 102, 282–307 [1964b].

GRANIT, R. Sensory mechanisms in perception, in: *Brain and Conscious Experience* (ed. by J. C. Eccles). New York: Springer-Verlag [1966].

HODES, R., and W. C. DEMENT. Depression of electrically induced reflexes ("H-reflexes") in man during low voltage EEG "sleep," *EEG Clin. Neurophysiol.*, 17, 617–629 [1964].

HUBEL, D. H. Single unit activity in striate cortex of unrestrained cats, *J. Physiol., 147,* 226–238 [1959].

———. Single unit activity in lateral geniculate body and optic tract of unrestrained cats, *J. Physiol., 150,* 91–104 [1960].

JASPER, H. H. Pathophysiological studies of brain mechanisms in different states of consciousness, in: *Brain and Conscious Experience* (ed. by J. C. Eccles). New York: Springer-Verlag [1966].

JOUVET, D., P. VIMONT, F. DELORME, and M. JOUVET. Etude de la privation sélective de la phase paradoxale du sommeil chez le chat, *C.R. Soc. Biol., 158,* 756–759 [1964].

JOUVET, M. Recherches sur les structures nerveuses et les mécanismes responsables des différentes phases du sommeil physiologique, *Arch. Ital. Biol., 100,* 125–206 [1962].

———. Étude de la dualité des états de sommeil et des mécanismes de la phase paradoxale, in: *Aspects Anatomo-fonctionnels de la Physiologie du Sommeil* (ed. by M. Jouvet), 397–449. Paris: Ed. du C.N.R.S. [1965a].

———. Discussion Générale, in: *Aspects Anatomo-fonctionnels de la Physiologie du Sommeil* (ed. by M. Jouvet), 613–650. Paris: Ed. du C.N.R.S. [1965b].

——— (ed.). *Aspects Anatomo-Fonctionnels de la Physiologie du Sommeil,* Colloque Int. du C.N.R.S., Lyon, Paris: Ed. du C.N.R.S., 657 pp. [1965c].

———, D. JOUVET, and J. L. VALATX. Etude du sommeil chez le chat pontique. Sa suppression automatique, *C.R. Soc. Biol., 157,* 845–849 [1963].

KETY, S. S. Sleep and the energy metabolism of the brain, in: *The Nature of Sleep.* Ciba Foundation Symposium. London: Churchill, pp. 375–385 [1961].

KLEITMAN, N. *Sleep and Wakefulness.* Chicago: Univ. Chicago Press, x + 552 pp. [1963].

KUBOTA, T., Y. IWAMURA, and Y. NIMI. Monosynaptic reflex and natural sleep, *Experientia, 20,* 316–317 [1964].

MAGOUN, H. W. *The Waking Brain.* Springfield, Ill.: C. C Thomas, viii + 138 pp. [1958].

MARCHIAFAVA, P. L., and O. POMPEIANO. Pyramidal influences on spinal cord during desynchronized sleep, *Arch. Ital. Biol., 102,* 500–529 [1964].

MORUZZI, G. Synchronizing influences of the brain stem and the inhibitory mechanisms underlying the production of sleep by sensory stimulation, *EEG Clin. Neurophysiol.,* Suppl. 13, 231–256 [1960].

———. Active processes in the brain stem during sleep, *The Harvey Lectures,* 58, 233–297 [1963a].

———. The physiology of sleep, *Endeavour, 22,* 31–36 [1963b].

———. The historical development of the deafferentation hypothesis of sleep, *Proc. Amer. Philos. Soc., 108,* 19–28 [1964].

———. See General Discussion in Jouvet [1965c].

———, and H. W. MAGOUN. Brain stem reticular formation and activation of the EEG, *EEG Clin. Neurophysiol., 1,* 455–473 [1949].

PHILLIPS, C. G. Action of antidromic pyramidal volleys on single Betz cells in the cat, *Quart. J. Exp. Physiol., 44,* 1–25 [1959].

RASMUSSEN, G. L. The olivary peduncle and other fiber projections of the superior olivary complex, *J. Comp. Neurol., 84,* 141–219 [1946].

———. Further observations of the efferent cochlear bundle, *J. Comp. Neurol., 99,* 61–74 [1953].

———. Efferent fibers of the cochlear nerve and cochlear nucleus, in: *Neural Mechanisms of the Auditory and Vestibular Systems.* Springfield, Ill.: C. C Thomas, pp. 105–115 [1960].

———, and W. F. WINDLE, eds. *Neural Mechanisms of the Auditory and Vestibular Systems.* Springfield, Ill.: C. C Thomas, xiv + 422 pp. [1960].

ROSSI, G. F. Brain stem facilitating influences on EEG synchronization. Experimental findings and observations in man, *E.E.G. Clin. Neurophysiol., 18,* 529–530 [1965].

———, and A. ZANCHETTI. The brain stem reticular formation. Anatomy and physiology, *Arch. Ital. Biol., 95,* 199–435 [1957].

RUCKEBUSCH, Y. Etude poligraphique et comportementale de l'évolution postnatale du sommeil physiologique chez l'agneau, *Arch. Ital. Biol., 101,* 111–132 [1963].

SCHLAG, J. D., and F. CHAILLET. Thalamic mechanisms involved in cortical desynchronization and recruiting responses, *EEG Clin. Neurophysiol., 15,* 39–62 [1963].

SHERRINGTON, C. S. *Man on His Nature.* Cambridge: Cambridge University Press, 413 pp. [1946].

STEFANIS, C., and H. H. JASPER. Intracellular microelectrode studies of antidromic responses in cortical pyramidal tract neurons, *J. Neurophysiol., 27,* 828–854 [1964].

TARCHANOFF, J. Quelques observations sur le sommeil normal, *Arch. Ital. Biol., 21,* 318–321 [1894].

WHITLOCK, D. G., A. ARDUINI, and G. MORUZZI. Microelectrode analysis of pyramidal system during transition from sleep to wakefulness, *J. Neurophysiol., 16,* 414–429 [1953].

WILLIAMS, H. L., J. T. HAMMACK, R. L. DALY, W. C. DEMENT, and A. LUBIN. Responses to auditory stimulation, sleep loss and the EEG stages of sleep, *EEG Clin. Neurophysiol., 16,* 269–279 [1964].

WOLSTENHOLME, G. E. W., and M. O'CONNOR, eds. *The Nature of Sleep.* Ciba Foundation Symposium. London: Churchill, xii + 416 pp. [1961].

16

Changing Concepts of the Precentral Motor Area

by C. G. PHILLIPS

Trinity College, Oxford, England

INTRODUCTION

We are nearing the centenaries of the discoveries that muscles can be made to move by giving electric shocks to the pericruciate area of the cerebral cortex of the dog [Fritsch and Hitzig, 1870] and to the Rolandic region of the cortex of the monkey [Ferrier, 1873].

If the electrical excitability of the brain was first revealed in terms of muscular contraction, this was the only index the early experimenters possessed. The result was sensational, and hopes of a rapprochement between mind and brain were plainly stirred. Ferrier supposed that he was mapping the centers of willed movement. His descriptions of results are permeated with this interpretation, for example, "Point 1. The opposite hind limb advanced as in walking"; and he used the same system of numbering for points on the brains of different species, as if to assert their homology. Others considered that the stimuli activated sensory centers: for muscle sense (Hitzig) or touch (Schiff); or centers for memories of movements (Munk). François-Franck [1887], reviewing these and other theories, was unconvinced, and himself concluded that the areas were "points de départ et non des centres de mouvement" [1887, p. 376]; "le faisceau moteur, recueillant à la surface du cerveau les incitations motrices volontaires, les transmet aux organes d'execution bulbomédullaires" [1887, p. 299]. He summed up in favor of the *fact* of cortical localization which others had doubted [1887, p. 416]. Sherrington [1885] had already tried to introduce the purely descriptive term *cord area*; he wished to be free of the functional overtones of the word "motor," and merely to denote that region of cortex so intimately connected with the spinal cord that lesions of it cause degenerations in the cord.

Today we know from the statements of conscious patients, made during stimulation, that this area is not the seat of the will [Penfield, 1936–7]. We know also that it is not the repository or, at any rate, that it is not the sole repository of stored skills and memories of movements. Lashley [1924] trained monkeys to open three types of problem boxes containing food. After bilateral destruction of the "motor" areas, paralysis was followed by considerable recovery. When the problem boxes were again presented it was found that the monkeys had not lost the secrets, but, in spite of their clumsiness, went correctly about the task of getting out the food.

In reading this literature it is helpful to follow François-Franck's lead and to distinguish always between facts of localization and concepts of function. The fact of *localization* was of the first importance for medicine and surgery. In 1883 Ferrier [1888] was criticized by *The Lancet* for suggesting that focal cerebral lesions should be explored by the surgeon. In 1884 Godlee successfully removed a tumor from the Rolandic region through an opening exactly overlying it and but little larger than it [Trotter, 1934].

The experimental neurophysiologist has always found much of his inspiration in clinical neurology. The study of human motor *function*, which was begun by Hughlings Jackson before the era of experimental stimulation, ablation, and electrical recording, is being pursued as profitably as ever in our own time [Denny-Brown, 1950, 1958, 1962]. It has been guided all along by Jacksonian concepts, which Walshe [1943] has re-expounded in language of great beauty and clarity. These concepts, for example, "levels," "representation," and "rerepresentation," are essentially functional concepts, whose discussion can be usefully sustained without, in the first instance, a too close preoccupation with possible anatomical substrates—as in the Black Box of modern jargon. The concepts have abundantly justified themselves as a stimulus to, and a framework for, accurate observation at the bedside. But to confuse anatomical and functional language, as in the old controversy whether movements *or* muscles are "represented" in the brain, is to misunderstand Jackson's position. One of the facts on which the Jacksonian concept of "representation" is founded is that cerebral lesions cause loss of some categories of movement, with preservation of others [Walshe, 1943; Denny-Brown and Botterell, 1947]. "Movements" in this sense may be translated "items of cerebral function"; they are *intracerebral processes,* and are not to be simply equated with "contractions of muscles." Thus one can conceive that *identical* contractions of an anatomical muscle could form part of the eventual exteriorization of *different* items of cerebral function. "To speak figuratively" [Jackson, 1889], "the central nervous system knows nothing of muscles, it only knows movements. . . . There are, we shall say, thirty muscles of the hand; these are represented in the nervous centres in thousands of different combinations—that is, as very many movements; it is just as many chords, musical expressions and tunes can be made out of a few notes." Today, the physiologist conceives that these "notes" are Sherrington's [1931] motor units, rather than the muscles of the morphologist. He wishes to discover how fluctuating aggregates of motor units can be excited, and others inhibited, by the selective operations of suprasegmental levels of the central nervous system. Such physiological aggregates need not always coincide with anatomical muscles.

Jackson, of course, was interested in the fact of localization as well as in the analysis of disorders of movement in terms of functional concepts. He followed with close attention the pioneer mappings of the monkey's brain. He distinguished between "minute localization," in which he believed, and "abrupt localization," which he rejected [Jackson, 1886]. Because, "in some of the cases I have to narrate, the disease has been ill-defined, coarse and widespread" [Jackson, 1875], he thought that "clinical knowledge is not yet precise enough for minute localization" [Jackson, 1886].

Although electrical stimulation of the cortex has been from the first a valuable tool in the study of localization in the projection pathways [Walshe, 1953], it has become clear that it does not evoke natural functioning of the cortical neuronal apparatus within the effective orbit of the stimulating electrodes [Burns, 1958]. The movements evoked from the precentral gyrus are not "willed" [Penfield, 1936–7], and are presumably not "movements" in Jackson's sense. Stimulation of the postcentral gyrus does not normally arouse natural sensation of the peripheries to which the sensation is referred, but "numbness, tingling, or a feeling of electricity" [Penfield and Jasper, 1954, p. 72; cf. also Libet, Alberts, Wright, Delattre, Levin, and Feinstein, 1964]. Stimulation of speech areas never evokes articulate speech: the characteristic effect is to interfere with or to arrest speech, if the patient is speaking at the time of its application [Penfield and Jasper, 1954, p. 110].

Stimulation of the temporal lobes may arouse dreams and memories, but only in patients in whom these psychical experiences are already part of an epileptic pattern [Penfield and Perot, 1963]. In the case of speech arrest, it is natural to suppose that disorganization of neuronal activities is a paralyzing act: that function must be disrupted if a population of neurons is forced to fire in step with a rhythmic stimulus. The case of the psychical experiences cannot be taken to mean that local neuronal mechanisms of memory may be set into action by direct electrical stimuli [Penfield and Perot, 1963]; and the relationship between the epileptic or artificially evoked "hypersynchrony" [Penfield and Jasper, 1954, p. 193], on the one hand, and the psychical experience on the other, still awaits elucidation. It is hard to see how the hypersynchronized discharge could itself be the basis of an *unfolding* hallucination. The unfolding pattern of discharge would have to take place outside the boundaries of the cell population preempted by the hypersynchronized discharge. It could be triggered by this discharge, but would have to evolve independently of it.

It is, of course, true that we have no right to assume that the motor performances of normal human subjects are wholly effected by the Rolandic cortex [MsI of Woolsey, 1958] and the corticospinal system. For the apparent integrity of this system does not avail those patients rendered akinetic by lesions of the basal ganglia [Denny-Brown, 1962]. Further, paralysis sometimes results from bilateral anterior chordotomy performed for the relief of pain, in spite of verified sparing of the lateral corticospinal tracts [Bernhard, Bohm, and Petersén, 1955]. But until very recently, the "motor" area and its projection pathway loomed so large in neurological thought that the fact of partial recovery of motor function following injury to it in man and primates seemed quite baffling. How could a man or a monkey move at all after the stimulable area had been destroyed? The discovery of "supplementary" areas [Woolsey, Settlage, Meyer, Sencer, Hamuy, and Travis, 1952; Penfield and Jasper, 1954; Woolsey, 1958] has shown that the Rolandic area is not the only sink for cerebral motor outflow. We see today that nerve impulses destined to initiate movement may leave the cerebral cortex by pathways of more extensive topographical origin and of varying synaptic complexity. In the corticospinal and corticobulbar pathway the axons are long, traveling without interruption from the cortex to the segmental apparatus. Although the corticosegmental link is thus direct, many spinal synapses may be interposed between the initial cerebral activity and the eventual excitation and inhibition of fusimotor neurons and motoneurons. In the macaque the cortical field of origin of corticospinal axons extends beyond area 4, which contributes only 31 per cent; area 6 contributes 29 per cent and the parietal lobe 40 per cent [Russell and de Myer, 1961]. In the remaining corticofugal motor pathways the axonal links are shorter, being interrupted by synapses in basal ganglia [Denny-Brown, 1962], red nucleus [cf. in cat, Nyberg-Hansen and Brodal, 1964; Rinvik and Walberg, 1963], reticular formation, etc. The cortical fields of origin of such axons may be even more extensive. We need not, therefore, be surprised if the results of stimulation and of ablation confined to area MsI are not exactly complementary. For stimulation would only be expected to have visible motor effects when applied to a cortical field whose axonal outflow was dense, and connected to the spinal motoneurons by a dense synaptic linkage. On the other hand, ablation of such a field need not deprive the cortex as a whole of more than a fraction of its available outflow. Inadequate density in the surviving projections would explain Leyton and Sherrington's [1917] failure to discover new stimulable areas after recovery of motor function.

In spite of such facts it is natural to turn first to the corticospinal system of neurons, whose axons traverse the medullary pyramids, when planning experiments on the neuronal basis of motor function. The experimental physiologist of today finds his position, perhaps, closer to that of François-Franck and Sherrington than to that of Hitzig and Ferrier [cf. Bates, 1957]. His ambitions are realistic. He tries to follow into the cortex, and to trace within it those afferent systems which excite and inhibit the corticofugal neurons. He tries to find out how fine or coarse is the grain of localization at the headward end of the cortico-spinal projection. He times and measures synaptic actions exerted by the corticospinal terminals on motoneurons [Preston and Whitlock, 1960, 1961; Landgren, Phillips, and Porter, 1962b]; on fusimotor neurons [Mortimer and Akert, 1961]; on the interneurons and presynaptic arbor-izations of reflex arcs [Carpenter, Lundberg, and Norrsell, 1963; Lund-berg and Voorhoeve, 1962; Lundberg, Norrsell, and Voorhoeve, 1962]; and on the neurons and presynaptic arborizations of ascending afferent systems [Lundberg, Norrsell, and Voorhoeve, 1963]. In all this work, the many differences between the corticospinal systems of different mammalian orders must always be stressed and not glossed over, not merely to avoid confusion but as a positive contribution to evolutionary biology.

NATURE OF CORTICAL MOTOR LOCALIZATION AS REVEALED BY ELECTRICAL MAPPING OF THE BRAINS OF PRIMATES

It is clear *a priori* that the results of electrical mapping of area MsI are likely to be complex. Not only corticofugal neurons, but also intracortical systems afferent to them, will be stimulated; and the relative importance of each of these factors in eliciting corticofugal discharge will have to be assessed. The muscular responses observed may be due to complicated actions of corticofugal discharge on spinal interneurons, fusimotor neurons, and alpha motoneurons which still await experimental analysis.

Again, it is certain that corticospinal neurons will not be the only corticofugal neurons discharging from the stimulated areas. If it may be assumed that all corticospinal fibers traverse the medullary pyramid, stimulation of the cortex after pyramid section will unmask the motor effects contributed by the commingled corticostriatal, corticorubral, corticoreticular, etc., projections. Recent experiments on baboons have revealed a larger residue of differentiated motor responses than the coarser synergies described by earlier investigators [Brindley and Lewis, 1964, 1965, with references]. Thus the 100 c/s sinusoidal stimulus still finds in the cortex of MsI the area from which movements of the limbs and tail are most easily obtained. Although the responses now have a higher threshold by a factor of 1.5–3.0, and are more fatiguable, "almost every kind of movement that can be obtained by near-threshold stimulation before section has been obtained from at least one of our animals after section"; and the pattern of localization was generally similar to that found before section.

It would not be possible, even if it were necessary, to summarize in this review the well-known somatotopic maps that have been published for the brains of different primates. The responses that are mapped are supposedly those determined by structure, and are repeatable at the same and at later explorations [Bates, 1957]; we are not here concerned with the functional instability of cortical points [Graham Brown and Sherrington, 1912]. The problem of presenting the very voluminous results of the explorations within a manageable compass is a formidable one.

In man, it would clearly be impossible to subject neurosurgical patients to the many hours of stimulation and restimulation that the experimentalist finds necessary for the drawing of a complete and confident map for an individual brain. Penfield and Boldrey [1937] therefore produced maps composite of the fragmentary results from many cases. To summarize the general pattern of localization they introduced the now familiar "homunculi," to which Penfield and Jasper [1954] later ascribed "the defects, and the virtues, of cartoons, in that they are inaccurate anatomically and yet they call attention to differences in the character of areas." The composite maps and homunculi are supplemented by a diagram indicating the relative number of motor responses of each part elicited by stimulation of pre- and postcentral gyri [Penfield and Rasmussen, 1950]. From the individual protocols (for example, those given by Penfield and Boldrey [1937]) one sees in close-up the nature of some of the detailed fragments of evidence that go to make up the maps and diagrams which summarize in a manageable form this uniquely valuable corpus of human observation.

The problem of summarizing and presentation is different in the case of subhuman primates. For each individual specimen it is here possible to produce a complete map. Differences in detail of the motor responses, and variation in cortical landmarks (sulci and blood vessels), make it difficult to constrain the results into composite maps, in which the (possibly important) variability is suppressed. Different authors have tackled this practical problem in different ways. Leyton and Sherrington [1917] presented their results on near-threshold unifocal faradic stimulation of chimpanzee, orangutan, and gorilla as a list of 445 numbered primary movements, not all seen in each specimen, and individual maps with points numbered to correspond with the list. Woolsey et al [1952] have mapped the precentral and supplementary motor areas of macaques and Java monkeys with a degree of refinement that is not likely to be exceeded. They stimulated unifocally with 60 c/s alternating current, which probably elicits a larger range of minimal muscular responses than any other form of electrical stimulation [cf. Hines, 1944]. They introduced a novel and successful pictorial method of presentation, the "motor figurine chart." On an enlarged tracing of the cortex, each point (and each was stimulated three or more times) is indicated by a diagram of the responding part with shading to indicate the locus of the movement. Such shading can be used to indicate flexion or extension of large joints, but not the direction of digital movements. Thus, some of the fine detail that was actually observed is missing from the charts. Different shadings indicate prompt and strong, intermediate, or weaker movements. Such charts are given for individual experiments, and also a composite chart which needed but little "tailoring" or "editing," except in the face area, in order to give a fair summary of the whole series. The general pattern is also summarized in two "simiusculi," with the strong warning that these are "an inadequate representation of the localization pattern, since in a line drawing one cannot indicate the successive overlap which is so characteristic a feature of cortical representation."

The motor figurine charts beautifully illustrate this "successive overlap," and the authors conclude that "foci for different muscles, or groups of muscles" are not "discrete entities, as in a mosaic. Rather there is very extensive overlap in the cortical motor patterns. . . . Nevertheless, the centres of the foci form a pattern which reflects in general the arrangement in the periphery." Hines [1944], whose experience is also very great, says that a particular muscle need not be the only muscle "represented at a specific cortical point, but that it is the one predominantly represented there"; thus weak stimulation "permits restriction of responses to single muscles."

The word "mosaic," which was in use in this context as early as 1888 [Mills, 1888], has sometimes stood for a hypothesis which has been well stated (in order to refute it) by Chang, Ruch, and Ward [1947]: "a mosaic pattern of strictly isolated subareas of the motor cortex, each dedicated to a single muscle." This, from the quotation above, is clearly not Hines' standpoint. Foerster [1936] also had come to the conclusion that "the foci of the different parts of the body were not like the stones of the mosaic to which they were compared, but they overlap to a more or less considerable degree." In another passage in which Hines [1952] states: "Those who found the mosaic considered it the result of observations, rather than the basis for an hypothesis," she is evidently not referring to the mosaic rejected by Chang et al [1947], which may be equated with the "abrupt localization" rejected by Hughlings Jackson [1886]; she is referring to the ability of 60 c/s sinusoidal current "to elicit contraction of single muscles and parts of muscles." Confusion can be avoided if we abandon the word "mosaic" as a description of this result and adopt instead Jackson's term *minute localization.*

That the corticospinal projection is not a strict anatomical mosaic is shown by the observations of Sherrington [1889], Glees and Cole [1950] and Barnard and Woolsey [1956]. Small lesions in the "hand area" caused degeneration diffused evenly throughout the cross-section area of the pyramidal tract, and extending down to the lumbosacral level. Barnard and Woolsey, however, have reservations about the possible, though not demonstrated, subcortical extension of their small lesions.

Chang et al [1947] investigated the minute localization of cortical foci by simultaneous quantitative myography of the muscles acting about the ankle joint in the macaque. Stimulation was unifocal, by 60 c/s pulses of 0.5 msec duration. Responses confined to a single muscle were not typical, appearing "only under favorable conditions," and then usually in the distal muscles, extens. digitorum longus and extens. hallucis longus. The usual finding was that several muscles contracted simultaneously. Some gave more tension than others, and contracted with a shorter summation period (up to 3 sec); these criteria enabled the optimum cortical area to be mapped for each muscle. Stimuli were sometimes strong enough to evoke epileptiform after-discharge. The muscles were not "equally available to cortical stimulation": it was very difficult to get any contractions from mm. gastrocnemius, soleus, flex. digitorum longus, flex. hallucis longus, or tibialis posterior; and none was ever obtained from m. peroneus longus. The hamstring and femoral nerves were cut, so there was no evidence whether hamstring or femoral motoneurons were ever activated. The intrinsic muscles of the foot were also discarded. No mention is made of small movements of the hand, which could have occurred unnoticed unless a special watch had been kept for them.

Interpretation is complicated by the fact that the responses got from the same point in the same individual sometimes varied with the strength of stimulation. In the example illustrated, m. extens. hall. long. gave a larger response than m. flex. dig. long; when the stimulus was weakened, the responses were equal; when strengthened, m. ext. hall. long. responded alone.

The mapped foci were all within a grid measuring about 5×7 mm in the angle between the sagittal and Rolandic fissures. The three methods—solitary responses, tension ratios, and summation periods—gave the same topographical relationship between the foci for those muscles that responded in each type of test. The foci were separated by inert patches, which were silent even to stimuli of epileptogenic strength. The results were interpreted in terms of a diagram of overlapping fields of Betz cells for each muscle, each with a denser focus and a more diffuse fringe; in the diagram "the degree of overlap is minimized for the sake of simplicity," and it was concluded that "the representation of muscles stands midway between a strict mosaic pattern and diffuse representation."

This paper, with its exemplary description of experiments and its clear discussion of the problems of interpretation, may be taken as a culminating effort to map the minute localization in the corticospinal projection by repetitive electrical stimulation lasting up to 4 sec, and working within the limitations set by these particular muscles as the indicators of response. The problems it raises, however—of the blurring of boundaries by physical and physiological spread of stimulus, and the complication that the projection arises from the walls of the fissures as well as from the stimulated convexity—cannot be solved without further special experiments. The finding that not all the muscles were equally available to the stimuli foreshadows the concept of "differential accessibility" (see below). With regard to physiological spread, Adrian [1937] had found that a weak single shock to the motor area of the macaque, strong enough to elicit a "deep response" (a surface-positive wave), caused no response of muscle. Repetition of such weak shocks increased the amplitude of the deep waves, and caused muscular contractions. (In the unfolded cortex of the rabbit, it was easier to show that the deep waves also spread in widening circles away from the stimulated point.) These experiments proved for the first time that an active response could be provoked in the motor area without any breakthrough to the spinal motoneurons. Some degree of facilitation was thus shown to be necessary even for the fixed, "repeatable" responses of the simplest maps.

In recent years the use of electronic stimulators has provided experimenters with what must sometimes seem an embarrassing wealth of parameters (variable pulse duration, amplitude and wave form; variable repetition frequency and train duration). Lilly, Austin, and Chambers

[1952] pointed out that a family of different "threshold maps" could be drawn by choosing different parameters of stimulation. Some of these maps may depend on direct stimulation of corticospinal neurons, others on stimulation of intracortical mechanisms lying upstream of the cortico-spinal neurons, and others on these effects mixed in different proportions. If the map of "repeatable" responses can be thus altered, what is to be done in pursuit of the goal of minute corticospinal localization? For studies of the evolution of localization in the mammalian series [Wool-sey, 1958], it is rational to stick, as Woolsey and colleagues [1952] have done, to a type of stimulation that gives a large range of motor re-sponses; and it is clear that 60 c/s alternating current is ideally suited to this work. But research is also needed to determine the extent to which this particular method maps corticofugal neurons, and the extent to which it maps other cells and axons which play upon their dendrites.

Lilly et al [1952] and Mihailović and Delgado [1956] were primarily interested in surveying the range of electrical stimuli able to call forth particular movements. Liddell and Phillips [1950, 1951] were interested in two types of maps that can be drawn for the brains of individual baboons, and in the strikingly different thresholds for the motor responses of different parts of the body. Using single rectangular cathodal pulses of 5 msec duration, they found that the region of lowest threshold (1.0–1.2 mA) was on the intermediate part of the precentral gyrus. The response was a flick of contralateral thumb and index in response to each shock. At this strength, no other area of the exposed cortex gave any muscular response. With increased strength, the thumb-index area was enlarged, and part of the medial part of precentral gyrus now gave a flick of the contralateral big toe. Slightly stronger shocks were needed to reach threshold for a flick of contralateral angle of mouth and of tongue from the lateral part of the gyrus. With every increase in pulse amplitude, the finger and other areas grew larger and overlapped more and more, until with the strongest shocks employed (about 5 mA), all these parts were moved together from a large part of the Rolandic area, including part of the postcentral gyrus. Such flick movements have also been seen in man by Glusman, Ransohoff, Pool, Grundfest, and Mettler [1952], Lewin and Phillips [1952], and Libet et al [1964].

The result with single pulses is a very remarkable one. With the stronger pulses, most of the precentral gyrus and some of the adjacent postcentral gyrus are overtly responsive; yet the repertory of motor responses is confined to distal parts—as it happens, to the parts that are commonly the first to move in Jacksonian epilepsy; "clotted" con-tractions of all parts of the body, which might have been expected *a priori,* were never observed. It is evident that the spinal and bulbar motoneurons governing these peripheries are *preferentially accessible* to cortical stimulation. The concept of differential accessibility was introduced by Liddell and Phillips [1952], who adopted the working hypothesis that larger numbers of corticofugal neurons project toward some motoneurons than toward others, and that the projection has a high synaptic density; spatial summation of the impulses discharged by single cortical stimuli would thus stimulate these motoneurons selectively. Recent experiments to test this hypothesis will be described below.

Where were all the familiar responses of the "classical" motor maps? By merely increasing the frequency of the stimulating pulses to 50 c/s a whole rich repertory of motor responses could be called forth. The highly significant observation with repetitive stimulation is that the more numerous foci revealed by it are not of equal area (all maps agree that the areas for hand, foot, and face are the widest), and are not equally "excitable"; the differences in "excitability" being evident in measurements of two kinds. First, the threshold current is lowest for the foci for toes, thumb, and mouth [Boynton and Hines, 1933] and fingers [Woolsey et al, 1952]. Second, when current strength is adjusted so that a large number of foci become effective, the lowest-threshold foci require shorter summation periods [Cooper and Denny-Brown, 1927] than the remaining foci [Liddell and Phillips, 1950]. Thus temporal summation is important in these conditions, and it is clear that motoneurons other than those for hand, foot, and face are less directly accessible to the cortex; but the experiments do not discriminate between the direct corticospinal and the indirect corticostriatal, corticorubral, etc., projections, and do not indicate whether the necessary summation is taking place in the cortex or at subcortical or spinal levels, or at all of these.

When repetitive stimulation is used, and the dorsal roots are intact, the maps differ according to the initial positions of the limbs [Gellhorn and Hyde, 1953]. This is another source of difficulty in getting at the underlying corticospinal localization.

The conclusions from this survey must be that repetitive electrical stimulation, combined with the detection of minimal muscular response, cannot be accepted as a tool which maps nothing other than the grain of localization at the headward end of the corticospinal projection [cf. Walshe, 1953]. The relative importance of direct and indirect excitation of the corticospinal cells [Patton and Amassian, 1954], and of other corticofugal cells, is still unknown. The underlying localization might be blurred by spread of stimulus, or by physiological spread of excitation in the superficial cortical laminae; it might, on the other hand, be spuriously sharpened by coincidental stimulation of inhibitory systems in the superficial laminae. Nor can the near-threshold, single pulse maps be taken as outlining the fields of origin of the projection to motoneurons of hand, foot, and face. Though the complicating factor of temporal summation is here avoided, the unknown errors introduced by physiological and physical diffusion of stimulus have first to be assessed. Thus the method of stimulation of the pia-covered cortical surface with currents adequate to provoke muscular contraction has already been pushed to the limits of its resolving power.

Fortunately, modern microelectrode techniques make possible a finer unraveling of the complex totality of the corticospinal system. By an investigation of the monosynaptic corticospinal projection, a beginning has been made to sample motoneurons of some muscle groups of the baboon's forelimb. The existence of a monosynaptic corticospinal connection in monkeys was proved by Bernhard, Bohm, and Petersén [1953], Bernhard and Bohm [1954] and Preston and Whitlock [1960, 1961], and in the baboon by Landgren, Phillips, and Porter [1962a] and Phillips and Porter [1964]. We owe to Bernhard and his colleagues the useful concept "corticomotoneuronal system." It is obvious that the simplest conceivable type of cortical motor localization that can exist is to be found by mapping the areas occupied by *colonies* of pyramidal neurons which project monosynaptically to single spinal α motoneurons. The α motoneurons can be functionally isolated by intracellular recording, and identified by antidromic stimulation of their axons in the peripheral nerves. The cortical field occupied by the appropriate pyramidal colony can then be mapped. Since the central nervous system manages muscle in terms of its motor unit organization, the colonies thus mapped must be conceived as functionally significant fragments from which the corticomotoneuronal system is built up. Selective stimulation of the cell bodies or axons of the corticospinal neurons, bypassing the complexities of the outer layers of the cortex, can be achieved by unifocal anodal stimulation of the pial surface by brief single pulses [Hern, Landgren, Phillips, and Porter, 1962; Phillips and Porter, 1962]. These weak stimuli were always below the threshold for movement. Each discharged a well-synchronized corticospinal volley which traveled at about 60 m per sec [Phillips and Porter, 1964].

Exploring the cortical surface with a roving focal anode, Landgren et al [1962b] did not map discrete cortical "points" for minimal monosynaptic actions on test motoneurons. They mapped areas which overlapped one another, and might measure several millimeters across. Somewhere within each area was its "best point," from which the largest quantity of monosynaptic action could be evoked in the test motoneuron. As the focal anode was moved away toward the edges of the area, the quantity of monosynaptic action fell to zero.

It cannot, of course, be assumed that the areas thus mapped are co-extensive with the distribution of the cells of the colony. Those cells might all be packed together near the "best point." There are about 18,000 pyramids in layer V in a cortical cylinder of 1 mm^2 cross-section area in this region in the baboon, and of these about 90 are conspicuously large cells. Stimulation near the edge of the area might excite cells near the best point by physical spread. To measure the transcortical distances across which shocks of different strengths could spread, Landgren et al [1962b], in separate experiments, plotted the thresholds for sample pyramidal units, stimulated from points at measured distances from the approximate positions of the pyramidal units. The curves thus plotted were used in analyzing the maps of the corticomotoneuronal colonies. From the curves, the effective spread of the strength of current used to map the colony could be read off. In about half the experiments, the currents used had been strong enough to spread from the edges of the area inwards to the "best point." In these cases the whole of the corticomotoneuronal colony could have been confined near the "best point." But in the remaining cases the currents would not have "covered" the best point from the edges of the area. The central area thus delimited was the true map of the minimum spatial extent of the colony. The largest example measured 8 × 2.5 mm. Landgren et al [1962b] confined their attention to colonies projecting to motoneurons of the ulnar, median, and deep interosseous nerves. The "true maps" of the colonies of motoneurons of the different nerves overlapped in individual brains, that is to say, their corticomotoneuronal colonies were intermingled.

Phillips and Porter [1964] used a different method to map the true extents of the colonies. They plotted curves of quantity of monosynaptic excitatory action evoked in the test motoneurons against increasing currents applied to the best points. The curves flattened, showing the strength of current needed to stimulate the whole colony. The spread of current horizontally and in the depth of the Rolandic fissure was estimated from separate experiments on sample pyramidal units and on populations of units. The largest corticomotoneuronal colony commanded its maximum monosynaptic action at a shock strength which would have been stimulating corticospinal neurons at 10 mm distant in all directions horizontally and also in the depth of the fissure (about 10 mm).

Landgren et al [1962b] found that shocks of identical strength, which they assumed to excite corticospinal *populations* of equal sizes, evoked different quantities of monosynaptic excitatory action when applied to the best points of different corticomotoneuronal *colonies*. The concept of differential accessibility is thus necessary even at this elemental level. Phillips and Porter [1964] extended the investigation to motoneurons of proximal muscle groups in order to compare their corticomotoneuronal colonies with those of the distal groups. Their general conclusion was that the "distal" colonies tended to occupy smaller cortical areas and to command larger total quantities of monosynaptic excitatory action: the "proximal" colonies tended to occupy larger areas and to command smaller quantities of action. About half of the triceps motoneurons exhibited no monosynaptic excitatory action, even with stimuli strong enough to reach corticospinal cells in the depth of the central fissure. They showed, however (as did the monosynaptically connected motoneurons), good polysynaptic excitatory and inhibitory potentials, sometimes clearly differentiated by stimulating at different cortical loci.

The picture which emerges from this work is one of intermingled corticomotoneuronal colonies, with the larger monosynaptic actions being commanded by the colonies controlling the "distal" motoneurons, and especially, one presumes, those controlling the hand [Phillips and Porter, 1964]. The refined degree of minute localization that is evidently possible in voluntary control, as in Basmajian's [1963] experiments in which human subjects learned to call up chosen spinal motoneurons, does not depend (if it depends on the corticomotoneuronal system exclusively) on a fine-grained anatomical mosaic at the head of the corticospinal outflow; it must, instead, require a marvelously subtle routing of activity in the outer cortical layers to pick up, in significant functional groupings, the required corticofugal neurons, which are scattered and intermingled with unwanted ones which may be suppressed. It remains an open question for experiment whether any parameters of electrical stimulation, as for example 60 c/s alternating current, can awake, even in crudest form, any manifestation of this fantastic selective property of the cortical neuropil.

Inputs to the Corticofugal Neurons

The corticofugal neurons are the key to the organization of the "motor" as well as of other cortical areas [Phillips, 1961]. In the impulse trains which they discharge through the subcortical white matter to adjacent or remote regions of the central nervous system, they encode the balance of synaptic excitation and inhibition brought to bear upon their dendrites by incoming axons and by the horizontally running axons of cortical interneurons. Their apical dendrites form a dense forest in which the finest presynaptic arborizations intertwine profusely with the finest dendritic branches to form the cortical neuropil [Herrick, 1948] in which, presumably, occur synaptic activities as subtle as any to be found in the central nervous system.

The corticofugal level includes corticocortical, corticocallosal, corticostriate, corticothalamic, corticorubral, corticoreticular, etc., neurons, in addition to the corticospinal (pyramidal tract) neurons. Of these cells, pyramidal tract (PT) neurons [Phillips, 1956a; Patton, Towe, and Kennedy, 1962] and callosal neurons [Asanuma and Okamoto, 1959] have already been identified in microelectrode experiments by antidromic stimulation of their axons. The synaptic actions of intracortical afferent systems on PT neurons can be shown by weak focal surface-cathodal stimulation of the cortical surface close to the cells, where the afferent systems are converging on them. In cats, one can record intracellularly from antidromically identified PT neurons, and can detect excitatory synaptic depolarization and inhibitory synaptic polarization [Phillips, 1956b, 1961]. In baboons, one can record from single axons in the lateral corticospinal tract, and investigate excitatory synaptic convergence by observing the different latencies of discharge. Focal surface-cathodal or bifocal stimulation stimulates the neurons with alternative preferred latencies (cf. Watson and Amassian [1961], in cats); as would be expected with a physiological intracortical transmission process, the latency lengthens progressively with increasing distance from the probable location of the cell [Phillips and Porter, 1962].

In the cat, electrical stimulation of median and lateral thalamic nuclei [Lux and Klee, 1962; Purpura, Shofer, and Musgrave, 1964] and of the head of the caudate nucleus [Klee and Lux, 1962], combined with intracellular recording from antidromically identified PT cells, has yielded valuable new evidence of the varied mixture of excitatory and inhibitory postsynaptic mechanisms acting upon these cells. But in the present context, interest centers more on the sources of impulses afferent to the PT cells, and whether these better-differentiated inputs from the periphery would exercise mainly excitatory or inhibitory control of the PT cells.

Work on inputs to single neurons in the precentral motor area MsI of primates has hardly begun. Albe-Fessard and her colleagues (personal communication) have tested the responses of unidentified single neurons in the precentral motor area of macaques to electrical and mechanical stimulation of the limbs. Chloralose was the anesthetic in most cases, but a few awake animals were also used, prepared with tranquilizer and receiving analgesics regularly. Most neurons responded to electrical stimulation of more than two limbs. To mechanical stimuli they were typically slowly adapting. Some responded to local stimulation of joint capsules, others to pressure on skin, others to pressure on deep tissues. Over half responded to movement of a limb, and to pulling on the tendon of a dissected muscle, or to very localized pressure on its belly; these were inhibited by "antagonistic" passive movements or by pulling on an antagonist's dissected tendon. Thus this largest group came from intramuscular receptors, probably from spindles. Further evidence for this projection from muscle spindles came from experiments in which the threshold for a minimum evoked potential in the precentral motor area was measured in terms of the electrical threshold for a minimum volley in the deep radial or medial gastrocnemius nerve. It was 1.35 for three shocks, strongly supporting the existence of a Group I projection to the cortex. If, as we must assume, this afferent projection exists also in man, it certainly arouses no conscious kinesthetic sensation [Merton, 1964].

Most of the work on inputs to the "motor" area has been done on the cat, and some of this will now be reviewed, bearing in mind that "encephalization" is less advanced than in the primates, the area MsI being small and the repertory of muscle contractions it can command being limited; there is no monosynaptic corticomotoneuronal system [Bernhard et al, 1953; Hern, Phillips, and Porter, 1962]; and decorticated cats still have a considerable repertory of performance [Bard and Rioch, 1937; Dusser de Barenne, 1920].

Oscarsson and Rosén [1963, with references] have now shown, under barbiturate anesthesia and with refined methods and controls, that excitation of Group Ia fibers in forelimb nerves, either by an electric shock or by a brief 60 μ muscle stretch, sends an afferent volley into the rostro-lateral part of the primary somatic receiving area SmI (which, in cats, overlaps the motor area) with a latency of about 5 msec; this volley then evokes a localized surface-negative potential. Little spatial summation was evident at the cuneate and thalamic junctions. Oscarsson and Rosén quote other experiments showing an absence of any such projection from the hindlimb, which is more purely a locomotor, reflex and postural organ, in contrast to the forelimb which is used in a greater variety of manipulative and exploratory behavior. That this projection is probably not concerned with kinesthesis is shown by Giaquinto, Pompeiano, and Swett's [1963] experiments in which 200 c/s tetanization of Group I afferents in the forelimb by implanted electrodes (thresholds being measured in terminal experiments) produced neither behavioral change nor EEG arousal in unrestrained cats. Oscarsson and Rosén [1963] therefore suggest that the system is important in the automatic control of movement. However, the muscle nerves in the experiments of Giaquinto et al [1963] were cut peripheral to the stimulating electrodes, so that it would not have been possible to observe the effect of stimulation on movements in progress in which those muscles were taking part.

Other peripheral sources of signals causing *discharge* of single neurons in the cat's motor area have been investigated by Buser and Imbert [1961]. Although the neurons were not identified antidromically as PT or non-PT cells, most of those located in the motor area were found at a depth appropriate for corticofugal cells. The stimuli were shocks to the skin of each of the four limbs, or brief clicks or flashes. Ninety-two per cent of the neurons in the pericruciate region were "polysensory." Compared with those of the muscle afferent projection, latencies were long: 12–29 msec from the skin, 25–45 msec for the clicks, and 45–90 msec for the flashes. The question whether the polysensory convergence occurred actually at the membranes of these neurons or at some lower neural level, possibly the center median nucleus, could not be settled. In the case of the long-latency visual input, the primary visual area is not necessary for the reflex pyramidal discharge that is evoked by a flash in chloralose anesthesia [Wall, Rémond, and Dobson, 1953].

Patton, Towe, and Kennedy [1962] compared the responses of identified PT cells to electrical stimuli to the central toe pads of contralateral and ipsilateral forepaws of cats under chloralose. Contralateral stimulation evoked more impulses in the response train and at a shorter latency. The mean difference in latency was 14 msec. (Asanuma and Okuda [1962] found that 15 out of 24 PT cells fired 6–8 msec after a shock to the opposite motor area.) When the corpus callosum was cut, the first component of the massed "reflex" discharge [cf. Patton and Amassian, 1960] to ipsilateral stimulation, recorded in the medullary pyramid, was abolished, and the response to stimulation of the contralateral motor cortex was also lost.

Brooks, Rudomin, and Slayman [1961a, 1961b] found that the peripheral fields from which 51 PT cells could be excited were of three types: 17 were "fixed local" fields (that is, confined to part of a contralateral limb, and were specific for hair movement, touch, pressure or joint movement), and 15 were "fixed wide" fields (usually bilateral, with discontinuities; only half were specific for the stimulus used). The remaining 19 fields were "labile"; they enlarged if stimulation was prolonged, and then responded to fresh modalities of stimulation. The discharges could sometimes be suppressed ("inhibited") by stimuli of another type. For example, the response to skin touch might be suppressed by joint movement. The sharpness of the edges of the "fixed local" fields was due to "surround inhibition"; the same specific stimulus suppressed the discharge from the center of the field when applied to a surrounding area. Another type of suppression ("inhibition") was found when a distant field (sometimes on a different limb) was stimulated.

In all these studies with extracellular recording, excitatory actions leading to the discharge of the target cells are more conspicuous than the inhibitory actions which are so prominent in the intracellular studies quoted above. In cases in which mere absence of response is noted, and in which continuous "spontaneous" firing happens to be absent, inhibition would inevitably be missed. This consideration should encourage fresh efforts to combine selective peripheral stimulation with intracellular recording, whose feasibility has now been sufficiently demonstrated by several workers.

Work of Bremer (Chapter 12) and Sperry (Chapter 13) has created renewed interest in the functions of the corpus callosum. Asanuma and Okuda [1962] have found that discharge of PT cells can be evoked only from an extremely circumscribed area on the opposite cortex, apparently the homologue of the region containing the cell under observation. In intracellular recording, the discharge is seen to arise from an excitatory postsynaptic potential (EPSP). The excitatory point is surrounded by a zone whose stimulation suppresses the discharge evoked from the center with a latency of about 3 msec and a duration of about 60 msec. In intracellular experiments the EPSP is reduced or delayed; no record of an inhibitory polarization (IPSP) in response to stimulating the surround zone is shown. This result shows that extremely localized traffic between corresponding motor regions is possible; *a priori* one would expect such traffic to be functionally important.

In conclusion, it is interesting, as supporting the concept that the corticofugal neurons are "common paths" leading out of the cortex, that so many differentiated peripheral inputs are brought to bear on their surface membranes for integration. Such inputs may initiate movement by a cortical "reflex," and also influence the course of the movements initiated and controlled by the intracerebral storage systems whose nature and location still elude us.

There is recent evidence of "plastic" changes in these inputs, which would have obvious importance for motor learning. Morrell [1961] found that during prolonged weak (2–10 μA) surface-anodal polarization of the motor forelimb area of rabbits and cats, visual or auditory stimuli, which were subliminal without the background polarization, could evoke discharges of single (unidentified) cells. (The discharges of some units were suppressed.) Surface-anodal polarization should have a depolarizing action on the somas and axons of corticofugal cells, and this would explain the facilitating effect observed during polarization. The effects, however, outlasted the polarization by about 20 min. Bindman, Lippold, and Redfearn [1964] found that surface-anodal polarization of the rat's cortex caused an increase in unit firing frequencies which outlasted the polarization by 1–5 hr. The explanation of this "plastic" change is quite unknown, but it is possible that the surface polarization caused a persisting hyperpolarization of the activated presynaptic arborizations lying superficially in the cortex, which would sum with their afterhyperpolarizations with a resulting increase in their transmitting potency [cf. Eccles, 1964]. Morrell [1961] confirmed Rusinov's [1953] discovery that during polarization the visual or auditory stimulus could actually evoke movement of the limbs, but with a latency measured in seconds. The motor effect again outlasted the polarization by 20–30 min, and this was specific for the stimulus applied during the period of polarization; thus, when auditory stimuli, but no visual stimuli, were presented during polarization, the auditory stimuli continued to be effective, whereas visual stimuli had no motor effect. As Morrell [1961] observes, "the anodal current appears to confer upon these cell populations the property of retaining, at least for a short period of time, a representation of the stimulus imposed during the polarization."

CONSIDERATIONS OF FUNCTION

Observations on human subjects testify to the probable functional importance of the various afferent signals to the cortex of area MsI which the neurophysiologist is discovering in his work on the synaptic inputs to the corticofugal cells. Guidance of movement by vision is the most obvious example. But the gaze and the hand can also be directed in the dark, although not, according to Merton [1961], very accurately. How is this done? Brindley and Merton [1960] and Whitteridge [1960] have revived, and have strengthened the evidence for, Helmholtz' belief that there is no position sense in the eye muscles, and that our awareness of willed movement of the visual axis depends on a "sense of effort" [Merton, 1964]. In Butt, Davies, and Merton's experiments on the thumb [Merton, 1964], ischemia limited to the tendons and joints, and not affecting the muscle bellies in the forearm, deprived the subjects of all awareness of position and of passive or active movements of the terminal phalanx. With eyes closed it was still possible for the subject to move a pointer, which was attached to his thumb, over a measured distance along a scale. Thus, "sense of effort," and not position sense, enabled the subject to measure out his movement; but he could not tell if the movement had been allowed to take place or if it had been resisted by the examiner. This very recent strengthening of the evidence for "sense of effort" invites a renewed interest in the actions of the recurrent axon collaterals of corticofugal and other neurons. Position sense derived from the joints is necessary, however, for knowledge of the starting point of the movement, and of the fact that it has been carried out.

If the input from the muscle spindles to MsI does not make us aware of passive movements, and if it cannot, by itself, inform us that a movement that we have willed has, or has not, been actually executed, what is its function? Oscarsson and Rosén [1963] have suggested that it is a necessary feedback concerned in the automatic governing of movement.

Section of the dorsal roots might be expected to throw light on this matter, since the operation must deprive the subject of the spindle input, for which no compensation would be possible; on the contrary, the associated loss of input from joints, skin, etc., should be substituted by vision.

Mott and Sherrington's [1895] observations, confirmed by Knapp, Taub, and Berman [1963], certainly show that a monkey's limb deprived of afferent innervation is permanently useless. The servotheory [Merton, 1953] would predict some degree of paralysis as a consequence of the breaking open of the segmental servoloops. But Mott and Sherrington also tested the cortical motor map of the paralyzed arm and found it normal; in some experiments the electrical threshold was even lowered. If the segmental reflex arcs are thus unnecessary for the motor effects of corticofugal discharge, it is tempting to suppose that the paralysis is due to the deafferentation of the cortex. Nathan and Sears [1960], however, have drawn attention to some points of disagreement between Sherrington and other experimentalists with regard to the degree of paralysis. Knapp et al [1963] have since found that under chronic restraint of the normal arm, the monkeys could learn to reach for food with the deafferented arm, but that movement was abrupt in onset and exaggerated in range. Nathan and Sears [1960] have searched Foerster's extensive writings without finding a full account of the effects of posterior root section in man; "observations and interpretations are inextricably mingled" and "it is difficult to sort out when Foerster is discussing tabes dorsalis and when he is referring to patients with proved division of posterior roots." It seems clear that there was no paralysis, not even immediate, but there was ataxia, worse at fingers than at proximal joints. There is no description of the patients' subjective statements about their disability. In one of Nathan and Sears' [1960] own cases, in which section of the first four cervical dorsal roots had been performed, the diaphragm was at first paralyzed for forced voluntary inspiration, but it recovered partially in 17 days. At the same time, the levator scapulae, which had at first been electromyographically silent in voluntary movements at shoulder, began to give weak responses. Thus, since the immediate paralysis of voluntary movement can be later compensated, particularly if motivation is strong, as in the experiments of Knapp et al, it is clear that the spindle input is not an essential condition for effective motor discharge, although all evidence points to its being essential for accurate control.

In singers and string players it is hearing that adjusts the extremely fine movements that procure accurate intonation.

Basmajian [1963] has published a preliminary report of experiments in which auditory and visual inputs enabled human subjects to train themselves to discharge selected motor units at will, mostly in the abductor brevis pollicis muscle. The subjects identified the characteristics of the unitary potentials by their sound in the loudspeaker or by their shapes on the face of the oscilloscope. In the course of training lasting up to half a day, some even learned to call up their familiar units without the aid of the auditory or visual feedback. They found it hard to say how they managed to do this without any conscious awareness other than the assurance (after the fact) that they had succeeded; they "thought about" a motor unit as they had seen and heard it previously [Basmajian, personal communication]. Is this memory of "sense of effort," refined by training? Some subjects, guided by auditory feedback, could regularly reproduce particular rhythms of motor unit discharge. These experiments are of the greatest interest from two points of view: they disclose the possibility of extremely selective and circumscribed conscious control of human motoneurons, and show that some, but not all, brains can establish this refined control in a short time and in circumstances which can never have arisen in the previous life of the individual.

Although the human brain is often exposed at operation, we still lack methods subtle enough to trace its activities in the course of even the simplest voluntary movement. Penfield and Jasper [1954] recorded the β rhythm from the precentral gyrus. When the patient gripped an object in response to a command, or even if he was merely warned to prepare to do so, the β rhythm disappeared. The effect was confined to the hand area in some cases, but spread beyond it in others. The local neurons were doubtless thrown into activity in executing the patient's will, but their activities were so desynchronized that nothing could be detected by the surface lead. The observations are of the highest importance, however, in proving that the precentral motor area is indeed involved in the initiation of willed movement. Bates [1951], recording through the intact human skull, found a tendency, in 20 per cent of trials, for sudden voluntary grasps to be initiated in phase with the α rhythm. No potential wave preceded the movement.

In conditioned motor reflexes in monkeys, Ricci, Doane, and Jasper [1957] also found that the surface electrical rhythm of the motor arm area was blocked. Sampled single neurons within the arm area showed every possible variation in impulse frequency, indicating that a complex reorganization of activity was taking place under cover of the blocking reaction.

SUMMARY

This paper has briefly reviewed the various concepts of the precentral motor area (Woolsey's MsI) and willed movement that have held sway between 1870 and the present time. It has gradually become clear that electrical stimulation does not, as some of the pioneers seem to have supposed, evoke natural functioning of the cortical neuronal apparatus within the effective orbit of the stimulating electrodes. An attempt has been made to assess the nature of the localization revealed in the different types of motor maps that can be drawn by different electrical stimuli. These maps are probably composite of the effects of direct stimulation of corticospinal and other corticofugal neurons, and of their synaptic excitation and inhibition by stimulation of cells and axons which converge upon them. The simplest conceivable type of motor localization can be mapped in terms of the areas of cortex occupied by colonies of corticospinal neurons which make monosynaptic connection with some single spinal motoneurons. These colonies are intermingled. Localized action within the corticomotoneuronal system thus requires a highly selective channeling of activity in the horizontally running intra-cortical networks which excite and inhibit the corticofugal neurons. Nothing is known of the locus or nature of the repository of motor skills or of the proportion in which these are normally exteriorized through the corticospinal and through other projection systems. Something is known, however, of the peripheral origin of inputs which converge on the neurons of MsI and could therefore initiate "cortical reflexes" and influence the course of other movements. An important part of this input appears to come from the muscle spindles. This large input does not arouse conscious sensation.

DISCUSSION

Chairman: PROFESSOR MOUNTCASTLE

ADRIAN: May I just ask about the last example that you were quoting. I did not quite understand it. You said these people could turn on the single unit in muscle without any feedback because they were not looking at the oscilloscope or hearing the thing going. But wouldn't they be feeling things from their skin, and from their muscle spindles and all the rest of it?

PHILLIPS: Yes, that is an objection which has not perhaps been completely controlled. There could be feedback from the responding part, even if only one motor unit is thrown into action. It was only after they had had some practice with the visual or auditory feedback, having learned to call up unit A, B, or C with the aid of the oscilloscope or loudspeaker, that they could then call them up without the visual or auditory aids. And in some cases they could even produce particular rhythms of discharge if they had already trained themselves to produce them. It is an extraordinary performance that they were able to learn during the course of a morning. But, of course, the very great motor skills that we can develop must obviously depend on the possibility of an equally high degree of selectivity.

SPERRY: On the same topic, how much of this learning is just learning to make an ordinary movement at a certain very critical threshold that just happens to pick out the unit that is being tapped?

PHILLIPS: Yes, I think that is what happened, but I am very eagerly awaiting the full publication of these experiments. There was only a preliminary report so far.

SPERRY: I thought the important point of this study was that with an electrode simultaneously recording from two adjacent units, the subject can differentially activate one or the other.

PHILLIPS: Yes, that was the point. The electrodes were so positioned that two or three characteristic unitary potentials were recordable and the subject was asked to select from these.

SPERRY: This would come down to a matter, then, of which muscle the electrode was in and whether a slight shift of direction in the implicit move-ment would bring out this unit and not that one—or a matter of different degrees of tension. In other words, the cortex is not thinking of individual units, so to speak, but thinking of the ordinary movements that we have and adjusting them to the particular electrode pickup.

PHILLIPS: Yes indeed. But in this context I wanted just to draw attention to the fantastic degree of selectivity within the different levels within the Jacksonian black box, whose neural basis will eventually have to be discovered by experimental neurologists.

THORPE: Did I understand you to say that you were investigating inherited structures in the nervous system? If so I would like to ask how you can be certain that the structure is really included in the original material and not acquired by early experience. I feel that this is a crucial question because, in the light of modern research on coding mechanisms, it is most important to know how much of the incredibly complex and detailed organization of the central nervous system has to be coded in the genome by DNA or some other system, and how much can be reasonably accounted for on the basis of individual experience.

PHILLIPS: Yes, I should have spoken only of structure. I was deliberately leaving aside instability of the kind which Sherrington began to study with Graham Brown in 1912. I was trying to get at what Bates has called the fixed, repeatable aspects of motor maps and to leave aside the facilitations, deviations, and reversals of response that were the first beginnings of an attempt to understand cortical function. But some, at least, of the fixed, re-peatable map must depend on inherited structure, for Hines has demonstrated "pyramidal-type" motor projection by electrical stimulation of the precentral gyrus of foetal and new-born monkeys.

PENFIELD: I think this type of critical, careful scholarly approach that Dr. Phillips is making may begin to tell us what the cortical areas actually do. Stimulation of the cortical area does not tell you the purpose of that area at all: it tells you what corticopetal activation can do and that gives you some reason to assume what the cortex may have been doing. But if, as in the precentral gyrus of man, the activation comes from a subcortical source (which it does), it is not easy to be sure what the cortex adds. What it adds to the messages that are coming up from that subcortical area and passing on to the muscles, is the function of that cortical area.

We can get some light by comparing man to the other animals. Looking back, there has been an extraordinary increase in the cortical representation, so-called, of different parts: in the human cortex the great enlargement of the thumb and the forefinger, and the other fingers to a lesser extent, is important. If one considers what a man does with those parts that the animal does not do, one might surmise what the cortex adds. The amount of paralysis that results from cortical removal is directly in proportion to the amount of representation. In man you can remove the leg area (it is comparatively small) completely, using a stimulator to make sure that you have got it all, and still that man will walk and walk quite well. We have done this in order to get rid of a small infiltrating tumor. He has some tonic difficulties, but his walking will be almost without a limp and without deficiency in a fairly short time. On the other hand, removal of the large area for the forefinger and thumb will leave a permanent paralysis for fine discriminating movements that will never recover.

The appearance in man of vocalization control from the cortex is a rather extraordinary thing. In no other animal that I know of does stimulation of the cortical motor area produce vocalization. I refer to the classical sensorimotor and the supplementary motor. In man there is not one area but there are four areas (right and left precentral and right and left supplementary area) of vocalization. The response to stimulation is the same, no matter whether it is right or left supplementary motor, or the right or left classical motor area. The vocalization sounds the same. (Perhaps it is a little more rhythmic in the supplementary area, but that is of no importance.) Vocalization requires the action of the whole mechanism, including diaphragm, lips, mouth, everything, so that it is quite clear that the cortex is utilizing a neuron mechanism which is in the brain stem lower down. I suppose it is that upward migration of the bark representation that makes possible the extraordinary voluntary performance during speech.

I may say I do not believe that the use of changing parameters is going to change our conception of the fundamental succession of movement in the precentral gyrus. We have used different parameters of course, often moving from 10 per sec up to 100. We settled on 60 per sec, quite independently of Woolsey. But we found no contradiction to the previously determined succession of representation. Let me say, in conclusion, that I know "representation" is a poorly chosen word! We must hope to discover what the true function of the motor cortex is, what it adds to the stream of potentials as they come through on the way to the voluntary muscles. When we learn that, it will be possible to choose a better word. My question to Dr. Phillips is: What happens in the motor cortex? What is its function?

PHILLIPS: I wish I could answer it. But I think that as far as *localization* is concerned, one can usefully state one's questions in terms of what quantity of axonal and synaptic density the cortex can command in its downward projection and how widely the origin of this projection is distributed over the cortical surface. This is a fact of structure, of anatomy, which changes as one climbs the phylogenetic ladder so that there is greater density, clearly, for the hand than there is for the leg in your example of the patient.

With regard to cortical *function*, should we not seek it upstream of this corticofugal level with its different quantities of axonal and synaptic density? The corticofugal projections define the boundaries of "committed" and "uncommitted" areas, but function may not respect these boundaries; one can picture activity weaving to and fro among the dendritic forests of corticofugal cells, exciting and inhibiting them in ways we all wish we understood.

TEUBER: Professor Phillips, do you have any information from your own work or that of others about what happens in individual Betz cell units during movements that the animal "initiates itself," as against either electrically or reflexly induced movement?

I think, if we take the outflow theory seriously, there should be a conspicuous and demonstrable physiological difference, depending on whether a movement is voluntary in that sense or not. I believe Dr. Evarts has some intriguing data on single units in the precentral gyrus (I believe in the fifth layer) that are activated during voluntary movement, a spontaneous movement, say, of a monkey's forelimb. Apparently, as movement starts, some of these units fall silent while other units fire when the monkey sits quietly in the restraining chair. That is, they do the opposite of what has been alluded to by Professor Moruzzi when he reported on the earlier findings by Lord Adrian and himself on what happens in the anesthetized animal when the motor cortex is thrown into action by electric stimulation.

PHILLIPS: I am very interested to hear about that. I was thinking in terms of collaterals, as I think we must when we are thinking about the sensation of innervation. If messages leave the cortex then something is fed back by the collaterals into it and that feedback, of course, is inseparable from the discharge of the corticofugal cell, however its discharge is stimulated.

ECCLES: That possibility of the feedback from axon collaterals of pyramidal cells could be tested, I presume. Perhaps Professor Penfield could tell us if there is any evidence of conscious sensations produced when the pyramidal tract is stimulated in conscious subjects.

PENFIELD: There is no evidence of any awareness of stimulation excepting the awareness of the movement, and the patient will often say in the end, "you made me do that." He recognizes the fact that it is not a voluntary movement of his own.

I never had a patient say "I just wanted to do that anyway."

ECCLES: I think this is a very important observation and I wonder how Dr. Phillips would reconcile that with the idea of feedback from axon collaterals.

PHILLIPS: I suppose that I would reconcile it in this way. I would say that the stimulating electrode has, as Penfield says, disorganized the normal functioning in this area so that the feedback from the discharging corticofugal cells arrives into an area of such confusion that no "sensation of innervation" is aroused.

PENFIELD: May I ask you one question? I was very pleased to hear your discussion of the problems of mosaic with the abrupt and minute localization. But one important observation that would help would be the reciprocal of the one you described. Is there any evidence as to whether a single cortical motoneuronal fiber may terminate by its branches in more than one motoneuronal nucleus at the spinal cord level? If it should terminate in but one, we may have the ultimate in minute localization.

PHILLIPS: No. One must think of the large number of corticofugal cells that are involved here. My colleague T. P. S. Powell estimated that in the arm areas of our baboons a cylinder of 1 mm square cross-section area would contain about 18,000 fifth-layer pyramids, of which about 80 are large and would be recognized by any student as Betz cells, although we don't allow ourselves to use that name any more. Many of the 18,000 must, of course, be corticocallosal, corticostriatal, corticorubral, and other corticofugal cells. And the question is whether, from a larger area than this, the axons of all the corticospinal neurons going to a particular motoneuron contribute synapses to that motoneuron only, or whether they branch and ramify along the spinal cord, contributing a lot of synapses to that motoneuron and fewer to some others. I don't believe we know the answer to this, but I was very struck last year by Szentágothai's pictures of fibers, whose origin I think he did not know, wandering along the spinal grey matter, giving off a bead here and then giving some beads to another cell and so on. We need to know if pyramidal axons do this.

ANDERSEN: I would just like to ask Dr. Penfield whether in patients with Jacksonian epilepsy there is a short period, just before the seizure starts, in which the patients are aware of movement before the actual movement is there? I am thinking of some kind of subliminal stimulation of the cortex.

PENFIELD: No, I don't think so. I think the patient who has a typical Jacksonian motor march is not aware that it is coming, before movement begins. If the discharge begins in the postcentral gyrus, then he probably has either a tingling in the finger or a sense of movement followed by actual movement. But if it starts really in the precentral gyrus, he notices the movement first; and, there again, he never thinks that he wished to make that movement.

Discharge in the second sensory area sometimes produces awareness of the desire to move.

MAC KAY: I would like to ask about the case of the paralyzed finger. I understood that there was no sense of effort, no awareness of movement, and that frustration of the movement did not give rise to any awareness that movement had been frustrated. Is this true?

PHILLIPS: The subject had no awareness of passive movement and did not know whether he had carried out a movement or not because you could prevent the movement without his knowing that you had done so. What I said was that he could measure out accurately a certain angular movement with this terminal joint of the thumb without vision, having trained himself to do it with vision.

MAC KAY: So he must presumably have been aware of a sense of effort, but he did not know whether it had succeeded or not.

PHILLIPS: Merton [1964] wrote: "If the movement is restrained by holding the thumb, the subject believes he has moved it just the same."

MAC KAY: This does not seem to me to lay you open to the criticism that was being made in terms of feedback from the axon collaterals. Recurrent axon collaterals need not give rise to consciousness of motion.

PHILLIPS: Not consciousness of motion, but consciousness of having put forth the correct effort.

SCHAEFER: Concerning the discussion of Professor Penfield and Professor Phillips, I should like to ask them: Is not the question of whether the patient is aware of a voluntary movement simply a matter of the context of his consciousness? We will feel always forced to do something if what we are doing is not the result of a long train of considerations which puts this movement into a framework which is intimately connected with our self-understanding. For example, I always make a very funny experiment with my students in that part of the lecture which concerns movement. I take two of the students and put them before the class and I ask them to do something completely free on a certain signal. Sometimes they do something very curious; for example, once I had a boy and a girl standing before the class and the boy suddenly kissed the girl! I then make a very serious investigation into what is really behind the story, and in all cases you find a complete development of what was going on: for example, here the boy who kissed the girl said: "Well, the professor is guilty of that mistake which I made here; and, since I have to do something quite extraordinary, this would be the best thing to do." And so he put this, so to speak, completely free and undetermined action into a very fine, elaborated framework of his consciousness!

CHAIRMAN: Dr. Schaefer has brought the discussion to a new and higher level, but I feel we must go on!

PENFIELD: We have the second sensory cortex in man as in animals. Stimulation there sometimes has caused several patients to say "I want to" make a certain movement. We have not enough examples to put very much reliance on this. I checked carefully, however. The movement did not occur. It seemed rather different from the result of stimulating either in the classical sensorimotor or the supplementary motor cortex.

PHILLIPS: I think I ought to have made it clear that in all these experiments with the corticomotoneuronal system the shocks were always far below the threshold for movement, so that you can have a discharge of corticofugal cells without any movement, as indeed we know from Adrian and Moruzzi's experiments. And I wonder if in your case there was some discharge of corticofugal cells as a result of physiological spread of excitation into the motor area, and that the feedback from those caused a feeling of the desire to move or even the belief that he had moved, perhaps without having actually moved.

PENFIELD: I don't know, of course, but there is a considerable distance— 5 or 6 cm certainly—between the second sensory area (which runs down into the fissure of Sylvius) and the area of the cortex that would have to be used to carry out the voluntary movement through the classical motor gyrus.

REFERENCES

ADRIAN, E. D. The spread of activity in the cerebral cortex, *J. Physiol.*, 88, 127–161 [1937].

ASANUMA, H., and K. OKAMOTO. Unitary study on evoked activity of callosal neurons and its effect on pyramidal tract cell activity on cats, *Jap. J. Physiol.*, 9, 473–483 [1959].

ASANUMA, H., and O. OKUDA. Effects of transcallosal volleys on pyramidal tract cell activity of cat, *J. Neurophysiol., 25,* 198–208 [1962].

BARD, P., and D. McK. RIOCH. A study of four cats deprived of neocortex and additional portions of the forebrain, *Johns Hopkins Hosp. Bull., 60,* 73–157 [1937].

BARNARD, J. W., and C. N. WOOLSEY. A study of localization in the corticospinal tracts of monkey and rat, *J. Comp. Neurol., 105,* 25–50 [1956].

BASMAJIAN, J. V. Control and training of individual motor units, *Science, 141,* 440–441 [1963].

BATES, J. A. V. Electrical activity of the cortex accompanying movement, *J. Physiol., 113,* 240–257 [1951].

———. Observations on the excitable cortex in man, *Lectures on the Scientific Basis of Medicine.* London: Athlone Press, Vol. 5, pp. 333–347 [1957].

BERNHARD, C. G., and E. BOHM. Cortical representation and functional significance of the cortico motoneuronal system, *Arch. Neurol. Psychiat.* (Chicago), *72,* 473–502 [1954].

———, E. BOHM, and I. PETERSÉN. Investigations on the organization of the corticospinal system in monkeys, *Acta Physiol. Scand., 29,* Suppl. 106, 79–105 [1953].

———. An analysis of causes of postoperative limb pareses following anterolateral chordotomy, *Acta Psychiat., Kbh., 30,* 779–792 [1955].

BINDMAN, L. J., O. C. J. LIPPOLD, and J. W. T. REDFEARN. The action of brief polarizing currents on the cerebral cortex of the rat (1) during current flow and (2) in the production of long-lasting after-effects, *J. Physiol., 172,* 369–382 [1964].

BOYNTON, E. P., and M. HINES. On the question of threshold in stimulation of the motor cortex, *Amer. J. Physiol., 106,* 175–182 [1933].

BRINDLEY, G. S., and R. P. LEWIS. Movements of single limbs and joints produced by stimulation of the baboon's motor cortex after section of the medullary pyramids, *J. Physiol., 170,* 25–26P [1964].

———, and R. P. LEWIS. The extrapyramidal cortical motor map, *Brain, 88,* 397–406 [1965].

———, and P. A. MERTON. The absence of position sense in the human eye, *J. Physiol., 153,* 127–130 [1960].

BROOKS, V. B., P. RUDOMIN, and C. L. SLAYMAN. Sensory activation of neurons in the cat's cerebral cortex, *J. Neurophysiol., 24,* 286–301 [1961a].

———. Peripheral receptive fields of neurons in the cat's cerebral cortex, *J. Neurophysiol., 24,* 302–325 [1961b].

BURNS, B. D. *The Mammalian Cerebral Cortex.* London: Arnold, 119 pp. [1958].

BUSER, P., and M. IMBERT. Sensory projections to the motor cortex in cats: A microelectrode study, in: *Sensory Communication* (ed. by W. A. Rosenblith). Cambridge, Mass. and New York: MIT Press and Wiley [1961].

CARPENTER, D., A. LUNDBERG, and U. NORRSELL. Primary afferent depolarization evoked from the sensorimotor cortex, *Acta Physiol. Scand., 59,* 126–142 [1963].

CHANG, H. T., T. C. RUCH, and A. A. WARD, Jr. Topographical representation of muscles in motor cortex of monkeys, *J. Neurophysiol.*, *10*, 39–56 [1947].

COOPER, S., and D. E. DENNY-BROWN. Responses to stimulation of the motor area of the cerebral cortex, *Proc. Roy. Soc. B.*, *102*, 222–236 [1927].

DENNY-BROWN, D. E. Disintegration of motor function resulting from cerebral lesions, *J. Nerv. Ment. Dis.*, *112*, 1–45 [1950].

——. The nature of apraxia, *J. Nerv. Ment. Dis.*, *126*, 9–32 [1958].

——. *The Basal Ganglia and Their Relation to Disorders of Movement.* Oxford [1962].

——, and E. H. BOTTERELL. The motor function of the agranular frontal cortex, *Res. Publ. Ass. Nerv. Ment. Dis.*, *27*, 235–345 [1947].

DUSSER DE BARENNE, J. G. Recherches expérimentales sur les fonctions du système nerveux central, en particulier sur deux chats dont le néopallium avait été enlevé, *Arch. Néerland. de Physiol.*, *4*, 31–123 [1920].

ECCLES, J. C. *The Physiology of Synapses.* Berlin: Springer, p. 99 [1964].

FERRIER, D. Experimental researches in cerebral physiology and pathology, *West Riding Lunatic Asylum Med. Rep.*, *3*, 1–50 [1873].

——. Discussion on cerebral localization, *Trans. Congr. Amer. Phys. Surg.*, *1*, 337–340 [1888].

FOERSTER, O. The motor cortex in man in the light of Hughlings Jackson's doctrines, *Brain*, *59*, 135–159 [1936].

FRANÇOIS-FRANCK, C. E. *Leçons sur les fonctions motrices du cerveau.* Paris: Doin [1887].

FRITSCH, G., and E. HITZIG. Über die elektrische Erregbarkeit des Grosshirns, *Arch. Anat. Physiol. Wiss. Med.*, *37*, 300–332, 1870; (transl. by G. von Bonin) in: *The Cerebral Cortex.* Springfield: C. C Thomas [1960].

GELLHORN, E., and J. HYDE. Influence of proprioception on map of cortical responses, *J. Physiol.*, *122*, 371–385 [1953].

GIAQUINTO, S., O. POMPEIANO, and J. E. SWETT. EEG and behavioural effects of fore- and hindlimb muscular afferent volleys in unrestrained cats, *Arch. Ital. Biol.*, *101*, 133–148 [1963].

GLEES, P., and J. COLE. Recovery of skilled motor functions after small repeated lesions of motor cortex in macaque, *J. Neurophysiol.*, *13*, 137–148 [1950].

GLUSMAN, M., J. RANSOHOFF, J. L. POOL, H. GRUNDFEST, and F. A. METTLER. Electrical excitability of the human motor cortex. I. The parameters of the electrical stimulus, *J. Neurosurg.*, *9*, 461–471 [1952].

GRAHAM BROWN, T. and C. S. SHERRINGTON. On the instability of a cortical point, *Proc. Roy. Soc. B.*, *85*, 250–277 [1912].

HERN, J. E. C., S. LANDGREN, C. G. PHILLIPS, and R. PORTER. Selective excitation of corticofugal neurones by surface-anodal stimulation of the baboon's motor cortex, *J. Physiol.*, *161*, 73–90 [1962].

——, C. G. PHILLIPS, and R. PORTER. Electrical thresholds of unimpaled corticospinal cells in the cat, *Quart. J. Exp. Physiol.*, *47*, 134–140 [1962].

HERRICK, C. J. *The brain of the tiger-salamander.* Chicago [1948].

HINES, M. Significance of the precentral motor cortex, in: *The Precentral Motor Cortex* (ed. by P. C. Bucy). Illinois, 1st ed. [1944].

HINES, M. The somatic function of the central nervous system, *Ann. Rev. Physiol.*, *14*, 391–408 [1952].

JACKSON, J. H. Cases of partial convulsion from organic brain disease, bearing on the experiments of Hitzig and Ferrier, *Med. Times & Gazette*, *1*, 578–579 [1875].

————. Discussion of brain surgery by V. Horsley, *Brit. Med. J.*, *2*, 674–675 [1886].

————. On the comparative study of diseases of the nervous system, *Brit. Med. J.*, *2*, 355–362. Reprinted 1932, *Selected Writings of John Hughlings Jackson*, *2*, 393–410 [1889].

KLEE, M. R., and H. D. LUX. Intracelluläre Untersuchungen über den Einfluss hemmender Potentiale in motorischen Cortex. II. Die Wirkungen elektrischer Reizung des Nucleus caudatus, *Arch. Psychiat. Nervenkr.*, *203*, 667–689 [1962].

KNAPP, H. D., E. TAUB, and A. J. BERMAN. Movements in monkeys with deafferented forelimbs, *Exp. Neurol.*, *7*, 305–315 [1963].

LANDGREN, S., C. G. PHILLIPS, and R. PORTER. Minimal synaptic actions of pyramidal impulses on some alpha motoneurones of the baboon's hand and forearm, *J. Physiol.*, *161*, 91–111 [1962a].

————. Cortical fields of origin of the monosynaptic pyramidal pathways to some alpha motoneurones of the baboon's hand and forearm, *J. Physiol.*, *161*, 112–125 [1962b].

LASHLEY, K. S. Studies in cerebral function in learning. V. The retention of motor habits after destruction of the so-called motor areas in primates, *Arch. Neurol. Psychiat.*, *Chicago*, *12*, 249–276 [1924].

LEWIN, W., and C. G. PHILLIPS. Observations on partial removal of the postcentral gyrus for pain, *J. Neurol.*, *15*, 143–147 [1952].

LEYTON, A. S. G., and C. S. SHERRINGTON. Observations on the excitable cortex of the chimpanzee, orang-utan and gorilla, *Quart. J. Exp. Physiol.*, *11*, 135–222 [1917].

LIBET, B., W. W. ALBERTS, E. W. WRIGHT, L. D. DELATTRE, G. LEVIN, and B. FEINSTEIN. Production of threshold levels of conscious sensation by electrical stimulation of human somatosensory cortex, *J. Neurophysiol.*, *27*, 546–578 [1964].

LIDDELL, E. G. T., and C. G. PHILLIPS. Thresholds of cortical representation, *Brain*, *73*, 125–140 [1950].

————. Overlapping areas in the motor cortex of the baboon, *J. Physiol.*, *112*, 392–399 [1951].

————. The cortical representation of motor units, *Brain*, *75*, 510–525 [1952].

LILLY, J. C., G. M. AUSTIN, and W. W. CHAMBERS. Threshold movements produced by excitation of cerebral cortex and efferent fibers with some parametric regions of rectangular current pulses (cats and monkeys), *J. Neurophysiol.*, *15*, 319–341 [1952].

LUNDBERG, A., and P. VOORHOEVE. Effects from the pyramidal tract on spinal reflex arcs, *Acta Physiol. Scand.*, *56*, 201–219 [1962].

————, U. NORRSELL, and P. VOORHOEVE. Pyramidal effects on lumbosacral interneurones activated by somatic afferents, *Acta Physiol. Scand.*, *56*, 220–229 [1962].

LUNDBERG, A. Effects from the sensorimotor cortex on ascending spinal pathways, *Acta Physiol. Scand.*, 59, 462–473 [1963].

LUX, H.-D., and M. R. KLEE. Intracelluläre Untersuchungen über den Einfluss hemmender Potentiale in motorischen Cortex. I. Die Wirkung elektrischer Reizung unspezifischer Thalamuskerne, *Arch. Psychiat. Nervenkr.*, 203, 648–666 [1962].

MERTON, P. A. Speculations on the servo-control of movement, *Ciba Foundation Symposium on the Spinal Cord.* London: Churchill, pp. 247–255 [1953].

———. The accuracy of directing the eyes and the hand in the dark, *J. Physiol.*, 156, 555–577 [1961].

———. Human position sense and sense of effort, *Symp. Soc. Exp. Biol.*, 18, 387–400 [1964].

MIHAILOVIĆ, L., and J. M. R. DELGADO. Electrical stimulation of monkey brain with various frequencies and pulse durations, *J. Neurophysiol.*, 19, 21–36 [1956].

MILLS, C. K. Cerebral localization in its practical relations, *Trans. Congr. Amer. Phys. Surg.*, 1, 184–284 (p. 237) [1888].

MORRELL, F. Effect of anodal polarization on the firing pattern of single cortical cells, *Ann. N. Y. Acad. Sci.*, 92, 860–876 [1961].

MORTIMER, E. M., and K. AKERT. Cortical control and representation of fusimotor neurons, *Amer. J. Phys. Med.*, 40, 228–248 [1961].

MOTT, F. W., and C. S. SHERRINGTON. Experiments upon the influence of sensory nerves upon movement and nutrition of the limbs. Preliminary communication, *Proc. Roy. Soc.*, 57, 481–488 [1895].

NATHAN, P., and T. A. SEARS. Effects of posterior root section on the activity of some muscles in man, *J. Neurol.*, 23, 10–22 [1960].

NYBERG-HANSEN, R., and A. BRODAL. Sites and mode of termination of rubrospinal fibers in the cat, *J. Anat.* (London), 98, 235–253 [1964].

OSCARSSON, O., and I. ROSÉN. Projection to cerebral cortex of large musclespindle afferents in forelimb nerves of the cat, *J. Physiol.*, 169, 924–945 [1963].

PATTON, H. D., and V. E. AMASSIAN. Single- and multiple-unit analysis of cortical stage of pyramidal tract activation, *J. Neurophysiol.*, 17, 345–363 [1954].

———. The pyramidal tract: Its excitation and functions, *Handbook of Physiology-Neurophysiology II.* Washington, D. C.: Amer. Physiological Soc., pp. 837–861 [1960].

———, A. L. TOWE, and T. T. KENNEDY. Activation of pyramidal tract neurons by ipsilateral cutaneous stimuli, *J. Neurophysiol.*, 25, 501–524 [1962].

PENFIELD, W. *The Cerebral Cortex and Consciousness*, Harvey Lectures, 32, 35–69 [1936–7].

———, and E. BOLDREY. Somatic motor and sensory representation in the cerebral cortex of man as studied by electrical stimulation, *Brain*, 60, 389–443 [1937].

———, and H. H. JASPER. *Epilepsy and the Functional Anatomy of the Human Brain.* London: Churchill [1954].

PENFIELD, W., and P. PEROT. The brain's record of auditory and visual experience, *Brain*, 86, 595–696 [1963].

———, and T. RASMUSSEN. *The Cerebral Cortex of Man*. New York: Macmillan [1950].

PHILLIPS, C. G. Intracellular records from Betz cells in the cat, *Quart. J. Exp. Physiol.*, 41, 58–69 [1956a].

———. Cortical motor threshold and the thresholds and distribution of excited Betz cells in the cat, *Quart. J. Exp. Physiol.*, 41, 70–84 [1956b].

———. Some properties of pyramidal neurones of the motor cortex, in: *The Nature of Sleep*, Ciba Foundation Symposium. London: Churchill, pp. 4–24 [1961].

———, and R. PORTER. Unifocal and bifocal stimulation of the motor cortex, *J. Physiol.*, 162, 532–538 [1962].

———. The pyramidal projection to motoneurones of some muscle groups of the baboon's forelimb, *Progress in Brain Research*. Amsterdam: Elsevier, Vol. 12, pp. 222–242 [1964].

PRESTON, J. B., and D. G. WHITLOCK. Precentral facilitation and inhibition of spinal motoneurons, *J. Neurophysiol.*, 23, 154–170 [1960].

———. Intracellular potentials recorded from motoneurons following precentral gyrus stimulation in primate, *J. Neurophysiol.*, 24, 91–100 [1961].

PURPURA, D. P., R. J. SHOFER, and F. S. MUSGRAVE. Cortical intracellular potentials during augmenting and recruiting responses. II. Patterns of synaptic activities in pyramidal and non-pyramidal tract neurons, *J. Neurophysiol.*, 27, 133–151 [1964].

RICCI, G., B. DOANE, and H. H. JASPER. Microelectrode studies of conditioning: Technique and preliminary results. IV. Congr. Inter. d'Electro-encéphalographie et de Neurophysiologie Clinique, Bruxelles. Réunions plénières, pp. 401–415 [1957].

RINVIK, E., and F. WALBERG. Demonstration of a somatotopically arranged cortico-rubral projection in the cat, *J. Comp. Neurol.*, 120, 393–407 [1963].

RUSINOV, V. S. An electrophysiological analysis of the connecting function in the cerebral cortex in the presence of a dominant region area, *Abstr. XIX Int. Physiol. Congr.*, 719–720 [1953].

RUSSELL, J. R., and W. DE MYER. The quantitative origin of pyramidal axons of Macaca rhesus, with some remarks on the slow rate of axolysis, *Neurology*, 11, 96–108 [1961].

SHERRINGTON, C. S. On secondary and tertiary degenerations in the spinal cord of the dog, *J. Physiol.*, 6, 177–191 [1885].

———. On nerve-tracts degenerating secondarily to lesions of the cortex cerebri, *J. Physiol.*, 10, 429–432 [1889].

———. Quantitative management of contraction in lowest-level coordination, *Brain*, 54, 1–28 [1931].

TROTTER, W. A landmark in modern neurology, *Lancet*, 227, 1207–1210 [1934].

WALL, P. D., A. G. RÉMOND, and R. L. DOBSON. Studies on the mechanism of the action of visual afferents on motor cortex excitability, *Electroenceph. Clin. Neurophysiol.*, 5, 385–393 [1953].

WALSHE, F. M. R. The mode of representation of movements in the motor cortex, with special reference to "convulsions beginning unilaterally," *Brain*, *66*, 104–139 [1943].

———. Some problems of method in neurology, *Can. Med. Ass. J.*, *68*, 21–29 [1953].

WATSON, D. E., and V. E. AMASSIAN. Synaptic organization of motor cortex, *Physiologist*, *4*, 131 [1961].

WHITTERIDGE, D. Central control of eye movements, in: *Handbook of Physiology-Neurophysiology II*. Washington, D. C.: Amer. Physiological Soc., pp. 1089–1109 [1960].

WOOLSEY, C. N. Organization of somatic sensory and motor areas of the cerebral cortex, *Biological and Biochemical Bases of Behavior*. Madison: Univ. Wisconsin Press, pp. 63–81 [1958].

———, P. H. SETTLAGE, D. R. MEYER, W. SENCER, T. P. HAMUY, and A. M. TRAVIS. Patterns of localization in precentral and "supplementary" motor areas and their relation to the concept of a premotor area, *Res. Publ. Ass. Nerv. Ment. Dis.*, *30*, 238–264 [1952].

17

Cerebral Organization and the
Conscious Control of Action

by D. M. MacKay

University of Keele, Staffordshire, England

Specifying our Problem

Our aim in this symposium, as Sir John Eccles has reminded us, is to "search for new insights" into the cerebral basis of consciousness. This is an opportunity to take stock of our armament and strategy as well as of our prizes; and the present paper sets out to contribute mainly to the first of these activities.

In the present phase of science, understanding normally means being able to point to a theoretical model of the process that baffled us, and say "this is how it works." The search for understanding thus generates three tasks in cyclic interaction:

(*a*) Elaboration of an adequate specification of what the model must do, and also, incidentally, of what it *need not* do. It is at this stage that philosophical thinking can make its most important contribution to science, particularly in ridding our specification of mistaken demands which might on the face of it have seemed essential.

(*b*) Discovery of a model (or more than one) that will meet the specification without making any physically unrealistic assumptions. Here, incidentally, the familiar appeal to "simplicity" can be treacherous, especially in a biological context. There is no virtue in producing a model of nervous activity using only one standard type of "neuron," for example, if physiological histology assures us of the existence of several radically different types.

(*c*) Invention of crucial tests in the light of which to refine the model and/or the specification.

In relation to the conscious control of action, we meet our first obstacle at the stage of specification. Our understanding of what consciousness entails, even behaviorally, is totally inadequate for the framing of an exhaustive catalogue. At the minimum, however, we can say that any model must have a correlate for *my* ability to control my action, as distinct from the many unconscious homeostatic capacities of my body. My capacity for conscious action, whatever it may mean in mechanical terms, is one of the least dubitable of data, at least for me.

The question immediately raised is whether any model to account for conscious human action must therefore be "detector controllable" in the sense that a ground-guided missile is, but sensitive to mental "signals" instead of physical ones. Must some links of the physical causal chain mesh be *open-ended?*

This is not the place for full discussion of the philosophical issues, but the whole principle of any scientific model of conscious action is bound to be affected by our answer, which in turn depends on our concept of "mind." I must therefore declare my own view [MacKay, 1954, 1965c], that to think of the brain as subject to nonphysical forces is at least unnecessary, and perhaps mistaken, as a way of admitting the reality and causal efficacy of human decision for human action.

Briefly, it seems possible to do full justice to our experience as conscious agents (and, I believe, to the Biblical doctrine of man) on the view that mental activity is not an additional *force* over and above those physically detectable in the brain, but an additional *internal aspect* of the total human activity, of which brain (and body) activity is the complementary "external" aspect. On this view, the two-way "interaction" of brain events and conscious experience which Professor Penfield and others in this symposium have discussed would follow automatically; but the interaction would not be like that of force on force; it would be more like the interaction, or rather interdependence, of a mathematical problem and the computing machine in which it is set up. The physical setup of a computing machine determines its subsequent behavior; yet at the same time and equally, the mathematical conditions so expressed determine the solution expressed by the machine's behavior. With this kind of relationship there is no need to doubt the reality of the one in order to do justice to the other; and to dismiss one as "nothing but" the other would be simply to miss the point.

Similarly (although the analogy is far from complete), if it were the case that the physical setup of an agent's brain and body (including sensory inputs) determined completely their physical behavior, this would give no reason for denying that the mental deliberations of the agent (including what he perceived) determined the action he took. On the present view, these could both perfectly well be valid accounts, describing respectively the external and internal aspect of the complex unity that we know as a human decision. Of the agent's responsibility for his decision we shall have more to say anon.

INFORMATION AND CONTROL

For the study of human behavior there are various conceptual levels at which the business of specification, model making, and testing can be carried on. Traditionally, a great gulf has separated the approaches of psychology and physiology. In both, it has been possible to draw up theoretical models in which entities found themselves linked by causal pathways to form systems. The difficulty has been that the entities and paths of the psychologist's models have classically had few pretensions to anatomical significance, while those of the physiologist, for reasons of sheer complexity, have been correspondingly vague in their predictions of gross human behavior. On both sides, a need has been felt for some intermediary conceptual level—for a language in which specifications could be framed and hypotheses made vulnerable to both physiological and psychological data. In the event, the concepts that physiological psychologists have found themselves using turn out to have a close kinship with those developed by engineers in what has come to be called "communication science." The common link is in fact their joint concern with the *organization of action*.

The organization of action can be studied at two levels. One of these concerns problems of "energetics"—the acquisition and application of the necessary *energy*. The other concerns what Norbert Weiner [1948], following Ampère, called problems of "cybernetics"—the acquisition and application of the necessary *information*.

The science of communication and control [Shannon and Weaver, 1949], though it owes much of its impetus to the need for artificial devices to replace human agents, is framed in sufficiently general terms to cover both natural and artificial systems in their cybernetic aspects. Not surprisingly, many of the ideas so formalized have been current for decades, at least in embryo, not only among neurologists and students of animal behavior, but also, for that matter, among economists and political theorists as well. In seeking to apply them to our present problem of the conscious control of human action, we shall in no sense be arguing by analogy. Our aim will merely be to sketch a formal conceptual model which may have sufficient anatomical as well as psychological implications to serve as a bridge between the data of physiology and of conscious experience, while being as open as possible to correction from either side.

Informational Requirements of Action

When a stone floor reacts passively to the impact of a ball, or a de-nervated muscle under tension reacts passively (as distinct from reflex-ively) to a sudden stress, we do not speak of the reaction as "controlled." When a thermostat reacts actively to a drop in temperature, or a spinal reflex to an increase in muscle tension, we do; but we would not regard the control so exercised as *conscious*.

Between simple passive or "Newtonian" reactions of the first sort, and reflexive or "feedback controlled" reactions of the second, it is possible to draw a sharp formal distinction. Reflexive reactions require "infor-mation" to determine their form (in space and/or time). In its absence, they could be otherwise [1]; whereas in Newtonian cases both the form and the energy of the reaction are uniquely derived from the impact of the event eliciting it. Reflexive reactions are characterized by the separ-ability of the flow of information (that which determines form) from the flow of energy (that which embodies form).

The question that concerns us is whether any distinction in similar terms can be found between unconscious reflexive reaction and con-scious action. In particular, what kind of "information flow map" might begin to do justice to the complexities of intelligent human choice be-havior? It need hardly be said that our answer in the present state of knowledge will be woefully incomplete, but perhaps we now have enough clues to attempt a first approximation.

The Concept of Control

The concept of control (as we shall use it here) implies the idea of a norm or goal with respect to which the action controlled can be termed successful or unsuccessful, convergent or divergent. In "unconscious" regulative activities such as the control of body temperature against ambient fluctuations, the requisite information flow map assumes the familiar form of Fig. 17.1, in which the essential features are:

E, an effector system capable of a range of activities (for example, heat-ing or cooling);

S, a selector which determines the form of activity selected from E's repertoire, according to information received from

[1] See MacKay [1962a] for a discussion of the difficulties behind this superficially simple statement.

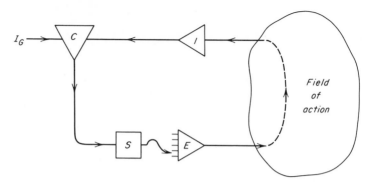

Fig. 17.1. Simple feedback control loop.

I, an indicator of the quantity or state of affairs under control (for example, temperature);

C, a means of calculating the "value" (positive or negative) of the indicated state of affairs in terms of a given criterion, and of selecting from
E's repertoire, activity calculated to maximize positive or minimize
negative evaluation.[2]

In many cases the criterion of evaluation, and hence the norm or goal
of control, may be fixed and implicit in the structure of *I*. In others,
and particularly in artificial regulators, this criterion may be determined
explicitly by an informational input (for example, the setting of a
thermostat). This input is shown in Fig. 17.1 as a signal I_G (indication
of goal) supplied to the evaluator *C*.

A well-known neurophysiological arrangement believed to function
on this principle is the skeletal muscle control system as elucidated by
Granit and others [Eldred, Granit, and Merton, 1953; Granit, 1955; Merton, 1951]. For a recent review see Matthews [1964]. According to their
"servo-theory," the sensitive fibers known as muscle spindles, which discharge into the spinal cord, serve as combined indicators and evaluators
of muscle length in a control loop similar to Fig. 17.1, in which *E* is the
main muscle fiber system and *S* is the spinal neuron pool. The resulting
tendency is to maintain the muscle at a given equilibrium length, actively resisting effects of muscle fatigue or changes in load. To complete
the resemblance to Fig. 17.1, control signals from higher centers via
the spinal cord, and along the so-called gamma efferent pathway, are
believed to determine this equilibrium length by varying the tension in

---

[2] Terms such as *evaluating, calculated,* and the like are here used elliptically. What
is meant is that, granted the *significance* of incoming signals as *betokening* information
about the field of action, the resulting internal activity, at the same level of interpretation, has the *significance* of evaluation, calculation, etc. [MacKay, 1962a].

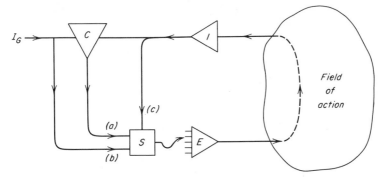

Fig. 17.2. Simple loop with feedforward. (*a*) Feedback. (*b*) Feedforward from indication of goal. (*c*) Feedforward from indication of field state.

the muscle spindles, and so acting as the "indication of goal," I_G in our figure.

One further refinement should perhaps be mentioned here. In the simple system of Fig. 17.1, whenever the goal signal I_G changes, the full signal to evoke the response from E must come by way of C. It is often possible to increase speed and accuracy by arranging that in addition to the "feedback" signals from C, the selector system S receives an input computed directly from I_G itself, together with any other relevant advance indications obtainable via auxiliary sensors. This "feedforward" need only roughly approximate to the required form, but will leave C more free for the task of fine adjustment, on which it still has the last word (Fig. 17.2). It seems not unlikely that feedforward of this sort (by "alpha innervation") plays a part in the control of muscle movement [Matthews, 1964].

HIERARCHIES OF CONTROL

A simple "servo-loop" on the lines of Fig. 17.1 or Fig. 17.2 could obviously be used in its turn as the effector in another, higher-order, control system. In that case the signals I_G determining the criterion of evaluation would play the role of the selector S in the higher-order system. A familiar example is the use of power-assisted steering in motor cars, where the steering wheel serves mainly to set the criterion for the servo-loop which determines the direction of the road wheels. Here the driver, steering by information received visually from the road, can be regarded as the evaluator in a second-order control loop for which the whole steering servo acts as effector (Fig. 17.3).

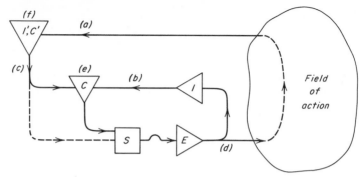

Fig. 17.3. Second-order control of steering. (*a*) Information from road. (*b*) Indication of wheel angle. (*c*) Angle of steering wheel (dotted line shows optional feedforward). (*d*) Angle of road wheels. (*e*) Mechanical comparator. (*f*) Driver (combining functions of second-order indicator, comparator, and norm setter).

Examples of more complex hierarchic control abound in the higher nervous system. The study of animal behavior, surveyed by Professor Thorpe, has shown that not only isolated acts but whole subroutines of goal-directed activity may be switched by releaser mechanisms triggered at a level which is "higher" at least in the sense of being able to override the current goal settings of the organism.

It would be implausible in the extreme to suggest that the presence of hierarchic organization on these lines could suffice to distinguish conscious from unconscious control; but the ability to set one goal aside in favor of another, and to evaluate goal priorities, is certainly one key feature of our own experience as conscious agents.

COGNITION AND ACTION

A goal-seeking and norm-holding system of the kind we are discussing comes up against the external world in two ways. On the one hand, it suffers stimulation of sensors; on the other, it finds limits set to its range of action. Where some degree of stability or regularity (in space or time) is present in the pattern of stimulation or limitation, or in the relations between them, there is scope for action of a new kind, which we call *intelligent*. This makes use of the correlations and regularities observable, to improve the strategy of control of adaptive action. In the jargon of information theory, the presence of "redundancy" (roughly, predictability) in the pattern of demand means that a given degree of performance can always, in principle, be achieved with a smaller amount of incoming information—or a higher degree with a given amount. The great achievement of Claude Shannon [Shannon and Weaver, 1949] was to give a precise quantitative expression to the foregoing statement. It is this redundancy which, as we shall see, invites the special kind of adaptation that we call perception and cognition.

Without going into details here [MacKay, 1956, 1959, 1961; Barlow, 1961], it may be seen that the principal elaboration required in order to profit from redundancy will be in the "feedforward" system. Repetitive demands on the effector system E, for example, may be efficiently met by evolving internal "organizing subroutines," subsequently stored, to supply the bulk of the necessary control signals on behalf of the evaluator as soon as their particular rhythm crops up.

Any patterning in the demand for different subroutines can in turn elicit, in ways discussed in the papers cited above, the spontaneous formation of higher-order matching subroutines, operating on selectors of lower-order organizers in the same way that they in turn operate on the repertoire of the external effector system. The patterns concerned may be spatial or temporal or both; and they may be determinate or merely statistical, defining perhaps the rank order in which various response mechanisms should be held in readiness for spontaneous trial. Detailed evidence on the structure of such organizing hierarchies in human beings is accumulating from studies of remembering and forgetting [see, for example, Conrad, 1959].

The behavior resulting from this simple but all-important elaboration begins to show many of the features that we recognize as intelligent. Not only overt anticipatory behavior, but the preparation of indefinitely complex conditional strategies based on abstract conceptualization, are within the scope of an active information system that is equipped to build up a hierarchic internal repertoire to match the coherent, and hence cognizable, features of the impact of the world upon it [MacKay, 1956, 1959, 1961]. In this picture, *perception* is represented by the activity of updating the "conditional state of organization" to match current sensory data. The focus of *attention* has its correlate in the region of the field of incoming data against which the state of organization is currently being evaluated and updated. Perception of *change* is the alteration of this state of organization, brought about by signals indicating inadequacy or "mismatch" in the existing state, judged by the current criteria of the evaluator.

VOLUNTARY CONTROL OF EYE MOVEMENT

To see how this kind of approach works out in practice, we may consider the problem of voluntary eye movement. When the direction of gaze changes, the optical image moves over the retina. If the change is imposed on the eyeball from without—say, by gentle pressure on the corner of the open eyelid—the visual world is seen to move. When the same change results from voluntary use of the eye muscles, however, no movement of the visual world is seen. What is it about voluntary control, we may ask, which makes this difference?

If we were to think of perception as an internal witnessing of incoming signals, we might be tempted to invoke the idea that the signals resulting from voluntary eye movement must be "canceled" in some way, presumably by signals derived from the oculomotor system.[3] If so, however, the accuracy of "cancellation" is remarkably high, and it is difficult to imagine how this could be achieved on the basis of either the "outflow" signals to the eye muscles or any "inflow" signals from proprioceptors, unless visual acuity for field movement is much lower than it seems.

The problem takes on a different complexion, however, if we ask what part a consciously controlled eye movement is calculated to play within the *total* information system. Informationally its function, like that of exploratory hand movements in the dark, is to steer the receptor surface to a fresh sample of the sensory world. If we are right in supposing that the perception of *change* results only from a significant *mismatch* between the signals received and those which the action was calculated to bring about, then the changes resulting from voluntary movement in a stable environment should generate no such mismatch. They are, in fact, precisely what the action was calculated to bring about on the basis of the *existing* internal world map [MacKay, 1962b].

As the case of tactile exploration makes abundantly clear, there is no question of having to *cancel* the resulting motion signals. What is wanted is not cancellation, but *evaluation,* in the light of the objective of the action. The sense of rubbing friction as the hand explores a stationary surface is part of the object of the exercise, and gives positive evidence that the surface is stationary. If it were absent or abnormally weak, this would be evidence that the surface was moving with the hand.[4] Because the eye normally explores in saccadic jumps, smooth motion of the image over the retina is *not* part of the calculated evidence of stability; but progressive displacement of the image certainly is, and in its absence, as with a stabilized retinal image [Ditchburn and Gins-

---

[3] A cancellation method of this sort is often used with a ship-borne radar display, to keep the radar map from rotating as the ship's head turns; but in that case there *is* an operator witnessing the display.

[4] We are not here speaking of intellectual interpretation, but of primary information processing, such as might take place in the computer of a radar system. See footnote 2.

borg, 1952], or with paralysis of eye muscles [Kornmüller, 1931], the visual world seems to move.

An important piece of evidence on the mechanism concerned comes from an elegant experiment by N. Bischof of the Max Planck Institute, Seewiesen (personal communication). If a lamp is flashed briefly in a darkened room during the course of a voluntary eye movement, it is seen as displaced from its true position. Moreover, this illusory displacement is observed with flashes occurring even several milliseconds before the eyeball begins to move. This suggests that the new criteria of evaluation are supplied to the evaluator from the *outgoing* signals to the eye muscles. On the other hand, Gurevitch [1959] has produced strong evidence that if a subject has been conditioned (in the light) to point his eyes in a given direction, he can still do so in the dark with surprising accuracy; and his eye movements, recorded electrically, exhibit self-corrective "hunting" of a kind which seems to imply the existence of feedback at some level.

Whatever the source of its information, however, it will be seen that the accuracy required by the evaluator in our present model need be no greater than the accuracy with which the *action* responsible can be executed. It is in this quantitative respect that the model most clearly differs from the cancellation theory of visual stability in the form advanced by von Holst [1957]. His feedback (*reafferenz*) model [von Holst and Mittelstaedt, 1950] has almost the same gross flow map as our Fig. 17.2; but the process of evaluation is replaced by one of subtraction. In its original context of sensorimotor coordination in fish and insects, this was unexceptionable, but in his later application of the model to the problem of *raumkonstanz* [von Holst, 1957], it seems to have been presupposed that what is perceived is the residue of the subtractive process; and this implies that perceptual stability should depend to a much higher degree on the accuracy of the *efferenzkopie* supposed to be subtracted. The issue still waits on physiological evidence.

ACTION ON THE SPRINGS OF ACTION

A major part of the activity of the system we have been developing is now internal. As with external reactions, we may distinguish between passive and active internal adaptation. Some internal changes, in sensory systems for example, may be as purely passive as those worked in the face of a mountain by the winter torrents. Others, however, may be highly complex active projects—building subroutines, conducting trial runs to evaluate probable future outcomes, or modifying both subroutines and the priorities of the various goals and norms that they are built to subserve. The internal field of action may in principle become as complex as the external.

Embodying as it implicitly does the current answer to any question that is relevant to action, the total organizing system may be regarded as an implicit representation or "cognitive map" of all those features and aspects of the world with which it has had to deal. Any change in it has the operational significance of a change in *belief* regarding the field of action.

For the intelligent control of the internal field of action, a cognitive system is required on the same general lines as for the external field; only now the objects of perception and cognition for this supersystem are the elements and structures of the organizing system itself. The developmental aspects of such "metaorganization" will not, however, be discussed here [MacKay, 1956, 1959, 1961], except to point out that development cannot be expected to happen spontaneously at anything like the rate of the primary organizing system; at this level, *education* (at least in the sense of dialogue with others) is necessary for efficiency.

Once constituted, the internal cognitive supersystem could in principle take its data not only from the subsystem concerned with external action, but from the whole internal field *including its own activity* [MacKay, 1952, 1953, 1963a]. Once this happens, as we might imagine, its logic develops some significant peculiarities, which are in fact suggestively parallel to those of human first-person language [MacKay, 1963a]; but we will not now pursue the parallel. The point which does need emphasis is that at this level of organization the hitherto clear separation of normative from representational function tends to disappear. At lower levels it was possible to treat as independent the setting of the goal or norm (by signals such as I_G) and the development of a suitable feedforward system to match (and so, implicitly, to represent) the state of the world. Now, however, we are at or above the level where signals such as I_G *originate*. This supersystem, by generating its own goal signals, becomes its own master.

The logical distinction between indicative and normative functions does not, of course, disappear; but activity that functions indicatively in one respect may here inevitably have normative consequences in another. Certain basic metabolic and other norms may be virtually immovable, but over wide areas of action our supersystem can present us with the same difficulty in disentangling its "facts" from its "values" as those which attend what Sir Geoffrey Vickers [1964] calls the "appreciative process" in human policy making. Decision making in a system of this sort, as in common human experience, is no longer always reducible to deduction from given premises, for the premises are among the variables of the process. This is not to say that an external computer supplied with complete information on the state of the system could not predict the outcome (see below), but it does mean that no computer could do *for the system* what it does for itself in that process.

It should be noted that in none of these respects have we had to engineer *ad hoc* the resemblances that have emerged between our information flow model and a self-conscious human agent. All we have done is to press towards their limits the informational principles of feedback and feedforward in the organization of adaptive and purposive action. If an organism whose information system embodies an adaptive organizer may be said to "know" the fact to which the organizer is adaptive, then it would seem that one which embodies a metaorganizing system on the foregoing lines could be said (other things being equal) to "know that he knows." This, more than any other feature of our information flow model, we might guess to be the main discriminant of systems capable of sustaining consciousness as we know it; but as always, we can at best hope one day to prove it a necessary feature, never a sufficient one.

CONSCIOUS CHOICE

We turn last to the question deferred from section 1: the implications of our model for the concept of responsibility. The determination of human action frequently entails choosing between courses, all of which are believed by the agent to be *open* to him. The essential paths of control in our hypothetical information flow maps, on the other hand, have all formed *closed* loops, either internally or by way of the field of action. Does not this, it may be asked, raise a basic objection to any such map as a model of conscious human control? Or do we have to conclude that our awareness of freedom in making our choices is in fact illusory?

In the present context it seems particularly important to do justice to possible objections on this score. Following a line of thought pursued in more detail elsewhere [MacKay, 1960, 1963b, 1964a], I hope to show briefly that we can do so without invoking any failure of physical determinacy in the linkages of the cerebral information system.

Our whole discussion has tacitly presupposed that all conscious human activity and experience—choosing, seeing, believing, or whatever —has a correlate in corresponding neural activity. No change in the content of awareness can take place without a corresponding cerebral change: such is the postulate whose implications we are considering. It would follow from it that if all cerebral changes were physically determined by prior physical factors, including other cerebral changes, then the future content of conscious experience would in principle be predictable from these factors. Granted this, the conclusion is often drawn that the agent is bound to choose what he does, that he is mistaken to believe his choice to be undetermined, and that the outcome is really forced upon him by his brain.

I believe this conclusion to be itself mistaken, for it overlooks a curious and far-reaching logical implication of that same postulated connection between brain and consciousness, irrespective of the particular form that the connection takes. The key point is that if what a man believes affects correspondingly the state of his organizing system, no complete up-to-date account of that organizing system could be believed by him without being *ipso facto* rendered out of date.[5]

By the same token, even given the most complete current data, no complete prediction of the future state of his organizing system is deducible upon which both agent and observer could correctly agree.

A prediction made *secretly* by a totally detached (nonparticipant) observer may well be valid for him (and his fellow nonparticipants), but upon the agent himself it has no logical binding force. On the contrary, he would be mistaken if he believed it, even though the nonparticipants were correct to believe it.

In this curious situation we have to face a kind of logical relativity principle [MacKay, 1960, 1964b, 1965a]. In order that the nonparticipants may validly believe what they do about the agent's brain, it is necessary that the agent should believe something else, for if he believed what they do, it would not be valid for him or for them. Accordingly, his own belief—that no determinative specification of his choice exists which he would be right to believe—*is not challenged* by the existence of a prediction valid-only-for-a-nonparticipant. He may even, in retrospect, com· pare notes and assent to the validity of the prediction *for a nonparticipant*, without thereby impugning the validity of his own belief that he,[6] as agent, chose freely.

Towards a Structural Criterion of Responsibility

If this argument is correct, it would seem to have some practical implications for the forensic evaluation of responsibility for an action. It

[5] This is merely a particular case of the general proposition that no information system can embody within it an up-to-date and detailed representation of itself, *including that representation*. A closely reasoned discussion of this in connection with the limits of computing machines was given some years ago by Professor Karl Popper [1950].

[6] The logic of personal talk about "him" is thus irreducibly different from that of physical talk about objects—ultimately because in the personal case one has to face the question "would he be correct if he believed this?" whereas in the physical case no parallel question arises.

hints, indeed, at a possible *structural* criterion, in terms of the information flow map of the organizing system [MacKay, 1960, 1963b, 1964a].

Central to our argument has been the claim that no prediction of a typical choice could be believed by the agent without affecting its own validity. Let us now ask under what circumstances a prediction of an act *could* be validly believed by the agent. From our theoretical standpoint, these would have to be cases in which the cerebral activity of his believing did not significantly affect the conditions on which the prediction was valid. In other words, there must be insufficient coupling between the agent's cognitive system and the subsystem which in the event determines the form of the act or action. By this criterion, acts performed as a result of uninhibitable seizures, direct stimulation of motor nerves, and the like are obviously excluded. Diminution of responsibility for acts performed under the influence of drugs and similar factors could in principle be estimated according to the degree to which, and the form in which, a prediction of the act could have been believed as certain by the agent without self-invalidation.

By the same criterion, however, responsibility would be undiminished by any evidence of "physical causation" that did *not* imply the existence in principle of a prediction beliefworthy by, and so mandatory upon, the agent, whether he knew it or not and liked it or not.

Our logical-structural criterion thus seems to draw a similar dividing line between free and unfree acts to that which has long been recognized intuitively in typical cases. Its merit, if valid, lies in the replacement of counterfactual hypotheticals ("If he had wished, he could have chosen otherwise") by statements of fact, ascertainable at least in principle, concerning the structure of the agent's information system.

Stock Taking

Our general approach in this paper has been to ask: If we had to design an information system to control adaptive purposeful behavior intelligently, what minimal features would we find necessary for efficiency? We have indeed taken hints along the way from both psychological and physiological data, but the logic of the features we have introduced has had to stand on its own feet. It may be appropriate now to look back and take stock. If our model, even in a formal sense, were to correspond to what goes on in the central nervous system, what answers would it suggest to the questions that chiefly concern us in this symposium?

The basic suggestion is that conscious experience is the correlate of what might be called metaorganizing activity—the organization of internal action upon the behavioral organizing system itself. A nervous system insufficiently complex to embody such metaorganizing activity would, as far as one can see, be deficient in the kind of behavior we recognize (rightly or wrongly) as evidence of consciousness.

The *unity* of consciousness would on this basis reflect the integration of the metaorganizing system, rather than the degree of anatomical proximity or interconnectedness of the various subsystems through which disturbances of equilibrium reach it or stem from it.

At this point it behooves an outsider to tread delicately, sobered by Sir Francis Walshe's scathing condemnation [1957] of "intellectual exercise carried out in the dark void of contemporary ignorance of cerebral functions." It may be legitimate, however, to ask whether any fresh light is thrown by our analysis on the vexed question of functional localization. In particular, how plausible is the currently orthodox argument for considering the cerebral cortex as the "dominant level" of the human nervous system?

Our discussion, in fact, brings out a troublesome and apparently unnoticed ambiguity in this question. It stems from the assumption, evident in much of the literature, that the dominant level of the nervous system can be equated with the region of maximum "integrative activity." If we are right in principle in distinguishing normative metaorganizing activity from the integrative activity of the main behavioral organizing system, it is clear that the foregoing assumption is at least questionable. It would admittedly be possible for both functions to be exercised by different subsystems in the same geographical population; but as with the government of a human organization, it might be both physically and administratively advantageous to have the metaorganization segregated in a compact community. This would facilitate the maximum of interaction between the elements of the normative system through which the balancing of current priorities and the selection and evaluation of different integrative activities must take place.

If, then, by the dominant level we mean the region in which the most detailed ongoing integration takes place, our model would suggest no better location for this activity, in respect both of capacity and of connectivity with other areas, than the cerebral cortex. In subserving this function it would not have to *initiate* voluntary action, except insofar as the action was a component of a subroutine already established. It would be concerned chiefly with (a) the elaboration of all the detailed feedforward necessary to keep the pattern of action matched to current sensory (including proprioceptive) data, in obedience to normative signals (like our I_G) from the metaorganizing central system; (b) the feedback to that central system of condensed indications of cortical activity, including activity which (as we saw) would amount operationally to a *categorized* representation of the external world. This feedback would, of course, influence in turn the ongoing computation of the normative signals, so that to this extent the two systems would function as one.

If, however, in speaking of the dominant level, we have in mind the "final arbiter"—the normative metaorganizing system which embodies the appraisal and evaluation of what the main organizing system is about— then it is difficult to find any grounds for giving this a cortical location. On all counts (unless contrary evidence were forthcoming) it would seem more natural that the metaorganizing function should be exercised by more central regions of the system.

The upshot of this is not, of course, any suggestion that consciousness can meaningfully be localized in one central department of the normal waking brain [MacKay, 1962a]. The content of conscious experience may be presumed (on our working assumption of one-to-one correspondence) to depend on all the ongoing cerebral activity reflected in the feedback loops to and from the metaorganizing center, as well as on those within it. What is suggested, however, is that we should be still more unwise to attribute the minimal functions necessary for consciousness to the cerebral cortex, even in the operational sense of assuming that removal or in-activation of cortex must abolish consciousness; and that, conversely, we should be prepared to find consciousness abolished even by central lesions which did not interfere with sensorimotor integration at the cortical level.

On this basis one might wish to take issue with both sides in the current debate over cortical function. Certainly it would not follow from our suggested model that "no major function remains for the cerebral cortex," that "the precentral cortex itself has no power of integrating im-pulses," or that the various cortical areas are "no more than way stations" for impulses to and from more central regions; and insofar as Walshe [1957, pp. 525, 527, 536, 529] was right in attributing such consequences to Penfield's theory of centrencephalic function (though I am not sure that he was), one might echo his objections. On the other hand Walshe's own argument, for all its pungency, seems greatly weakened when we distinguish the notion of sensorimotor dominance from that of normative metaorganization.

Detailed discussion would here be out of place, but one question raised by Walshe [1957, p. 537] is clearly pertinent to our present model. Could what he calls the "meagre collections of cells in the 'old brain'" suffice to mediate the complexities of conscious experience? Does not Hughlings Jackson's aphorism, "the more movements the more grey mat-ter" (quoted by Walshe) make this seem quite implausible? It is here, however, that information theory introduces a new twist with its concept of *redundancy* (see section on cognition and action, above). If all signals to be handled by a network are statistically independent, then its size may indeed be determined by their number, as Jackson implies; but as soon as the signals concerned are highly correlated, the number of elements needed to handle them is in principle correspondingly reduced. The signals are said to be "redundant," and the network capacity required depends mainly on their "information rate" rather than on their complexity.

Now the significant thing about conscious experience, as quantified by psychologists [see, for example, Miller, 1956], is the extremely low information rate which it represents. By contrast with the thousands or even millions of "bits" per second which could be handled by the human sense organs, the average information rate of conscious perception seems to be more like a few hundred bits per second. High rates and high capacities may be needed in the early stages of signal analysis, before the input has been reduced to familiar categories; but once redundancy has been taken into account, it is far from obvious that the meager *information* flux of final conscious awareness should be beyond the capacity of the millions of cells in subcortical structures.

On this view, the cortex, so far from being left without any major function, would have the most laborious and complex task of all, transforming and condensing the informational traffic of the body into a minimally redundant form from the standpoint of the organism. In this respect it might be likened to a vast contracting agency and labor pool—finding or assembling the right subroutine for the right job and vice versa. For this purpose a far greater information capacity (in the technical sense) would be required in it than in the controlling headquarters.

Ablation of parts of the primary organizing system, according to the present model, would affect the dimensional content, but not necessarily the persistence, of consciousness (metaorganizing activity). On the other hand, damage to the metaorganizing system could result in the release of complex automatisms at the behavioral level without conscious awareness or control. The notable absence of perceptual signs of the splitting of the visual cortical map,[7] as well as the relative paucity of psychic effects of commissural section reported by Professor Sperry [1961] and others and discussed here by Professor Bremer, would also seem to fit well with this suggestion.

Finally, what of Sherrington's famous question: Does mind have working contact with matter? What we have been sketching is a system in which no physical action waits on anything but another physical action. Analyze it physically, and mind will slip through our net as readily as

[7] Almost the only reported sign that the visual map has two widely separated halves is Gengerelli's observation that "phi" apparent movement is more readily seen along rather than across the midline [Gengerelli, 1948]. Using spatiotemporally random optical patterns (visual "noise") as a neutral test stimulus, one can observe a number of fugitive signs of anisotropy, including a fountain or firework effect reported by some subjects to be visible about the midline [MacKay, 1965b].

the mathematical aspect of the problem embodied in an electronic computing machine slips through the net of electronic analysis. Physically indeterminate events may or may not play a significant part in the dance of cerebral activity, but any unpredictability they might contribute would seem radically inadequate as a model of the responsible freedom of sober decision.

Our suggestion has been that we see mind at work, not by finding unexplained details of physical analysis but by making a fresh start; by *reading* the significance of brain and body activity. If this be correct, then indeed mind has "working contact" with matter, more intimate than that of one form of energy upon another; for they are complementary aspects of one and the same situation—the mysterious unity that we know as personal agency.

It is not that control by mind or consciousness is an exclusive *alternative* to control by a physical system—something which takes over where physical control leaves off. It is rather (we are suggesting) that a particular kind of complexity of control mechanism in an organism is (without detriment to its explicability in physical terms) the expression or embodiment of the personal agency of consciousness and mind.

Finally, regardless of the degrees of physical determinateness obtaining in such a mechanism, we have seen that no amount of physical knowledge of its state can generate a prediction of a typical decision which has binding logical force upon the agent whose brain it is. In short, our belief that we are normally free in making our choices, so far from being contradictable, *has no valid alternative* from the standpoint even of the most deterministic pre-Heisenberg physics (nor, a fortiori, of psychology). In this vital sense we must remain irreducibly responsible for the conscious control of action.

Abstract

By formalizing the general requirements for the organization of action in terms of the necessary flow of information and control, it has proved possible to throw some fresh light on the controlling function of the brain in voluntary agency.

From the elementary information flow map for goal-directed activity, a hierarchic organizing system is developed which can account for some key features of consciously controlled behavior. As a simple illustration of the concepts involved, the mechanism of the voluntary control of eye movement is discussed in the light of recent findings. It is shown that efficient adaptive behavior requires the development of an internally active metaorganizing system to determine the current norms and goal priorities of the main organizing system. The suggestion emerges that such metaorganizing activity may be a specific correlate of conscious awareness.

It is characteristic of such information flow maps that the path of control forms a *closed* loop. This might be thought to raise a doubt whether any model on these mechanistic lines could apply to human behavior in which we are conscious of a measure of freedom of choice.

The second part of the paper is devoted to meeting this objection. The argument hinges on a singular logical consequence of the assumed correlation between conscious experience and brain activity, which does not seem to have received sufficient attention. It is shown that in the case of a typical choice, even if the human information system were physically determinate in a pre-Heisenberg sense, it is impossible in principle to deduce, from the prior state of the world including the agent's brain, a prediction of his choice upon which agent and observer would be right to agree. More strongly, but for similar reasons, no prediction of it exists which is binding equally upon the observer and upon the agent whether the agent knows it or not. In this sense, typical human choices would be "logically indeterminate" even if the flow system that mediated them were physically determinate.

It is therefore suggested that the invocation of Heisenberg indeterminacy, though potentially relevant to our picture of spontaneous human activity, is logically unnecessary in order to make room for the kind of freedom that goes with responsible choice, and that objections a priori to a closed-loop model of the conscious human control of action are without foundation.

DISCUSSION

Chairman: PROFESSOR MOUNTCASTLE

TEUBER: I do think that Professor MacKay does himself and his scheme injustice if he keeps stressing that it is a general scheme into which new facts can hopefully be fitted, because I think it does have some considerable generative powers if we only look for them. We have a tendency to exploit information theory in physiology and psychophysiology primarily from the standpoint of rather elementary feedback notions, and the one thing that became particularly clear in today's presentation of your approach is the tremendous emphasis on what you call here "feedforward." This is what was, of course, very much on my mind when I commented on Professor Phillips' presentation earlier today.

I think one of our great embarrassments in coming to terms with the physiology of movement is that we always approach it from the wrong end. We are so constrained by classical spinal cord physiology that we always start at the sensory end and try to come out at the motor side. I very much agree with the late von Holst when he suggests that we start at the other end and work our why back toward sensation. I think that voluntary movement has physiologically distinctive properties that could fit into these feedforward notions, from motor to sensory, so exactly that we would suddenly see them after they have been before our eyes all along. It requires some different way of looking.

THORPE: Your scheme appears to me remarkably illuminating in relation to Professor Polanyi's ideas about knowledge being obtainable only by personal commitment. It seems to me to constitute just the right kind of physiological approach to a philosophical idea. Maybe I am looking at this in the wrong way: but if you have anything further to say on this subject I, for one, shall be most interested.

May I ask a further question which is perhaps a very naive one? You say that you have been sketching a system in which no physical action waits on anything but another physical action. That being so, supposing tomorrow absolutely conclusive proof of extrasensory perception was presented, what would your reaction to it be?

MAC KAY: I am inclined to wait until tomorrow comes before committing myself! If we had evidence of information flow that did not involve physical pathways, the *detailed* application of this model would be out of date; but since an information flow model need pay no regard to the nature of its channels, in principle the game could go on. We could seek to include extrasensory flow paths in our models of interpersonal interaction, and could ask perfectly good empirical questions: is this extra information coming into the cortical setup, or the midbrain organizing system, or where? So in principle, the game would go on, but we should perhaps speak of "informational action" rather than "physical action."

GOMES: Professor MacKay has remarked on the course of his exposition that there is a sort of similarity between the principle of physical relativity and a principle of logical relativity which, according to his views, one must resort to when considering the problem of free action. Although this remark was made only in passing, and might not seem specially important for him, it nevertheless provides a convenient starting point for the statement of what I consider to be an insuperable difficulty with his conception. Indeed, two observers situated in two differently moving systems will have different descriptions for the movements occurring in each of the systems. However, there are quite definite transformations for the formulas which adequately apply to the movements in relation to one of the systems and those about the same movements in relation to the other system; and, of course, there is also an invariant core of relationships which holds good in the two cases. There is nothing of this sort, however, when a movement is interpreted by a supposed agent as resulting from his own free deliberation, and, at the same time, by an external observer as absolutely inevitable because of the physical state of the supposed agent and the action of the physical environment on him. There is a change in the relationships among the several elements involved in the processes which no formula of transformation could account for. My point is then that in any case of that sort, the voluntaristic point of view of the so-called agent would be ultimately illusory. The point of view of the other, on the contrary, would be grounded on facts which the pretended agent would be unable to grasp directly.

MAC KAY: I mentioned physical relativity only to remind us that two accounts can differ without logically contradicting one another: indeed that the accounts of two people may *have to differ* in order that both be valid. With the agent and the observer, however, although there is a rigid transformation between the accounts, the transformation, oddly enough, is from a deterministic to an indeterministic one. It must be so, because no deterministic prediction could validly be believed by the agent; so the analogy with physical relativity departs at that point, and I did not mean to *argue* from it at all.

The important point is that we are dealing here not with statements about things but with statements about people. There is a kind of agreement possible in principle between observers of things, which would be invalid in principle for people discussing other people; and this is not meant as a mystical statement, but a statement of logical fact. If you simply ask "would the agent be right to believe this?" the answer is "no."

This marks the main point of contrast with arguments for free will based on Heisenberg indeterminacy. In the case of the electron, there is no self-contradiction in imagining the *existence* of a universally valid prediction of what it will do, even if no human being could ever know it. In the case of a free choice that you have not yet taken, however, *no prediction of it exists* (whether anyone knows it or not), which you would be right to believe, until *you* make the choice; that is what makes the choice your own.

BREMER: I wonder if it would not be interesting to test your organizing system hypothesis by the study of pure cases of apraxia, ideomotor apraxia. Pure, means unaccompanied by gross motor, sensory, or mental disturbances. In such cases the striking thing is that there is an obvious mismatch between what the subject desires to do and what he does really. In some cases that I have personally followed, which were neurosurgical ones, the mental condition of the patient appeared to be normal, and yet the incongruity was an enormous one, as if the organizing system you postulate was grossly disturbed. The interest of such cases of ideomotor apraxia is that one knows the cortical region which is affected. It is the supramarginal gyrus. Thus we have here a very definite situation where something is located in the brain which is neither sensory nor motor, which is organization *à l'état pur*.

MAC KAY: This is indeed what I would love to see. What I have sketched here is not so much a theory as a program, and it is exactly in such cases that the model could be useful in generating questions: for example, is this the result of a distorting operator in the normative system? is it the result of a failure of feedback from the monitoring system? etc. All these are operational questions.

CHAIRMAN: Could I enquire your reasons for making this tentative assignment of the metaorganizing system to the midbrain?

MAC KAY: In the first place, the metaorganizing system could be expected to be phylogenetically ancient, because the need for it would arise as soon as goal priorities had to be flexibly modifiable. Developmentally, one could think of this as coming before such things as the storage of subroutines and the need for a "labor exchange" to match subroutines to incoming demands. Both in terms of topography and the capacity required, I think that cortex offers itself in the latter rôle, and the midbrain-plus-limbic system in the former.

My second reason is, of course, the encouraging coincidence with the clinical picture that Professor Penfield and others have been uncovering, together with the split-brain discoveries of Professor Sperry.

CHAIRMAN: In the sense of communication engineering, would the meta-organizing system require a large number of elements?

MAC KAY: The metaorganizing system does not have to handle the highly redundant signals that the main organizing system does, so it would not require nearly as many elements as the detailed "labor market."

HINSHELWOOD: I would entirely agree with Professor MacKay that indeterminacy does not provide any analogy with free will. In physics, statistically, the course of events is perfectly determinate. The indeterminacy principle merely means that the phase structure of space and time has to be finite and not infinitesimally fine-grained: otherwise the structure of reality would collapse. I think the analogies, as you say, are quite unfair.

On the other hand, I am not quite happy about the relativity argument, because, of course, two observers do, in fact, agree in relativity provided they use the correct kinematics and not the incorrect pre-Einstein kinematics. Another point I would like to ask about is this: at a certain stage of your exposition you closed a circuit—an open-ended system. Could you just say a little more about the nature of that closing arm? It seems to me that it might contain something very important.

MAC KAY: The relativity analogy is limited; but, of course, agreement of a kind is possible between agent and observer. In retrospect, the agent could accept a movie of his own brain (taken before his choice) as validating the expectations of the observer. What he could not do, without self-contradiction, is to regard this as negating his own previous view.

The simplest example of a closed circuit setting a goal or norm might be a thermostat in which the target temperature setting was mechanically linked to some indicator, say, of fuel economy, or of overload. Here we have a situation where the job of goal setting is part of the function of the system itself. It is in a sense in command of its own goals.

JASPER: Some ten years ago during a comparable discussion in Canada, Professor Lashley objected to placing the metaorganizing system in the simpler parts of the brain stem by the statement that he felt that there were not enough cells here to provide for such a complex function. Essentially you are implying that this is a misconception of the problem. That the emphasis by many neurophysiologists on complexity in the brain has seemingly overlooked completely the fact that the brain is the greatest simplifier of any organ you can think of— that its real function is simplification of complexity—and I would ask you, if the information that you would assume was necessary to be transmitted to the metaorganizing system would necessarily be complex information? Could it not be extraordinarily simple to act as executive to the subcompartments of complexity which were the executors of the action?

MAC KAY: It would be sufficient for the metaorganizing system to receive a highly condensed representation—as, for example, a few graphic words can often suffice to delineate a whole scene. I would not, however, suggest that the cortex should be thought of as merely a simplifying "way station." The function of "advertising" and calling up subroutines to meet demands is important in its own right. For this, incidentally, it would require a far greater capacity than that of its metaorganizing monitor, which could treat the corresponding control signals as the "words" identifying the content of awareness.

REFERENCES

BARLOW, H. B. Possible principles underlying the transformation of sensory messages, in: *Sensory Communication* (ed. by W. A. Rosenblith). Cambridge, Mass. and New York: MIT Press and Wiley, pp. 217–234 [1961].

CONRAD, R. Errors of immediate memory, *Brit. J. Psychol.*, 50, 349–359 [1959].

DITCHBURN, R. W., and B. L. GINSBORG. Vision with a stabilized retinal image, *Nature*, 170, 36 [1952].

ELDRED, E., R. GRANIT, and P. A. MERTON. Supraspinal control of the muscle spindles, *J. Physiol.*, 122, 498 [1953].

GENGERELLI, J. A. Apparent movement in relation to homonymous and heteronymous stimulation of the cerebral hemispheres, *J. Exp. Psychol.*, 38 [1948].

GRANIT, R. *Receptors and Sensory Perception.* New Haven: Yale Univ. Press [1955].

GUREVITCH, B. Possible role of higher proprioceptive centres in the perception of visual space, *Nature*, 184, 1219–1220 [1959].

VON HOLST, E. Aktive Leistungen der menschlichen Gesichtswahrnehmung, *Studium Generale*, 10, 234 [1957].

———, and H. MITTELSTAEDT. Das Reafferenzprinzip, *Naturwiss.*, 37, 464 [1950].

KORNMÜLLER, A. E. Eine experimentelle Anästhesis der äusseren Augenmuskeln am Menschen und ihre Auswirkungen, *J. Psychol. Neurol.*, 41, 343–366 [1931].

MACKAY, D. M. Mindlike behaviour in artefacts, *Brit. J. Phil. Sci.*, II, 105–121 [1951]; also III, 352–353 [1953].

———. Mentality in machines, *Proc. Aristot. Soc. Suppt.*, XXVI, 61–86 [1952].

———. On comparing the brain with machines, *The Advancement of Science*, 40, 402–406 [1954]; also *Amer. Scientist*, 42, 261–268 [1954]; and *Ann. Report of Smithsonian Inst.*, 231–240 [1954].

———. Towards an information-flow model of human behaviour, *Brit. J. Psychol.*, 47, 30–43 [1956].

———. Operational aspects of intellect, *Mechanization of Thought Processes* (N.P.L. Symposium No. 10, 1958), H.M.S.O., 37–52 [1959].

MacKay, D. M. On the logical indeterminacy of a free choice, *Proc. XIIth Int. Congr. Phil.* (Venice), *III*, 249–256, 1958; also *Mind, 69*, 31–40 [1960].

————. Information and learning, in: *Learning Automata* (ed. by H. Billing). Munich: Oldenbourg, pp. 40–43 [1961].

————. The use of behavioural language to refer to mechanical processes, *Brit. J. Phil. Sci., XIII,* 89–103 [1962a].

————. Theoretical models of space perception, in: *Aspects of the Theory of Artificial Intelligence* (ed. by C. A. Muses). Plenum Press, pp. 83–104 [1962b].

————. Communication and meaning—a functional approach, in: *Cross-Cultural Understanding: Epistemology in Anthropology* (ed. by Northrop and Livingston). New York: Harper [1963a].

————. Freewill and causal prediction, in: *Cross-Cultural Understanding: Epistemology in Anthropology,* pp. 356–364 [1963b].

————. Brain and will, *The Listener* [May 9 and 16, 1957]; also (rev.) in: *Body and Mind* (ed. by G. N. A. Vesey). London: Allen & Unwin, pp. 392–402 [1964a].

————. Indeterminacy, uncertainty and information-content, *Nachrichtentechnische Z., 16,* 617–620 (in German) [1963]; also (in English) *NTZ-Communications J., 3,* 99–101 [1964b].

————. Information and prediction in human sciences, in: *Information and Prediction in Science* (ed. by S. Dockx and P. Bernays), Symposium of Int. Acad. for Philosophy of Science, 1962. New York: Academic Press [1965a].

————. Visual noise as a tool of research, *J. Gen. Psychol., 72,* 181–197 [1965b].

————. A mind's eye view of the brain, in: *Cybernetics of the Nervous System* (ed. by N. Wiener and J. P. Schadé), Progress in Brain Research, *17,* Amsterdam: Elsevier [1965c], pp. 321–332.

Matthews, P. B. C. Muscle spindles and their motor control, *Physiol. Rev., 44,* 219–288 [1964].

Merton, P. A. The silent period in a muscle of the human hand, *J. Physiol., 114,* 183–198 [1951].

Miller, G. A. The magical number 7 plus or minus 2, *Psychol. Rev., 63,* 81–97 [1956].

Popper, K. R. Indeterminism in quantum physics and in classical physics, *Brit. J. Phil. Sci.,* I, Part I, 117–133; Part II, 173–195 [1950].

Shannon, C. E., and W. Weaver. *The Mathematical Theory of Communication.* Springfield: Univ. of Illinois Press [1949].

Sperry, R. W. Cerebral organization and behaviour, *Science, 133,* 1749 [1961].

Vickers, G. The psychology of policy-making and social change, *Brit. J. Psychiat., 110,* 465–477 [1964].

Walshe, F. M. R. The brain-stem conceived as the "highest level" of function in the nervous system, *Brain, 80,* 510–539 [1957].

Wiener, N. *Cybernetics.* New York: Wiley [1948].

18

The Brain-Consciousness Problem in Contemporary Scientific Research

by A. O. GOMES

Universidade do Brasil, Rio de Janeiro, Brazil

THE TWO-WAY ASPECT OF THE PROBLEM

Among the different formulations of the brain-consciousness problem in the modern scientific world, Sherrington's has become the most widely known—and, if we can say this of the statement of a puzzle, the most cherished one. Sherrington's exceptional stature as a scientist, allied to the sincerity, directness, and wise humility of spirit so vividly revealed in his writings, easily explains the success of his formulation of the problem. How can physical sense receptors affect sense? he asks. How can a reaction in the brain condition a reaction in the mind? How can the (often quoted!) "enchanted loom" of nerve impulses in the brain, which always weaves meaningful, but never abiding, patterns—how can this "loom" evoke such rich mental experiences as the vision of everything we see, all the sounds we hear, all the bodily sensations we may ever become aware of? Mind is not physical energy such as compose the electrical impulses, Sherrington proceeds, and no process occurring only with physical energy could produce "mind out of no mind." Yet, "unless mind have working contact with energy, how can energy serve it?" "The energy-scheme brings us to the threshold of the act of perceiving, and there . . . bids us good-bye." The difficulty with sense, Sherrington also recognizes, is the same difficulty from the converse side, as besets the problem of the mind as influencing our motor acts. The extent and moment of this question, he acknowledges with another very cogent, almost pathetic expression: "Physics tells me that my arm cannot be bent without disturbing the sun. Physics tells me that unless my mind is energy it cannot disturb the sun." Yet, the theoretically impossible happens; and despite the theoretical, as Sherrington [1955] puts it, the mind does bend the arm and thus disturbs the sun.

Of course, the question of a reaction in the central nervous system affecting a reaction in the mind is not restricted to the case of perception, which Sherrington more closely insisted on. The relation of the complex interweaving of electrical impulses in the brain to other types of mental experience defines no less challenging puzzles for us. Since the time of the height of Sherrington's career, scientific research has disclosed a whole wealth of new facts pertaining to that relationship, the most striking of which may have been those obtained by the technique of artificial stimulation of the brain by means of either chronically implanted electrodes that penetrate to the most central regions of the organ, or by means of mere contact probes that survey the exposed surface of the cortex. The behavior of the animals with which the chronic electrode experiments are conducted is reported to indicate most significant alterations of emotional experience—enhancement, for instance of a mood of meekness or, on the contrary, of anger, even changes from one to the other—as well as sensations such as hunger, thirst, and sexual appetite. As to the electrical exploration of the exposed cortex, which has been performed during cerebral surgery in human subjects affected with epilepsy—we actually have in this congress the greatest authority in the world on this technique—it has yielded, besides vague experiences of sounds, lights, and colors, when the appropriate regions are stimulated, recollections and approximate relivings of past events, as well as definite interpretations of the experiences which, of course, should also be counted among their significant features.

The widely known facts referred to here up to this point have all come to light in the laboratory or the hospital room, and have all been elicited by the specialized work of experts. They are thus the facts of the most immediate interest for a scientific review of the general problem with which they are connected, but it seems convenient and pertinent to supplement their mention with that of other events which frequently come about in the current life of nearly everybody, but which ultimately have the same meaning as the phenomena specified above. Sometimes there is again the work of the scientists, or of the expert, in some other sense, behind the events: for instance, when we take a tranquilizer pill which may change a feeling of anxiety or restlessness into one of calm and relief; or when we resort to some analgesic in order to put an end to some uncomfortable pain. Other times, the phenomena are still simpler, as in the case of the profound changes in our mood which may—and often do—follow the ingestion of alcoholic drinks; or even in the case of a more drastic, though fortunately less frequent transformation of mental state as, for instance, the one that may result from a vigorous blow in the head—which is no less than a change from full consciousness to the complete cessation of it.

Of course, there is no difference, for our problem, between the action of physical and of chemical stimuli, since, at the level in which the phenomena must be investigated in the nervous system, that distinction does not ultimately hold in any sharp form. However, the explicit mention of chemical stimulation immediately brings up at least two other cases beside those few already specified here: hallucinogenic drugs and medical anesthesia.

The second general aspect of the brain-consciousness problem is that which Sherrington has dramatically stated with the reflexion of how could his mind move his arm and, thus, affect the sun itself. Scientific research has on the whole been rather biased against this side of the problem, and more often than not has tended to reduce it either to the first aspect, or simply to another problem that is not so puzzling; it has tacitly or explicitly admitted that the mental processes apparently at the origin of the physiological or bodily changes are merely the result, in turn, of some former physiological courses of events. As a result of this, research is frequently conducted as if the whole occurrences under study were ultimately nothing more than the transformations of some physiological events into others; the mental phenomena involved are either ignored or given only a secondary importance. They are thus regarded as no more than apparent relays between physiological occurrences or, more exactly, as epiphenomena of the initial part of these occurrences. Of course, there are several cases of the control of bodily action—mostly those of the demonstrably simplest reflex nature—where physiological processes are in truth nearly everything worth being investigated. But this is very far from being the general case, since, more usually, the problem of that control coincides, to a very significant extent, with the problem of free action, which, for multiple and obvious reasons, is at the very core of a host of other questions about individual and social life in general—including the fundamental question of communication of ideas between persons. Thus it is no wonder that Sherrington should have been so impressed with the momentous character of that problem, that he preferred to admit that what for him was theoretically impossible—that is, his mind moving his arm and thus affecting the sun—actually happens.

Owing to the scientific nature of the present symposium, I shall not develop the last remarks into any discussion of philosophical matters. Nor shall I even simply mention the immense and complex catalogue of topics that the subject of brain-consciousness relations also evokes in the specific field of philosophy. Suffice here to say—and this only as a partial explanation of the divergence of interpretations frequently found among scientists concerning many facts that they disclose and analyze in the field now under revision—suffice here to say that the significance of our general problem is also so great for philosophy, when translated into its specific terms, that practically all the chief currents of the philosophy of nature, and even some of the main conceptions of the theory of knowledge, can be fairly characterized in their outlines by the particular conception which each of them entertains about it—either explicitly or by implication.

As a matter of fact, it is not only the interpretation of the phenomena which is open to wide variability and, with it, to some arbitrariness. It is also the very questions that spontaneously define themselves by the disclosed facts: they may take for granted what is not definitely established, or elucidated, either by science or by philosophy.

THE QUESTION OF INDETERMINATE ORDER

The nervous control of action has so far been systematically and detailedly studied only with the application of the principles of prequanta physics. Of course, there is still an almost inexhaustible wealth of material to be significantly explored with the application of only those principles —and hardly any opportunity yet for the specific employment of quantum physics to any branch of the empirical investigation of the nervous system. Yet, the idea that the great novelty that came to light in quantum theory —microphysical incertitude—might play a significant role in the nervous control of action, and, on account of this, might allow a great and decisive advance in the scientific understanding of the steerage of free action—that idea, I say, was to some degree entertained by several scientists shortly after the development of quantum mechanics and the establishment of the uncertainty relations. Bohr himself was one of the first to sketch some conjectures about the subject [Bohr, 1932]. Eddington discussed it [1928, 1935]. Pascual Jordan devoted a great deal of attention to the topic and elaborated the conception of amplification of results of discrete, uncertain events [*La Physique et le Secret de la Vie Organique*]. Herman Weyl, James Jeans, and, for a time, Louis de Broglie [Weyl, 1949] have at least occasionally considered the new ideas. Elsasser has more recently returned to them [Elsasser, 1958]. And Eccles conducted some brief computations about the subject and made a short review of it [Eccles, 1953, Chapt. VIII], which was perhaps the first and only instance of discussion of these matters in the context of a work of neurophysiology. The author of the present paper has also made an approximate quantitative analysis to verify the amplitude of uncertainty to which some of the chief components of the physiology of neurons could be subject, and he has found that that amplitude may be in different cases quantitatively compatible with the possibility of the occurrence of differentiable processes of amplification of discrete, uncertain events.[1]

However, the criticism raised from different quarters against the incipient conceptions very soon became more intense and widely accepted than the new attempts themselves. Several arguments have been forwarded in opposition to the novel ideas, the least tenable, but not the least frequent of which, stating that according to the new physics, physical indetermination can hold good only in the microphysical level, and never be translated into macrophysical processes. Another argument is, however, apparently very pertinent; it stresses the complete inadequacy of the resort to phenomena that are characterized above all by randomness—such as discrete microevents—for the elucidation of processes as elaborate and rich of order, significance, and motivations of several sorts as those of free action, or of life in general. Yet this argument takes for granted that whoever speculates about a possible relation between micro-incertitude and free action necessarily commits the gross mistake of attempting simply to reduce the latter to the former, or explain the one by the other. Schroedinger has unfortunately been one of those who developed a criticism based only on that unfair assumption [Schroedinger, 1952]—and he tried to strengthen his position with references to a very powerful thinker, Cassirer, who made suppositions to the same effect [Cassirer, 1937]. However, it seems only too obvious that what can be logically expected of microuncertainty in the physiological control of action is only the establishment and the maintenance of conditions different from those which would impose a completely deterministic work for the nervous system, which can thus become, in principle, favorable for the occurrence of free action—never the whole key to this action. Schroedinger [1952] again expressed another objection to the same hypothesis, which would seem much more pertinent than the former; and approximately the same argument has also been stated by Eddington [1928]. It says that there is certainly no determinism, according to the quantum theory, in the occurrence of discrete microevents; yet, when these repeat themselves in the same circumstances, the resultant series of events obey statistical laws which, of course, are not much more compatible with free action than the deterministic laws of classical physics; as a consequence, free action could only profit by microphysical incertitude if it violated the statistical laws of those series, so ultimately there would be no smaller interference with the regularity of the physical world than a break with the classical, deterministic laws. However, this is once more an objection that oversimplifies the hypothesis against which it is directed. It would

---

[1] A part of these computations has appeared in a paper [Gomes, 1955, 1956] which also incorporated other reflections on the subject.

be decisive if that hypothesis stated that free action is directly and almost exclusively controlled in each living organism by microphysical indeterminate controls—that is, amplifying systems with output not completely and uniquely determined by the input, or a series of discrete microphysical events with effects amplifiable within a macrophysical structure and somehow connected by this structure, which, in the case of a living being, would be some part of the organism. If, on the contrary, we suppose, as we should, that such controls—preferably, but not even necessarily in a very large number—are coupled to other controls of physically determinate nature (that is, with the output completely and uniquely determined by the input), the coupling of all of them can be such that the steerage of which the whole set is capable results in macrophysical work that is at the same time ordered and indeterminate, without this requiring either the violation of the statistical regularity of each indeterminate control or the translation of the statistical character of that regularity into any output of the steered system that is not an exceedingly long run.

A MERELY PHYSICAL ILLUSTRATION

In truth, if a machine is steered by a complex interlocking of several units of indeterminate and determinate control, the number of states it can come to under the determining influence of the overall controlling situations of the steerage system can be as large, in principle, as the number of the combinations among the differentiated indeterminate configurations possible for each unit of indeterminate control. Yet, while planning the system, we can easily do it in such a way that only the controlling situations which can be interpreted as orderly are allowed to work out their influence. But the selection among these would still be indeterminate, because dependent on physically uncertain processes. This principle can be true both of the final situations of the machine considered statically, and of the successions among them—which means that these successions themselves can also be made at the same time well ordered and indeterminate.

It would be convenient to introduce a concrete illustration of a case of this nature. To this effect, let us imagine, as a unit of indeterminate control, a cylindrical vacuum chamber with a very tiny aperture in the center of one of its transversal walls, and a ring with a certain number of differentiated parts electrically insulated from one another and each of them connected to a high-sensitivity detector amplifier capable of responding to discrete manifestations of electrons of very low energy over the corresponding area of the ring. Let us also suppose a source of low-energy electrons before the aperture in the first wall, and a low accelerating difference of potential between the two ends of the chamber. If the aperture is small enough, each electron which penetrates the chamber will have its spatial localization very sharply defined, and will consequently suffer a physically indeterminate disturbance of momentum, with the magnitude given by the uncertainty relations of Heisenberg. The chamber can be so constructed that the medium diameter of the ring in the second transversal wall coincides with the region of the most probable manifestation of the indeterminately disturbed electrons. The place where each electron will appear upon this ring—and thus upon one or other of its several differentiated parts—is completely indeterminated, and the laws of microphysics require only that in sets of relatively large numbers of individual manifestations their distribution be uniform along the circumference of the ring, and thus that the number of the discrete arrivals upon each part of it be approximately equal for all of them. There is, however, absolutely no law for the localization of a particular manifestation upon the ring or for the step-to-step successions.[2]

If we connect some macrophysical gadget to each of the detector

[2] Processes of amplification of discrete, indeterminate microphysical events come about in several laboratory experiments, and even in some gadgets of current use in some sectors, such as Geiger counters. The device proposed here affords a sharper and more cogent illustration of them.

In a chamber 10 cm long, with an aperture 1.55×10^{-5} cm in one of the transversal walls, the ring of maximum probability of manifestation of perturbed electrons on the opposite wall will have a diameter of nearly 2.5 mm, if the accelerating difference of potential is 0.1 volt.

In fact, the wavelength of the so-called de Broglie wave associated to each of the disturbed electrons is defined by the expression:

$$\lambda = \frac{12.2 \times 10^{-8}}{\sqrt{U}} = \frac{12.2 \times 10^{-8}}{\sqrt{0.1}} = 38.4 \times 10^{-8} \text{ cm}$$

and the corresponding angle of perturbation of moment by

$$\sin \alpha = \frac{\lambda}{\Delta l} = \frac{38.4 \times 10^{-8}}{1.55 \times 10^{-5}} = 0.0248$$

which angle defines a ring of maximum probability of manifestation of uncertainly disturbed electrons nearly with the dimension specified above.

The chief difficulty with the unit proposed here might be the maintenance of a really discrete rhythm of electronic emissions of very low energy, through the tiny aperture of the chamber. If we admit higher accelerating differences of potential, the diameter of the ring of maximum probability of manifestations of disturbed electrons will shrink (at a given distance from the point of perturbation) and the construction of the chamber will become more difficult. Yet, we might in this case employ the second or the third ring of probability (corresponding to values of n higher than 1, in the Heisenberg relations), with the added advantage of a more discrete rhythm of arrivals of electrons upon the ring. Photonic radiation could also be resorted to, in principle, instead of electrons. A radiation of, say, 5,000 Å would have its ring of maximum probability with a diameter of nearly 1 cm at a distance of only 20 cm from an orifice 10^{-3} cm wide. And, of course, we can also think of some adaptation of the systems of high-energy electrons employed in the current experiments of diffraction.

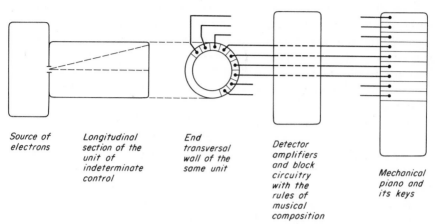

Source of electrons

Longitudinal section of the unit of indeterminate control

End transversal wall of the same unit

Detector amplifiers and block circuitry with the rules of musical composition

Mechanical piano and its keys

Fig. 18.1. Plan for an orderly but physically indeterminate machine.

amplifiers coupled to the several elements of the ring, and have those gadgets performing some macrophysical operation under the switch-on, switch-off command of the detector amplifiers, in such a way that they are put to work or to rest every time that a disturbed electron manifests itself upon the corresponding part of the ring, the assembly as a whole will constitute a macrophysical system completely undetermined in the order of its final operations. We can imagine, for instance, a jukebox with the selection of its records commanded by a unit of indeterminate control, or some sort of roulette under the same guidance.

So far, our device illustrates only physical indetermination in a series of macrophysical processes which can be in themselves either very simple —the case of the roulette—or very elaborate—the case of the reproduction of a record in the jukebox. With the further purpose of illustrating order which is significantly indeterminate all along its development, let us now imagine a piano Fig. 18.1 with a certain number of keys—say, 100—and the activation of each of these keys decided by the output of one indeterminate control with a corresponding number of possible different states. Let the connection between this device of indeterminate control and the final mechanism of activation of the keys pass through circuitry specially designed to switch it off every time that the message started a unit that does not conform to a set of rules of musical composition which can be translated into the intermediary circuitry.[3] This circuitry may, of

[3] The construction of any such circuitry would define only a relatively easy task for the contemporary technique of design of computers, automata, and systems of control in general.

course, incorporate a recording mechanism for all the operations of the system; and the rules of composition may accordingly state that after the successful activation of one key of the piano, only a few other keys—say, 5 among the 100—may follow. The rules may also be such that in certain special cases they condition the activation of a new key in a sequence, not only to the immediately preceding element, but also to whole previous passages of the sequence; and they may as well comprehend other factors of musical composition such as rhythm and harmony of simultaneously sounding notes. Yet, as long as each new step in the musical succession admits more than one possibility which is in turn decided by the indeterminate control, the output of the instrument will also remain undetermined, irrespectively of the high degree of order and organization which it can maintain.

Now, if elaborate and ordered, but physically uncertain and, in not very long runs, statistically irregular work is thus possible for merely physical machines, it is clearly also possible, in principle, for living beings —very specially for those with a highly developed nervous system. Such a nervous system may house millions or billions of nearly simultaneous processes equivalent to those described in connection with a unit of indeterminate control, and have all these connected according to the most elaborate interlocking; hence it can afford the opportunity for the accomplishment of sequences of meaningful, organized, and not-statistically monotonous behavior, very far exceeding in length of time the span of individual life.

In exceedingly long stretches of work, certain statistical regularities would in principle be rediscovered. But they would ultimately mean nothing more than, say, the statistical regularity of biological or social phenomena in their broadest scale, which, important and significative as they may be to the study of those phenomena in that scale, do not in the least account for a host of events that, for one reason or other, may be of the greatest possible significance, not only for nonstatistical sciences but also for other forms of interpretation of phenomena extremely meaningful and important for us.

During the last decades, certain devices have been designed and constructed which harness what are apparently indeterminate variations, or trial-and-error processes, into well-ordered sequences of behavior, or which simply associate the two by means of the employment of the so-called random generators. The work of Ross Ashby, Grey Walter, and other cyberneticians in that field is already widely known. However, the type of system and processes outlined above is like the reverse, in a very important sense, of what those other devices accomplish and exemplify —in spite of all the significant points of contact between the two cases. In fact, in the system proposed here as an illustration of the basic compatibility between physical indeterminacy and elaborate organization, the indeterminacy is ultimately real and absolutely irreducible to any sort of implicit physical laws; and the influence which the indeterminate events have on the system is not merely a restricted interference with what would otherwise be a completely defined determinate work. It is much more than that, since the indetermination actually occurs between the input and the output of the system; and, thus, contrary to the case of the cybernetic devices which incorporate "random-generators," does not manifest itself only in processes which can be ultimately regarded as a part of the input of the devices. Each new indeterminate step in the musical sequence "composed" by the piano outlined here is most significantly decisive for the whole rest of the sequence; and no sign of randomness properly could be discovered in the sequence. Music itself would be its order.

"Order-from-Disorder"

However, although it is thus clearly possible to put randomness and statistical regularity at the service of elaborate order in macrosystems significantly affected by discrete microevents, we should not overlook what is actually random, or merely statistically regular, in life, when we speculate about the possible role, or presence, of microincertitude in the steerage of living organisms. Schroedinger supposed that the transition from randomness into regularity or, as he calls it, the "order-from-disorder" principle, was an exclusive feature of the inanimate world, and that living matter might even be distinguished from inorganic matter by its observance of the different principle of "order-from-order" [Schroedinger, 1944]. There are, however, too many striking and ponderous exceptions to this rule for it to be attributed such an importance. Let us initially remark, in passing, that the semblance of a change of indetermination into order, in the work of devices such as those designed by Ashby and Walter, is exactly one of the chief reasons why they are often regarded as remarkably similar to living beings. Let us then notice that few things can look more haphazard than, for instance, the behavior of a unicellular organism, which, nevertheless, accomplishes what it must in order to survive or to fulfill the tasks it has to serve. No less random in aspect are also the variations of the physical shape of different intracellular structures which perform definite, ordered functions, among different specimens of a same species, and even in the same unicellular specimen along different moments of its life. The development of plants within a genus is again subject to a very wide random diversity. And once more liable to the same type of variation are the most typical behavioral patterns of several animals. The detailed study of some bird species, for instance, has led Professor Thorpe to remark "puzzling irregularities, uncertainties, and differences in individual and specific behavior" [Thorpe, 1961], an observation which certainly falls in with that made by other members of the ethologist school.

The research work of this school has, in fact, disclosed that the instinctive behavior of many vertebrates, which so often looks like a set of functional wholes very well ordered in all their several stages of development and completely predetermined from the start in all their chief features, is, as a matter of fact, open to a number of fortuitous variations. There are indeed well-determined innate action patterns, but these are often far from covering whole instinctive and behavioral functions, and thus also far from coming already mounted in broader schemes adapted to the functions—no matter whether or not they are among the most important which the animal will have to perform. The functional wholes are the later product of complex combinations, sometimes called "instinct-training interlockings," among innate and acquired patterns—such random flexibility prevailing in the shaping of the second of these patterns as well as in the processes of their compounding with the first ones that individual cases not infrequently arise quite out of harmony with what would be the normal rule, or the normal function. Many a most bizarre situation may then be defined. Let us just remember, at this juncture, the extremely curious—and sometimes delightful—observations of such phenomena which Lorenz has so vividly recorded and analyzed. Referring to the work conducted with chimpanzees by another ethologist, Schiller—a scientist of as strong behavioristic tendencies as Lashley—has textually said the following: "Playful manipulation is the instinctive response to objects. The acts are performed with no prescience of usefulness, and in the problem situation the very acts which might solve the problem may be performed in such way as to prevent success. The appropriateness of the act for such a task as getting food is discovered only by chance" [Lashley, 1957].

The shaping and the maintenance of order in conjunction with fortuity is thus something very currently accomplished in the biological domain with much ampler random variation and an even more unmistakable resource to haphazard procedures than in the merely physical machines of the type conjectured above, which can be made to work at the same time orderly and indeterminately. And if, on the one hand, we may suppose —without lapsing into simple fantasy—that microphysical incertitude affects the nervous system according to schemes in many points physically equivalent to those outlined here, we have to admit, on the other hand, that there is not even an invariably direct proportionality between degree of development of nervous system and ordered complexity of behavior physically controlled by it. This fact is more frequently and strikingly apparent during the early stages of individual life, but not always only then. The behavior of some insects is at the same time extremely more elaborate and regular than that of a very large number of fully grown vertebrates which, nevertheless, are endowed with incomparably more developed nervous systems.

If we consider, in addition, that no other transformation of haphazard, trial-and-error methods into rich and advanced order is accomplished between extremes as far apart as those defined by the behavior of human babies on the one side, and adult human behavior on the other, we shall certainly tend to conclude logically and realistically that the fully developed nervous system must be much more apt to work on the disorder-to-order principle than on the order-to-order one. If things are really so, the matchlessly intricate organization of the system provides us, not only with examples of striking coordination of all-the-time determinate functions —which are unmistakably always present, from the very start of individual life—but with no less remarkable instances as well, of a gradual fashioning of order against a background of randomness.

The systematic study of behavior of human infants furnishes indications basically in agreement with those we can get from the investigation of animal behavior—in spite of the very significant fact that the behavior of human beings is much more rudimentary, at its individual beginnings, than that of so many other animals species. The poverty of early human behavior does not exclude, of course, a number of definite reflex and automatic action schemes; but these, as in the case of the animals studied by the ethologists, do not come organized into broad, elaborate, instinctual, or functional wholes. Before this organization takes shape and acquires enduring structures, the accomplishment of some basic functions depend, to a significant extent (that is, in nearly all that is not achieved with learned external guidance), on random activity. This activity at best, but not always, betrays only the semblance of a purposeful groping, and no more than a monotonous statistical regularity. As a matter of fact, a theory has already been advanced which asserts that the adaptation of the human infant to the different circumstances that he will have to live with is fundamentally effected by means of trial-and-error methods, that is, groping. Piaget, who does not subscribe to the "groping" theory in its simplest and most radical form, does not fail, however, to recognize explicitly the occurrence and the importance of random activity in the early development of infants [see, for instance, Piaget, 1959].

It might also be pertinent, at this moment, to make just a general reference to the role of play in the behavioral and mental development of the child. I would not attempt, of course, to identify play with random activity. Yet, there is no denying that one of the basic modalities of play—and one widely practiced by infants, as well as by animals—presents a characteristically random element in its development. It is the kind of a mere exercise of activity, which Piaget calls "practice games" [Piaget, 1951]. Besides, if there is not anything properly random in the other modalities of play, there is nothing there either, which denotes strictly determined order. Play is always characterized as a reverse of compulsion. Even in the case of games with definite and complex rules, these rules are there as if to define a structure within which, or around which, free variation can manifest itself; so that play actually provides a very cogent illustration for the conception of free order.

THE SCIENCES OF THE INDIVIDUAL PAST AND GROWTH

Now, it is also very important to stress the obvious fact that the substitution of order for haphazard in the life of organic beings is a process essentially dependent on the past achievements and experiences of each specimen in its environment. To recognize this fact is to recognize also that the study of that substitution must have the form of a genetic theory. In turn, just a simple reflection on the truth that a finite, individual life in a certain environment identifies itself to a great extent with the history of its mental and motor activity in its environment—just a simple reflection on this and, of course, merely on the chief structural features of the several types of experience and of motor action, is sufficient for the establishment of a general conception of genetic science comprehending and unifying all the different branches of genetic studies which are separately developed today.

Some chapters of ethology, which are exerting a strong influence upon other types of animal research, investigate the relatively quick establishment of some previously undecided marked features of animal behavior and psychism (let us just remember the study of "imprinting") and the no less quick growth of order in them, as well as the deep connections which prevail between the characteristic types of action by means of which an animal asserts its specific presence in the environment, and the perception which this animal must have of the world. Genetic psychology in its stricter sense, such as developed by Piaget and his associates, conducts approximately equivalent research about the human infant, where, of course, the shaping of order is much slower and more complex, and the initial indetermination in many points correspondingly much broader. It also investigates how the intellect develops on the basis of the food provided to it by the senses; and how the perception of the external world, and of the body itself, is gradually defined and enriched by means of relationships with motor actions no less profound than in the case of animals. In turn, theoretical psychoanalysis concentrates its attention upon the effects that the emotional components of experience—which so often, though not always, may, once more, have a fortuitous appearance on the scene—work on the development of human personality. Animal psychology again is starting on a course of research which reproduces, in principle, the chief task of theoretical psychoanalysis—allowing, however, for the immense differences between the two cases. Of course, the field of study in this case is much less ample and interesting, but it profits by the advantage that in it we can tamper with the functional factors under observation to an extent that would be inadmissible in the study of human beings.[4]

We should only not fail to notice, when referring to psychoanalysis as a tool for the elucidation of the genetic processes of the mind—and of some organic phenomena as well, as psychosomatic medicine clearly discloses—that it is regrettable that the discipline should still be fragmented into a number of different currents which are often vainly engaged in warring against each other on the basis of gratuitous or exaggerated assumptions and of the no less artificial exclusion and denial of the more reasonable points that each rival school stresses. It is, however, not difficult to discern what is the product of bias in the several currents, and which are the contributions that we can—and should—accept from each of them. The degree of harmony that ultimately prevails among those contributions is remarkable—and it should not surprise us at all, since it very understandably derives from the unified nature of the human mind.[5]

If we now also stress the fact that the several branches of the genetic studies point to, and very often fully accept, the necessity of investigating action and experience together, and not as if they were sharply separate functions, we immediately become aware of an additional weighty reason for the fundamental importance of the genetic sciences for the general brain-consciousness problem. Indeed, it seems clear that any joint

[4] I am now referring, of course, to the investigation of the influence of emotional factors in animal development. As a matter of fact, this type of investigation is not so new. It has ultimately been amply conducted by Pavlov, for instance, who, nevertheless, was narrow mindedly concerned with only the physiological aspects of the phenomena, and stubbornly bent on ignoring—if not on explicitly denying—the mental side of them. Even the study of "imprinting" conducted in ethology may have some relations to the present subject. Lorenz himself has not failed to notice this (in an article which appears in Schroedinger [1944], p. 104); and Fletcher [1957] has also indirectly dwelt on the question.

[5] Only Jung's conception is more refractory on account of the insistence on collective factors in individual minds. It is not either difficult or gratuitous, though, to propound schemes of individual genesis to the facts that have particularly attracted Jung's attention.

study of experience and action disclosing and analyzing their interweaving should be regarded ultimately as an integral part of the study of the relations between nervous system and mind. While some branches of genetic investigation disclose the most direct aspects of the compounds —for instance, between perception and motor activity, both in the cases of animals and of human infants—others reveal only more indirect and variable connections; however, the latter are scarcely less significant. Adler's analysis of individual somatic peculiarities as genetic factors in the development of personality, for instance, illustrates that second type of relations.

The forms of prevalence of the connections between mind and experience indicate, in addition, that we should not even regard the two chief aspects of the general brain-consciousness problem, specified with the help of Sherrington's cogent terms at the beginning of this paper, as reflecting, in principle, a sharp dualism. The traffic between mind and action is in truth so complex, and it also develops itself along such deep and tortuous channels, that it is often not possible to distinguish clearly between two definitely opposite directions in it. This is a situation of which neurology, neurophysiology and general experimental psychology have also become sharply aware; and which resulted, among other things, in, for instance, the abandonment of the old notion of a sharply defined separation between sensorial and motor areas in the cortex. The specific contribution of the genetic sciences to this topic is, of course, the insistence on the absolutely decisive role of the past experience of a living being in the molding of the compounds between action and experience; it is also the converse revelation that this process remains at the very core of the general transformations of the innate capabilities determined by the specific structure of the sensorial, nervous and motor systems peculiar to each species into complex actualities by far richer and more organized —very specially in the case of man—than those that constitute inaugural experience and behavior.[6]

MEMORY, A CENTRAL TOPIC

The last considerations about the genetic sciences of mind and action spontaneously introduce the final topic to be explicitly dealt with in this

---

[6] There would be no point in repeating here the brief indications about this fact already forwarded in this paper. Nor is the dimension of this work compatible with the reproduction of more detailed illustrations. The literature on the subject is abundant. Above all, the different works by Piaget and his associates should be consulted for the case of individual human development. Besides the two other books specified in previous notes, The Child's Construction of Reality [Piaget, 1955] is among the most helpful and elucidating of his monographs.

brief survey. It could also have been no less naturally arrived at from the area of neurophysiology and neurology, and even from the area of psychology again, for all of which the topic—memory, of course—is scarcely less important than for the specifically genetic sciences. On memory hinges all that is not just the simple beginning of a finite, individual life. And in the light of it—or, if we so prefer to say, with the due consideration of it—it is necessary to make a revision of the facts that more strikingly and urgently define our general problem in the domain of science.[7]

Let us very briefly consider just a few examples such as the following: a hallucinogenic drug is ingested and rich sensorial experiences are induced, without correspondence with the normal external stimulation; the result would certainly not be the same in a child with only a poor stock of individual experience; the hallucination provoked by the drug is not a sort of simple product of it, but much rather an elaboration of individual past experiences. An electrode penetrates a central region of the brain of an animal and transmits an electrical stimulus; as a consequence of it, the animal may be compelled to go through an intricate maze in the experimental grounds where it is placed in order to reach a place where it can drink water, and, there, compulsively drink it out of proportion with its normal needs; once more the reaction is not merely an epiphenomenon of the artificial stimulus; the past experience of the animal—even that which becomes past during the very development of the reaction—informs and guides the whole process, from its beginning to its end. Some abnormal organic state provokes a crisis of mental depression in us: everything we then think and do depends on what, in our individual past, is behind the new, organically induced difficulty we have to face; even the pitch of the crisis will depend, among other things, on the way in which we have reacted to similar critical situations we may have come through in the past, on the memories we may seek in order to fortify ourselves against the onset of the depression, or, on the contrary, on those of even more unfavorable nature than the new crisis, which may compulsorily present themselves to heighten it. We may also profitably resort to a chemical stimulant which will help the restoration of our emotional balance: what the drug ultimately does then is to introduce a new basic component into our experience which, in turn, facilitates the intervention of invigorating recollections to which we may have appealed in vain before, but which will now have the chance to substitute themselves for the gloomy, obsessive ideas that were previously emerging from our store of experiences.

No experience is in truth instantaneous—every experience carries por-

---

[7] Let us just remark, in passing, that the philosophical moment of the topic of memory is not smaller.

tions of the past along with it, or, conversely, is carried on by those portions. Reasoning is obviously inconceivable without the presence of at least some recent past; without it no argument—nay, no simple, bare statement —can acquire meaning. Perception, which may at a first inspection seem more independent from the memory of previous experiences, is ultimately not less dependent on it. Very often, in the current phenomenon of "constancy," some privileged feature of an experience is asserted, or maintained as such, out of proportion with the corresponding physical stimulation. This phenomenon, which usually passes unnoticed, is so important for the structure of our mental life in general, and has understandably so vividly attracted the attention of researchers, that, referring to it, Professor Granit has pertinently asked whether we could have ever succeeded in intuiting the very conception of constancy in general—that is, in the sense that it has in current and philosophical language—if the phenomenon were lacking [Granit, 1955]. Constancy of perception obviously illustrates, not only the presence of the recent past in it, that is, of the past not yet separated in time from the experience that is being lived, but also the role of the more remote individual past [8]—as seems to be indicated by the facts that in very young children, who still have a relatively poor accumulation of past experience, the phenomenon is less intense,[9] and that deliberate training may sometimes modify the function [Hirst, 1959].

If, thus, in practically all cases of the mutual influences between nervous system and experience—including those in which there is manifestly no direct relationship between an experience and the corresponding physical stimulation—the most significant mediation of individual past experience is to be found, the topic of memory can indeed be only thoroughly challenging to that crucial science of the relations between brain and mind, neurophysiology—for which it also ultimately is the problem of learning, habit, training, and conditioning themselves.

[8] The orthodox followers of the Gestalt theory, who have often conducted such remarkable research work on the constancy of perception, have stubbornly tried to deny the participation of past experience in the phenomenon, possibly because it might amount, in their view, to an instance of mechanical associationism—the conception they so tenaciously and justifiably oppose. Yet, since the orthodox Gestaltists themselves admit the presence of different elements in the Gestalts, there is no a priori reason, it seems, why past experiences could not be equally present in the wholes. Their contribution would certainly not represent a necessary contradiction to the chief features of the Gestalts. The main objections of the Gestaltists to the idea of a participation of past experience in the constancy phenomenon disappears if—just as we should do—we admit the influence of the remote past too and recognize that the influence of the past does not require an intervention of intellectual functions (which makes room for the presence of the phenomenon in animals too).

[9] See, for instance, Piaget [1955], pp. 149, 156, 157, 171; [1951], pp. 76, 267, where also Piaget expresses his disagreement with the Gestalt thesis about "constancy" discussed in the previous note; Piaget and Inhelder [1956], p. 12. The problem has also been referred to by Professor Teuber [Teuber, 1959–1960].

Thus, we should not feel surprised at all to see that in spite of the impressive amount of work which neurophysiologists have devoted to the question of memory, of all the ingenuity with which they have devised experiments for its investigation, and of all the extraordinary wealth of collateral material that has been brought to light with that work, we should still see one of the greatest and boldest laborers in the field—Lashley—state that we do not seem much nearer to an understanding of it than the man who, three hundred years ago, defined what was "perhaps the earliest attempt to explain memory in terms of the action of the brain"—Descartes [Lashley, 1960]. For the very same reasons we should not feel astonished at the ultimately equivalent assertion which another researcher, Halstead, forwarded in the chapter on memory, which he wrote for the colossal *Handbook of Physiology* of the American Physiological Society: "There is no known way, compatible with life by which an individual memory trace can, with certainty, be erased from the neural pool once it has been laid down" [Halstead, 1959–1960].

DISCUSSION

Chairman: PROFESSOR CHAGAS

MAC KAY: I am very much in sympathy with Dr. Gomes' insistence on the usefulness of spontaneous activity in the nervous system, in that this relieves the animal from the sort of dilemma of which Buridan's donkey died, being unable to choose between two equally tempting bundles of hay. On the other hand, I am not sure that I have properly understood his connection of this with freedom of action. In exploring the idea of spontaneous processes in the nervous system, it has seemed to me that the effect of a random change in my neuron net would be something I would experience as *happening to me* rather than *being done by me*. In references [MacKay, 1951, 1952, 1953] in my paper, I have suggested that changes in the order in which ideas occur to one, for example, might be produced by processes which a physicist would describe as partly random; but I imagine that one would experience this as "an idea popping into one's head unbidden." I wonder if Dr. Gomes would agree that this field where spontaneous activity can be invoked is really quite separate from the domain of conscious sober control of action, without caprice?

GOMES: The main purpose of the part of my paper dealing with the possible role of microphysical incertitude in voluntary action is the proof of a rather negative aspect (because it chiefly aims at the removal of objections) that there is no inevitable antagonism between what necessarily are the physical characteristics of free action and the regularity of the physical elements of the world, such as the science of physics sees it today after the introduction of the uncertainty principle. I have not intended to proceed with my discussion to the core of the problem of free, responsible action, because I would then have to go very far into problems and hypotheses, the nature of which lies outside the scope of this Study Week. The point that it was my purpose to stress is that if anything equivalent to the system I have now described actually exists in the brain, the actions controlled in this organ may have the physical characteristics of free action—that is, they may be ordered and physically indeterminate at the same time. Let me add now that if the human will exerts a control over a system of that nature, it can do it without any violation of the physical regularity of the physical elements of the brain.

As to the question of randomness itself, I have shown in the subsequent part of my paper that the more advanced is the place of a species in the animal scale, the more does the behavior, and probably the mental experience, of a specimen begin at a rudimentary level. Randomness is then often a very obvious feature; and it is only gradually during life that this randomness is changed into order.

MAC KAY: Perhaps I did not make my question clear. I was not discussing this theory in particular, but rather the nature of our freedom to control our actions. Would you not agree that if an element of randomness came into the chain of control of my action, this would tend towards *excusing* me from responsibility for it, rather than crediting me with responsibility for it?

GOMES: That I sharply distinguish between randomness and freedom should have become sufficiently clear in several passages of my exposition, though I have purposely avoided the philosophical question of their detailed characterization. However, I do believe that randomness has a decisive role in the genesis, though not properly in the full exercise, of freedom and responsibility. This is a point which, owing also to the shortage of time, I have now only very hurriedly referred to. Its full exposition would require the development of a whole genetic theory of individuality, which, of course, I cannot do now.

I shall nevertheless advance this: when a human baby is born, his mind, and, with it, his capacity to control his behavior, are practically nonexistent; they gradually grow and take shape only with the accumulation of experience, which, in the beginning, owing to the nondeveloped state of the brain, can only be extremely rudimentary too. The most frequent among these experiences must be those of motor processes of several sorts accompanied by vague—though not necessarily weak—sensations and emotions of pleasure or displeasure. And they must succeed themselves in a quite haphazard way, owing to the fluctuations of their causal factors that are originated either externally or internally. These may be either apparently or actually random, that is, random because really provoked by the amplification of discrete microphysical events occurring in the centers of control of the motor actions. With the passing of time, the experiences begin to constitute a stock of memories that provide motivations for the incipient will: the desire to repeat or to maintain what is pleasurable, and to avoid what is unpleasurable. It is only then that the individual will comes into definite existence by beginning to exercise itself in the matter of the selection of experiences and the actions associated with them. It will begin at this time to try to substitute itself for what was previously random. And the initial randomness is in truth very important, for the following chief reasons: first, because it is apt to provide the greatest variety of elementary experiences, with the motor associations; second, because when really provoked by microphysical events—as I conjecture that it must often be —it defines a field which is physically plastic to will; last, but not least, because elaborate order from the beginning would leave no room for the subsequent free creation of this order, in which case, will would be greatly determined and thus stunted. Randomness is thus a very suitable antecedent of freedom.

During its first stages of development, individual will must know no fewer failures than successes in its attempts to control actions and experiences, but this very situation provides further experiences of the greatest instructing value. Random variations exhibited in ever more minute details of the incipient mental life will subsequently extend the voluntary control to these details too. And it is also the stock of ever more elaborate memories which provides the ground for the later refinements of the emotions of pleasure and displeasure, with the corresponding further voluntary discriminations.

But, of course, we have to supplement this view of the gradual development of individual will with the hypothesis that it is ultimately able to control the coordinated output of the millions or billions of microindeterminate processes conjecturally going on within the nervous system. We do not have to experience the minute processes which we affect in our nervous system when we exercise our will over it—it would be the most encumbering experience— any more than we do those going on in our digestion, or in the circulation of our blood, or in any other physiological process which is currently going on in our bodies.

MOUNTCASTLE: I believe there is a simple example which would fit very beautifully with the model that you have outlined on the board (Fig. 18.1). In recent years, extensive studies have been made of this spontaneous activity of the brain to which you and Dr. MacKay have referred. When one looks at the temporal ordering of discharges in this spontaneous activity, it is obvious that it is under a restraining device of the type that you postulate. Certain intervals of time are forbidden in the sequence, some have higher probabilities than do other intervals. A regular order is frequently discernable. Most commonly, for example, the orders which are discernable are quite similar in frequency to the slow wave activity of the brain. So, assuming a random series of events at the microphysical level in the cells, one could explain the temporal order of discharge by postulating such a harnessing mechanism as you indicated by the detector amplifier in Fig. 18.1. Interestingly enough, this harnessing mechanism is also itself under the influence of external events such as stimulation, because the temporal ordering of impulses is frequently directly correlated with, for example, intensities of stimulation. I wonder if you have any comments to make about this idea.

GOMES: Of course, external stimulation can have a decisive role in the systems which participate in the control of action. I must, however, say that the chief purpose of the model I have presented is the demonstration of the basic compatibility between indeterminacy and organization. I would not propose it as a concrete, direct model for the nerve cell, though of course I suggest that this model illustrates general principles equivalent to those actually at work within, or between, the neurons. The crucial part of the concrete test of my conjectures would depend on the demonstration of the differentiated amplification of discrete microevents in the molecular structure of the neurons or of the synapses themselves. But this is something that cannot be contemplated yet at the present state of neurophysiological research, since it would require a degree of detail which has not yet been reached. So at present I would rather abstain from looking for empirical evidence for the type of processes I have not described among the neurophysiological processes already identified. I have, however, already developed computations for the purpose of discovering whether that differentiated amplification of microevents could actually occur within the microstructures and processes of the cell, or of the synapses. I have concluded that in respect of their magnitudes, indeed, they can. It seems even significant that the dimensions and other magnitudes of those structures and processes should be critical in that respect—that is, that they should be on the limit of dimensional compatibility, but still within it.

ECCLES: Would it be fair to summarize Dr. Gomes' thesis by saying that some kind of amplification of random events on the microscale could give rise to a series of events on the macroscale which were apparently not determinate?

GOMES: Quite certainly.

ECCLES: If so, I would still raise the question that I think Professor MacKay was raising: wouldn't that on perhaps a longer time scale be determinate statistically except insofar as some agency which we call free will could direct the microevents themselves?

GOMES: In truth, it is ultimately necessary to develop the supplementary hypothesis of an action of will over the physically indeterminate processes. Microindeterminacy alone could not account for free action; it only defines a situation where the action of will over physical elements or processes is possible without the violation of physical regularity. This can be seen even if we concentrate our attention upon only one unit of indeterminate control such as I have proposed here, but is much more apparent if we consider the case of millions or billions of controlling processes of similar type interconnected within a system of extreme complexity such as the brain. In any such system the will can achieve its results by means perfectly compatible with the regularity of the physical world. It can cause the outcome of an indeterminate process to be this or that without violating the statistical regularity which must prevail in many series of such processes, exactly because this regularity is only statistical. There are so many different ways of maintaining a statistical regularity, because the selection to be effected by the will is a selection on a field where no physical factor could achieve it, that is, where no physical factors can be determinatingly at work—although it is a physical field. It is not only that the will would not require physical energy to achieve its presumable influence on the microphysical level of the nervous system; physical energy could not effect any influence of that kind—this is what physics itself assures us.

MAC KAY: In relation to the processes mentioned by Professor Mountcastle, I think Dr. Gomes would agree that the sort of randomness required can be very easily, and I think more plausibly, put down to thermodynamic fluctuations in and around the neurons concerned, rather than to microphysical indeterminacy of the Heisenberg sort.

GOMES: But have I not already said to Professor Mountcastle that I would not yet look for evidence for the kind of processes I am postulating among any of those which have already been discovered and systematically studied in the context of present—say, neurophysiological research?

ECCLES: I think one should begin to think about the size of objects involved in triggering the discharge of the nerve cell. For example, Kuno * has shown that synapses in the central nervous system probably do not operate by the discharge or liberation of the synaptic transmitter contained in more than one or two synaptic vesicles; that is, we are down to a kind of unitary operational characteristic of the synapse. Moreover, there have been several suggestions that small interneurons may be concerned in the cerebral activity giving rise to consciousness, and these may have relatively few synapses on their surfaces, so that the contents of very few synaptic vesicles would be sufficient to trigger off a cell. Synaptic vesicles have a size indicating a mass of rather less than 10^{-16} g; so we are down to microphysical levels under these conditions. We may, therefore, have a possible explanation of the random firing described by Dr. Mountcastle, because there is always a random spontaneous emission of vesicles at synaptic junctions, both at the neuromuscular junction, and, as Katz and Miledi have now shown, at synapses in the spinal cord.

MOUNTCASTLE: Yet the output of that cell is never, or scarcely ever, observed to be random, so what I have said and what Dr. Gomes has said fit together in suggesting that a random series of events producing excitation of the cell does not result in a random discharge of the cell. There is a harnessing mechanism with certain intervals forbidden, which seems quite comparable to the drawing on the board.

SPERRY: Ever since people started to make brain lesions experimentally the most surprising outcome has always been the tremendous amount of material you can remove or destroy and still have functional order preserved. An alteration in a single cell or in hundreds of cells is not going to change much the tremendous coherence and inertia in brain organization that seems to be specifically designed to counteract any caprice or randomness.

GOMES: I would completely agree that one single cell or even a few hundred or thousand cells might not be enough. But there is no reason why the hypothesis I have expounded should be restricted to any relatively small number of cells, when in principle it can be extended to practically all neurons in the brain.

SPERRY: It is difficult to find a flaw in your argument because you have both factors—determinacy and indeterminacy.

CHAIRMAN: I would just like to say about Dr. MacKay's references to thermodynamic fluctuations, that I do not think they could mainfest themselves with the order of magnitude of the phenomena studied by Dr. Mountcastle; I

* M. Kuno. Quantal components of excitatory synaptic potentials in spinal motoneurones, *J. Physiol.* (*London*), *175*, 81–99 [1964].

suppose they could become apparent only in much lower levels of energy, such as are involved in molecular movement—if I understood his observation.

MAC KAY: I would only say that if KT does not apply, then *a fortiori* the quantum uncertainty, which is much smaller than the thermodynamic, should not.

CHAIRMAN: You then agree that the thermodynamic fluctuation is of a lower magnitude than the seemingly random processes which Mountcastle has reported.

MAC KAY: Yes, though I would not be surprised if one could take nerve cells near the threshold of excitation and "titrate" them up to a point at which you would have to attribute their firing at one instant, rather than another, partly to thermodynamic fluctuation.

CHAIRMAN: I would like to discuss briefly the concept of energy in cells, in connection with the puzzling experiment recently conducted by Dr. Bensley, which indicates the possibility of mutations with absorbed energies of the order of 10^{-5} to 10^{-8} erg, that are much lower than any other known before to provoke similar effects—and which may be attributed to protonic processes. We must be very careful when drawing conclusions about minimum energy levels in biological systems, because new techniques may reveal new facts that exemplify and elucidate what seemed impossible or unexplainable for us before.

REFERENCES

BOHR, N. *La Théorie Atomique et la Description des Phénomènes.* Paris: Gauthier Villars, pp. 94, 95, 109–111 [1932].

CASSIRER, E. *Determinism and Indeterminism in Modern Physics.* New Haven: Yale Univ. Press, Chapt. 13 [1937].

ECCLES, J. C. *The Neurophysiological Basis of Mind. The Principles of Neurophysiology.* Oxford: Clarendon Press, Chapt. VIII [1953].

EDDINGTON, A. S. *The Nature of the Physical World.* New York: Macmillan [1928].

———. *New Pathways in Science.* Cambridge, Eng.: Cambridge Univ. Press [1935].

ELSASSER, W. M. *The Physical Foundation of Biology—An Analytical Study.* London: Pergamon Press [1958].

FLETCHER, R. *Instinct in Man.* London: Allen & Unwin [1957].

GOMES, A. E. *Os movimentos dos seres vivos* (The movements of living beings), *Revista Brasileira de Filosofia* (São Paulo), No. 20 [Oct. 1955]; No. 21 [Jan. 1956].

GRANIT, R. *Receptors and Sensory Perception.* New Haven: Yale Univ. Press, p. 9 [1955].

HALSTEAD, W. C. Thinking, imagery and memory, in: *Handbook of Physiology, Section I, Neurophysiology.* Washington, D. C.: Amer. Physiological Soc., Vol. III, p. 1675 [1959–1960].

JORDAN, P. *Die Physik und das Geheimnis des organischen Lebens.* Braunschweig, F. Vieweg [1941].

LASHLEY, K. S. In search of the engram, *The Neuropsychology of Lashley* (ed. by D. O. Hebb, C. T. Morgan, H. W. Nissen). New York: McGraw-Hill, p. 478 [1960].

———. Introduction, in: *Instinctive Behavior* (ed. by C. S. Schiller). London: Methuen [1957].

PIAGET, J. *Play, Dreams and Imitation in Childhood*. London: Heinemann, Chapt. V [1951].

———. *The Child's Construction of Reality*. London: Routledge [1955].

———. *La Naissance de l'Intelligence chez l'Enfant*. Neuchatel: Delachaux et Niestlé, Chapt. I and Conclusions (Sect. 4, 5) [1959].

———, and B. INHELDER. *The Child's Conception of Space*. London: Routledge [1956].

SCHROEDINGER, E. *What Is Life?* Cambridge, Eng.: Cambridge Univ. Press, Chapt. VIII [1944].

———. *Science and Humanism; Physics in Our Time*. Cambridge, Eng.: Cambridge Univ. Press, pp. 60–62 [1952].

SHERRINGTON, C. S. *Man on His Nature*. New York and London: Penguin and Pelican Books, pp. 187, 216, 219, 249, 257, 258 [1955].

TEUBER, H. L. Perception, in: *Handbook of Physiology, Section I, Neurophysiology*. Washington, D. C.: Amer. Physiological Soc., Vol. III, p. 1649 [1959–1960].

WEYL, H. *Philosophy of Mathematics and Natural Sciences*. Princeton: Princeton Univ. Press, pp. 279, 282 [1949].

19

Ethology and Consciousness[1]

by W. H. Thorpe

Cambridge University, Cambridge, England

The C.I.O.M.S. symposium volume on brain mechanisms and consciousness was published just ten years ago. Several of those who took part in that conference are here today. I have found the volume a valuable basis for assessing the ideas of physiologists as to the type of physiological mechanism which may plausibly be regarded as necessarily giving rise to consciousness. Of course, there are widely differing views among physiologists on this; and, indeed, there was a good deal of disagreement among members of the conference of ten years ago. Nevertheless, all the states and mechanisms there discussed can at least be regarded as important in, if not essential to, the production of consciousness.

In order to take the first step in limiting the scope of this discussion, I had better say what I mean by "ethology." The original meaning of this word in English was "the interpretation of character by the study of gesture," though it was also extended to cover "the art of mime." The word became obsolete in general English usage during the nineteenth century, but towards the end of the nineteenth or in the early years of the twentieth was revived to signify *"the scientific study of animal behavior";* and it is in this broad sense that I shall use it today.

The ancestry of the word "ethology" indicates another essential characteristic of the science: that is, it is a study which tries to understand the animal's nature by interpreting its "gestures." In other words, we study its movements both under natural and experimental conditions in as great detail as possible. (By movements here I mean to include all types of movement, whether simply locomotory or whether concerned

---

[1] Dedicated to Professor Dr. Otto Koehler on the occasion of his seventy-fifth birthday.

470

together with food getting, display and sex, social behavior, and organization; all kinds of signal production and emotional expression.) To make this kind of study acceptable, one must as far as possible take into account the whole behavioral repertoire, both innate and acquired, of the animal. This in its turn involves looking at the animal with the eye of the naturalist and the physiologist combined, seeking to understand both the function and the causation (in an evolutionary as well as a physiological sense) of its behavior. That is tantamount to saying that the ethologist tries to view the animal as a whole but that in so doing he is ready to employ, or at least give full weight to, any and every scientific technique which gives promise of being useful. Thus the ethologist has to be ready to use and interpret all types of physiological data, for example, neurophysiological, endocrinological, etc., as well as to employ many types of electronic and other techniques for recording, analyzing, and interpreting animal actions.

The term *consciousness,* although having innumerable overtones of meaning, involves, I think, three basic components. First, an inward awareness of sensibility—what might be called "having internal perception." Second, an awareness of self, of one's own existence. Third, the idea of consciousness includes that of unity; that is to say, it implies in some rather vague sense the fusion of the totality of the impressions, thoughts, and feelings which make up a person's conscious being into a single whole. As Lashley put it, the process of awareness implied in the belief in an internal perceiving agent, an "I" or self which does the perceiving, leads inevitably to the conclusion that this agent selects and unifies elements into a unique single field of consciousness. This belief in a perceiving self has two other important consequences: (*a*) it transcends time and space since memory brings into immediate relation events remote from one another in these dimensions; (*b*) it creates aesthetic and ethical values held to be absolute.

These, then, as I see it, are the basic constituents of the ordinary educated man's conviction that he is a conscious, thinking, being—in fact, his conviction that he has a mind. Before going on to the physiological and then the ethological implications of this, I want to say a little more about the general, one might say the nontechnical, implications of such common-sense ideas.

First it is obvious that if the conscious self has the capacity to know what is going on inside its own mind, the intelligent human being should be able to report at least some of this. This is the self as a perceiving agent; and this idea of a perceiving agent is, I think, always linked with the belief that this agent is also a causal agent, to some extent at least, in control of the situation. As a psychologist, Hebb [1954], has put it, consciousness is supposed to involve or imply the existence of processes in the brain that are not sensorily dominated. Not only are these processes not sensorily dominated, there is also (it almost comes to the same thing) interaction between them; that is to say, there is a capacity for ideation—a freedom or ability to manipulate ideas. This freedom to manipulate ideas, together with the concept of the central agent having a causal function, leads to at least some form of the belief in free will. This of course inevitably, in its turn, implies the ability to have purposes and to express those purposes in behavior. Thus, if we can see purposive behavior in animals or men, we have provisional grounds for believing that there is within the organism some sort of expectancy of the future which entails or implies a capacity for ideation, an integration of ideas about past and future, and a temporal organization of ideas [Hebb, 1954].

Now everybody knows that such a concept of consciousness has been assailed from many sides, and I wish to consider one or two of these criticisms insofar as they bear upon the kind of evidence we look for, whether in animals or men, in our attempt to get to grips with this baffling problem. Thus in what follows I shall of course omit at least some of the general philosophical arguments for consciousness and free will—such as the epistemological one, according to which the alternative (that consciousness and free will are illusory) inevitably implies that all knowledge, including all the results of science and every other activity of man, is illusion. It seems to me that arguments of this kind and the facts upon which they are based provide a quite overwhelming *a priori* reason for believing in consciousness as a distinct kind of event very much in the way in which it is understood in ordinary speech. I need say no more on this topic, perhaps, than to note the recently expressed opinion of a distinguished Oxford logician [Kneale, 1962] that, "we must retain the Platonic notion of mental events which are distinct from anything in the physical world and manifest a special kind of connectedness. The occurrence of such events is part of what we ordinarily intend to assert when we speak of the existence of mind and a presupposition of all the more interesting things we want to say about them."

But to return to some of those criticisms which are the concern of the ethologist. These, of course, grade imperceptibly into the criticisms of the physiologist.

William James [1890] pointed out that there is no direct knowledge of an experiencing self. The self, as known, reduces to the physical self—largely as kinesthetic sensations from the head and throat. The knower as an entity is, according to James, an unnecessary postulate. Any process which will account for the characteristics of the content of experience fulfills all the requirements of the process of awareness.

Physiologists have a comment to make here which I think is important. Thus Lashley [1954] points out, as have many others before him, that *there is never awareness of the integrative activity of the brain while it is in progress.* The perceived items are always the product of preceding and complex integrative processes. Visual distance is a good illustration of this. Things are seen as near or far, yet this distance is actually determined by a number of variables, binocular parallax, estimates of relative size, texture, etc., which are not separately perceived but are only revealed by experimental isolation. To sum up, "our thoughts come in syntactical form, without effort and without knowledge of how that form is achieved. So in every case, that of which we are aware is an organized structure; the organizing is never experienced." And again: "Awareness, as we know it, is not a state distinguished by any single specific character, but is a sequence of events which may be organized in various ways and which do not necessarily have any character in common." As a matter of fact, such psychophysical objections as they may be called—or rather, psychophysiological objections—can be, and indeed have been, under valid attack, particularly from those concerned with the higher mental processes of man and of the higher animals. Thus the implications of much of the work of the Gestalt school by no means completely supports James' pronouncement.

The first physiological question is that of self-regulation; in the conscious human being, self-regulation of course creates the impression of the self as a causal agent. But everyone knows that there are an enormous number of self-regulated actions which occur in ourselves far below any conscious level, and the natural presumption is that in animals a far higher proportion must be below this level. In many animals indeed there is no reason to believe that all of them may not be below the conscious level. In this connection, James has an interesting remark. He says, *"Consciousness is what we might expect in an organ, added for the sake of steering a nervous system grown too complex to regulate itself."* If this is true, it implies that simpler nervous systems and simpler examples of structural organization may well be self-regulating, in the same manner that so many machines incorporating cybernetic principles are self-regulating, and that there may be no need whatever to bring in any concept of consciousness. It follows that if self-regulation as such is evidence for consciousness, all animals and plants are conscious! And why not machines too? I think the matter need not be disscused further here.

Another physiological aspect of the problem is brought to the fore by the problem of attention. The fact of attention and the shifting of attention, like the beam of a searchlight, from one aspect of the perceptual world to another is one of the most obvious features of human conscious mental organization. Next comes the question of the integration of the present. Fessard, in the volume just mentioned, defined conciousness as "the integrated perception of the present"; and some physiologists have supposed that this process of integrated perception necessarily involves the matching or comparison of incoming current information with previously stored information. That is, we have to have a coincidence or congruence between an incoming pattern of impulses and what may be called a "filing card" of past experience. It is interesting and I think significant that essentially this same idea is involved in the theories of von Holst and Mittelstaedt [1950], which comprise the so-called "reafference principle." This postulates that any orienting mechanism, any "taxis" device, which ensures that an animal when stimulated turns to the correct quarter, involves the concept of an *expected* reafferentation which prevents abnormal or inappropriate reaction. Details of this physiological principle were worked out primarily in insects, especially certain Diptera and in the praying mantis (*Mantis religiosa*). If, then, consciousness is a necessary outcome of this mechanism, all animals down to at least the lower metazoa, including all the insects (except perhaps a few degenerate parasitic forms), are conscious. There is, however, a form of anticipation or of expectancy which seems to involve something much more than this; and Rioch has said that anticipation of one or other of several possible responses is a necessity for consciousness. Again there is a group of learning theorists, principally in the U.S.A., who have established what they call the principle of expectancy on the ground that they believe such a principle is unavoidable if we are to obtain a full explanation of the efficiency of certain types of reward in facilitating and consolidating a learned response. These views, and with them the views of Berlyne [1960] and a number of modern Russian workers on anticipatory arousal (for example, Sokolov) are much more relevant because, although anticipatory arousal or something like it occurs far down in the animal scale, the cases where real expectancy, in anything like the human sense, are found in the animal kingdom are clearly associated with very elaborate behavior indeed.

Ethology is the scientific study of animal behavior, and I propose now to look at some of these physiological theories and their implications in the light of ethology in the hope that it may get us some way further in understanding the essential nature of the conscious process. It is, however, important to make clear that if there is a one-to-one correspondence between mental and neurophysiological events, then *any* piece of behavior could *in principle* be accounted for in mechanistic terms if physiology itself is purely mechanistic. Thus we can never say that a given piece of behavior, however elaborate it appears and however much it suggests the presence of consciousness, cannot possibly be the unconscious result of a physiological mechanism. This is merely to stress the apparent impregnability of the solipsist position—that we only "know" consciousness in ourselves. Solipsism is at least refutable to the extent that nobody believes it. But some other theories are in little better case. The sense datum theory and the common-sense theory and the representative theory all run into great difficulties, though as defended by physiologists such as Lord Brain, the last seems to be more promising. Perhaps as modified into the modern "aspect theory" [Wyburn et al, 1964] it will prove to have staged a real advance. At least this seems to do least violence to the work and views of present-day physiologists and psychologists. But our concern here is with consciousness in animals. While, then, we cannot give final proof of consciousness in animals, we can bring evidence to bear which is cumulatively highly impressive and does, I believe, give powerful reasons for concluding that consciousness is a widespread feature of animal life.

Let us turn now to the ethological aspects of some of these physiological and philosophical ideas.

ATTENTION AND THE INNATE RELEASIVE MECHANISM

Innumerable species of animals, many of them far down in the scale among the lower metazoa, show evidence of attending selectively to particular stimuli, responding to them, and ignoring others which must assuredly be capable of detection by their sensory systems. Where these stimuli are of extreme simplicity, consisting often of the commencement or change of intensity of a simple sound or of the general illumination, the response can be regarded as a reflex in the sense of the term as usually employed in the physiological laboratory. But very often the "stimulus" is something far more complex than this, and may involve perception of color, speed of movement, distance, relative size, shape, and even complexities of visual pattern. Stimuli which have this character are usually called *releasers* and it is possible, by appropriate experiment, to isolate the particular element of a releaser (for example, the flight overhead of a female butterfly which serves as a stimulus to sexual pursuit by the male) into a number of component parts known as "sign stimuli." These sign stimuli are in themselves often relational in the sense that they depend upon the relation of one patch of color to another, on the proportions of the outline, or upon the distribution of light and dark areas over a given shape. Releasers of this kind are very well known in the insects and have been, perhaps, more thoroughly studied in this group than in any other. Yet even though they may be relatively complex, the response of the lower animals to them tends to occur quite automatically and often to be rather independent of the physiological state of the animal concerned. That is so say, whenever the releaser happens to appear, the organism is activated. This works well enough in many simple creatures, and the overall effect is very like that of a reflex, except that the nature of the stimulus is much more complex than that usually employed in the physiological laboratory. When we come to the higher animals, however, the response, although it may appear to be of the same kind, is often far more closely dependent on the internal state of the animal. In other words, it is evident that there is some internal activity within the nervous system, or linked with it, which is exerting a good deal of control upon its selectiveness. The animal is no longer passively responding to the stimuli which it encounters but is actively selecting from among them.

In recent years it has become abundantly clear that, in vertebrate animals, the selectivity of the creature for the meaningful features in its environment is physiologically of considerable complexity. The present picture provided by ethological and physiological work on the problem of the innate releasive mechanism (IRM), and of selective attention in animals, shows us a series of what may be called provisionally "physiological filtering mechanisms." The highly complex environmental pattern of stimulation has to encounter and secure a passage through these filtering mechanisms before the animal can respond. It is supposed that there are three types of such filtering devices: (*a*) that imposed primarily by the receptors themselves—in the case of vision, by such things as color responsiveness, brightness discrimination, movement sight, flicker fusion frequency, visual acuity, binocular fixation, etc.; (*b*) the filtering effected by the receptor's afferent pathways and the central nervous system as they function together in normal perception; (*c*) a central filtering or matching mechanism (which is perhaps equivalent to the original rather crude concept of the IRM). It is the existence of this last central mechanism, with its powers of selective discrimination (which apparently confers on the animal the ability to switch the process on or off "at will" and to pay attention now to one part of the environment, now to another), which may give us ground for supposing that animals having this ability thereby possess powers of conscious choice. As an example of the kind of behavior that can be observed in birds, even a bird rather low in the avian scale, I would mention the herring gull (*Larus argentatus*). Many ground nesting birds will roll back an egg which has been accidentally removed from the nest until it is again being safely brooded. In the herring gull there are many characters of the egg which determine whether or not it, or objects in some way similar to the normal egg, will be retrieved. It is clear that the birds are capable of responding to size, shape, color, and degree of speckling. In this series of characters, it is speckling, size, and color which are of major importance, and shape which is of minor importance. If the herring gull is given eggs that are larger than normal, it may accept them and even try to incubate objects too large for brooding to be possible. Moreover, eggs that are darker than normal are preferred to normal ones, and eggs that have more spots and darker spots than normal are also preferred. But it is the amount or intensity of speckling which is the major factor, and this is integrated with the other characteristics in such a manner as to ensure that under normal conditions all "good" eggs which may be lying a little way from the nest are collected and rolled in, but no other objects such as stones, etc.

So when we come to organisms of this degree of development in the vertebrate scale, it is inadequate to suppose that, with behavior of any degree of complexity, the animal is passively filtering the stimuli impinging upon it [Hinde, 1966]. Mechanical analogies solely based on such a concept tend to give a dangerously simple view of the animal's neurophysiological and "mental" organization. Whether, at this level, behavior of such complexity is reasonable evidence for consciousness or not is another matter; but certainly, as we go up the animal scale and as we investigate more and more closely the higher learning abilities of birds and mammals, the stronger becomes the overall impression that here we are dealing with choice-mechanisms which it is only reasonable, at any rate as a preliminary hypothesis, to class as conscious. Of particular interest in this connection are the experiments of Horn [1960] upon the potential evoked at the cat's visual cortex, when the animal is exposed to repeated light flashes, other peripheral changes being controlled. This evoked potential was reduced if the cat was distracted by nonvisual stimuli, *but only when this distraction involved visual searching behavior.* If there was no visual searching component in the distracting stimulus, the evoked response was not altered. This seems to imply that the reduction in potential evoked at the visual cortex is not so much to the cat's paying attention to stimuli arriving via another nonvisual sense organ, but to searching behavior in the same sensory modality. There is a considerable amount of neurophysiological evidence on such matters. Thus it has been found [Evarts, 1962] that the response of single cells in the cat's visual cortex to flashes of light is reduced when the cat is shown a mouse. Similarly, Hubel and Wiesel [1959] have located cortical cells in cats which are responsive to sound stimuli only when the cat is paying attention to a sound source. These results and many more like them serve to show how complex the whole problem is.

Ideation and the Manipulation of Abstract Ideas

The most characteristic thing about human speech and other human communication devices is the enormous extent and power of our ability to symbolize. By this I mean the ability to represent, by words or other symbols, completely abstract or general ideas, which in themselves have nothing of the essential characteristics of the concepts which they denote. This seems to be preeminently a conscious process, at any rate in its developmental stages in the individual human being. Can we find anything resembling it among the animals? As far as we yet know for certain, no animal language, however much information may be conveyed, involves the learned realization of completely general abstractions. However, animals can evidently go a very long way towards this. Thus Otto Koehler and his pupils, in their famous studies of the recognition of number, showed that animals, and especially birds, can "think unnamed numbers"—that is, they have a prelinguistic number sense; to some extent they think without words. To give one or two examples: A raven (*Corvus corax*), confronted with a series of boxes with a varying number of spots on the lids, was taught to open only that box which had the same number of spots as there were objects on a key card placed in front of it. This bird eventually learned to distinguish between five groups indicated by two, three, four, five, and six black spots on the lids of the boxes, the key being one of those numbers lying on the ground in front. The raven learned to raise only that one of the five lids which had the same number of spots as the key pattern had objects. As a control, every other factor was changed in a random manner from one experiment to the next. Thus there were 15 positions of the five boxes, and very many different positions of the key patterns. The number of units in the key patterns was changed with each experiment, and there were five places for the positive number of spots on the lid corresponding with that of the key. Moreover, there were 24 permutations of the four "negative" numbers; also the relative situations of the spots were changed by the experimenter with absolute irregularity. In the final series of experiments for each trial, the experimenter broke afresh a flat plasticine slab into pieces of highly irregular outline, the area of a piece varying from 1 to 50 units, care always being taken to make the arrangement and general appearance of the positive number on the lid as unlike that of the key pattern as possible. Nevertheless, in spite of all extraneous clues having been eliminated with such care, this raven solved the problem by choosing the positive lids according to the only item which was not changed throughout all the experiments, that is to say, the "number" characteristic of the particular key pattern presented. The minimum ability which it seems necessary to attribute to birds in order to account for such experimental results is that which we might employ if we were to give, or think of giving, one nod of the head for one, two for two, three for three, and so on. We can call this "thinking unnamed numbers."

Lögler [1959] has carried the investigation of the problem of number sense in animals a step further by his extremely thorough and painstaking work on counting in the gray parrot (*Psittacus erithacus*). Extending the kind of investigation which had been carried out earlier, he found that the parrot was able to recognize that the successive presentation of a number of optic stimuli was a signal for the task of performing the same number of actions. The bird having been shown, say, four or six or seven light flashes, was then able to take four or six or seven (as the case might be) irregularly distributed baits from a row of food trays. Not even numerous random changes in the temporal sequence of signal stimuli impaired the percentage of correct solutions. Having learned this task, a signal of successive light flashes was replaced by successive notes of a flute. The further training, the change from light flashes to flute notes, had no effect on the number of correct solutions. Nor was the accomplishment hindered by the completely a-rhythmic presentation of stimuli or by a change of pitch. Although this parrot was not able to accomplish a task which represented a combination of the two faculties of learning numbers presented successively and simultaneously—that is to say, he would not respond to visually presented numbers after hearing the same number of acoustic stimuli—yet when he had learned to act upon two or one, after hearing two sounds simultaneously or a single sound, he was spontaneously able to open a lid with two spots on it or a lid with one spot according to the same acoustic signals. That is to say, he was able to transpose from the simultaneous-successive combination to the simultaneous-simultaneous in 20 experiments without relearning.

It seems then that this remarkable work shows the counting achievements of birds to be nearer those of man than was thought, though still not true counting ability in the full human sense. True human counting offers a completely general solution to the problem of transfer, that is to say, the transfer of a number from one quality to another, and also combining successive and simultaneous. Only this can be regarded as satisfactory evidence of true counting. For unequivocal evidence of true counting in animals it would be necessary to train an animal to combine simultaneous and successive counting and at the same time to respond to a given number in quite diverse circumstances; as, for instance, the recognition of four blasts of a whistle after training to four dots on a paper as standing for four grains to be eaten. We may, therefore, say that although the ability of animals to count does not appear to have reached the point at which it can be equated with human counting, it has certainly gone a very long way toward it in animals which, in social organization, rate so immeasurably inferior to man that it is surprising to find the ability present at all. But however deficient the counting ability of animals may appear to us when compared with that of man, I think we must concede that we have here extremely strong evidence that animals can perform the mental abstraction of the quality of number which in human children can only be accomplished by conscious cerebration.

ANTICIPATION OR EXPECTANCY

There is evidence for the existence of expectancy in many sub-mammalian forms, for example, in relation to the feeding behavior of birds. Thus jays (*Garrulus glandarius*), once they happen to find a well-camouflaged "stick caterpillar" of a geometrid moth and have experienced its good eating qualities, will go on pecking at similar looking sticks for some time afterwards. Tinbergen [1960] adapted the concept of a "searching image," previously employed, to account for this kind of behavior, and placed it on a more precise basis as a result of his study of titmice (Paridae). It seems that the proportion of the bird's diet made up by a given prey species may be expected to depend upon the probability of the bird encountering that prey while foraging—that is to say, on the prey density. The small number of certain prey species taken at low densities is ascribed to the insufficient experience of the birds with the prey; with increasing density they learn to find a given species of prey more efficiently. The explanation offered for this is that the bird has a "specific searching image" which it can only adopt, or arrive at, at a critical prey density, and a certain frequency of encounters is necessary for the maintenance of such a searching image. Gibb [1962], again working with tits preying on insect larvae, provides evidence that birds learn what prey density to expect in a given general area, and slacken their searching when the expected number of larvae has been taken from (in this case) pine cones. Here again is work that suggests the operation of a specific searching image.

But perhaps expectancy is more strongly evidenced in those higher animals which are capable of using tools even in the wild. Thus Goodall [1963, 1964], in her study of the feeding behavior of wild chimpanzees (*Pan satyrus*), frequently observed that sticks are used in order to enable the animal to extract termites from their nests in the ground. A stick or twig is poked into an open passage and after a short pause is withdrawn—the termites, which are holding on with their mandibles, being pulled out with it. The stick is then drawn sideways through the mouth and the termites licked off. There seems to be some general agreement among a band of foraging chimpanzees as to the prey which is to be sought on a given day. If the expedition is to be for termite gathering, then the chimps will go to a particular type of bush or tree to pick twigs, strip them of their leaves, and carry them to the termite hills. It seems impossible to account for such behavior without supposing that definite anticipation and intention accompany the act. Chimpanzees will also crush up certain leaves which they use as sponges to absorb water from small hollows, the water being sucked out and the sponge used again a number of times. They also use leaves for wiping themselves as we use handkerchiefs, napkins, or toilet paper.

A similar impression emerges from recent studies of the tool-using behavior of the California sea otter (*Enhydra lutris nereis*) [Hall and Schaller, 1964]. This animal feeds upon crabs, sea urchins, and mollusks, all of which have a stout shell, carapace, or other covering which has to be broached before the food can be obtained. Food objects are gathered on the sea bed, and after finding a satisfactory sample, the otter reappears on the surface of the sea carrying, say, a clam under one arm and a stone under the other. He then floats on his back, resting the stone on his chest, and bangs the shellfish against the stone until the shell is broken. When the meal is finished he discards the shell but often retains the stone and dives again, returning with another specimen but the same stone. The retention of the stone in this manner would seem to imply anticipation of use which goes beyond the immediate situation. The tool-using habit appears to be present in the behavioral repertoire of the animal and is elicited during feeding only when the ecological situation requires it. It is probable that the young learn the various methods of collecting and opening food items by following and observing their mothers during the long period of dependence. But whatever the means of acquiring the perfect act, it seems impossible to understand its regular use under appropriate conditions without postulating conscious anticipation and attention.

There is much hunting behavior, particularly in lions and wolves and hunting dogs (*Lycaon pictus*), which gives a very vivid impression of carefully prearranged and planned cooperation. Such observations tend of course to be anecdotal, and are apt to grow with the telling, but many of them are sufficiently precise to inspire a good deal of confidence (lions [Moorehead, 1959]; tigers and Indian wild dogs [Anderson, 1954]; hunting dogs [Hillaby, 1964]). Perhaps the most convincing and certainly the most precisely studied and observed behavior of this kind is that recorded by a most careful and experienced observer, Goodall [1963, and personal communication, 1964]. She observed a concerted attack by members of a chimpanzee group upon a Colobus monkey (*Colobus polykomos*). The evidence seemed to point to one or more individuals attracting the monkey's attention from the front while another stalked silently up from the rear and leapt upon the monkey which was then seized by all, torn to pieces, and eaten.

But perhaps the most striking evidence for anticipation comes from work with captive monkeys in the course of experiments designed to reveal what has been called "reward expectancy." If a rhesus monkey (*Macaca mulatta*) is allowed to see some food placed under one of two or more containers, for example, under inverted cups, and is subsequently allowed access to these cups, it shows a high ability to choose the correct one. If, in an experiment, a piece of banana is hidden under one cup while the monkey is watching, then if, with a screen placed in front of the monkey, the experimenter quickly substitutes for the banana a less desirable food such as a lettuce leaf—the monkey will go to the cup where he expects to find the preferred food, and on finding not banana but lettuce may not only reject the lettuce (though normally, in the absence of banana, he would have eaten it) but may even throw a temper tantrum as a result of his disappointment [Tilkelpaugh, 1928]. Very similar results have been obtained with rats [Elliott, 1928] and chimpanzees [Cowles and Nissen, 1937]. They seem to provide overwhelming evidence for a learnt searching image, a definite and precise expectancy, and a disappointment at failing to find what is expected and sought.

SELF-AWARENESS AND RECOGNITION OF OTHER SELVES

The study of the social behavior of animals provides much evidence for individual recognition of associates, in particular, in relation to the development of highly organized play and of elaborate imitation; facts which strongly suggest if they do not prove the existence of self-awareness.

There are many examples in both fish and birds of large groups or flocks of many species in which individual recognition seems to be lacking. The anonymous swarm or troop as seen in schools or shoals of fish, and probably also in certain very closely coordinated flocks of birds, may be regarded as a primitive form of social life. In this kind of organization there are no leaders and no followers, in fact, no individuality. The whole body is coordinated by fixed responses to releasers of one kind or another —releasers which have been evolved over long periods by the action of natural selection. The more numerous the individuals, the more intense is the herd cohesion and herd instinct. But there is no mutual recognition. There is a very illuminating experiment by von Holst (quoted by Lorenz [1963]) in which operations were carried out on the brains of minnows (*Phoxinus laevis*). The result was that the normal social responses were eliminated. Consequently, those fish with no social responses became the leaders, since they were responded to but no longer responded themselves. Previously, in the normal fish school, as in the normal ant swarm, there were no leaders. With a primitive social organization of this kind, that is, troops or schools or swarms, any one comrade is as good as another and there is not the slightest evidence of individual recognition among them.

The next point to remember is that all animals with bond behavior also have aggressive behavior. In animals with very primitive social organization this bond behavior can give rise to the phenomenon of individual distance. Where there is constant conflict between the tendency to scatter and the tendency to keep contact, the former mediated by the innate releasers and the latter by the aggressive tendency, "individual distance" is determined by the point at which the two normally balance. In birds during the breeding season, however, any one individual has to maintain much closer contact with one other individual, namely, the mate. So in many species the breeding contact is closer than the contact in shoal, or flock, and something has to be done to assuage the aggression which otherwise would manifest itself and break up the breeding cycle and organization. As a result, we find a number of mechanisms apparently fully explained by the need to redirect the male fury released by the presence of a female (first viewed as an intruder) from the female to rival males. This has been called "abreaction" and is primarily a means of getting rid of aggression. By the courtship and other displays of birds, the aggressive reaction is checked or limited or dispersed by greeting ceremonies and appeasement ceremonies at the nest. Nevertheless it is still there, waiting to be redirected against the rival male.

When one comes to mammals and to those birds in which individual recognition *is* fully developed—that is to say, in which the individuals recognize one another personally and in which long-maintained attachments are developed—then the social organization is different. In many species of birds (notably in geese), as in many mammals, the family, clan, or group (most or all of the members of which are known to one another personally) becomes the basis of the social organization. Mammals, in contrast to birds, are "contact animals" with few devices for the maintenance of individual distance. In fact they tend to huddle. Therefore, if strangers are introduced into this situation, in a cage, in which they cannot flee from the owners or hide, disaster will supervene. The same is true to an even greater extent of domesticated or tame animals introduced into a wild population, since these domesticated individuals may have lost the appropriate appeasement responses—responses which we see in dogs in the form of cringing or presenting the neck (the most vulnerable part) to the dominant animal. Lorenz in a recent book describes the terrible lot of a rat, artificially provided in a cage with "foreign kindred": it will be slowly torn to pieces by its associates.

Now nearly all these observations give clear evidence for some kind of individual recognition. In some highly social birds it is clear that upwards of 90 different individuals can be independently recognized and there is no reason to think that it is less in mammals. Although much of this could be accounted for by simple conditioning procedures, the overall picture is such as to leave very little doubt of the recognition of other members of the species as beings in some respects similar to oneself.

At the time of going to press, particulars of some very remarkable work on the concept-forming abilities of the pigeon have been published by Herrnstein and Loveland [1964]. Pigeons were trained to respond to the presence or absence of human beings in photographs. The precision of their performances and the ease with which the training was accomplished suggest greater powers of conceptualization than are ordinarily attributed to animals. Unless there is something extraordinary about the conceptual capacities of pigeons, these findings show that an animal readily forms a broad and complex concept when placed in a situation that demands one. The results are so remarkable in view of the difficulty that animals, and even primitive human beings, have in understanding complex pictures, that one will wait with keen interest for confirmation. It must be said, however, that the methods employed were highly sophisticated and every care taken against misinterpretation. The graphs published summarize a large mass of data and on every count the work appears to merit confidence.

In the higher birds and mammals, with a family or social organization, play is often particularly evident and is found in highly complex forms. In this play, as in the play of children, all the social inhibitions are maintained even when the game is violent and passionate. It may on occasion change to serious fighting, particularly when a predatory animal such as a cat or ichneumon (*Herpestes ichneumon*) is playing with real prey. But normally, as in playful combat between two young dogs, there is a clear and obvious difference from serious fighting. However fierce they may appear, they do not bite each other seriously. It is difficult to avoid saying that "they are not in earnest." Careful studies of mammalian play have shown that it includes innate behavior patterns, acquired behavior patterns, and combinations of the two. It appears to be performed for its own sake and is often correlated to an object which may be the animal's body as a whole or its parts. Very often there is a social component, as in play with a partner or partners, using an intermediate object; and play is often repeated a very large number of times in succession. True play is often even more indefatigable than the instinctive acts upon which it is based.

In the past it has been seriously argued that the ability to play is one of the most characteristic and distinctive of human attributes; yet the play of some mammals, where it may take the form of relatively elaborate or even "organized" games, seems to be on a par with children's games such as "touch" and "hide and seek." Here again, is it reasonable to suppose that these could have developed without some form of self-awareness? This subject brings us back again to the question of communication. Human language can be defined as a communication system which is propositional, syntactic, and clearly expressive of intention. Now I do not think we can find any single example of animal communication which fulfills all these requirements. Yet all these features can be found separately (at least to some degree) in the animal kingdom. Consequently, distinguishing between man and the animals on the ground that only the former possesses true language seems far less satisfactory and logically defensible than once it did.

Further, and perhaps more convincing, evidence for self-awareness is provided by the imitative abilities of mammals. By the word "imitation" I here mean the ability to copy a novel or an otherwise improbable act or utterance or some act for which there is clearly no instinctive tendency. Defined in this way, we see that true visual imitation becomes something which apparently involves self-consciousness and an intent to profit by another's experience. My definition of imitation does not at this stage include the vocal imitation of birds, remarkable though it is. This is because the action of uttering a sound is unique among all actions in that, whereas action of any other kind cannot be perceived by the actor in the same way in which it is perceived by his fellow creatures and in which he perceives their bodily movements, the *sounds* he and they utter are presumably perceived by him and them in much the same way. "Observational learning" has been effectively established as occurring in birds [Klopfer, 1961], rats [Miller and Dollard, 1945], rhesus monkeys [Darby and Riopelle, 1959], and the domestic cat [Herbert and Harsh, 1944].

More elaborate learning of manipulation is well known for chimpanzees in captivity, but perhaps the most remarkable example concerns the origins of new habits, and their propagation, in groups of rhesus monkeys living under seminatural conditions in Japan. In recent years, Dr. Miyadi and his associates have succeeded in luring several monkey groups to artificial feeding places. First they met with resistance and found the monkeys suspicious of new food materials. But the monkeys became gradually accustomed to them and then started to establish new food habits for the group. The experimenters found that the new-born babies did not seem to distinguish between artificial and natural foods. In this case it was usually the baby that first tried to feed on the new food and the mother interfered with the adventure of her baby. Meanwhile, however, the mother imitated her baby and the behavior propagated itself to other individuals who had intimate relationships with each other, until the whole group acquired the new habit. While the first male of one particular group was reluctant to try new foods, the first male of another group was quick in learning, and was imitated by other members very soon. Once established, the habits appear to be handed down from mothers to babies or from older monkeys to younger ones, but the reverse route is taken in cases of new habits.

In a group on one of the islands, the authors discovered another kind of new habit, namely, the washing of sweet potatoes before eating them. This processing method was first started in 1953 by a young female and was imitated by other monkeys in a definite order. It was first learnt by the monkey's mother and playfellow, then by her sisters and brothers. Now many other monkeys, especially the younger ones, already show the same behavior, which is expected to become a new cultural habit of this group in the future. In this case, however, there seems little chance of the propagation of new habits from one group to another, except possibly by solitary males, because Japanese monkey societies are closed to members of other groups [Miyadi, 1959].

Aesthetic Values

The existence of genuine artistry among animals has often been suggested but is hard to prove. Nevertheless, there is now plausible reason for thinking that something like true art, at least in its first glimmerings, is shown by birds as well as mammals.

Birds, in fact, show artistry of a type which leads both to visual and auditory satisfaction. The bower birds (Ptilonorhynchidae) of Australia and New Guinea establish display grounds consisting of variously constructed bowers to which they eventually entice females and in or near which mating takes place. Nests, however, are built away from the bowers. These bowers are decorated in various and often highly elaborate fashions, some with an avenue approaching the bower, containing objects such as bleached bones, pieces of stone, metal, or (if they can get them) shining coins or other objects produced by man. Some will arrange brightly colored fruits or flowers which are not eaten but are left for display and replaced when they wither. Yet other species paint the walls of the bower with fruit pulp or with charcoal, using dried grass as a brush; and another species manufactures a painting tool out of a small wad of spongy bark. Some species not only select, and maintain in an attractive state, objects which seem beautiful to us; they also stick to a particular color scheme. Thus a bird using blue flowers will throw away a yellow flower inserted by the experimenter, and a bird using yellow flowers will not tolerate a blue one. It seems impossible to deny that a well-adorned bower may give the bird a pleasure that can only be called aesthetic.

We get the same impression from much precise modern work on the analysis of bird song. Szöke [1962] has argued that birds with the most highly developed song show a general similarity in the structure of their song. This seems to have been originally determined by the peculiar nature of the vocal apparatus of the primitive birds, and the overtone series which it can produce. Within these inherent limitations, some of those few species of birds which have been critically investigated in this regard show evidence of spontaneous rearrangement of phrases and the invention of new material which suggests something similar to real musical invention [Thorpe, 1961; Hall-Craggs, 1961]. How right was Robert Bridges when he said (*Testament of Beauty*, Book III, 1, 393–394):

> *Verily it well may be that sense of beauty came*
> *to these primitive bipeds earlier than to man.*

Indeed, it is now seriously argued by Szöke [1962] that insofar as man uses intervals of the natural series of overtones, these must have been learned from the environment, since they are not necessitated by the nature of our vocal equipment. It seems plausible that the intervals which are acceptable to the human ear as normal and natural for music are, in fact, those intervals which were first offered to the ancestors of man by bird song. Other animals do not have much in the way of song, but the fundamental intervals of human and bird song are the same; and highly developed bird song was presumably audible at man's first appearance on earth. Since man always had bird song all around, impinging on his ears, is it not reasonable to suppose that he developed a musical signal system by imitating the birds? This bird song was palaeomelody. Human premusic gradually developed, according to this theory, to be the component of the total art of primitive society and later to be a differentiated musical art, always "in the closest relationship to the development of society, under its influence and its interest" (Szöke).

It is again plausible to think that at least some of man's artistic activities, notably his dances and displays involving headdresses and other ornaments, may have been stimulated by watching the ceremonial displays of birds. Here, perhaps, the really fundamental problem is why, in so many cases, the patterns which have been produced in evolution as recognition marks for sexual behavior (quite apart from bird song) strike us as beautiful. (Quite apart also from beautiful sound patterns, one must remember the display plumes of many birds and the subtle and magnificent colors and patterns of Lepidoptera.) Does it all imply some fundamental unity between the mind and perceptual systems of groups as far apart as the Insecta, the Aves, and mankind?

There are many instances of bird songs which seem to transcend biological requirements and to suggest that the bird is actively seeking new auditory and vocal experience—"playing with sounds," so to speak —and this may represent the beginnings of a true artistic activity. Thus the twilight song of the wood pewee (*Myochanes virens*) appears to have no territorial function and is said to be independent of the breeding cycle, and the daytime song also continues long after the end of the breeding season. Experienced observers state that the song of late summer and autumn is, in many American song birds, superior to that of the breeding season. The duration of the skylark's (*Alauda arvensis*) song in Europe is greatest in September and October. Similarly, in many species of American song birds, the lengthening, elaboration, and sometimes complete change in the song after the end of the nesting period is noteworthy, and these changes often seem, to our ears, to take the form of aesthetic improvement. It has been suggested that the song can be improved at this time of year because it no longer is biologically necessary for it to retain the simpler form of the territorial song.

These instances refer particularly to development in the pattern of a song. Another aspect of the matter is the tonal purity of bird voices. Lorenz has suggested that purity of color in some visual social releasers —as in the duck's speculum—could be of selective value just because they have to be seen against a complex, inanimate or non-animal background containing every shade of color. Song, he argues, encounters virtually no nonbiological competition, since there are practically no sounds of inanimate origin which are of such frequency or form as to compete for the ear of the hearer. Here, however, there seems to be a possible flaw in the argument, for surely once a bird vocalization has acquired a specific signal function, vigorous interspecific competition for the available frequency range will be initiated [Thorpe, 1963]. Thus purity of tone will at once become a potentially advantageous feature since, in common with the tendency to elaborate the pattern of the sound, it will provide an additional dimension for distinctiveness, and therefore should lead—as the international agreement on the allocation of radio frequencies should have led—to an economic and peaceful utilization of the available spectrum. But even admitting this, it is hard to imagine any selective reason for the extreme purity of some bird notes, since the releaser function does appear to have been transcended in many cases. It is hoped that further study and analysis of bird sounds by modern methods will in due course yield further facts relevant to these problems.

The investigations of what may be called protoaesthetic phenomena in animals have been followed up by Rensch [1957], who offered experimental animals (monkeys and birds) choice of pieces of white cardboard, differently patterned, as materials for play. The animals showed preferences for symmetrical and rhythmical patterns, and for those with steady rather than faltering lines. But, by comparison with the achievements of wild birds, the artistic abilities of subhuman mammals seem meager in the extreme. I am indeed impressed by the sense of unity and of design shown by some of the "paintings" which chimpanzees can be induced to produce in captivity. However, they are to our eyes feeble, in comparison with some of the apparently biologically redundant performances of the bird vocal organs as they appeal to our ears. I shall be more impressed by the evidence for ape art if I learn of examples of its occurrence in the wild. It may be that the drawings of chimpanzees have been, in some subtle and at present undetermined way, affected by the unconscious predilection of the experimenter (in the same way as the famous calculating horses were in fact responding to the unwitting signals given by the trainer) [see Thorpe, 1963]. Perhaps, too, the order in which the painting materials were presented to the apes, and the way in which this was done, may have affected the result.

ETHICAL VALUES

Here, in this last section, we find ourselves on still trickier ground, but nevertheless, I think, ground which is not incapable of bearing some weight. If we are seeking examples of genuine altruism in animal behavior, we shall naturally look for it in those species where long-lasting personal friendships seem to be formed. It is common knowledge that, in many animals, separation from a close partner of long standing may give rise to what appear to be expressions of grief and moping, and a reunion may result in gestures of intense joy. One would expect porpoises to establish friendships, since the social cohesion and high activity of the porpoise school would seem likely to provide excellent conditions for its development. An extraordinary friendship between two male bottle-nosed dolphins (*Tursiops truncatus*), even though they had long been rivals for the attentions of a female which was sexually receptive and with which they had been confined, is described by a worker at the Oceanarium in Florida [McBride, 1940]. After a period of some weeks separation, the reuniting of these two males caused a tremendous amount of excitement. The author says: "No doubt the two recognized each other and for several hours they swam side by side rushing frenziedly through the water. For several days they were inseparable but neither paid any attention to the female." From the nature of the case it is extremely difficult to investigate porpoise behavior except in captivity. It appears that there are clear expressions of dominance; and vicious attacks without any apparent reason have been observed. On the other hand, there is elaborate and apparently nonmalicious teasing, and clearly marked cooperation and social play. In the wild it is presumed that the female gives birth in isolation. A female giving birth in captivity proved to be very exciting to the males, some of which became aggressive. The other females gathered round the one in labor and helped to ward off the attacking mate. When the new-born infant began its first gradual ascent to the surface to breathe, another female accompanied the mother, swimming just below the infant as if in readiness to support it [McBride and Hebb, 1948]. Recently the distinguished big game naturalists [Grzimek and Grzimek, 1960] described how a full grown male lion (*Panthera leo*) was completely incapacitated by a broken shoulder, due, it is supposed, to the kick of a giraffe, so that it had obviously been unable to hunt for some time. Nonetheless it was well nourished, the implication being that another male who accompanied it had kept it adequately supplied with food. Similar highly cooperative behavior has been described for the African elephant (*Loxodonta africanus*), particularly in connection with the protection and care of the young by both the mother and other adult female members of the group. With captive chimpanzees, although most of the behavior may seem entirely selfish, strong personal friendships are formed. Nissen [1951] has given an amusing description of the effect of begging by one chimpanzee upon another. This seems to be both an unpleasant yet also a very compelling stimulus. "Often it appears that the chimpanzee cannot tolerate this. Reluctantly or even with some show of irritation or anger, he hands over some of the food or throws it violently at the beggar." Although this response seemed the reverse of generous, the very reluctance to make the gift shows how strong the compulsion behind it must be. There are also examples in chimpanzees of one animal temporarily putting herself in a position where she was in danger of attack, apparently solely for the purpose of shielding a less experienced or more foolhardy animal from danger. Miss Goodall's studies of wild free-living chimpanzees suggest that under these natural conditions the behavior is even more social and gives even more evidence of personal attachments than do observations of captive animals.

The process of taming and domestication often reveals unsuspected subtleties in the behavior of animals. This may happen in two ways. First, the process of taming may lead to the adoption of the experimenter as a fellow member of the species by the animal being studied, and so (in at least some respects) the experimenter begins to get an inside view —an intraspecific view—of the species behavior. Second, once an animal becomes attached in this way and sensitive to the emotional expression of its human associate, it becomes exposed to the more elaborate social and mental life of the human. In consequence, its emotional and mental nature can sometimes be developed to a higher pitch than is possible in the normal wild environment. Nearly all the higher animals have, I believe, potentialities in this way, which only training by man can fully bring to view. Thus it is possible that the performance of a well-trained sheep dog surpasses in certain respects anything of which even the most highly socialized wolf (*Canis lupus*) is capable, though we still know too little about the fascinating organization of the wolf pack to be sure. Those who have reared rats as pets say that they display a charm, affection, and intelligence that the worker who is only acquainted with the laboratory rat of the psychologist finds hard to believe. Much careful observation of a pet African civet cat (*Viverra civetta*) and a pet lion cub by Hubbard [1963] revealed much humanlike behavior. It seems quite clear that the affection of this civet for its human companion was nonsexual. The lion cub, like the famous Elsa of Mrs. Joy Adamson, showed extraordinary forbearance with its human playmates, as if realizing the dangers of its own strength. In one case the young lion was actually found protecting a human child from its angry parent. Another remarkable characteristic of the pet civet cat was its jealousy, or at least behavior that it is extremely difficult to describe in any other terms. The question of jealousy in pet animals is in some ways the most interesting and yet the most difficult of all. If the observations, which are now quite extensive, can be taken at their face value—and I personally think they can—it is difficult to disregard them as evidence not only of high-level ideation, but also for elaborate self-awareness and something like ethical values.

The most remarkable instance of what is *apparently* jealous behavior in mammals that has come my way was repeatedly observed in my own laboratory by my colleagues Professor R. A. Hinde and Miss Y. Spencer-Booth. We have a number of groups of rhesus monkeys (*Macaca mulatta*), each consisting of a male, a number of females, and the resulting young, each group being housed separately in a compartment of the monkey house, the compartment consisting of a large outside enclosure and an indoor shelter with a window between, and a communicating swing door which the monkeys can work themselves. When a baby is born in one of these groups it is always the object of intense interest on the part of the various "aunts," and their possessiveness may give rise to a good deal of squabbling. In the latter half of 1962 a female, Rosie, at the bottom of her group's hierarchy of females, produced a baby. This infant seemed particularly attractive to Eliane, the favorite wife of the male, Tom, and thus at the top of the hierarchy. Eliane actually succeeded, on two occasions, in getting the baby away from Rosie, and much effort was needed to restore it to its rightful owner. When Rosie had finally re-established possession of the coveted infant, Eliane was seen on many occasions going through a remarkable performance. When Rosie and her child were "indoors" looking out through the window, Eliane would come and "gacker" at them from outside. Sometimes she would shadowbox with Rosie through the window and would then run away squealing as if she had been attacked. The result was as might have been expected: Tom, the male in charge, went in and beat up Rosie. It is very difficult to avoid the conclusion that this was a carefully thought-out piece of behavior "designed" by Eliane to ensure that Tom punished her rival.

Among birds the most remarkable case that has come to my notice concerns a pet barn owl (*Tyto alba*) which belonged to Dr. Miriam Rothschild. The owl was hand-reared from the nestling stage. At the time of its capture, the owner was ill and the bird lived in a wastepaper basket at the end of the bed. It was, therefore, constantly in the company of its foster mother, to whom it became extremely attached. It was never pinioned and lived free in the house. It was also house-trained and returned always to the same perch on every occasion. Dr. Rothschild describes the bird's nature at this time as catlike—very independent, but affectionate and sensual. It particularly liked being stroked and tickled, and it would sidle up to its owner (say, on a writing desk) and solicit stroking and fondling. It would then close its eyes and show every symptom of enjoyment, swaying and purring. When the owl was seven months old, in 1945, the owner went to London for six weeks while her child was born. She returned with the baby in early February. The owl recognized her immediately and, when she first saw her, showed the same affectionate disposition as in the past. But directly the bird saw the baby, a sudden change came over its attitude. It savagely attacked the owner and from that moment onwards was unsafe. Dr. Rothschild found it difficult to believe the situation, for she says this greatly loved bird was the most affectionate tame animal she had ever possessed. Every effort was made to win back the owl. She continued to keep it in the living room and wore protection over her head and face. The owl never had the chance to get near the baby, and only rarely saw it, but its hostile attitude did not change. It was not nervous or afraid, but continued to launch unpredictable and savage attacks on the owner, *but on no one else.* For instance, the bird was docile and affectionate to the cook. If the owner approached it with food it was quite possible that the owl would strike savagely at her with its claws and beat at her with its wings. After trying for six weeks to win back the bird's affection, it was decided with extreme reluctance to part with it. On separation from the foster mother, this owl built a nest and laid sterile eggs. The story ended a few weeks later after some fertile eggs had been provided for the owl to sit upon, when some well-meaning but ignorant visitor gave the bird a moribund mouse to eat. It turned out that the mouse had been poisoned, and the owl died too.

I referred at the start to the possibility that consciousness might be a process essential for the steering of nervous systems when they get beyond a certain degree of elaboration. This implies that if the machine gets beyond a certain degree of complexity, if it reaches the fantastic degree of elaboration which we find in the brain of the higher mammals, then unconscious, and even subconscious, methods of control are no longer adequate and we enter the realm of conscious control. This suggests that consciousness is a necessary evolutionary step which natural selection *must* take before the more complex animals can become adequately adapted to their environment. This in its turn suggests that if we were to make a machine of the order of complexity that we find, say, in the higher mammals (a task which at present seems infinitely beyond the wildest projects of technology), we should in a very real sense have brought the machine "to life." But this, of course does not follow. As a geneticist has remarked [Sinnott, 1950], in discussing Norbert Wiener's book *Cybernetics,* "one may question whether these artefacts really give us more than an instructive analogy with protoplasmic regulation. After all, we are not made of electronic valves, or wires and gears but of protein molecules. Our bodies are a triumph of chemical, not mechanical, engineering." The upshot of this is, then, that the production of consciousness may have been an evolutionary necessity, in that it may have been the only way in which highly complex living organisms could become fully viable. Whether this view is right or wrong, it is therefore clearly of great interest to consider the evidence for consciousness in animals and to consider whether we can find grounds for thinking that consciousness is only present above a certain level of organization. The evolutionary justification for expectancy has been well indicated by Berlyne [1960], who refers to expectancy as the device which cuts down the cost of adjustment. If the event that calls for action is part of a regularly recurring sequence of events, its predecessors can serve as warning signals. Expectations open the way to preparatory and avoidance responses, or to prior selection of response by reasoning, if the animal is capable of such reasoning. Expectations, moreover, may diminish stress by making adjustment less abrupt. They will usually be accompanied by high arousal as well as by responses that identify the particular event that is expected. But there will be times when the precise nature of an impending occurrence cannot be anticipated, either because the appropriate clues are lacking or because their significance has not been learned. In such cases an executive response cannot be preselected. Those component processes of the orientation reaction that come into play in coping with any urgent situation, and that do not depend on the specific properties of the situation, can, perhaps, be mobilized in advance. This anticipatory mechanism may be called *anticipatory arousal.* It requires the presence of a pattern of cues indicating how arousing, how novel, how important, etc., the experience is, how crucial the next few moments are going to be, without telling exactly what they will contain. So this mechanism, although it will not afford all the advantages of a specific expectation, will permit speedier and more energetic action when the anticipated event has been detected as a result of the heightened sensitivity of receptor organs, etc. Moreover, if the anticipated event has unpleasant aspects that nothing can mitigate —if it is, for example (to take a human instance), a piece of irrevocable bad news—anticipatory arousal will make it easier to withstand the shock, perhaps by producing some anticipatory habituation. So again we are in the situation of finding evidence for something like anticipation far down in the animal scale; again we know of physiological mechanisms which control and organize behavior which certainly appears anticipatory and which, we have good reason to believe, is often associated in higher animals with intelligent awareness. Some of these anticipatory mechanisms we can certainly envisage as functioning without the necessity of anything we could call consciousness. On the other hand, as we have seen, the anticipatory behavior of some of the higher animals seems to any intelligent observer, or so I think, to give an overwhelming impression of conscious and deliberate foresight. Perhaps here again the evidence suggests that at the lower levels, consciousness, if it exists, must be of a very generalized kind, so to say, unstructured; and that with the development of purposive behavior and a powerful faculty of attention, consciousness associated with expectation will become more and more vivid and precise.

One final point: If the evolution of consciousness was indeed an evolutionary necessity as brains got larger, does this not imply that *consciousness is something other than* brain action—a real emergent?

SUMMARY

The various physiological mechanisms which have been regarded as the bases of consciousness are briefly reviewed, and the evidence provided by recent studies in animal behavior, for or against them, is assessed.

These ethological studies are grouped under a number of subheadings: (1) attention and the innate releasive mechanism; (2) ideation and the manipulation of abstract ideas; (3) anticipation and expectancy; (4) self-awareness; (5) aesthetic values; (6) ethical values. It is pointed out that there is a significant body of work under all except the first of these categories which points with increasing certainty, as we go up through the animal scale, to the existence of consciousness and self-consciousness in animals. This seems to apply with particular force to the more highly evolved amongst the birds, and applies widely among the mammals. In particular, the anticipatory behavior which we find among both these groups often gives an overwhelming impression of conscious and deliberate foresight. It is suggested that, as William James supposed, consciousness is what might be expected in an organ added for the sake of steering a nervous system grown too complex to regulate itself. The suggestion is made that at the lower levels of animal life, consciousness—if it exists—must be of a very generalized kind, so to say, unstructured, and that with the development of purposive behavior and a powerful faculty of attention, consciousness associated with expectation will become more and more vivid and precise. With this in mind, we have powerful reasons for concluding that consciousness at one grade or another is a widespread feature of animal life.

DISCUSSION

Chairman: PROFESSOR CHAGAS

HEYMANS: Professor Thorpe pointed to a very interesting series of facts, showing discrimination and awareness up to consciousness in various species of animals, and I think we have to agree with his suggestions and also his conclusion. Perhaps I could add one more observation of a very typical case of discrimination and awareness in a gorilla. While staying at the research laboratory in the Congo we planned to perform some observations on a male gorilla weighing about 400 lb, but nobody could approach this huge and very dangerous fellow, so I was asked how we could quiet down and thus approach the gorilla; and we suggested the injection of some reserpine—a quite powerful sedative—in one of the bananas given to the gorilla as food. The gorilla, being hungry, got a large bunch of bananas, including the reserpine-injected one (injected with a thin needle and syringe through the skin of the banana). So the gorilla peeled one banana after the other, and was eating them very nicely, until he got to the reserpine-injected banana. We were, of course, anxious to see what he was going to do, but he peeled this banana just as the other ones, put it quite close to his mouth and then immediately threw it away, seeming to be very disgusted, and then took the other bananas, peeled them and ate them very nicely. I am quite sure the gorilla could not taste the reserpine because he did not put the banana in his mouth; several people tried it, and, at least for human beings, reserpine has no smell. This observation at least showed that the gorilla has a very marked sense of discrimination; how he did it, I do not know. Anyway, this observation struck us very markedly, and, of course, we all came to the conclusion that the gorilla was not so stupid and seemed to be quite an intelligent fellow.

THORPE: I think we ought to be very careful about supposing that an animal cannot detect a strange object hidden in a banana. We have tried giving monkeys gentian violet pills in bananas, and the speed with which they detect these and take them out before they eat the fruit is quite astonishing. I think these monkeys may have a more acute sense of smell than is generally supposed and that by its means they detect that the food is strange or that it has been contaminated by human hands. In any case, they are very cautious about eating anything new without a thorough preliminary investigation.

ECCLES: I was going to make another suggestion: that the gorilla was watching the audience and drew the conclusion there that he was going to be doped!

HEYMANS: Would you agree that it had a very good sense of discrimination, anyway?

GOMES: I would like to ask Professor Thorpe whether his long and detailed experience as a researcher of animal behavior and psychology would not incline him to believe that consciousness can always be associated with the independent behavior of an animal within its environment, that is, with behavior that is not completely and uniquely determined by the physical influence of the environment on the physical state of the animal. Is it not only behavior of this nature that puts the requirement of consciousness—and thus not the mere complexity of the system? I can still remember the remark—as realistic and impeccable as it is perplexing—which Professor Eccles advanced here some two days ago, to the effect that when confined to the strict status of a neurophysiologist, he could see no use and no motive for consciousness. He deals, however, with systems of extreme complexity, and this complexity has not induced him to entertain a different opinion. Is it not only the transference of a part of the responsibility for the control of behavior of a living being to this being itself that can throw light on the question of the appearance of consciousness?

THORPE: The difficulty with your question is that independence of the environment is characteristic, in some degree, of all animals. True, it is greater, on the whole, in the more highly evolved animals. But you cannot, in my view, use it, by itself, as a criterion of consciousness. And indeed it is not only animals and plants which display this "homeostasis"—many mechanical nonliving systems do so too. The question I am asking is whether the physiologist here can suggest that a machine of given complexity or a brain of given complexity would be more likely to be fully effective than a less complex physiological mechanism merely by virtue of the fact that it has acquired consciousness? Is that in itself likely to make it more effective? You see, I am impressed by the evidence that consciousness must have evolved certainly more than once, probably a number of times, in different animal lineages. One wants to know why this is. Is there a good selective reason for it or is there just no reason at all why the animal should not have got on quite as well without having developed this apparently strange and new faculty?

MAC KAY: In relation to these birds which perform selectively as if they recognized and so forth—I wonder what your comment is on computer programs which now exist and do the like? I certainly would hesitate to suggest that an artificial program, even with a complete metaorganizing system, could thereby be guaranteed to have consciousness, and I wonder whether behavior alone can ever offer an adequate criterion. I am sympathetic to the idea that protoplasm may be necessary, if only to provide the right information flow conditions.

THORPE: This is just what I wanted your opinion about. It seems to me that one has to ask oneself whether one can envisage the kind of computer which it would be necessary to postulate as being within the bird to enable it to do these things without having had, at some stage in the process of acquiring the ability to perform these feats, something like consciousness. I rather expected that you would be inclined to equate consciousness with the center or the organization that you are supposing to be in the brain stem or in a large part of the cortex. I thought, too, that you would consider this as in fact more or less equivalent to what we *introspectively* decide is consciousness. Having got that far you would naturally expect something like consciousness rather far down in the animal scale. I think one can sum it up by putting it like this—when the bird is learning to do one of these tasks, or when the species is acquiring the performance, do you think that consciousness adds anything to the computer design or not?

MAC KAY: We have to discuss one level at a time. The information flow level does not have any place for consciousness as a concept, but I would certainly say that from an evolutionary point of view *metaorganizing activity* would have an advantage—it would enable the prefabrication of matching subroutines which could not be prefabricated in any other way, and so on. And I am prepared to believe that in the biological kingdom the evolution of a metaorganizing system has had as its correlate the development of conscious experience in these other organisms, but I don't know, of course; I only know of myself and other human beings.

THORPE: From that point of view, are you quite happy to regard it as an epiphenomenon?

MAC KAY: Not as an epiphenomenon in any derogatory sense, but as a complementary aspect and, indeed, for us, the most important aspect of all.

THORPE: But not as important selectively? That is the point. Is it important selectively?

MAC KAY: Inasmuch as selection depends on behavior, organisms with a metaorganizing system would be differentially favored in an evolutionary struggle regardless of whether these organisms had internal conscious experience, as long as they behaved-as-if-conscious. If we are looking at it mechanistically, the personal, internal subjective aspect does not come into the picture at all. But by analogy I think it implausible to *deny* conscious experience to lower animals of a sufficient complexity to have metaorganizing activity.

JASPER: I would like to ask Professor Thorpe if he does believe the whole evolutionary argument of the emergence of a new phenomenon of consciousness, which I gather is his principal theme? At some level of this complexity would you say there emerges a new phenomenon which is the conscious aspect of behavior? Couldn't one argue quite the opposite way: that consciousness is given in a very simple form—of course, in a simple way relative to the complexity of the organism—and in evolution we don't have the emergence of a new consciousness, but rather the specialization of a large amount of computing machinery which is unconscious; and that this development of specialization is actually in the opposite direction—that it is a pushing aside of specific mechanisms into unconscious processes because their elaborate complexity would make it quite impossible for each one of them to be a unified conscious process. Maintaining the original simplified model, I should think I could reverse the whole argument you have presented: that we have in the beginning a very low level of what would be considered consciousness; and evolution is not the development of that, but the elaboration of a very complex machinery that feeds into it, but the processes of which are in themselves mostly unconscious.

THORPE: I think my difficulty there would be to see what evolutionary function such a very general kind of consciousness could have served. I find it very difficult to imagine a highly organized consciousness which could be of real use to the animal in its everyday life without a fairly elaborate mechanism behind it. And so it seems to me very improbable that it has gone the way you suggest, but of course I cannot state categorically that it has not.

PENFIELD: I want to ask Professor Thorpe why he questions these matters in wild animals which are hard to get at, and overlooks his companion the dog, for which there is so much more evidence? It is perfectly clear (if I may refer to my own little dog of no known breed) that he had a clear capacity for nonverbal perception that was quite as good as any little child's. He had verbal perception also. We could prove that he recognized between 30 and 40 words. It is quite impossible to have either nonverbal or verbal perception without assuming that there is consciousness. It does not seem to me that this is open to debate.

THORPE: I do not feel anything like as sure about it as that. Turning to your first question. I think that ethologists are rather cautious about domesticated animals, particularly the dog, because of two things: first, they feel that people tend to get biased about the performance of their dogs; and certainly many ordinary dog keepers will often read much more detail into the significance of their dog's behavior than is actually there. I am a dog keeper myself, so I realize this. It is, therefore, perfectly proper for the ethologist to be cautious about reports of the behavior of pet animals; although, I may say, it is possible to err on the other side and dismiss a lot of perfectly well-established facts as fairy tales. But, over and above this, there is a feeling that perhaps a good deal of this apparently intelligent behavior in domestic animals may have in some way resulted from the animal watching the behavior of its human associates and so becoming remarkably sensitive and attuned to extremely subtle human gestures or other modes of expression. So before one can be sure, the effects must be studied under very closely controlled conditions; as has been done in some of those experiments with monkeys and rats that have been referred to. As an example of this it has been argued that the tool-using achievements of chimpanzees do not really mean very much because the chimpanzees had long seen human beings using tools, and by this they were given a lead as to how to start. Till now the tool-using ability of chimpanzees has thus been regarded, in some quarters, as of doubtful significance because it was supposed that they could not do this in the wild. Now, as a result of Miss Jane Goodall's work, we know this to be untrue.

ECCLES: We have to face up to the fact that consciousness is not an invariable concomitant even of the fully organized human brain. We have, for example, states of sleep or of automatic states that, as far as we know on all tests, are not conscious. There can be much complex functional activity going on in the fully organized human brain and yet it does not reach consciousness. I think it is very important to appreciate that it is not just complex nerve structure that gives consciousness. On the other hand, consciousness seems to be related to certain features of the functional state, and to occur only under those conditions. The intense cerebral activity of an epileptic convulsion is associated with a loss of consciousness. But when there are more subtle, discriminative, variable functional states, then consciousness emerges. I am very chary about postulating that consciousness necessarily occurs at a certain level of complexity, not merely in computers but even in animals.

THORPE: Would you say that it is quite obvious that very elaborate perceptions may go on in the totally unconscious condition? That is to say, do you think those perceptions could have been achieved in the absence of consciousness? That is the key point. Could the human being have achieved that kind of discrimination if it had all the time been unconscious?

ECCLES: There is evidence that conditioned reflexes can be set up at quite low levels of the nervous system, in decorticate animals, for example—and even, it is claimed by some, in the spinal cord. Thus it appears that discriminative learning behavior is possible in regions of the nervous system that we would ordinarily think are unconscious.

HINSHELWOOD: Whatever be the ultimate status of consciousness in the scheme of things, it is clear that a very flexible physical counterpart is necessary. It would seem impossible that nature should ignore the almost infinite multiplication of degrees of freedom, so rendering possible the adjustment mechanisms which biochemistry affords with its tremendous complexity and variability of compounds and codings. I would have thought, therefore, that there was a very intimate connection indeed between the complexity of chemistry and the possibility of a vehicle for consciousness.

On the other question about the purposes of evolution, I almost hesitate to say this in a scientific gathering; but one does just wonder what would be the point or purpose of anything at all if there were no consciousness anywhere.

THORPE: I am inclined to agree with you. On the other hand, I suppose you could say that the strength of natural selection is that nothing succeeds like success and anything which can leave more offspring—whether it does this by conscious or by unconscious processes—will then inherit the earth. That seems to me the problem.

LIBET: I wanted to make a point along the line already developed by Professor Eccles. One cannot assume from behavioral evidence that subjective awareness has occurred in animals merely because one finds complexity or ability to handle symbols, etc., in their behavior. As I tried to indicate in my paper, even in awake and attentive human subjects we have some experimental evidence of differences in the nature of the two kinds of responses. It would seem to me that any behavioral or objective indices of conscious experience would have to be validated in man, as being sufficiently unique correlates of conscious experience, before we could apply them with confidence to other animals.

THORPE: I think that is most important. What we do want is some EEG or other method of deciding whether a conscious process is going on in the brain so that we can bypass behavior and have a direct and reliable criterion.

SCHAEFER: I should like to ask Dr. Thorpe whether this whole problem can ever be decided. Let us for example assume that, according to the book of Lorenz about the natural history of aggression, all behavior of animals is really the outcome of natural selection; then of course, all things could have been organized by nature on merely physical and biochemical methods, so that the behavior of the animal is adapted to his environment. I feel we are all convinced that no consciousness can happen without a physical and biochemical background provided by some structural properties of our brain; and so, if the structure of the brain is the result of natural selection, then so would be consciousness; and consciousness and brain would develop in two streams of selection which cannot be divided.

THORPE: Yes, but this then brings us back to William James and to my original question. Given a brain of a given degree of elaboration, is it likely to be a more effective mechanism—more effective in an evolutionary sense—if it has consciousness attached, than if it has not? Just because of my general approach to animals, I am inclined to feel that this very high degree of social behavior and personal affection (even something that appears to be like jealousy) is very unlikely to be merely the result of an extremely efficient mechanism at work and nothing more. But only *appears* to be very unlikely; I cannot, of course, say that it is not so. So can you really say: this brain will work better if its owner is conscious than if he is not?

GRANIT: The neurophysiologists have no tests for consciousness or unconsciousness. I think that is clear. But the evolutionary theory of consciousness that you propound is, of course, the one that Sherrington proposed in *Man on his Nature;* this theory was one of his main themes. I realize that you are forced by the theme of this study week to put the evidence the way you have put it, but my impression from reading the ethological literature has been that this is the great literature for fine mechanisms without consciousness. If you really want to find examples of most elaborate things which are likely to be done with very little consciousness, you have to go to these experiments of your own field, particularly those with birds. I can think of one, that of Tinbergen with the eggs of the herring gull which had rolled out of its nest, and the bird tries to get it back into the nest. It will take an oversized egg and try to roll it in, which seems extremely unintelligent; but if the normal egg is a little too far away, but is well within his field of vision, the bird will not get up and roll it into its nest.

This is to me a striking example of a very elaborate mechanism which is not in the least intelligent or conscious. If the bird had been conscious it would have realized that when the egg is that far, why not get up and roll it back slowly. But it is only when it is within a certain distance, and independently of its size, that the bird rolls it back.

THORPE: I agree with you that there is a great deal of ethological experiment which does suggest just that view; at any rate, it suggests that the animal cannot possibly have an understanding of the ultimate objective of what it is doing. For instance, I am quite sure that a bird, the first time it is building its nest, is not aware of the fact that this nest is to put eggs in and then that the eggs shall be sat on and young shall be produced. We need never suppose that degree of conscious purpose in birds in such a situation. On the other hand, when you go to the orientation of either birds or insects, you find very elaborate and much more flexible behavior. It is one of the fascinations of ethological study, particularly of birds, that in one aspect of the life you find very elaborate behavior which runs off mechanically without any suggestion at all that the bird understands what it is doing this for. Then in another context you find quite different behavior. There one gets the impression of real foresight. So you get these two rather conflicting impressions from modern ethological work. Because of the subject of this conference I have been choosing, of course, the more exciting, more elaborate, stranger examples to give you because they, at any rate in a *prima facie* way, seem to suggest that consciousness must be present. But I could have given you a whole host of examples which make the behavior, even in the same groups of animals, appear much more stereotyped and mechanical.

TEUBER: I am very happy that Professor Thorpe has stressed those features in ethologic studies that are usually underplayed, and that he did all this in 40 minutes without once using the word "instinct" which I think has stuck to all this like a burr and deterred many people from even looking at these phenomena. Of course, these achievements by animals were called instinctive merely in order to deny them certain features that we gladly grant to each other's behavior. It was an attempt to make a sharp division and to say that what we do by reason, foresight, and with full awareness of why and how we do it and what the goals are, the animals do by mere instinct, as automata if you will. In reality, we are not always so insightful, and higher animals are rarely as automatic as this old division implies. Professor Thorpe's compilation cites a great variety of prodromes of human-type consciousness in animals. While agreeing with most of this, I might quibble a bit with you, Professor Thorpe, with regard to the interpretation of the work of the Freiburg group— the work of Otto Koehler and his students.

The basic phenomena have been confirmed elsewhere and by people who are less inclined to think of true counting ability in birds, but I completely agree with Dr. MacKay that it is not at all difficult to program a machine to extract numerosity without, I think, having to say that this machine is able to handle number concepts in the sense in which I think this is possible for a child once he really learns how to handle numbers. What is required here on the human level is not just an awareness of three being less numerous than four and acting upon it, but an ability to generate a forward-going number series according to a law, the law of generating numbers; and there in fact is the great riddle of how this is ever learned, how you learn a rule rather than specific elements that you can then chain together. It is this generative rule that is lacking in the animals, and I would stress this difference rather than the similarities which are being stressed by Otto Koehler. As to Lögler's work, I agree that his experimental results would appear to approximate human counting, since he reports cross-modal transfer of numerosity on the part of his parrot between visual and auditory modes of presentation. However, just because this observation is so important, it would seem to me to require extensive checking in other animals. I recall that during a visit to Freiburg some years ago, Dr. George Ettlinger and I discussed this experiment with Dr. Lögler, and it seemed to us that this parrot might have had some earlier laboratory experience which may well have been crucial here. I believe that the animal was exposed to combined stimulation in the visual and auditory modes at some earlier stage. It is possible, therefore, that what seemed like cross-modal transfer was really the capacity to respond to parts of a series which had been learned originally through both modalities together.

THORPE: It is true there has been a paper written on this question of previous experience of that particular parrot, and I quite agree that the work does want doing again. On the other hand, as far as I can see from the account of this, it is very unlikely, but not impossible, that previous training was the explanation of this particular achievement.

But one general thing I should like to say is that of course there have been attempts, 60 or 70 years before the work of Otto Koehler and his pupils, to establish the counting ability of animals but they were always unsatisfactory methodologically; there has always been some snag in the design of the experiment. Koehler was the first to get what seems to be a flawless experimental design worked out. But one very remarkable thing is this: the "counting ability" needs a very long period of training to produce and there is not the slightest evidence, that I have been able to find, that it can be of any use to the animal in the wild.

There seems to be a latent ability which can be brought out by this experimental training. And there is a similar situation in regard to the imitative vocalization of many birds. After all, talking parrots have been known since before the time of Aristotle. Yet as far as I know, no one has ever heard either a myna, which is the best talking bird of all, or a parrot, imitate anything in the wild. But rear them in captivity they can perform these astonishing feats of vocal imitation. In this respect the performance is very similar to counting. But the function of this is still very problematical. Whether it is possible to regard it as having been produced without the faculty of consciousness I am much more doubtful.

BREMER: I apologize, Professor Thorpe, if the question I shall ask you may sound rather impertinent. I wonder if the most interesting and beautiful animal performances you described could not be analyzed and commented without any use of that word "consciousness," with the elusive content it covers?

THORPE: It could certainly be described; whether it is possible to regard these performances as having been produced without the faculty of consciousness I am much more doubtful. My problem is, how did they arrive either in the individual or in the race if there is not something like consciousness present?

SPERRY: You know the old saying that "ontogeny repeats phylogeny." I just want to point out that we have exactly the same problem in the early stages of human development that we have with animals: before the child can reason or calculate or tell you what it sees and feels, one is obliged to infer what is there in the way of consciousness, from its actions alone.

THORPE: I find great difficulty in supposing that the conscious awareness of a child suddenly leaps into being. That is why I stressed at the end the idea that the consciousness of a child must be a very simple affair compared with the elaborately structured consciousness of the adult. But both in ontogeny and phylogeny it is hard to know where to draw the line.

MAC KAY: May I attempt a short answer to Professor Thorpe's question, whether consciousness must, or could usefully, "come in" in order to exercise control? If he is thinking of consciousness as a nonphysical source of information to mold action, then I think this could be useful, but we lack any evidence that it happens! If consciousness does not mean that, I would say that the question is empty, because control in a conscious organism can then be fully specified by informational considerations without reference to the word "consciousness."

CHAIRMAN: Would not some of the experiments so beautifully presented by Professor Thorpe indicate that in several animal species, molecular biochemistry is constantly playing an important role in behavioral interactions? I would also like to know how much higher animals are losing the power to react to some apparently important stimuli from the outside world, and are acquiring the ability to elaborate their behavior from less active and seemingly less significant ecological factors.

REFERENCES

ANDERSON, K. D. S. *Nine Man-Eaters and One Rogue.* London: Allen and Unwin [1954].

BERLYNE, D. E. *Conflict, Arousal and Curiosity.* New York: McGraw-Hill [1960].

COWLES, J. T., and H. W. NISSEN. Reward-expectancy in delayed responses of chimpanzees, *J. Comp. Psychol., 24,* 345–8 [1937].

DARBY, C. L., and A. J. RIOPELLE. Observational learning in the Rhesus monkey, *J. Comp. Physiol. Psychol., 52,* 94–95 [1959].

ELLIOTT, M. H. The effect of change of reward on the maze performance of rats, *U. Calif. Pub. Psychol., 4,* 185–88 [1928].

EVARTS, E. V. Patterns of neuronal discharge in visual cortex during visual inspection, waking and sleep, *Proc. XXII Int. Congr. Physiol. Sci. Leiden., 1,* 448–450. Amsterdam [1962].

GIBB, J. A. L. Tinbergen's hypothesis of the role of specific search images, *Ibis., 104,* 106–111 [1963].

GOODALL, J. M. Feeding behaviour of wild chimpanzees, *Symp. Zool. Soc. Lond., 10,* 39–47 [1963].

———. Tool using and aimed throwing in a community of free living chimpanzees, *Nature, 201,* 1264–66 [1964].

GRZIMEK, B., and M. GRZIMEK. *Serengeti Shall Not Die.* London [1960].

HALL-CRAGGS, J. The development of song in the blackbird (*Turdus merula*), *Ibis, 104,* 277–300 [1961].

HALL, K. R. L., and G. B. SCHALLER. The tool-using of the California sea otter (*Enhydra lutris nereis*), *J. Mammal., 45,* 287 [1964].

HEBB, D. O. The problem of consciousness and introspection, in: *Brain Mechanisms and Consciousness,* pp. 402–417. (Ed. by J. F. Delafresnaye; E. D. Adrian, F. Bremer, H. H. Jasper.) Oxford: Blackwell Scientific Publications [1954].

HERBERT, M. J., and C. M. HARSH. Observational learning by cats, *J. Comp. Psychol., 37,* 81–95 [1944].

HERRNSTEIN, R. J., and D. H. LOVELAND. Complex visual concept in the pigeon, *Science, 146,* 549–51 [1964].

HILLABY, J. *Journey to the Jade Sea.* London [1964].

HINDE, R. A. *Behaviour: An Approach and a Synthesis.* New York. (In press) [1966].

HOLST, E. VON, and H. MITTELSTAEDT. Das Reafferenzprinzip. Wechchselwirkungen zwischen Zentral nervensystem und Peripherie, *Naturwiss., 37,* 464–76 [1950].

HORN, G. Electrical activity of the cerebral cortex of unanaesthetized cats during attentive behaviour, *Brain, 83,* 57–76 [1960].

HUBBARD, W. D. *Ibamba.* London: Gollancz [1963].

HUBEL, D. A., and T. N. WIESEL. Receptive fields of single neurones in cat's striate cortex, *J. Physiol., 148,* 574–91 [1959].

JAMES, WILLIAM. *The Principles of Psychology.* Vol. 1. New York: H. Holt and Co. [1890].

KLOPFER, P. H. Observational learning in birds: The establishment of behavioural modes, *Behaviour, 17,* 71–80 [1961].

KNEALE, W. *On Having a Mind.* Cambridge [1962].

LASHLEY, K. D. Dynamic processes in perception, in: *Brain Mechanisms and Consciousness,* pp. 427–443. (Ed. by J. F. Delafresnaye; E. D. Adrian, F. Bremer, H. H. Jasper.) Oxford: Blackwell Scientific Publications [1954].

LÖGLER, P. Versuche zur Frage der "Zahl"-vermögens an einem Grau Papagai, *Z. Tierpsychol., 16,* 179–217 [1959].

LORENZ, K. *Das Sogenannte Böse, Zur Naturgeschichte der Aggression.* Vienna: G. Borotha-Schoeler [1963].

McBRIDE, A. F. *Nat. Hist. Mag., 45,* 16–29 [1940].

———, and D. O. HEBB. Behaviour of the captive bottle-nosed dolphin (*Tursiops truncatus*), *J. Comp. Psychol., 41,* 111–123 [1948].

MILLER, N. E., and J. DOLLARD. *Social Learning and Imitation.* London: Routledge [1945].

MIYADI, D. On some habits and their propagation in Japanese monkey groups, *XV Int. Congr. Zool. Proc.,* 857–60 [1959].

MOOREHEAD, A. *No Room in the Ark.* London: H. Hamilton [1959].

NISSEN, H. W. Social behaviour in primates, in: *Comparative Psychology* (ed. by C. P. Stone). New York: Prentice-Hall [1951].

RENSCH, B. *Gedächtnis, Abstraktion und Generalisation bei Tieren.* Cologne [1957].

SINNOTT, E. W. *Cell and Psyche: The Biology of Purpose.* Chapel Hill: Univ. North Carolina Press [1950].

SZÖKE, P. Zur Entstehung und Extwicklungsgeschichte der Musik, *Studia Musicologica, 2,* 33–85 [1962].

THORPE, W. H. *Bird Song: The Biology of Vocal Communication and Expression in Birds.* Cambridge: Cambridge Univ. Press [1961].

———. *Learning and Instinct in Animals.* 2nd ed. London: Methuen [1963].

TINBERGEN, L. The natural control of insects in pine woods. I. Factors influencing the intensity of predation by songbirds, *Arch. Néerl. Zool., 13,* 265–343 [1960].

TINKLEPAUGH, O. L. An experimental study of representative factors in monkeys, *J. Comp. Psychol., 8,* 197–236 [1928].

WYBURN, G. M., R. W. PICKFORD, and R. J. HURST. *Human Senses and Perception.* London: Oliver and Boyd [1964].

20

Dopamine and Central Neurotransmission

by C. Heymans and A. de Schaepdryver

Pharmacological and Therapeutic Institute, Ghent, Belgium

In recent years it has been attempted to define the mode of action of drugs which act on the central nervous system in terms of the influence which they exert on the biosynthesis, storage, release, effect, or inactivation of various hypothetical neurotransmitter substances.

Several conditions should be fulfilled, however, before a substance can be regarded as having a transmitter function in the CNS [Lewis, 1963]: its presence in a relatively high concentration at the synapse or effector site, the occurrence of precursors and metabolites, as well as of ana- and catabolizing enzyme systems, the possibility to mimic or enhance its physiological actions by administering either the substance itself or its precursors, or by inhibiting its inactivation, the possibility to decrease its physiological actions either by preventing its synthesis or by speeding up its inactivation.

Among other substances, dopamine seems to fulfill these physiological and biochemical requirements. Dopamine or 3-hydroxytyramine is known as a natural product in certain plants [Guggenheim, 1951], many fruits and vegetables [Udenfriend et al, 1959], and insects [Östlund, 1954].

In 1950 Goodall [1950, 1951] detected dopamine in the suprarenal glands and heart of the sheep, and a year later Euler et al [1951] found it in relatively large quantities in human urine, as confirmed afterwards by Drujan et al [1959]. Schümann [1958] showed later that it was also present in extracts of splenic nerves. Relatively large amounts were found in cow's lung and bronchi [Euler and Lishajko, 1957]. In the suprarenal glands, dopamine represents about 2 per cent of the total catecholamines [Dengler, 1957], whereas in sympathetic nerves it makes up about 50 per cent of the total catecholamine content [Schümann, 1956]. From 1957 on, various investigators [Montagu, 1957; Weil-Malherbe and Bone, 1957b; Carlsson et al, 1958] reported the presence of dopamine in the brain, where it was found localized to a large extent in the corpus striatum, mainly the putamen and caudate nucleus [Carlsson, 1959; Sano et al, 1959; Sano et al, 1960; Bertler, 1961].

The typical distribution of dopamine in cerebral areas (Fig. 20.1), which contain only very small amounts of noradrenaline, and the different subcellular localization of both amines [Carlsson et al, 1962] suggest that dopamine is not only a precursor of noradrenaline but that it also exerts a central nervous function in its own right.

Both the biosynthesis and metabolism of dopamine have been fairly well studied (Fig. 20.2). Dopa decarboxylase, the enzyme responsible for the formation of dopamine starting from its amino acid precursor dihydroxyphenylalanine or dopa, has been found in many types of nervous tissue, including the brain [Holtz, 1960; Holtz and Westermann, 1956]. It should be mentioned that the biosynthesis of dopamine occurs much more rapidly than the biosynthesis of noradrenaline, since hydroxylation of the dopamine side chain, under influence of dopamine-β-oxidase [Udenfriend and Creveling, 1959], is a very slow process. The rapidity of the biosynthesis of dopamine is demonstrated by the fact that a significant increase in brain dopamine levels occurs as early as ten minutes after administration of a monoamine oxidase inhibitor [Holzer and Hornykiewicz, 1959].

Besides this dopamine-anabolizing enzyme, the brain also contains dopamine-catabolizing enzymes, namely, monoamine oxidase [Bogdanski et al, 1957] and catechol-O-methyl-transferase [Axelrod et al, 1959].

The study of the function of brain dopamine has been approached in different ways. Since dopamine does not easily cross the blood-brain barrier, the dopamine content of the brain cannot be substantially increased by systemic injection of the amine. Injection of dopa, however, which readily crosses the blood-brain barrier and which is rapidly decarboxylated in the brain, leads to a significant increase in cerebral dopamine [Carlsson et al, 1957; Murphy and Sourkes, 1959]. This increase will be more pronounced if a monoamine oxidase inhibitor is administered in addition to dopa, thus preventing the enzymatic destruction of the dopamine formed. This treatment was found to provoke hypermotility and arousal [Everett, 1961; Smith and Dews, 1962].

Using dopa, deserpidine, and the monoamine oxidase inhibitor pargylline, alone or in combination, with the purpose of separating the various amine profiles for correlation with behavior, Everett and Wiegand [1962] reported a very good correlation between dopamine brain levels

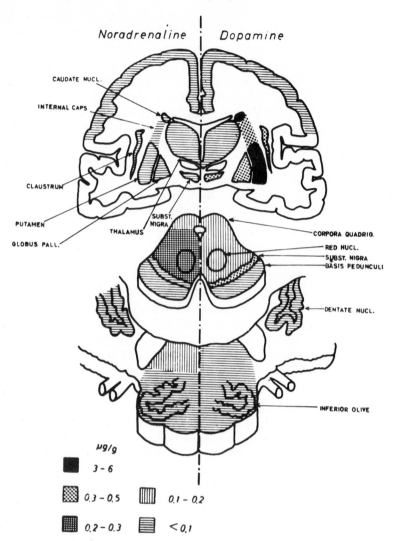

Noradrenaline   Dopamine

CAUDATE NUCL.

INTERNAL CAPS

CLAUSTRUM

PUTAMEN

GLOBUS PALL.

THALAMUS

SUBST. NIGRA

CORPORA QUADRIG.

RED NUCL.

SUBST. NIGRA

BASIS PEDUNCULI

DENTATE NUCL.

INFERIOR OLIVE

μg/g

3 - 6

0.3 - 0.5   0.1 - 0.2

0.2 - 0.3   < 0.1

Fig. 20.1. Noradrenaline and dopamine in the human brain, according to Bertler [1961].

and central excitement. These observations also tend to corroborate the view that brain dopamine is involved in the control of alertness. One should be cautious, however, in attributing these changes exclusively to an accumulation of dopamine in the brain, since monoamine oxidase inhibitors are known to produce other biochemical effects as well.

Mantegazzani and Glässer [1960], avoiding the use of monoamine oxidase inhibitors, observed an arousal reaction in the *cerveau isolé* preparation after a countercurrent injection of dopa into the lingual artery. It was further observed that at the moment of the appearance of the electroencephalographic signs of the arousal reaction the dopamine levels in the caudate nucleus and in the hypothalamus showed a very significant elevation—up to 100 per cent and more of control levels—whereas hypothalamic noradrenaline levels remained unchanged [Bertler and Rosengren, 1959; Dagirmajian et al, 1963]. The same alerting effect of dopa was also observed in the reserpine treated animal [Carlsson et al, 1957; Everett and Toman, 1962].

These observations suggest that the arousal reaction described above is related to an accumulation of dopamine in the brain, without permitting, however, a precise anatomic localization of the area where this reaction has its origin.

In contrast to the stimulating effect of systemically administered dopa, intrathecal injection of high doses of dopamine produces sedation. This difference is not necessarily of a qualitative nature, but may be due to the fact that much higher concentrations of dopamine occur in the ventricle after intrathecal than after peripheral injection.

A decrease of brain dopamine levels, on the other hand, may be induced either by substances which inhibit the conversion of dopa to dopamine, such as α-methyldopa and α-methyl-m-tyrosine [Weil-Malherbe and Bone, 1957a; Murphy and Sourkes, 1959; Sourkes et al, 1960] or by reserpine, which releases practically all dopamine from the brain [Holzbauer and Vogt, 1956; Brodie et al, 1957; Carlsson et al, 1958], together with the other amines, noradrenaline and serotonin. In contrast to reserpine, some noradrenaline-releasing substances, such as β-tetrahydronaphthylamine, have at first sight no influence on the dopamine levels in the caudate nucleus. The fact, however, that the level of homovanillic

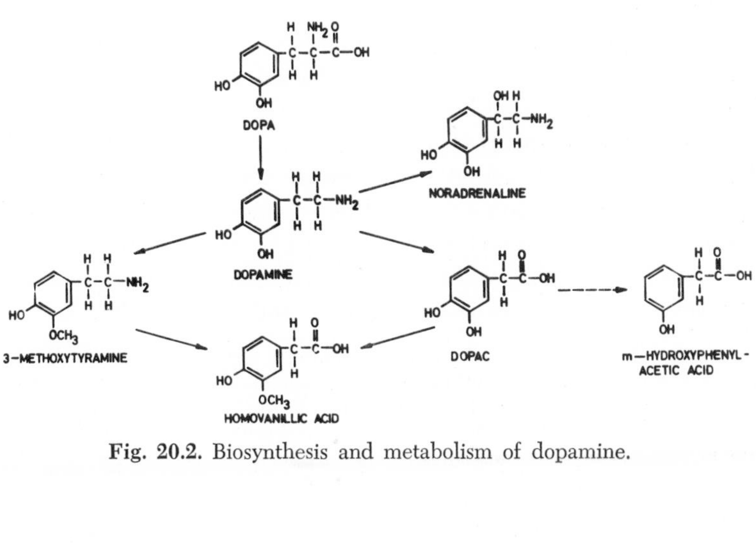

Fig. 20.2. Biosynthesis and metabolism of dopamine.

acid (3-methoxy-4-hydroxyphenylacetic acid), a dopamine metabolite, increased in these circumstances from 2.8 to 7.7 μg per g on an average, suggests that these substances influence brain dopamine in the same way as they do with regard to brain noradrenaline, but that the increased release of dopamine is masked by a more rapid resynthesis of dopamine as compared with noradrenaline [Laverty and Sharman, 1963]. It is of special interest that reserpine, when given in rather high doses, may provoke Parkinsonism.

Following up the physiological and biochemical evidence cited above, additional experimental evidence that dopamine has a transmitter function in the central nervous system has been obtained by the use of a recently developed electroshock technique, which permits a more accurate analysis of the effects of pharmacological substances on both electroshock threshold and convulsion characteristics.

Our experiments were performed in 304 unanesthetized rabbits with intracranial electrodes. The electrodes were implanted one week prior to the first electroshock application, according to the previously described technique [Delaunois et al, 1962]. Using a Grass S4B stimulator, rectangular DC pulses with a duration of 2 msec and a frequency of 125 per sec were applied for 0.5 sec. Application of these stimuli at an energy level of 0.2 W per sec provokes in intact rabbits a typical convulsive seizure characterized, after a latency period of 3.0 sec ± 0.9 sec, by the occurrence of a tonic phase, including a flexion and extension of both fore- and hindlegs, accompanied by a hyperextension of the trunk with a duration of 16.4 sec ± 3.5 sec, ending in a shorter lasting and less pronounced clonic phase.

Control electroshocks were applied one week before administration of drugs.

By means of various drug combinations, the serotonin, noradrenaline and dopamine brain levels may be manipulated somewhat independently from each other, thus permitting a correlation of these different amine brain levels with the electroshock threshold [De Schaepdryver et al, 1962; Piette et al, 1963; Heymans et al, 1964].

A decrease of the levels of brain amines was obtained by means of reserpine,[1] dimethylaminobenzoyl-methylreserpate (Su-5171) [Brodie et al, 1960], α-methyldopa [Hess et al, 1961], and α-methyl-m-tyrosine [Brodie and Costa, 1962], whereas a selective increase of brain serotonin and a combined increase of brain serotonin and noradrenaline were pro-

[1] Reserpine (Serpasil ®) and Su-5171 were kindly supplied by Ciba A.G., Basle; iproniazid (Marsilid ®) and l-dihydroxyphenylalanine (l-dopa) by F. Hoffmann-La Roche & Co., Ltd., Basle; JB-516 and JB-835 by Lakeside Laboratories, Inc., Milwaukee, Wisconsin; α-methyldopa and α-methyl-m-tyrosine by Merck Sharp & Dohme Research Laboratories, Rahway, New Jersey; imipramine [N-(γ-dimethylaminopropyl)-imino-dibenzyl hydrochloride, Tofranil ®] by Geigy A.G., Basle.

voked by pretreatment with 5-hydroxytryptophan and β-phenylisopropyl-hydrazine (JB-516), and by pretreatment with β-phenylisobutyl-hydrazine (JB-835), respectively [Brodie et al, 1959]. A selective increase in brain dopamine was obtained by means of a combined pretreatment with reserpine, iproniazid, and l-dopa, as described by Carlsson [1962].

Our experimental observations have been summarized in Tables 1 and 2.

Table 1

Drug	Brain Serotonin Noradrenaline (% of Normal)		E. S. Threshold (Changes, %)
Reserpine	10	9	−62
α-CH$_3$-m-tyrosine	100	0	−50
Reserpine	25	20	−50
Reserpine	65	25	−42
Su-5171	35	30	−35
Su-5171	60	30	−30
α-CH$_3$-dopa	25	50	−32
α-CH$_3$-dopa	80	50	−30
Su-5171	85	55	−25
5-HTP	270	100	0
JB-516	169	104	−10
JB-516	183	140	0
JB-835	332	182	0

Table 2

Drug	E. S. Threshold (Changes, %)
Reserpine + iproniazid + l-dopa	+300
Reserpine + iproniazid + α-CH$_3$-dopa	−50
Amphetamine	+900
Reserpine + amphetamine	0
Iproniazid + amphetamine	+1,300
Reserpine + iproniazid + l-dopa + amphetamine	+2,500
Imipramine	+5,900
Reserpine + imipramine	+75
Iproniazid + imipramine	+13,750
Reserpine + iproniazid + l-dopa + imipramine	+15,000

Table 1 shows, first of all, a marked decrease of electroshock threshold in reserpinized animals.

Since reserpine lowers brain serotonin as well as brain catecholamines, the question arises whether this decrease of electroshock threshold, which is also prevented by monoamine oxidase inhibitors, such as JB-516, may be attributed more precisely to one or another of these substances.

Using reserpine, the reserpine analog Su-5171, α-methyldopa and α-methyl-m-tyrosine, more or less selective decreases of either brain serotonin or brain noradrenaline levels may be obtained with well-defined doses and at well-defined periods of time after administration of these drugs.

It can be seen that there is no parallelism between the decrease of electroshock threshold and the decrease of brain serotonin, whereas a fairly good relationship holds between the decrease of electroshock threshold and the decrease of brain noradrenaline.

As shown further in Table 1, selective or combined increases of brain serotonin and noradrenaline, provoked by pretreatment with 5-hydroxytryptophan and JB-516 or JB-835 respectively, were found not to modify significantly the electroshock threshold.

Selective increases of brain dopamine, however, provoked by pretreatment with reserpine, iproniazid, and l-dopa, were followed by a very pronounced increase of electroshock threshold (Table 2), which appeared to be dose-dependent for l-dopa, whereas substitution of α-methyldopa for l-dopa, resulting in a decrease of endogenous dopamine, provoked a clear-cut decrease of electroshock threshold.

Table 2 shows further that amphetamine and imipramine provoke a very marked increase of electroshock threshold, which is completely prevented by pretreatment with reserpine.

Since reserpine lowers the serotonin as well as the noradrenaline and dopamine levels in the brain, the question again arises whether one or another of these amines is more specifically involved in this effect of amphetamine and imipramine. Our experimental observations show that this effect is enhanced after pretreatment with iproniazid, that is, in presence of a combined and moderate increase of all brain amine levels, whereas a very marked potentiation occurs after combined pretreatment with reserpine, iproniazid, and l-dopa, that is, in the presence of selectively increased brain dopamine levels.

It may be concluded from our experimental data that reserpine markedly lowers electroshock threshold, thus confirming previous observations, in which, however, 2–8 times higher doses of reserpine were used [Chen et al, 1954; Everett et al, 1955; Bros, 1957; Prockop et al, 1959b]. A similar reserpine effect was also observed in the case of metrazol convulsions [Jenney, 1954; Chen and Bohner, 1956; Kobinger, 1958b; Weiss et al, 1960].

Conflicting observations have been reported with regard to the effect of monoamine oxidase inhibitors on the convulsive seizure provoked by electroshock or metrazol. Some authors claim that these substances have anticonvulsant properties [Prockop et al, 1959a, 1959b; Chow and Hendley, 1959; Weiss et al, 1960; P'An et al, 1961a, 1961b], whereas others report that monoamine oxidase inhibitors do not influence or may even facilitate convulsive seizures [Kobinger, 1958a, 1958b; Hertting, 1958; Everett et al, 1959].

In our experiments, a slight facilitative effect on electroshock convulsions was observed shortly after pretreatment with JB-516, at a time when the level of noradrenaline in the brain was unchanged and the level of brain serotonin nearly doubled. Pretreatment with 5-hydroxytryptophan, with or without previous administration of JB-516, thus producing a selective increase in brain serotonin, did not influence or slightly increased the electroshock threshold. The combined increase of brain serotonin and noradrenaline levels, elicited by pretreatment with JB-516 or JB-835, was without any effect on the electroshock threshold.

It is of particular interest that a selective and marked increase of brain dopamine, induced by pretreatment with reserpine plus iproniazid plus l-dopa, was found to provoke a very pronounced increase of electroshock threshold, amounting to as much as 300 per cent of control values, when 75 mg per kg of l-dopa was given. This increase was less pronounced but still very significant when 25 mg per kg of l-dopa was given.

These experimental observations show that the electroshock threshold is not very much influenced by an increase in both serotonin and noradrenaline in the brain, but may be markedly increased by selectively increased levels of brain dopamine.

The data derived from the amphetamine and imipramine experiments, on the other hand, produce additional experimental evidence for the assumption that changes in electroshock threshold are mediated through changes in brain dopamine levels.

It should be mentioned here that Balzer et al [1960] observed that hydrazide-induced seizures were abolished when the dopamine content of the brain was raised by the administration of iproniazid and l-dopa, corroborating the view that brain dopamine is of importance in determining the sensitivity to electroshock.

These experimental observations may have practical implications.

First, it is known that various side effects may occur as a consequence of electroshock application, such as electroencephalographic alterations, psychic disturbances, and amnesia. These side effects have been attributed not only to the convulsive seizure as such but also to the total electrical energy applied in order to provoke a seizure [Piette, 1959]. Thus the possible pharmacological lowering of the electroshock threshold and consequent reduction of the minimal electrical energy required to provoke a convulsive seizure may be helpful in avoiding these side effects of electroshock therapy.

Second, the experimental study of the role of dopamine in the CNS may provide a new and fruitful approach to the elucidation of the pathogenesis of certain central nervous diseases and, accordingly, to more rational methods of treatment.

Thus the association of extrapyramidal motor disturbances with anatomical lesions of the corpus striatum led Ehringer and Hornykiewicz [1960; Bernheimer et al, 1963] to the observation that the brain of Parkinsonian patients shows a distinct deficiency in dopamine (Table 3).

Table 3

Mean Dopamine Content in μg per g
[According to Ehringer and Hornykiewicz, 1960]

	Controls (17)	Morbus Parkinson (2)	Postencephalitic Parkinsonism (4)
Caudate nucleus	3.5	1.1	0.2
Putamen	3.7	0.8	0.3
Globus pallidus	0.5	—	0.1

Barbeau et al [1961] reported, on the other hand, subnormal urinary excretion figures of dopamine in Parkinsonism (Table 4).

Table 4

Excretion (mean $\pm$ S. E.) of Urinary Dopamine (μg per 24 hr)
[According to Barbeau et al, 1961]

Controls (24)	316 ± 14.6
Parkinsonism	
all types (16)	241 ± 21.5 *
idiopathic (8)	297 ± 36.2
postencephalitic (6)	177 ± 41.8 *
arteriosclerotic (2)	212

* $P < 0.01$

These changes are more pronounced in postencephalitic than in idiopathic Parkinsonism.

In line with these observations, Parkinsonian patients have been treated with l-dopa (50–100 mg, i.v.) alone or in combination with monoamine oxidase inhibitors.[2] Various authors reported encouraging therapeutic results, consisting in a complete abolition or marked reduction of the akinesia, which reached a peak between the second and third hours and lasted for about 24 hours, and an electromyographically shown reduction of tremor and rigidity, which set in more rapidly but persisted for 20 to 30 minutes only [Gerstenbrand and Pateisky, 1962; Hirschmann and Mayer, 1964], subsiding gradually when the antikinetic effect became fully manifest.

A similar antiakinetic effect of dopa was observed in reserpine-induced Parkinsonism [Degkwitz et al, 1960].

It is interesting to note that the monoamine oxidase inhibitor harmin has been used previously [Behringer and Willman, 1962] with good results for the treatment of akinesia, although this substance is most suitable for producing experimentally a Parkinsonlike tremor. As pointed out recently by Hirschmann and Mayer [1962], the reciprocal action of dopa on tremor and rigidity on the one hand and on akinesia on the other hand, and the fact that the symptom triad of Parkinsonism, tremor-rigidity-akinesia, may not be explained by precise morphological alterations, such as a degeneration of certain cells in certain nuclei, suggest that a more functional approach of the pathogenesis of extrapyramidal motor disturbances might be more rewarding than a purely morphological one.

The biochemical and clinical pharmacological observations with regard to dopamine in the central nervous system are thus not only of therapeutic interest in the treatment of Parkinsonism, but may also contribute to a better understanding of this disease.

In conclusion, the prediction seems justified that further experimental research, largely based on neurochemical and pharmacological investigations will considerably broaden perspectives in both neurology and psychiatry in the years to come.

As Philip Abelson stated recently in a paper published in *Science*, "The area in which most vital advances are being made today is molecular biology. Perhaps in this area the greatest research frontier of our times is investigation of the human mind and the way it functions."

Acknowledgment

Our experimental work reported in this paper was supported by a research grant (H-3393) from the National Heart Institute, National In-

---

[2] Lauer et al [1958]; Pare and Sandler [1959]; Bernheimer et al [1961]; Birkmayer and Hornykiewicz [1961]; Pollin et al [1961]; Barbeau et al [1962]; Friedhoff et al [1963].

stitutes of Health, U. S. Public Health Service, Bethesda, Maryland, and by a grant from the Fund for Collective Fundamental Research, Belgium.

DISCUSSION

Chairman: PROFESSOR MORUZZI

GRANIT: The catecholamines are a very popular theme in Stockholm. These results with Parkinsonism are exceedingly striking and interesting. You have here raised the question of whether one might not be able to do a more detailed analysis of the nervous function with the aid of these substances. I will just draw your attention to the fact that Professor Lundberg (Gothenburg) has started a very rewarding piece of research on reflexology under the control of catecholamines.

HEYMANS: I agree with Professor Granit's statement; my feeling is, however, that morphology and also electrophysiology have been very important areas for the investigation of function of the central nervous system; but I think we ought to switch, perhaps a little bit more at least, to the area of the biochemistry of the central nervous system, and to the influences of changes in levels of what we may call the biological transmitters in the central nervous system having action on excitability and transmission. In addition, we should consider the mechanism of action of a number of drugs on the central nervous system. Perhaps it may be possible to throw light on the disorders in Parkinson postencephalitic disease, and some other pathological situations.

LIBET: In connection with the question of the nature of the action of these substances, as I understand it, you got an arousal effect with increased dopamine in the brain; on the other hand, you got a rise in electroshock threshold with increased dopamine, which appears to be somewhat contradictory. Do you have some idea of whether these substances are inhibitory or excitatory, or both, but at different sites? Is this latter possibility the way to explain the apparent contradiction?

HEYMANS: In many points we are indeed just on the surfaces of the problems. Much more work is needed on molecular biology and the general field of biochemical pharmacology.

CHAGAS: Although I really believe with Professor Heymans that much work is still needed in the field of molecular biology we are now discussing, I, on the other hand, firmly think that significant results can be obtained only with the concurrence of several techniques and, thus, that the biochemical or pharmacological approach is not exclusive of a good many others of the greatest significance too. We have been discussing here the difficulties of localization of specific functional structures in the central nervous system when we employ microelectrophysiological techniques. This difficulty becomes, of course, much greater in the molecular approach; for example, even the most refined isotope methods which we have been using have completely failed to give results similar to those obtainable on the peripheral structures. However, new developments based on the combination of techniques are very promising; for instance, the combination of autoradiography with electron-microscopy is capable of giving us extremely precise localizations.

HEYMANS: With Professor Chagas, I think that a combination of different techniques may provide more information concerning the central nervous system. I quite agree that the technique of electroshock threshold is a rough method because it induces a stimulation of the whole brain. But we had to start the investigations with this method before we could go further ahead.

BREMER: Quite apart from the obvious practical and biochemical interest of the experiments described by Professor Heymans, there is again the controversial question of the catecholamines and their precursors as synaptic transmitters in the central nervous system. Professor Heymans is inclined to believe in this quality, but, as far as I see, the general trend seems to be actually against that conclusion.

The controversy was raised after the well-known experiments of Dell and Bonvallet, producing arousal in the cat by catecholamines, especially adrenaline, and, interestingly, by endogenous adrenaline. At first sight this last fact seemed to be a definitive proof that, at least for some central structures, notably the reticular formation, the catecholamines could act as real trans-mitters and that the cells there should be adrenoceptive and even adrenergic.

Yet, experiments conducted independently in Moruzzi's and in our laboratory led to the conclusion that it was not the explanation; that the catecholamines—and notably adrenaline—did not act directly on the reticular or other brain cells, but produced their effects indirectly by stimulating hemodynamically receptors located perhaps even outside of the brain.

Therefore, the question is still open.

HEYMANS: I quite agree with your statement that the question is still open. I think, however, that we have to be careful when using the word "transmitter" to signify the function of transmitting the stimulation in the central nervous system.

Some of these compounds may also have a pharmacological action of their own, not correlated with a function of transmission or mediation. It is a difficult field, anyway.

MOUNTCASTLE: Although it is true that the direct microphysiological evidence for the existence of these substances as transmitters is not available as it is for the neuromuscular junction, for example, it certainly is clear that the adrenergic system is contained within the synaptic vesicles of the central nervous system; it seems to me at least a working hypothesis that these substances are transmitters.

SCHAEFER: I should like to ask Dr. Heymans whether there is some informa-tion available of an influence of dopamine on the membrane properties of these cells, and I should like to add a remark concerning our own experiments. We were deeply disappointed when we made expriments with adrenaline on the central nervous system, and found at the beginning good actions, but later realized that these effects, with some exceptions, were indirect. When keeping the blood pressure constant by a special device, adrenaline had almost no action. Though adrenaline has very marked influence on the membrane properties, I do not know whether this is clear for ganglionic cells, though at least it is clear for cardiac muscle cells. And so my question is now: is anything known about any change in the membrane properties under the influence of dopamine, such as action potentials, membrane potentials, afterpotentials, and so on?

HEYMANS: I quite agree with your observations. Adrenaline may, indeed, induce some changes in central nervous activities which are not related to adrenaline itself, but to the changes adrenaline produces in blood pressure and blood flow. Circulatory changes may affect the activities of some nerve centers. I am sorry I do not have any information about the action of dopamine on membrane potentials. Perhaps some other members of the group may have some information about this.

CHAGAS: May I reply to Dr. Schaefer that work conducted in my laboratory with adrenaline has shown results in line with the observations he has now reported. Indeed, we should not neglect a more careful verification of the effects of dopamine either; but I have not yet tried it as thoroughly as adrenaline.

SCHAEFER: May I add that adrenaline in the muscular tissue of the heart has no effect on membrane potential either, but it restores very much the membrane properties if they have been lost by treatment with high potassium concentrations, and so on.

TEUBER: I want to make a tentative suggestion to Professor Heymans, somewhat in line with Professor Moruzzi's proposal that you might want to use in addition to the ECS threshold some other indicator of interference with caudate function. In the monkey, and we now know in the rat, there is a rather specific and easily measured aspect of behavior in a test situation that is influenced by stimulation or lesions in the caudate. This behavior is called alternation; the animal is simply going from one lever to another lever, back and forth. Alternation is disrupted by caudate stimulation and is permanently impaired by caudate lesions. This symptom is quite separable from other behavioral changes. This might be another way of assaying these central drug effects, and it would be, I think, of very great interest to see whether it behaves in the same way as your seizure threshold does. But surely no apology is needed for working on these catecholamines if one is interested in certain clinical entities, as we all are.

HEYMANS: Thank you very much for the suggestion. I hope electrophysiologists are going to work in this field also and give us more precise information with different techniques. The arousal reaction seems, however, to be related to an accumulation of dopamine in the brain. Perhaps someone more specialized in this field could find out if this suggestion is right or wrong.

REFERENCES

AXELROD, J., W. ALBERS, and C. D. CLEMENTE. *J. Neurochem.*, 5, 68 [1959].
BALZER, H., P. HOLTZ, and D. PALM. *Biochem. Pharmacol.*, 5, 169 [1960].

BARBEAU, A., G. F. MURPHY, and T. L. SOURKES. *Science, 133,* 1706 [1961].

——, T. L. SOURKES, and F. MURPHY. In: *Monoamines et Système Nerveux Central* (ed. by J. de Ajuriaguerra), Symposium Bel Air, Geneva, Geneva: Georg, p. 247 [1962].

BEHRINGER and WILLMAN. Cited in Gerstenbrand and Patersky [1962].

BERNHEIMER, H., W. BIRKMAYER, and O. HORNYKIEWICZ. *Klin. Wschr., 39,* 1056 [1961].

——. *Klin. Wschr., 41,* 465 [1963].

BERTLER, A. *Acta Physiol. Scand., 51,* 97 [1961].

——, and E. ROSENGREN. *Experientia, 15,* 382 [1959].

BIRKMAYER, W., and O. HORNYKIEWICZ. *Wien. Klin. Wschr., 73,* 787 [1961].

BOGDANSKI, D. F., H. WEISSBACH, and S. UDENFRIEND. *J. Neurochem., 1,* 272 [1957].

BRODIE, B. B., and E. COSTA. In: *Monoamines et Système Nerveux Central* (ed. by J. de Ajuriaguerra), Symposium Bel Air, Geneva, Geneva: Georg, p. 13 [1962].

——, K. F. FINGER, F. B. ORLANS, G. P. QUINN, and F. SULSER. *J. Pharmacol., 129,* 250 [1960].

——, J. S. OLIN, R. KUNTZMAN, and P. A. SHORE. *Science, 125,* 1293 [1957].

——, S. SPECTOR, and P. A. SHORE. *Ann. N. Y. Acad. Sci., 80,* 609 [1959].

BROSS, R. B. *Amer. J. Psychiat., 113,* 933 [1957].

CARLSSON, A. *Pharmacol. Rev., 11,* 490 [1959].

——, B. FALCK, and N.-A. HILLARP. *Acta Physiol. Scand., 56,* Suppl. 196 [1962].

CARLSSON, A., M. LINDQVIST, and T. MAGNUSSON. *Nature, 180,* 1200 [1959].

——, M. LINDQVIST, T. MAGNUSSON, and B. WALDECK. *Science, 127,* 471 [1958].

CHEN, G., and B. BOHNER. *J. Pharmacol., 117,* 142 [1956].

——, C. R. ENSOR, and B. BOHNER. *Proc. Soc. Exp. Biol. Med., 86,* 507 [1954].

CHOW, M. I., and C. D. HENDLEY. *Fed. Proc., 18,* 376 [1959].

DAGIRMAJIAN, R., R. LAVERTY, P. MANTEGAZZINI, D. F. SHARMAN, and M. VOGT. *J. Neurochem., 10,* 177 [1963].

DEGKWITZ, R., R. FROWEIN, C. KULENKAMPFF, and U. MOHS. *Klin. Wschr., 38,* 120 [1960].

DELAUNOIS, A. L., A. F. DE SCHAEPDRYVER, and Y. PIETTE. *Arch. Int. Pharmacodyn., 136,* 242 [1962].

DENGLER, H. *Arch. Exper. Path. Pharmakol., 231,* 373 [1957].

DRUJAN, B. D., T. L. SOURKES, D. S. LAYNE, and G. P. MURPHY. *Can. J. Biochem. Physiol., 37,* 1153 [1959].

EHRINGER, H., and O. HORNYKIEWICZ. *Klin. Wschr., 38,* 1236 [1960].

EULER, U. S. VON, U. HAMBERG, and S. HELLNER. *Biochem. J., 49,* 655 [1951].

——, and F. LISHAJKO. *Acta Physiol. Pharmacol. Néerl., 6,* 295 [1957].

EVERETT, G. M. *Neuropsychopharmacologia, 2,* 479 [1961].

EVERETT, G. M., J. C. DAVIN, and J. E. P. TOMAN. *Fed. Proc.*, *18*, 388 [1959].

——, and J. E. P. TOMAN. *Biol. Psychiat.*, *1*, 75 [1959].

——, J. E. P. TOMAN, and A. H. SMITH. *Fed. Proc.*, *14*, 337 [1955].

——, and R. G. WIEGAND. *Biochem. Pharmacol.*, *8*, 85 [1962].

FRIEDHOFF, A. J., L. HEKIMIAN, M. ALPERT, and E. TOBACH. *J. Amer. Med. Ass.*, *184*, 285 [1963].

GERSTENBRAND, F., and K. PATEISKY. *Wien. Zschr. Nervenheilk.*, *20*, 90 [1962].

GOODALL, McC. *Nature*, *166*, 738 [1950].

——. *Acta Physiol. Scand.*, *24*, Suppl. 85 [1951].

GUGGENHEIM, M. *Die Biogenen Amine*. Basel: Karger [1951].

HERTTING, G. *Wien. Klin. Wschr.*, *70*, 190 [1958].

HESS, S. M., R. H. CONNAMACHER, M. OZAKI, and S. UDENFRIEND. *J. Pharmacol.*, *134*, 129 [1961].

HEYMANS, C., A. F. DE SCHAEPDRYVER, Y. PIETTE, and A. L. DELAUNOIS. *Commentarii Pont. Acad. Sci.*, *1*, No. 32, 1 [1964].

HIRSCHMANN, J., and K. MAYER. *Phenothiazine und neurologische Symptomatik*. München: Th. Intern. Gesellsch. f. Neuropsychopharmakologie [1962].

——. *Arzneimittel-Forschung*, *14*, 599 [1964].

HOLTZ, P. *Psychiat. et Neurol.*, *140*, 175 [1960].

——, and E. WESTERMANN. *Arch. Exper. Path. Pharmakol.*, *227*, 538 [1956].

HOLZBAUER, M., and M. VOGT. *J. Neurochem.*, *1*, 8 [1956].

HOLZER, G., and O. HORNYKIEWICZ. *Arch. Exper. Path. Pharmakol.*, *237*, 27 [1959].

JENNEY, E. H. *Fed. Proc.*, *13*, 370 [1954].

KOBINGER, W. *Arch. Exper. Path. Pharmakol.*, *233*, 559 [1958a].

LAUER, J. W., W. M. INSKIP, J. BERNSOHN, and E. A. ZELLER. *Arch. Neurol. Psychiat.*, *80*, 122 [1958].

LAVERTY, R., and D. F. SHARMAN. Cited in M. VOGT. *Actual. Pharmacol.*, Sér. 16, Paris: Masson, 164 [1963].

LEWIS, J. J. *Science Progr.*, *51*, 382, 551 [1963].

MANTEGAZZINI, P., and A. GLÄSSER. *Arch. Ital. Biol.*, *98*, 367 [1960].

MONTAGU, K. A. *Nature*, *180*, 244 [1957].

MURPHY, G. F., and T. L. SOURKES. *Rev. Can. Biol.*, *18*, 379 [1959].

ÖSTLUND, E. *Acta Physiol. Scand.*, *31*, Suppl. 112 [1954].

P'AN, S. Y., W. H. FUNDERBURK, and K. F. FINGER. *Fed. Proc.*, *20*, 323 [1961a].

——. *Proc. Soc. Exp. Biol. Med.*, *108*, 680 [1961b].

PARE, C. M. B., and M. J. SANDLER. *J. Neurol. Neurosurg. Psychiat.*, *22*, 247 [1959].

PIETTE, Y. *Acta Neurol. Psychiat. Belg.*, *59*, 1045 [1959].

——, A. L. DELAUNOIS, A. F. DE SCHAEPDRYVER, and C. HEYMANS. *Arch. Int. Pharmacodyn.*, *144*, 293 [1963].

POLLIN, W., P. V. CARDON, and S. S. KETY. *Science*, *133*, 104 [1961].

PROCKOP, D. J., P. A. SHORE, and B. B. BRODIE. *Ann. N. Y. Acad. Sci.*, *80*, 643 [1959a].

——. *Experientia*, *15*, 145 [1959b].

SANO, I., T. GAMO, Y. KAKIMOTO, K. TANIGUCHI, M. TAKESADA, and K. NISHI NUMA. *Biochim. Biophys. Acta, 32,* 586 [1959].

——, K. TANIGUCHI, T. GAMO, M. TAKESADA, and Y. KAKIMOTO. *Klin. Wschr., 38,* 57 [1960].

DE SCHAEPDRYVER, A. F., Y. PIETTE, and A. L. DELAUNOIS. *Arch. Int. Pharmacodyn., 140,* 358 [1962].

SCHÜMANN, H. J. *Arch. Exper. Path. Pharmakol., 227,* 566 [1956].

——. *Arch. Exp. Path. Pharmakol., 234,* 17 [1958].

SMITH, C. B., and P. B. DEWS. *Psychopharmacologia, 3,* 55 [1962].

SOURKES, T. L., G. F. MURPHY, and V. R. WOODFORD, Jr. *J. Nutrition, 72,* 145 [1960].

UDENFRIEND, S., and C. R. CREVELING. *J. Neurochem., 4,* 350 [1959].

——, W. LOVENBERG, and A. SJOERDSMA. *Arch. Biochem. Biophys., 85,* 487 [1959].

WEIL-MALHERBE, H., and A. D. BONE. *J. Clin. Path., 10,* 138 [1957a].

——. *Nature, 180,* 1050 [1957b].

WEISS, L. R., J. W. NELSON, and A. TYE. *J. Amer. Pharmaceut. Ass., 49,* 514 [1960].

21

Psychosomatic Problems of Vegetative Regulatory Functions

by H. Schaefer

Physiologisches Institut der Universität, Heidelberg, Germany

This conference deals with the linkage of two items of an essentially different character. To what an extent this is true may be elucidated by reading the last paragraph of the chapter devoted to the theme "brain and consciousness," in the green program book, where one finds on pp. 18–19 that,

> As to the meaning of the term "consciousness," the Study Week intends that it strictly designates the psychophysiological concept of perceptual capacity, of awareness of perception, and the ability to act and react accordingly.
>
> Consequently, the subject which the invited scientists are requested to discuss, has to be duly delimited by this semantic acceptation, which is of a strictly scientific character.
>
> It is obvious, that every extrapolation of the meaning of the term "consciousness" leading the subject into an extra-scientific field, would be contrary to the spirit of the Study Week.[1]

One could scarcely expect to find prescriptions of such a kind in regard to a definition of "brain."

I do not know what punishment stands on the violation of this somewhat dogmatic request. I hope it might not be the eternal fire, but I am nevertheless happy to find myself in a *general* agreement with this statement. It is, however, an old custom of scientists to test the validity of assumptions under such experimental conditions which bring the object

---

[1] As organizer of the Study Week I have to report that this statement with its strange linguistic usages was not referred to me for approval or even for comment before it was printed and circulated to all participants of the symposium! J. C. Eccles

under consideration into a borderline position, to look whether the laws thus far found will still be valid. But since man cannot be brought artificially and purposely into situations of a sufficient borderline character without some interference with his personal welfare, the only method to gain convincing results is, here as elsewhere in the science of human beings, to observe man under the conditions of disease. This has amply been done by many speakers on this conference.

Looking at the conventional way of analyzing our problem, we will see that the *classical* concept of mind-brain relationship, to which all previous papers were devoted, has preferably to do with what might be called the "standard conscious mind of the experimenting physiologist," who explains himself with some sort of self-denying attitude in terms of sensory input, sensory perception, concepts of an external world which really exists, and conscious logical operations to find out what his subjective feelings are good for in processes which to a certain degree seem to function well without our "self" or "ego" (and sometimes even better). The classical philosophy and the psychology behind the stage of our conventional physiology is a philosophy of rationalism and of the theory of recognition. My aim should be to invalidate to some extent these fundamentals on which we all are residing so full of glamor and with such pleasure. But as Dr. Sperry has denied my free will, I can always withdraw on his position to have my soul saved. I really must do what I now should like to do.

First of all I should like to start with the definition of words to be used in such an approach.

DEFINITION TABLE

Conscious. That which is given in the immediate experience (Protophenomenon).

Unconscious. Processes objectively testable (for example, action potentials, motoric or effectoric excitations) and having the same physicochemical and neurological structure as conscious processes, but not appearing in the consciousness. (Against this:

Unconsciousness. The simple vanishing of consciousness in blackout, or lack of consciousness, in lifeless material.)

Vegetative. All bodily events which, if able to be influenced by the nervous system, are influenced *directly* only by the autonomic nervous system. They are inaccessible to all direct voluntary influences. Under this heading, of course, all processes have to be subsumed which are not influenced by nerves.

Psychogenic. Expression for the hypothetical statement that a primarily mental process has elicited a bodily correlate, although an adequate physiological mechanism cannot be described.

Psychosomatic. Expression of the hypothesis that bodily and mental events are fundamentally inseparable, the apparent separability being simulated by the methods of observing mental and physical processes.

Mind, psyche (in German: *Geist, Seele*). Both words are synonyms and are only definable methodologically. The whole of all conscious subjective phenomena has the quality of mental or psychic (*geistig, seelisch*). From this definition a hypothetical agent may be deduced which carries these mental (psychic) phenomena in the same formal sense, as previously the agent matter (*materia*) carried the physical phenomena. This agent, acting as a carrier model, is called *mind* or *psyche*.

Let me develop now the first viewpoint of this paper, the modern psychosomatic concept in its earliest state.

The Early Time of Modern Psychosomatic Medicine

A look into the history of the so-called psychosomatic medicine and of the term *psychogenic disease* reveals a very surprising fact. A "psychogenetic mechanism" of abnormal bodily events is regarded today, in a clear majority of cases, as a hypothetic explanation in disturbances of those functions of the body which are commonly called vegetative functions. Though Charcot, in the beginning of modern psychosomatic medicine, analyzed first what was called "hystery," and which was predominantly some disorder of *behavior or movement*, diseases with disorders of heart function, respiration, intestinal disturbances, shifts in the regulatory homeostasis of some bodily servomechanisms such as blood pressure, came only much later to the importance they seem to possess now. It cannot be doubted that the phenomena of disease called later on "psychogenic disorders" have deeply changed their patterns.

As in all attempts to explain hitherto unknown phenomena, in the field of these (as we say today) psychosomatic processes, one tries to construct a model. If one looks through the early scripts of Sigmund Freud, one easily detects the structure of the model he made himself to describe what he called "hystery," and it is not by chance that he, in the beginning, found the *hystérie d'occasion* as he called it with Charcot's words.[2] The model of Freud really is one, in which the theories of neurology and conditioned reflexes of those times were applied to the mechanism of hysteric disturbances.

[2] S. Freud. *Gesammelte Werke*. Vol. 1, p. 4, London [1952].

Models of such a kind may simply be applied to distu
ment, and the literature of those days is full of descripti
like epileptoid reactions, "big movements" (as Freud
passionelles and, at the end, disturbances of consciou
Freud's writings, nowhere a token of surprise, *how* t
sibly act on the body. His technique, on the co
describe the history of the patient, so that, as he confesses nim..
descriptions read like a novel, and at the end of the story two effects may
be stated: the one on the side of the patient is, that in elucidating the
history of the case and bringing the disturbing emotions into the consciousness of the patient, the hysterical symptoms disappear.[5] The second
effect, on the side of the physician, is that, regarded with the eyes of a
philosopher of today, Freud himself found the case cleared up and no
degree of inquietude remained with him.

Evidently Freud believed to have found a *complete* model of what
we would call the psychosomatic relationship in his patients. He described, in his first book on hystery, a rhinitis in a case where some deep
emotions had been fixed to certain smells. A young governess realized
by chance the deep affection of some children for her, just at the moment
when an intense smell of burnt food came into her nose; and when
shortly after that event, a conflict of love between the father of those
children and herself arose, she developed the illness of the nose. Freud
invented the word *"conversion"* for this transformation of an emotionally
loaded conflict situation into a bodily disturbance. He obviously was
satisfied by having found the two points of the conversion line: the start
and the end. The physiological *machinery* which brings about such a conversion was, as it seems, not the object of his concern. This may be better understood if one regards the pattern of such conversion syndromes.
Freud's explanation was, formally described, that some "psychic" excitement (the physiological importance and effectiveness of which is nowhere controversial) is transformed into permanent symptoms of physiological or pathological character, taking place, so to say, within the
framework of well-known bodily events, mainly of reflectoric character.
All this was applied, at the beginning of the story, to processes, which
are called in German physiology *animalische Prozesse*: problems of
humor, of inhibitions in the sphere of voluntary movements, and in some
cases, the anorexia and pains of the stomach are already included.[6] This
means that the events, described in those early stages of the problem,
had mainly to do with that part of bodily functions which we all know

[3] *Ibid.*, p. 93.
[4] *Ibid.*, p. 227.
[5] *Ibid.*, pp. 85, 253.
[6] *Ibid.*, p. 142.

st *from our daily experience*. It obviously appears to everybody easy
to explain how *our* voluntary movement is inhibited, or how *we* get
pains in the stomach, experiences all of us have already had in our lives.
This was evidently the model underlying Freud's early work. We see, how
far an analogous understanding was active at this stage.

THE SITUATION TODAY

Change in the Scientific Reflection

Our situation has now changed in a twofold respect. The first change
affected the theory of science itself. It is characterized by the fact that
apparently obvious incidents are relegated to a reflection, by which very
soon the *questionability* just of the simplest models appears to be obvious.

In this phase of increasing reflection we also find ourselves in psy-
chosomatics. The apparently obvious becomes problematic. This one
realizes when one reads the scripts of Freud and finds that many
thoughts which to him were evident, today produce the biggest problems.
We may demonstrate that in a very famous example. Darwin had been
informed by a medical friend that man blushes preferably on the head
and neck. He took this to mean that these special places on the skin were
just those which attract the attention of the observer, and he states that
in this way the phenomenon is satisfactorily explained. We, however,
want on the one hand to look for the mental patterns by which blushing
is determined; on the other hand, we look for the mechanisms which
generate it at the site of the vessels.

Changes of Disease

The second change in our situation concerns the typology of the
psychosomatic diseases themselves. The classical hysteria has nearly disappeared. This may be due to a severe change in the general understanding of modern man, who regards hysterical symptoms as ridiculous. This
disease therefore is converted into patterns of a more or less *vegetative*
type. Perhaps the most common psychosomatic disease today is what
is called "vegetative dystony," a disease which increased in the last ten
years in the statistics of our insurance companies to 1,400 per cent of its
original frequency as a cause of preventive treatment. For such diseases
we have neither models nor do we know their mechanisms. The fact
that we regard them to be psychosomatic results from their beginning
and ending simultaneously with mental conflicts. Classical medicine is
so helpless in the situation that the majority of clinicians do not notice
even obvious facts, or even try to deny them. There exists, for example,

extensive literature on eczema in handbooks and reviews, which do not even mention the fact that eczema can be of psychological origin.[7]

Behind this clinical attitude stands the old belief that man is divided in body and soul, both being separated by the gulf Lord Adrian has spoken of. One tried to interpret in an inacceptable manner a *methodological* principle in an *ontological* manner, insofar as the introspective method of exploring psychical events was regarded as a guarantee that psyche is essentially different from the body, which is, on its side, investigated by the methods of counting and measuring. It will be very much the concern of this paper to show that such an ontological division of man into a bodily, unconscious half of his vegetative life and a spiritual half of his psychic events has no evidence in the facts of modern anthropology.

With these preliminary remarks we are already approaching our main problem, which we can define with the simple headline, that:

THERE ARE NO CLEAR BOUNDARIES BETWEEN CONSCIOUS AND UNCONSCIOUS IN BEHAVIORAL AND BIOLOGICAL EVENTS

Obviously our consciousness receives only a very small amount of the total sensory input, the majority of which remains *below* the "conscious level," as Dr. Thorpe put it. It remains unknown, and no contribution on this conference was able to clarify which factors condemn an input signal to remain unconscious. We all are convinced that simple patterns of organization, mostly in the thalamic and geniculate pathways, are responsible, and some experimental evidence has been given in this respect. Nevertheless, all unconscious information is evaluated in integrating systems, which operate by highly "intelligent" rules. Our clinical experience tells us a similar fact from diseases, in which external stimuli without any meaning to the patient arouse vegetative disorders in his body, which carry the character of a strong emotional disturbance; and no explanation of such disorders can be reached but by psychoanalysis in long sessions or deep hypnosis. At the end of such a treatment, a "displaced" emotionally loaded experience is brought back into the consciousness, by explaining the disturbance as an unconscious *analog* of otherwise well-known conscious emotional effects and so eventually curing the patient.

Perhaps, it is here already that the question raised by some speakers the day before may get an answer, namely, what consciousness might

[7] A critical review of the literature by: S. Morelli. *Med. Klin.*, 49, II, 1806 [1954]; F. Dunbar. *Emotions and Bodily Changes.* New York, Columbia Univ. Press [1949]; H. Schaefer. *Studium Generale, 17*, 500 [1964].

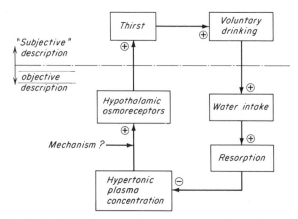

Fig. 21.1. Block diagram of a somatic regulatory function.

be good for: here its beneficial action is to dissolve the linkage between a stimulus and some unwanted reactions by making the causes of such reactions clear. How far, however, our consciousness is embedded in the total framework of our bodily life is shown by the role it plays in some somatic regulatory functions such as eating and drinking, functions which keep essential values of our metabolism on constant levels and which are operated by drives. These drives, however (hunger, thirst), act only over their conscious implications. One can even construct block diagrams of these processes which show all the characteristics of a servomechanism (Fig. 21.1), regardless of the fact that the machinery with which one works is still only partly known.

Such a block diagram is, in the sense of our definition, of psychosomatic nature. Possibly such a scheme may *one day* become completely somatic. For respiration this has already been nearly achieved. For eating and drinking we only know the hypothalamic centers, the destruction of which destroys the regulative functions, so that polyphagia, anorexia, and excess or lack of thirst result. The translation of the nervous function of these centers into the language of consciousness is not yet possible, but is nearly within reach.

One could of course imagine a perfect robot, with behavior identical to ours, and who eats, drinks, makes social contacts, etc., without any consciousness. It seems as if insects like bees would represent such robot-like creatures. In his last book, on the natural history of aggression, Lorenz [8] pictures such a world of consciousnessless behavior, in a nearly Cartesian manner, which has been created by nature only by means of

[8] K. Lorenz, *Das sogenannte Böse. Zur Naturgeschichte der Agression.* Vienna: Borotha Schoeler Verlag [1963].

Darwin's selection theory. We know nothing of the internal life of bees, we do not even know anything of the possible subjective events in our dominated half of the right hemisphere or of the spinal cord, as Dr. Sperry demonstrated. Any answer to the question what the subjective part of beings other than man might be, lies positively beyond the possibilities of our imagination. This is the reason why I regard every question concerning what consciousness might be useful for, and how and when it developed in phylogenesis, as an unlawful question, as unlawful at least as any attempt would be to extrapolate the meaning "consciousness" in the sense of the term defined by the fathers of this conference.

DISEASE AS A TOOL OF RESEARCH FOR PSYCHOSOMATIC PROBLEMS

As we stated in the beginning, in the field of psychosomatic theory, experiments are possible—on ethical or theoretical grounds—only within strict limits. The *observations* of diseases replace the experiment.

The strict methodologist here would make the objection that an experiment presupposes the voluntary variation of the experimental conditions, a variation which is naturally not realized in the case of diseases. We may, however, reply that in the case of diseases the variation of experimental conditions is replaced by the observation of coincidences. One makes a hypothesis on the nature of a disease just as one makes a hypothesis on the interdependence of physical phenomena. These hypotheses can be falsified by the observation that the phenomenological relations in question do not exist. If the relations are found, the hypothesis remains open, if one does not find it more and more probable. A strict *verification* of the hypothesis is not known anywhere in the natural sciences. In medicine, the method of testing the coincidences is called *epidemiology*.

As an example of such epidemiological methods we may quote the following. One can analyze the cause of hypertension of the circulation in testing, by means of extensive epidemiological investigations, which fate or which characters hypertensives have in common, and which separate them from the normotensives. Among others, one finds in hypertensives an accumulation of definite characteristics which could contain a model of the psychosomatic nature of the disease. All characteristics of hypertensive patients coincide with an increase of emotional and most probably also of sympathetic activity.[9] One can conclude that a model might be correct, in which the augmented sympathetic activity evokes the augmentation of blood pressure. One detects easily that this type of

[9] See F. H. Smirk, *High Arterial Pressure*. Oxford: Blackwell, p. 220 [1957].

illness analysis does not differ principally from the examination of scientific hypotheses. Hereby the legality of a research is proved, in which the disease is used as an experiment in the investigation of psychosomatic hypotheses. Such experiments give two types of result.

1. One detects what is phenomenologically possible. In Lourdes, for example, one can observe cures which are seen seldom or never at other places. I ask for forgiveness if I take out of brackets the question of a miracle. A miracle could not be defined.[10] But it can be stated that a severe tuberculosis can be healed in hours, if we can trust the careful reports in the bulletin.[11] Furthermore, in a few cases one can replace the experiment "illness" by an experiment of classical type, by a suggestion with or without hypnosis. The placebo experiments with sham medicaments belong here, but especially, deep hypnotic suggestion. One of the strangest experiments of that type is that in which it is suggested to a person that he is touched by a glowing iron rod or that a blister-producing plaster is applied. Strong reddening and, in some cases, burn blisters result. This experiment has been successfully repeated on many occasions. There exists a critical review on the literature.[12] I know personally of such a case, observed in Heidelberg by one of the young professors of anatomy.

2. One can learn the structure of psychosomatic interrelations by means of epidemiological observations. One can define which subjective phenomena are correlated with which objective phenomena. Not all that is physical can be influenced mentally.

The results of such investigations lead us immediately to the core of of our problems. Thus theoretical difficulties of the following type arise. When one has discovered the phenomena, for example the suggestive appearance of burn blisters, one must look for the physiological mechanism which makes the phenomenon possible. Here the nervous system causes the local change of the skin in the form of reddening and blistering. In the case of the suggestively originated blister, the difficulties in explanation are large, as we will see. In other cases they may be small.

GENERAL MECHANISMS OF PSYCHOSOMATIC TYPE

Allow me to discuss the theory of acute blood pressure changes as an example of comparative simple psychosomatic theory. Everyone knows that with excitement the blood pressure rises (*Situationshypertonie* of

[10] Ph. Frank. *Das Kausalgesetz und seine Grenzen.* Vienna, p. 73 [1952].

[11] H. Grenet. *Rapport sur la guérison de Mlle Malgogne, Bull. Ass. Méd. Inter. Lourdes,* No. 75 [Jan. 1, 1948].

[12] G. L. Paul. *Psychosomat. Med.,* 25, 233 [1963].

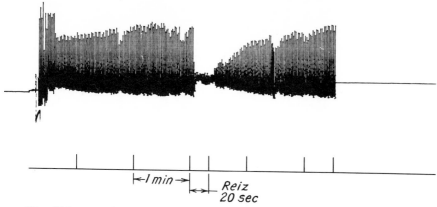

Fig. 21.2. Record of the finger pulse amplitude with a condenser pick up of mechanical displacement of the skin (method Boucke-Brecht, *Pflügers Arch., 257,* 410 [1953]). The pulse pressure is recorded in arbitrary units. Time in minutes. During the black bar at the bottom, the person hears a sound of 90 phon. (Unpublished experiment of Dr. Blohmke.)

Th. von Üxküll).[13] This pressure increase is obviously generated through an overall activation of the sympathetic, which contracts the blood vessels, expels the blood from the veins into the heart and increases the heart strength. The sympathetic is activated by two mechanisms: (1) By the impulses which arise from various sense organs of the skin or the muscles.[14] The muscle spindles especially seem to be very effective, as the muscular work activates the sympathetic so specifically (as Stegemann [15] found) that I cannot but interpret his results in such a way. (2) By an irradiation from higher parts of the brain. One can demonstrate that a conscious excitation as simple as reading, calculating or vigilance, dilates the pupil, lowers the skin resistance, increases the blood pressure, the heart rate, and the muscular tone and lowers (not always!) the finger pulse amplitude (Fig. 21.2). Those findings show that the sphere of the unconscious bodily events is nowhere separated from the conscious psychic sphere.

Local Effects

In contrast to the explicability of such general psychosomatic phenomena, it is very hard if not impossible to explain local effects, such as blisters, eczema, and numerous other skin diseases, which are psychoso-

[13] Th. von Üxküll. *Arch. Kreislaufforschg., 39,* 236 [1962].
[14] R. Sell, A. Erdely, H. Schaefer. *Pflügers Arch., 276,* 481 [1963].
[15] J. Stegemann. *Pflügers Arch., 276,* 481 [1963].

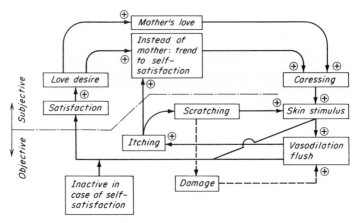

Fig. 21.3. Psychosomatic block diagram.

matic illnesses. In my opinion this assumption is emphasized by over-whelming evidence. With "psychosomatic" it is meant here—exceed-ing our nomenclature statement—that the origin of different skin diseases cannot be fully described without hermeneutics. As an example,[16] a block diagram tries to show the origin of an eczema in a child suffering with some lack of mother love (Fig. 21.3). In this case one detects that an ex-planation can be made without too complicated assumptions. It is ques-tionable, however, whether this very simple scheme is adequate.

Different, however, is the explanation of a suggestively induced burn blister. As it begins without any activity on the side of the patient, such as scratching, it must be produced by nerve impulses, which presents two difficulties in our explanation. First, it is unknown how the only nerve leading to the skin, the sympathetic, can above all originate a burn blister. We previously accepted the fact that such blisters occurred as a result of local destruction of cells and damage of the blood vessels through heat. These reasons do not apply here. Second, it is unknown how the sympa-thetic action may remain local. When we investigate it in animals, we always see that in all cases the sympathetic is active with a similar time and strength pattern in all branches of the system (Fig. 21.4). It may be, however, that those impulses which generate the blisters have not yet been found. They could be slowly traveling inmpulses which indeed be-have differently from the quick ones, and, for example, persist during inhibition of the latter, which really is the case in our most recent experi-ments.[17]

For the benefit of a broader discussion of our conference, I should

[16] F. Dunbar. *Mind and Body.* New York: Random House, p. 198 [1947].
[17] R. Hetzel, and F. Kirchner, unpublished.

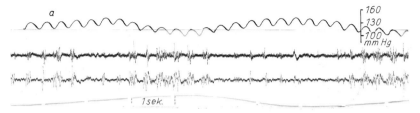

Fig. 21.4. Action potentials in the sympathetic branch to the heart (upper record) and to the kidney (lower record) in a cat. The discharge in both branches is nearly completely uniform. Record at the top: blood pressure, at the bottom: respiration (artificially driven by a pump, inspiration upward). Interruptions: 1 sec. Discharges synchronous to the heart beat and the respiration in both branches [from Weidinger, Fedina, Kehrel, and Schaefer, *Z. Kreislaufforschung, 50,* 229, 1961].

like to say only that the machinery able to produce *local* events on a psychosomatic basis is still unknown. The sympathetic nerve is the only organ linking the brain and the skin. That it evokes *general* responses like vasoconstriction or blushing is easy to explain. For *specific* local effects however, we have never found a sound physiological basis.

CONCLUSION

In looking back to our previous statements, we may say that the same objective inputs into the C.N.S. may lead to conscious as well as to unconscious effects; the same outputs come from conscious as well as unconscious central sources. On the other hand, is consciousness dealing with a group of other bodily events such as blood pressure,[18] wakefulness in the sense of an EEG pattern of "arousal," sympathetic activity, muscular tone [19] (which is always increased in every mental and conscious activity)? Consciousness regarded with the eyes of a pure physiologist appears then as a random effect, attached somewhere, and for unknown reasons, to some of the many happenings in our brain. The brain is a large network with network and membrane properties, both of which explain much of the conscious experience already and should explain–at the end of all scientific progress–*all* its phenomena. For the moment, every description of subjective phenomena in psychological language is of course permitted; it has its problems, if the behavior of *other* living beings is described by that same language, because such a description is methodologically based on *analogs* to ourselves and on conventions made by such analogizing procedures (we say, a man is sad, if we see his tears). We never

[18] W. Baust, H. Niemczyk, and J. Vieth. *EEG Clin. Neurophysiol., 15,* 63 [1963].
[19] H. Göpfert. *Psycholog. Beiträge, 2,* 439 [1956].

know of a foreign consciousness, neither in our dominated cerebral hemisphere, if it does not "speak" to us, nor in animals. Conclusions of the kind made by Dr. Thorpe are *analog* conclusions, with high probability I admit, but of a metaphysical character, insofar as (in the sense of Kant) they never can be tested by experience. We stated, that in the human body, reactions may occur with all characteristics of conscious and teleological character, of an apparent intelligence, which nevertheless are not concomitant with any conscious knowledge of their origin. We may take it for granted that consciousness must not necessarily be assumed in purposeful reactions, and we should be very cautious, therefore, in assuming, by mere analogy, that consciousness is acting in animals if we observe in them an apparently intelligent behavior. When consciousness appears in other beings is unknown. What we know is that every conscious behavior has floating boundaries to forms of behavior, which in ourselves are not linked to psychical events. There is no sharp boundary between conscious and nonconscious, and this is the reason why consciousness cannot be a *simple* phenomenon describable in a static terminology such as that of morphology or of an *all or none reaction*. It is a sliding phenomenon most probably without a "threshold" or a "level" and, as such, most probably difficult to associate to a *certain* event determined in the language of gr, cm, sec. Consciousness *perhaps* never disappears, and every apparent disappearance might be the consequence of fading memory—no theory of memory without a theory of consciousness and vice versa! However, this statement of an overall consciousness, too, has a positively metaphysical character.

One may, in the formal method of MacKay, try to construct an analog of the central machinery, and in trying to do so, we may come to the concept of Fig. 21.5, well knowing that every attempt to construct analogs of that kind has the scientific rank of making a hypothesis, which, by further investigation, might be either falsified or left open to further dis-

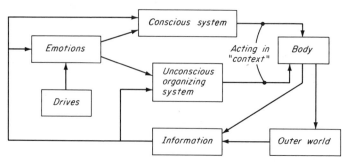

Fig. 21.5. Proposed analog of neural machinery.

cussion. Nor can we say anything about the neuronal pathways bringing about these most intricate effects.

This unconscious organizing system is self-conducting, pseudo-intelligent, purposeful, and emotionally driven. Its action is compulsory, as long as the consciousness has no information about its acquired patterns. However, as soon as consciousness is informed, the integrative action gets lost and becomes controlled by the conscious "context": this is what happens in a successful psychoanalysis.

THESES

There seem to be some special conclusions to be drawn out of these considerations.

1. Any theory of the unconscious as a cause of somatic effects is formally identical with the theory that somatic and psychical events belong to one unit, man, which cannot be divided into a somatic and a psychic half. Argument: If some effects similar to those stemming from conscious reactions can be observed without consciousness, then consciousness cannot be but an epiphenomenon [20] (a side or by-effect) of bodily processes.

2. There is no boundary between conscious and unconscious processes, each sliding in both directions, dependent on the state of apperception.

3. Somatic events reflect central excitations of an emotional character. Emotions are somatic and psychic events at the same time.

4. Body and mind result as abstractions from methodologically different observations, which in the case of man are concerned with the same object: with ourselves. This object cannot be analyzed further with respect to the linkage of these two concepts. The only possible statement is that both, mind and body, vary "in parallel" or, better said, in correspondence.

5. Mental items are always linked to somatic items. This means no devaluation of "mind," but only a revaluation of the body.

[20] The term *epiphenomenon* should, in this connection, not be taken as a valuing expression, depreciating the conscious experience. The term is used here in a strictly descriptive manner, expressing, that for one and the same neuronal process, consciousness may or may not be present without having any influence on the quality of the neuronal output, as far as it is observed with physiological (that is, scientific) methods.

DISCUSSION

Chairman: PROFESSOR MORUZZI

GOMES: My comment is on Professor Schaefer's doubts about the occurrence of consciousness in animals. Indeed, we may lack conclusive evidence of consciousness in animals; but ultimately only in the absolute, Cartesian sense, according to which each of us can doubt the occurrence of mental life even in other men. The communication of ideas and feelings by means of language is, of course, the best evidence we have for the conscious life of our fellow beings; and this is a type of evidence that is lacking in the case of animals. But it is also wanting for human babies, and even for some already developed, or half-developed people pathologically deprived of language, to whom, however, we do attribute conscious life. Nobody would have denied it in Helen Keller, for instance, before she at last acquired a form of systematized language for her communication with her teacher. Professor Thorpe has yesterday disclosed most remarkable instances of evidence for the occurrence of consciousness in animals. But even without considering the type of thoroughly convincing illustrations which he forwarded, I would see no reason for doubting the phenomenon.

SCHAEFER: I completely agree that it is highly probable; and also with all things that you and Professor Thorpe have said. I would accept this for my own belief, that we have at least something like consciousness in animals as well.

This is, nevertheless, a matter of a general theory of life. If we take the whole creation from animal to man as one unity, as one thing developing from primitive beginnings to what we are now, then of course we have no sound reasons for denying animals consciousness. But what I should like to say is only that we cannot have any definite test for this, and I wonder how one could, for example, contradict Descartes in his concept that an animal is just only a highly complicated machine. In his book *The Natural History of Aggression*, Lorenz tried to explain that the very complicated behavior of animals can more or less be understood by natural selection and by something which can easily be explained on the hypothesis of usefulness in the struggle for life. But of course he never could explain that this is really only machinery; and what such a little fish of the southern seas really feels internally is absolutely unknown to Dr. Lorenz as well as to everybody else.

THORPE: This of course raises again the problems that I was speaking of yesterday; and it seems to me that it all comes down to the first point I made concerning solipsism. I don't think that you have any *logically* better ground for assuming consciousness in other human beings than you have for assuming consciousness in other animals. To that extent solipsism is *logically* impregnable. But it is quite obvious that no one in this room is a solipsist. And when you come to those animals which are in many respects very similar to man, you have available the same kind of evidence—though not quite so strong—upon which you decide that human beings are conscious. So in this respect I agree entirely with what Dr. Gomes has said. I think it was D. O. Hebb who said that it is impossible to work with chimpanzees for more than a few days or weeks without becoming convinced that they are conscious beings in many respects similar to oneself. Moreover, once you admit that you are not a solipsist it becomes possible to argue that the evidences for consciousness that we have from the animal kingdom are to be taken seriously; and that these do, in a cumulative manner, provide very strong grounds for supposing that consciousness is a feature present not only in man but also in some, perhaps many, other grades of animal life. Of course it follows that I do not agree with you that the question of the function or otherwise of consciousness in evolution is an unlawful question. I consider it a most important question, one which it is for biologists to ponder and attempt to answer. It seems to me that you are in danger of falling into the kind of error referred to by Professor MacKay when he quoted Professor Popper's opinions about the nature of computer programing. According to him, it would be impossible for a computer to have, up to date, all the necessary information about programing and construction. These are the chief amongst a number of interesting points which you raise in your account. There is only one other matter I would like to refer to and that is where you say that obviously mental processes always have a correlate in neuronal excitation. That is a theory and a very useful theory, but we have no proof. So I fail to see your justification for saying that this is "obviously true."

SCHAEFER: I agree completely with you and I am grateful to you for the occasion once more of making my point clearer. Your assumptions are mine in practical life of course, and what I would like to say is only that every extrapolation from our mental experience in ourselves to other beings is the more valid the better the analog behavior is. If I meet another person, the evidence is striking that he is a man like me, and so it would be quite nonsense to suppose that he is merely a machine. If I play, for example, with my dog and I observe all his behavior including his attitude towards me, then I feel so many identifications between him and me that I am deeply convinced that he must feel something like me. But I will give you an example which showed me best the puzzle in the whole story.

I know this experiment from Lorenz (Ztschr. Tierpsychol., 5, 235–409, 1942, p. 253). He made the following experiment. He took goslings who never had any contacts with adult animals, and at the head of these goslings he let the image of a bird travel with a certain velocity. It was very interesting to see when these goslings showed signs of fear. It was only the case when this image gave a shadow which was more or less like the shadow of an eagle. If this shadow was small enough and the velocity low enough to indicate, as we would say with our intelligence, that this must be the image of an object very far away and therefore moving with a comparatively high velocity, the bird seems to conclude that this can only be an eagle. Now, we reconstruct the behavior of the animal by making very complicated mathematical assumptions of how the bird possibly could have interpreted this experiment, but I wonder what the bird really feels. All these concepts that we put into the experiment in explaining it are far too complicated to assume that they might have been present in the brain of a gosling.

MAC KAY: I think it was Bertrand Russell who said he was cured of solipsism for life by receiving a letter from a woman saying: "I am so glad you think there may be something in solipsism; I wish there were more of us."

It is useful, I think, to distinguish between two rational ways of arriving at belief, one being deduction from evidence, and the other being commitment that is judged reasonable (but not logically obligatory) on the evidence. In other words, there are cases where the burden of proof is on us, and cases where the burden of disproof is on somebody else; and I think that in recognizing consciousness we tend to work in the second mode. This is not to say that we cannot enumerate some of the things that convince us, but it does mean that we don't wait for 100 per cent deductive evidence of consciousness before committing ourselves. We may sometimes be fooled in this respect, as for example in some psychiatric circumstances, but we take this risk.

This brings me to the main difficulty I felt about Professor Schaefer's conclusion. He says: "If effects similar to those stemming from conscious reactions can be observed without consciousness, then it cannot be but an epiphenomenon." I want to ask: can we enunciate a demonstrably *sufficient* specification of the effects stemming from consciousness? I personally doubt it, and I don't see how this conclusion could be substantiated in our present state of knowledge, if indeed ever.

SCHAEFER: The difficulty is, of course, that we have no complete theory of the counterpart of consciousness in the body. I believe it might be possible to get such a counterpart; for example, a few years ago one could say that possibly in the EEG one could find such a counterpart, but unfortunately the paradoxical sleep and the atropine EEG, which shows a sleep EEG in a wakeful person, suddenly disturbed all our hopes. However, my first conclusion is drawn from clinical experiences. I have been deeply impressed by life histories which we discussed many times in Heidelberg with my colleagues of the psychosomatic clinics; and most of this paper comes out of this collaboration with the Heidelberg group. You find very curious things which in my opinion can be explained only by assuming that what we all believe to be completely originated by some purposeful conscious behavior may as well come out of the brain of a patient without any consciousness at all of what is going on; then the physician tries to explain to the patient what possibly had been at the root of his behavior, and as soon as these displaced experiences come back into his consciousness, he becomes suddenly aware of the reasons for his disturbances. The disturbances disappear and the patient comes to normality again. The expression "effects stemming from conscious reactions" means, therefore, something which can be tested only in self-experience. We realize that we behave in exactly the same way (movement e.g.), though in the one case we are conscious of our behavior, in another case we are not. This does not mean that we have any further specification of conscious reactions than just this statement: they were conscious.

ECCLES: With regard to the question of whether animals are conscious or not, I would suggest the following test. How do animals regard their dead companions? It seems probable that the development of ceremonial burial customs provides the first evidence for the dawn of self-consciousness in the developing hominids in the evolutionary process. I would suggest that the development of burial customs is the best evidence we can have that these human progenitors have both self-consciousness and also have rejected solipsism. Have any animals, other than man, got to that stage?

THORPE: This is certainly a difficult question. Nevertheless, there are one or two things one can say. First, that chimpanzees show an extraordinary fear, amounting to a sort of horror, of detached limbs or other parts of chimpanzee bodies, and also of stuffed chimpanzees. Again, there are some puzzling and remarkable accounts—I would not put too much weight on them at present—of what are known as "badger funerals." When a badger dies in the set, the dead body is brought out with curious mournful cries and is then taken and deposited in some litter or rubbish some distance from the hole. This has not been sufficiently well described to merit much reliance; nevertheless, I think it worth mentioning.

The question of ritual burial or ritual performances associated with the dead certainly goes back a very long way in prehistory. There is, in fact, overwhelming evidence that what you might, for the want of a better word, call "spirituality" was a striking quality of early man. This spirituality may manifest itself in animism, worship of the dead, and other similar characteristics of human stock. Magic and spirituality certainly antedate the appearance of Homo sapiens in Europe. Neanderthal man had some kind of a skull cult and also funeral rites. It has even been suggested that Pekin man, *Homo erectus Pekingensis*, may have engaged in ritual cannibalism; for here again skulls have been found with broken occipital parts—as if for extraction of the brain for ceremonial consumption. It looks as if this was some sort of attempt, by ritualization, to acquire the power and personality of the dead person. These cults are of such antiquity that one begins to wonder whether something similar was not present in what you might call prehuman primates. Perhaps one will never know at what stage these extraordinary rituals first appeared and what their original significance was. But that they were firmly established in many primitive cultures is clear beyond a doubt.

GRANIT: Dr. Schaefer brought up the Freudian psychoanalysis and what has come afterwards. It seems to me that psychoanalysis throws some light on this question because I think we can all agree that the cures which the psychoanalysts achieve by making unconscious events conscious, often relieve the patient of his trouble. So it seems that in these cases consciousness brings on a deeper insight and also a definite shift of bodily function because there is a change from being sick to being cured.

SCHAEFER: Of course one must have seen that in some cases there are facts which one can observe, which are so self-evident and striking that it is hard to deny the psychoanalytical conclusions. Such a fact is, e.g., if suddenly the patient loses all his symptoms, in that same moment when by very hard and very long psychoanalysis he is suddenly aware of what really is the source of his disturbance. In some cases perhaps the scientific test can be best given by some sort of statistics.

If you found that the cure and the developing of the conscious awareness of the disturbance occur at different times, then your criticism would be perfectly all right. But the evidence that these two are really linked is given by their coincidence in time. This gives such strong evidence that one should conclude that the basic theory of psychoanalysis is right, at least in this respect. There are some things which are still very unclear and I would not say that all assumptions that Freud made in his early papers are valid nowadays, but this is a very long story and it would take hours and hours to discuss it.

MAC KAY: Just one further point on your first conclusion. I understand now that Professor Schaefer is claiming not that *all* effects, but only that *some* effects similar to those stemming from conscious reaction, can be observed without consciousness. I would suggest that, if it is modified in this way, then this conclusion does not logically follow.

SCHAEFER: Why not?

THORPE: I would reply by referring again to the example Professor Schaefer has been discussing. In this particular case subsequent experiments have, as it happens, altered our views as to what it is that the animal is actually responding to. This is perhaps not important. But it is true that responses of this kind, relational responses which we call "releasers" and "sign stimuli" in ethology, are very characteristic of quite low animal groups—of the insects, for instance. That was part of my thesis yesterday. Here we have quite elaborate relational perceptions occurring in situations such that it seems quite *unreasonable* to assume they are correlated with conscious behavior or conscious perception.

Again, when you come to the birds, there is no reason whatever to suppose that the bird building its nest for the first time knows what the nest is for. The bird somehow has instructions within it to stop at one point making the main structural part of the nest and then to start putting in the lining. We are beginning to know the endocrinological basis of all this, thanks largely to the work of Professor Hinde. We do now have some understanding of how one set of actions is brought to an end and another comes in, to bring about the next step. The ultimate result is that in due course the nest is completed, the eggs are laid, the young are fed, and the whole breeding process goes off normally. All this—or much of it at least—seems to take place without the necessity of making any assumptions concerning conscious thought.

On the other hand, even in the same creatures, in birds and in insects, there is much behavior concerned with direction finding—finding the way about, remembering how to get back to the territory and so forth, which does appear to require something which it is difficult in my view, to suppose has been produced without some degree of consciousness.

SCHAEFER: I would now add that the reason for this is that you conclude from such types of behavior, which seem to be more or less analogous to our own behavior, that in such types consciousness is present. Whereas, to our misfortune, we have no analogs to be found in ourselves of instinctive behavior. I have read of possible innate instinctive behavior; but I think it is not very clear and I would like to hear something of that.

THORPE: It is true that the evidence for instinct (in the Lorenzian sense) in man is fairly meager. But there is one striking case where it does seem to apply fully: that is in the movement of the new-born baby searching for the breast. The new-born baby will execute side to side movements of the head and will go on doing this for a long time until one corner of the mouth touches the nipple. Dr. Gunther has shown that feeding in the neonate is an instinctive behavior evoked by the pattern of stimuli provided by the nipple and the areola tissues of the breast when these are in contact with the mouth. A bottle teat can also act as a releaser and can be supernormal to poorly formed breasts. However, once the mouth touches the right stimulus it fastens on to the nipple and sucking begins. But the characteristic head movement of the baby searching for the breast is internally driven and seems to me to be just the kind of instinctual movement that Lorenz was postulating as the key to his scheme of instinct.

There may be other aspects of human behavior that are truly instinctive in the same sense. Certainly with man it seems likely that erection, ejaculation in the male and perhaps the pelvic thrusts in both sexes are of an innate and probably reflex nature. But even if they are reflex in the ordinary sense of the word, they show the same type of internal drive which is by definition a feature of instinct. Be this as it may, such innate motor patterns as we have are very quickly overlaid with conditioned responses, so much so that it is hard to say much about them. Nevertheless, I think one must assume that there is a certain amount of crude instinct still left in human behavior.

SCHAEFER: Yes, that is really so, but we have all forgotten the time when we made this instinctual movement in our early life, and that is what I meant in saying that we have no analogs in our adult behavior. The sexual things might perhaps be the only possibility of explaining to ourselves a little bit of what an instinct is; but this is quite an uncertain story, and all certain instinctual behavior stems from the time from which we have no normal personal experience i.e. no traces of memory.

ECCLES: I made the statement in my second talk that conscious experience in all forms is the primary reality. Everything else, including brains and behavior and psychosomatic events, and so on, are derivate realities, interpretations, in fact, derived from our conscious experiences. I think this statement contradicts epiphenomenology.

SCHAEFER: It is perfectly true that you have two possibilities of approaching every experience. Of course, the first approach is always coming from an analysis of our internal feelings; that is definitely true, and this statement here has nothing to do with your statement, because you work much more at the bottom of the phenomena and I now go a little bit into the scientific theory. But as soon as we come to some sort of an image of the world, to models of the world, we realize suddenly that we have a body, and of course then we are forced to assume that this body is something which carries our psychical events, and in that sense I mean that the psyche is some sort of epiphenomenon of matter. You may easily put it the other way round and say that matter is something of an epiphenomenon of psyche. These statements I would say, radically speaking, are more or less the same.

GOMES: I am so very glad to hear these comments by Professor Eccles, because they increase the importance of the problem defined by his previous assertion about how the present state of the science would induce him to view consciousness. Of course, the evidence we have for consciousness is such that, if we are to escape at any cost the sharp dualism apparent in the classical formulation of the body-mind problem, we can only do it by asserting that the nature of the body—and of the world where it is—must be qualitatively homogenous with that of consciousness. Epiphenomenalism, on the contrary, is the last and the least reasonable hypothesis one could expect to see formulated.

From your paper, Professor Schaefer, I would not say that you are an epiphenomenalist unless you attributed reality to matter first and then deduce consciousness from it.

SCHAEFER: I suppose that you admit that body and mind are, as I say here in conclusion 4, abstractions from methodologically different observations.

GOMES: I would like to ask whether the attempt to escape the conventional dualism between brain and mind by regarding it as simply due to different types of observation is ultimately only a mere shift of the problem. Is not any such attempt equivalent merely to the substitution of a dualism between two mutually incongruent forms of knowledge for the original dualism which posed the original question? Is this not like simply giving a new name to the problem?

SCHAEFER: Perhaps, but there is no distinct dualism between the objects of these two methods of observation, which are insofar identical, as they both occur connected in ourselves. Is this not different from the conception of body and mind as two completely separate entities?

GOMES: Yes, but is this not simply a shifting of the problem?

SCHAEFER: Perhaps. But I don't see any other solution of the problem.

GOMES: Perhaps we could try monism of some sort. Like the so-called neutral monism of William James and others.

SCHAEFER: In my model of the world I would say that most probably things like consciousness come out of the development of matter. How this has been brought about is a completely different question, and has something to do with the organization of the gray matter of the brain and of his network properties. For example, we certainly know that consciousness cannot be a matter of single nerve cells because we have in many cases an abundant excitation of cells in the brain without any consciousness at all. So we must stick to the hypothesis that consciousness must be correlated with and must correspond to some very peculiar patterns of a neuronal network excitation; but how consciousness comes into play in the history of matter, in the development of the world, is completely unknown; and it is the more unknown the more we go back into ethology and phylogeny.

THORPE: Could we not just put it this way: that consciousness is a primary datum of existence and that as such it cannot be fully defined? It is what we all start with and assume, and it is an absolutely necessary assumption for all we do. If there were no consciousness, there could be no philosophy, no science, no art, no religion. There would be no life of any kind that we would regard as worth living. It is the basis of everything that we do, of every activity, and to that extent it cannot be defined; we have got to assume that we know, directly, enough about it to go ahead.

MAC KAY: I think this word "epiphenomenon" is causing us more trouble than it is worth. The difficulty with most of these terms is not what a man affirms by them but what he is thought to deny by using them; and epiphenomenon has the reductionist flavor of what I like to call "nothing buttery." (Nothing buttery is illustrated by the argument that you can ignore a NO SMOKING sign, because it is "nothing but" so much ink on paper.) I think we would all agree that if some effect similar to that stemming from conscious reactions can be observed without consciousness, then consciousness *need not be invoked in explanation* of these bodily processes. The suggestion that you have given priority to bodily processes is inherent in the traditional epiphenomenalist position, and that I think is causing us the trouble.

SCHAEFER: Yes. I feel that really this term *epiphenomenon* has been largely misunderstood here by the conference, and it is not meant in the sense of being just a denial. To put it in a simple way in which everyone who knows of these books will immediately understand, I meant it more or less in the same way as Teilhard de Chardin.

GRANIT: I merely wanted to rise in defense of Professor Schaefer. I think he really means what you other people mean, but he has emphasized the methodological aspect of science; and it is clear that if you do that you come up with a result that will not tell you much about consciousness. I think that if you take up this standpoint, the only one here who has really contributed to the theme of this week is Professor Penfield. When he stimulates certain parts of the brain and the people do complex things, they feel these things as if they were impressed upon them; they have no consciousness of them. On the other hand, there are things of which they are conscious. No one else has drawn such a clear distinction between conscious and unconscious experience as has Professor Penfield.

JASPER: In line with what Professor Granit just said, I think your definition does not mean to use the word epiphenomenon but "protophenomenon"; and I think this probably gives equal importance, perhaps, to the phenomenon. In your definition "what is given in the immediate experience," there is no indication of the nature, or quality, of this experience that is the definition of a conscious experience. And this seems to me to be an excellent point to make. You have made it over and over again in your illustrations, that complexity of behavior cannot ever be assumed as a criterion of consciousness. This seems to be lost, however, in discussions of Professor Eccles, who seems to imply that one cannot attribute consciousness to immediate experience unless one has a complex experience or an emotional experience such as devotion to other members of the species. I think this logical difficulty has gone through many of the discussions where the emergence of consciousness has been attributed only to animals who seem to have highly complex intellectual or affectionate behavior. This seems to be not a logical necessity at all. Consciousness may be a very simple immediate awareness rather than a complex intellectual process.

ECCLES: I would like to refer back to the minimum conditions that I think are requisite before one is justified in assuming consciousness for, say, an animal. I would suggest these conditions would be fulfilled if the death of a companion aroused reactions of a kind which you would interpret as indicating that this animal had felt there had been in this dead animal an existence somewhat like itself. Primitive burial customs have, I think, been found to occur at least 100,000 years ago in hominid development. Since animals are so imitative, valid evidence for burial customs can be obtained only in the wild state. Hence I would like to ask Dr. Thorpe if, with these wild chimpanzee colonies in Africa, Miss Goodall has found any evidence of mourning for a dead companion?

THORPE: No, she has not done this yet; for of course she is not able to be in contact with the chimpanzee group or colony the whole time. One or two chimpanzees have disappeared since she first commenced her work and she is pretty certain that one died of pneumonia. But she was not able to be present at the time it happened, so unfortunately no information was obtained. However, if the work goes on long enough it may be that a member of a troop will actually be found *in extremis,* and then it will be interesting to see what happens. It is, of course, well known that many female primates hold very tenaciously to the bodies of dead infants even, in some cases, after they have actually begun to putrefy and decompose.

GOMES: My present remark refers to Professor Jasper's observation to the effect that complexity of behavior should not be necessarily taken as a criterion for consciousness. I agree with this view. And it is not complexity, but something else—individual independence—which I look at in behavior as indicative of consciousness. This will become clear by means of a comparison between some insects and some developed vertebrates. The behavior of the members of a good many species of insects is much more complex than that of a good many vertebrates. Yet the elaborate, sometimes amazing, complexity and organization of behavior of some insects do not incline us to attribute a rich conscious life to them. There is something else in the extraordinary behavior of insects which very often more strongly impresses us, namely, its rigid patterns and semblance of automatism. On the other hand, we usually think of a dog, for instance, as currently living with a certain wealth of conscious experiences, though in many cases its behavior may be much less complex than with insects. We regard dogs as possessing a lot of independence in relation to the environment, but we regard bees and ants as possessing only the slightest independence in relation to their societies and milieu.

ANDERSEN: It seems to me that people around this table are discussing consciousness as a kind of unitary process, "yes" or "no." To me, it seems to be different. Is there not a continuous function of different degrees of consciousness? Certainly, there are states in my own life where I am aware of very little, some other times I am aware of much more, of myself and of the surroundings; and there are, of course, descriptions in the literature whereby people under the influence of certain drugs seem to be aware of much more than they are in usual life. And also, since this faculty is a nondimensional one, could this be the reason why we have such difficulty in describing it, or defining it, and also to describe the onset of it in phylogeny?

SCHAEFER: This is exactly my opinion and I said nearly the same words somewhere in the paper.

PHILLIPS: I would like just to make one further point about very highly complex behavior. It is true, I suppose, that the performances of musicians are the most complex human activities that we can imagine. Could one not say that a performance as complex as that of a pianist is always laid down by many years of conscious practice and application, but, having been laid down, can then be carried out unconsciously so that the man, for instance, can be playing the piano while he is talking to someone about something else? One could say that the motions in their final elaborated form can be carried out unconsciously. But surely it must be true that some performances are so complex that they could never have been learned without full concentration of consciousness during the learning period.

THORPE: I think the point here is that it is certainly true that it would be quite impossible for a pianist, or any other type of musician, to *learn* a complex performance without consciousness. Once he has got the general idea of the performance and what is required, then a great deal of unconscious practice can continue. I used to play the piano myself and I found that if, after having practised for a certain time, I then gave the piece a rest, next time I came back to the piano, two or three days later, I might have improved a good deal. There is evidence from many sources of something like unconscious practice taking place in situations such as this. Finally, I found that I could play a piece in at least a passable manner without thinking about it at all; even when thinking actively about other things and perhaps talking to people at the same time. But this, of course, does not mean that consciousness was not necessary in the initial stages. One can develop one's sight reading powers to such a pitch that whole themes, chords, and positions can be apprehended and translated into action subconsciously just as one can sometimes read aloud without having any idea of what one has been saying. But I do not believe that any human being could have reached the stage of playing a complex, or indeed a simple, piece on the piano without a great deal of conscious concentration in the first place.

SCHAEFER: Dr. Phillips raises the same problem which I tried to answer the other day. Assume or imagine what would happen if a very complex machine would be developed which you can describe with your wonderful methods of neurology in a more or less complete manner. Then, of course, you would be able to explain its operation without any assumption of subjective things in it, and this can perhaps be the end of scientific development—that eventually we will be able to describe the behavior of the brain with all its implications without any assumption of subjective association. But, of course, that says nothing about the role which your consciousness plays; and I do not see how one could bring consciousness into a position where it plays a decisive role beside any physical or chemical events because they are obviously intimately connected to each other. And so, I would say in a formal sense, both ways of explanation are identical; they only use different methods of approach.

PENFIELD: To get away from the question of definition of epiphenomena and other things, I have been thinking of the fact, as Dr. Jasper pointed out, that consciousness may be a very simple thing. Thinking of the individual lying on the operating table who has simultaneously two streams of awareness, that is, from two different periods of his life, the brain seems to have made the whole phenomenon a very simple one—so simple that he can be aware of what was happening 20 years ago, in a certain period of time, and what is happening progressively in this present period of time, aware of the fact that he is on the operating table and of what the surgeon is saying and asking him, and yet aware also of what seems to be going on in a previous period of time.

If that is the case, that two streams of consciousness are being appreciated, then there is something more than the awareness of conscious experience: there is something that is capable of appreciating two conscious streams simultaneously and judging their relations to each other. There is something more that we come here to consider and cannot even name! There is something more that is able to see, and reflect, and compare such simple things as two streams of awareness. I am not expressing that very well but I am sure you guess what I am driving at. There is something more than just the stream of awareness.

SCHAEFER: One could perhaps even define the patterns of these two streams; one would be what I call at the very beginning of this paper the standard consciousness of the experimenting physiologist, and there is a second stream which obviously is not covered by the conventional psychology of the last century, for example, and which we explore more and more in patients suffering from psychosomatic diseases. Perhaps that is the sort of thing which you mean with these two streams?

PENFIELD: I find it difficult to answer that question. I would like to avoid the question and express it differently. If one is writing a biography of a man he may describe the subject's conscious experience over the years. But he also has the problem of describing a character, a personality. He cannot do it in terms of mental capacity. There is something that he sets out to do besides describing experience; he sets out to describe a character different from the character of any other individual. There is something that looks out of the eyes of an individual. It changes through the years. It is what the biographer must make his readers familiar with. There is something beyond the stream of conscious experience that we still are not either naming or identifying or understanding.

JASPER: I am very pleased to hear Dr. Penfield bring in the question of several streams—at least two—which seem to join and yet be appreciated as separate. Dr. Schaefer has emphasized, and we must all emphasize, the impossibility of dissociating memory from our evidence of conscious experience. Memory comes into the comments of Dr. Penfield on the relation between the inmmediate operating room experience and the elicited experience which I think you would probably categorize as a memory, wouldn't you, Dr.

Penfield? And at least in our physiological work we are operating on a hypothesis that, although dissociable, there is a very intimate relationship between the physiological mechanism of permanent memory and what we assume is consciousness. This is a conjunction of the residual or past experience with present experience. This "comparator" function is an essential of any complex conscious process and it seems to me not impossible, Dr. Eccles, that we might get further in our thinking about physiological hypotheses if we worked on the assumption that it is this particular junction of past with present that is so critical for that new event of consciousness.

SCHAEFER: Dr. Jasper, I agree with you completely. No theory of consciousness without a theory of memory.

Final Discussion

Chairman: PROFESSOR ECCLES

CHAIRMAN: It has seemed expedient to organize this final discussion so that the principal topics of the symposium are reviewed in general terms by Professors Mountcastle, Moruzzi, MacKay, and Teuber, and after each of these introductory talks there can be a free discussion.

I call upon Professor Mountcastle.

THE FUNCTIONAL MEANING OF SPECIFIC AND NONSPECIFIC SYSTEMS

MOUNTCASTLE: The present operational point of view taken by neurophysiologists is that it is possible to define in rather precise terms the neural replications of the external world in the highly organized specific afferent systems. There is some confidence also that we will be able to define the transformations of that neural replica, that is, the results of integrative action, which occur at synaptic relays and in the cerebral cortex. If this is true, and if the work of the next few years is successful in this regard, we will then be able to define at least the neural discriminanda upon which the perceptive process operates. The perceptive process is presently only vaguely conceived as a detecting mechanism, itself composed of neurons. Very little is known of this perceptive mechanism at the present time, but it is possible that some of its properties can be inferred by learning more about (*a*) the neural substratum upon which it operates, as outlined above, and (*b*) the behavioral output which results from its action. This is the idea behind the type of correlative study of neural and psychophysical operations which I have described earlier this week. The steady closure of these two fields is likely, I believe, to reveal more and more of the qualities of the perceptive process, of the central detection and decision apparatus.

It is at this point—when these two fields begin to close—that the

548

neurophysiologist must make the assumption that conscious activities and processes are involved, that is, when sufficient numbers of nerve cells are involved in sufficiently complex interactions to allow *differential discrimination*. We should remember also that discriminations at this level of complexity include also the capacity to withhold response, a property which has been shown to depend upon the integrity of the cerebral cortex. It is at this level that I must take issue with many, and to some degree with the ideas of cortical action suggested by Professors Penfield and MacKay. I do so because I believe that studies of the cerebral cortex have so far revealed only the general framework upon which much more complex activities must depend. They have revealed only those aspects of function which are determined strictly by synaptic connections—connections probably continually renewed and susceptible to change during ontogeny, but static during any single acute experiment. These studies have produced a wealth of information concerning the neural substratum for place and quality, and have suggested that afferent inhibition is an important property of integrative action in sensory systems. Beyond this they have not yet gone, though the physiological revolution from the study of things static to things dynamic promises well for the future. Perhaps the finding of a columnar organization as a basis for function in the cortex has only added to what I regard as an excessively deterministic point of view concerning cortical function.

The truth is that so far physiological studies have only added to what we know of the anatomical substratum for function—and this is what I mean by the term *static properties*. The tide of experiment moves towards an elucidation of the time-dependent, dynamic aspects of cortical function. One may suppose, and indeed some observations already indicate, that the sequential forming and reforming of new and highly complex patterns of activity, occupying both the cortical cells activated initially by a sensory stimulus and others independent of it, result in functional patterns far more complex than those predicted by the columnar organization alone, and it is this aspect of neural activity to which I believe we must look for the neural correlates of the perceptive process.

It is, thus, I believe far too soon to close the possibility for an action in the cortex far higher in the scale of neural integration than is subsumed by the hypothesis of Dr. Penfield, or that indicated by Dr. MacKay's reference to the cerebral cortex as a "labor exchange." Indeed, the silencing of cortical function by the application of electrical stimuli is compatible with, if indeed it does not provide direct evidence for, my hypothesis. If the higher-order aspects of cortical function do depend in a sensitive manner upon the time-bound aspects of neural activity, then their artificial initiation by an electrical stimulus will most certainly result in temporal patterns which are functionally meaningless. All that will remain will be in the pigeonhole function—that which requires for its expression only the simple fact of a static anatomical connection.

Nonspecific Systems. Concomitant with the processing of the neural replication of the sensory event in specific systems, there occurs a widespread activation of nuclear groups of the brain stem, the mesencephalon, of the midline and intralaminar nuclei of the thalamus, and perhaps, but not certainly, of other structures of the basal forebrain as well, for example, the hypothalamus and limbic structures. Now it is clear that many of these very same structures are intimately concerned, in their multisynaptic upward projections upon the telencephalon, with maintaining levels of awareness. It is clear also that sensory convergence in these systems is widespread, that, as Dr. Jasper has said, stimulus novelty is frequently required for activation, that there is no neural replication in space or in time of any aspect of the stimulus other than that it has, in fact, occurred. All these facts I believe to support the point of view that this sensory inflow from nonspecific systems is itself concerned with an energizing action, with controlling levels of excitability of the forebrain, and thus setting the stage for that complex neural interplay from which some quantitative aspects of the external world can be derived—which depends upon action in specific systems. This second inflow will also, by virtue of its further projections upon the hypothalamus and other basal forebrain structures, give to the total sensory experience those subtle aspects which we subsume under the terms set, or affect.

To my surprise I find this a most unpopular, in fact a nearly unique, point of view. Others believe that the mere fact of convergence a priori results in integrative action. But how can there be integrated action when all aspects of the actions supposedly integrated are lost, save the mere fact of their occurrence? It seems to me more likely that the neural substratum for these higher-order integrations is to be looked for in the further elaboration of cortical activity.

Last, I would like to say that until positive evidence is available, the matter should be left open, particularly whether the neural decision apparatus I have referred to is localized, or not. Let us be free of a rigid geography, and yet retain what geography has to give. Over and beyond it, integrative action, neural discrimination, perception, and perhaps conscious action itself may be regarded as emergent properties of large populations of neurons, properties to be revealed only by continuing experiment.

CHAIRMAN: Dr. Jasper, would you like to continue on the theme of this discussion?

JASPER: I would be pleased to present a working scheme from evidence we have in this field, but I hesitate to suggest even a working hypothesis at this stage of our knowledge, for it is likely to be wrong. But we have to work with some hypothesis, and I must say the conception that Mountcastle has put forward is not far from the scheme I was drawing out on this paper for the neurophysiological processes that we know to occur. We know also a fair amount about where they occur. We may hope to discover those more critical processes related to awareness as opposed to those concerned with information processing as such. Dr. Mountcastle has raised the question of where to look. He would look in the cortex, I presume, and Dr. Penfield would look in the brain stem and diencephalon, others would look in the midbrain, and some may look in the hippocampus. It seems clear that we must consider more than those processes engaged in the transduction, conduction, and central processing of afferent inputs.

Dr. Penfield has emphasized repeatedly that it is an interaction between the cortex and subcortical structures, not something that occurs uniquely in subcortical structures. This interaction is capable of being studied and has been studied, of course, in Dr. Moruzzi's laboratory and in many other laboratories. But we have studied it in the wrong time scale, and I think if we study now the later interactions and the ones which have a different chemical sensitivity than the primary ones, we may find that there is a unique type of interaction regularly associated with what we call awareness. I feel that this will necessarily involve brain stem circuits. Dr. Sperry's work has made this problem more acute. How do you incorporate into your notion, Dr. Mountcastle, the unification of perception from the extraordinary diverse multiplicity of simultaneously active circuits in the great mantle of the cortex—the remarkable simplicity of what comes to conscious awareness?

This I think is the key to the selectivity from extraordinary multiplicity of activity. And this selectivity in awareness cannot be divorced from its selectivity in memory. To say that repetitive discharge in synaptic circuits produces memory or learning seems to me to be impossible to accept. One only has to place a few microelectrodes to see the great noise of continuous repetitive activity going on everywhere, most of which, I think, is not related to the memory. We have to add something. That "something" is removed by certain lesions in subcortical structures which abolish memory recording without an appreciable effect upon "conscious behavior" or awareness. I would not agree with the proposal of Penfield that memory therefore is located in these structures; but again I would return to an interaction process, as Dr. Mountcastle has implied. The characteristics of this critical mechanism of the limbic and mesial part of the brain for the "stamping in" processes are, I think, representative of an interaction, not a localization, of memory processes.

MOUNTCASTLE: An answer I cannot give, but I want to leave it open. I think there are many reasons for thinking that it cannot be wholly due to the activity of these central structures. I think it more reasonable to regard them as being supporting in nature. It seems to me that this integrated action which brings a perception into consciousness must first depend upon the extraction of universal signs of the parameters of the peripheral stimulus; and this has got to be due to a further elaboration of activity within the cortex and between the cortex and subcortical structures, but not localized initially in these nonspecific systems. I think you will not agree with this, but it is one of my major points. The fact that one loses this when a lesion is placed in the subcortical regions is not, I think, a telling argument. Of course you also remove this supportive action, which maintains levels of excitability in the cortex.

THORPE: I am not quite sure whether what I have to say, which is brief, is more appropriate to the present discussion or to one yet to come. Nevertheless, for convenience I will bring it in now. There are a number of recent papers—I recall the names of Landsell, J. C. Smith, and Pinto-Hamuy—which deal with the question of cortical localization in rat behavior. We all know the classic work of Lashley which led to his theory of equipotentiality. But this new work seems to show that if the rat is given experience of a much wider kind than that provided by the ordinary laboratory cage; if its environment is richer, more structured, in fact, more like the varied environment of the natural wild life—then the evidence for equipotentiality diminishes and, in contrast, we begin to get evidence for localization. These studies appear small-scale compared with Lashley's magnificent contribution. But obviously the conclusion, if correct, is most important and I would like to know whether others here consider it to be reliable.

MOUNTCASTLE: I would certainly agree with this, and I would like to make what is certainly a critical statement here. But I believe the original experiments of Lashley should be disregarded. They were all done before the specific receiving and motor areas of the rat had been determined. If you look at the maps, I believe it is fair to say there is no single lesion which totally removes any one area which does not involve more than another area. And the second point is, and I think that Dr. Thorpe will confirm me in this, that the brains were all infected.

BREMER: I think that for future progress in the understanding of the mechanisms underlying perceptual integration, special attention should be given to the study, at thalamic and cortical levels, of the arousal process resulting from the ascending impulses issued from the midbrain reticular formation. We know that failing these dynamogenic influences, even dense impacts of sensory impulses may remain without conscious integration and may leave no memory trace, although being clearly recorded as primary cortical responses. As our colleague Jasper has reminded us, the difference between the two functional conditions, associated with the presence or absence of the reticular energizing influence, is expressed electrophysiologically by the presence or absence in the cortical sensory reaction of the afterdischarge, and more generally of the late events, which follow the primary evoked potential of the receiving area.

It would be important to know with more precision what this after-discharge process exactly represents intrinsically and functionally. Does it reveal the processing of a short, lasting reverberatory or autorhythmic activity, which is the immediate condition of dynamic memory and of the temporal continuity of the psychic life? And, by lowering the threshold for associative irradiations of the primary reaction in the cortical mantle, does it allow the formation of the complicated spatio-temporal neuronal patterns which is the condition of perceptual integration?

Electrophysiological evidence exists for such cortico-cortical irradiations in reticular arousal. Their increase accompanies the changes of the primary-evoked potential and of the sensory afterdischarge in the cortical receiving area. But they are not directly causally related to these local responses. Rather, they betray mainly the subcortical effects of reticular arousal, which can be demonstrated in both specific and unspecific thalamic nuclei. Thus, here again, the "horizontalist" and "verticalist" concepts of cerebral integration are confronted.

The increase of amplitude, in barbiturate narcosis, of the cortical-evoked potential—an increase which is always a moderate one—is not the significant feature of that condition of functional depression of the activating reticular system. The fact that the evoked potential should still be there, at a time when all psychophysiological recording is abolished, is the important fact. On the other hand, depending from the experimental condition, reticular arousal may result, as I have shown in my report, in a spectacular augmentation of the voltage of the evoked potential or in an equally striking increase of its fast afterdischarge, to-gether—in the two cases—with a speeding of intracortical and subcortical transmission processes.

TEUBER: Quite a number of times throughout this week various speakers have referred to Karl Lashley and his work, and it has seemed at times as if he were right amongst us and we were arguing back and forth with him. I do in a sense agree with Professor Mountcastle that the evidence for the mass action concept of cortical function has to be reassessed. I think, maybe Lashley himself would say so now.

Some of Lashley's results may turn out to be limited to animals reared under the stress of living in small cages and unable to explore their environment in a normal fashion. If these animals are reared instead in an enriched environment, maze learning is more seriously impaired after removal of the posterior cortical areas, as contrasted with corresponding cortical removals elsewhere in the forebrain. The reason for the selectivity of this loss might be that these enriched-environment animals tend to rely much more on visual cues, but even for animals reared under the usual laboratory conditions, the statements about equipotentiality have to be seriously qualified. In fact, a careful reading of Lashley's own publications makes it apparent that he held what might be called a duplicity view of this situation, since he himself had devised tasks that were exquisitely sensitive to certain specific lesions, and other tasks which failed to pick up anything but general effects irrespective of the lesion site. Lashley preferred to think of these general effects as reflecting impairment in some of the highest cortical functions, while others elected to speak of vigilance. There certainly are tasks that can be designed which will bring out similarly general effects in brain-injured man, yet these effects coexist with extremely specific and localizable effects of the same lesions.

Lashley's evidence for cortical mass action in the rat, insofar as it was based on the particular maze he used, will have to be reexamined and, in fact, rejected. In this respect, I agree with Professor Mountcastle since the maze employed involved several distinct capacities which are separately disturbable by differently localized lesions. The task required orientation in a complex spatial environment, and this aspect of the task is selectively vulnerable to posterior cortical lesions. The task also involved rapid and repeated alternation from one side to the other, and such alternation behavior depends on the integrity of anterior cortex and caudate nucleus. Destroying anterior cortex or caudate nucleus thus impairs alternation but leaves spatial orientation intact, while posterior cortical lesions impair orientation without and trouble in alternation. Larger lesions that involve both areas will produce the more global deficits which Lashley obtained and interpreted as non-specific effects.

ANDERSEN: Dr. Mountcastle said that convergence a priori does not mean integration. But I hope he agrees with me that when we look upon a cortical cell, the convergence is the physiological prerequisite for its integration. Another thing I found puzzling was the time resolution. Is this not very much dependent upon your detector? If you have a detector that can determine whether or not a pulse is coming, then you have a tremendous resolution in a series of events. But the higher levels of the nervous system do not operate like that, I think. Most cortical cells do not pick up one incoming event, but they have to accumulate certain quite large numbers of events. Following this accumulation they discharge one or more impulses. The series of discharges will be quite different in different situations. It will be a property of the neuron network. The pattern will probably be much more complex than a set of impulses in a train along one line.

MOUNTCASTLE: Concerning your first comment, I would say, of course it is a prerequisite. Concerning the second, I would really take the position that there will be a whole spectrum. There are certainly some systems in the brain in which the unique presence or absence of an impulse may be of great importance, as for example, the single climbing fiber synapse in the cerebellum. Perhaps you are replying to Dr. MacKay that the singularly unique event of an impulse is of crucial importance.

To Dr. Teuber I would like to reply that his description of Lashley's attitude is precisely my own—that we specify geography in the midst of the absence of it. The patterns of the activity which are geographically determined may include those cells which also participate in the geographically determined activity. This is a point I was trying to make.

SPERRY: Memory has been mentioned several times, with considerable emphasis on possible synaptic factors. I would like to stress again that along with the synaptic possibilities, one can list a whole series of other possible types of changes involving endogenous physiological properties of neurons that would effect the temporal patterning in the networks and which I think would fit in with the comment of Dr. MacKay. But I think this is not the place to go into details of memory trace theory.

CHAIRMAN: In closing this session I would like to say that Dr. Mountcastle produced some most fascinating ideas on the neuronal basis of perception. It is important to remember that there is always a great background activity of the nervous system and upon that we superimpose the sensory inputs; nevertheless, out of all this immense complication we may derive a clear perceptual experience. This simplification is accomplished by the various types of collateral and feedback inhibition that any strong sensory signal exerts on all the surrounding background activity and on other weak sensory signals. In this way, strong signals can be lifted out of the background noise. It is important to emphasize the role that inhibition plays in integrated cortical activity.

I now call on Professor Moruzzi to introduce the subject of brain plasticity.

Brain Plasticity

MORUZZI: One day, a day which is certainly not near, we may be able to count the sensory impulses which impinge upon the cerebrum during any period of conscious activity; we might even know the functional significance of each of these impulses and of their spatial and temporal patterns; we might be able, finally, to understand how the spontaneous activity of brain neurons is modulated by the different patterns of sensory stimulation. I would certainly not try to predict how neurophysiology will appear to our sophisticated descendants. One prediction, however, I would dare to make now is that the percentage of brain activity which is *directly* related to perception will appear extremely small.

An impressive amount of data supports this prediction. The discovery of electroencephalography by Berger, in 1929, and the classical work of Bremer on the *cerveau isolé* (1935) had already led to the conclusion that an electrical activity is going on during sleep, when men or animals are unconscious. Microelectrode work, culminating in the fine investigations of Evarts (1964, 1965) on unanesthetized monkeys, clearly shows that the overall activity of the cortical neurons—those, at least, which have been recorded so far—is certainly not abolished. Neuron firing is frequently not even decreased, and occasionally is enhanced, during sleep. Only the patterns of neuronal activity are changed. Hence a considerable amount of neuronal firing is going on within the cerebrum quite independently from any conscious experience. We know, moreover, that a great amount of sensory information is never utilized for our perceptions. The discharge from the muscle spindles or from some labyrinthine receptors are the examples which are usually quoted in support of this statement.

These facts are naturally well known to every physiologist. But even when one considers the retinal activity, which is so important for our conscious experience, we are surprised to see how small is the amount of visual information which is utilized for visual perception. The retinal dark discharge is an impressive phenomenon, but there is now ample physiological evidence [1] that visual sensation in darkness (Helmholtz's and Hering's *Eigenlicht*) represents only a minor aspect of the physiological significance of the tonic firing of the retinal ganglion cells. Even during photopic vision only a small amount of the retinal information is utilized for our perceptions.

It is certainly difficult to draw conclusions about perceptions from animal behavior. The fine investigations carried out by Hinde (1954) on the mobbing response of the chaffinch to wooden models of owls [2] show, however, that only a few visual patterns are important for the

---

[1] See G. W. Hughes and L. Maffei. *Arch. Ital. Biol., 103,* 45–59 [1965], for original data and literature.

[2] See W. H. Thorpe. *Learning and Instinct in Animals.* London: Methuen [1956].

release of this inborn fear reaction. It is likely that only a few aspects of the complex retinal information which is undoubtedly reaching the brain of the chaffinch is utilized for the perception of the predator. Probably only those data which are most relevant for releasing the appropriate motor response are actually perceived by the bird. The same considerations apply, of course in a quite different degree, to our own visual perceptions. We walk in a garden, we look at the flowers and detailed information on their hues and shapes reaches our visual centers from the retina. And yet we know that so many details are entirely lost, and that the amount of losses is likely to be quite different from one man to another, and in the same person from one moment to the other.

Some penetrating considerations on this theme were made a long time ago by Henry Bergson, in his philosophical essay, "Le rire" (1900):

Entre la nature et nous, que dis-je?, entre nous et notre propre conscience, un voile s'interpose, voile épais pour le commun des hommes, voile léger, presque transparent, pour l'artiste et le poète. Quelle fée a tissé ce voile? Fut-ce par malice ou par amitié? Il fallait vivre, et la vie exige que nous appréhendions les choses dans le rapport qu'elles ont à nos besoins. Vivre consiste à agir. Vivre, c'est n'accepter des objects que l'impression *utile* pour y répondre par des réactions appropriées: les autres impressions doivent s'obscurcir ou ne nous arriver que confusément. Je regarde et je crois voir, j'écoute et je crois entendre, je m'étudie et je crois lire dans le fond de mon cœur. Mais ce que je vois et ce que j'entends du monde extérieur, c'est simplement ce que mes sens en extraient pour éclairer ma conduite; ce que je connais de moi-même, c'est ce qui affleure à la surface, ce qui prend part à l'action. Mes sens et ma conscience ne me livrent donc de la réalité qu'une simplification pratique. Dans la vision qu'ils me donnent des choses et de moi-même, les différences inutiles à l'homme sont effacées, les ressemblances utiles à l'homme sont accentuées, des routes me sont tracées à l'avance où mon action s'engagera. Ces routes sont celles où l'humanité entière a passé avant moi. Les choses ont été classées en vue du parti que j'en pourrai tirer. Et c'est cette classification que j'aperçois, beaucoup plus que la couleur et la forme des choses. Sans doute l'homme est déjà très supérieur à l'animal sur ce point. Il est peu probable que l'œil du loup fasse une différence entre le chevreau et l'agneau; ce sont là, pour le loup, deux proies identiques, étant également faciles à saisir, également bonnes à dévorer. Nous faisons, nous, une différence entre la chèvre et le mouton; mais distinguons nous une chèvre d'une chèvre, un mouton d'un mouton? *L'individualité* des choses et des êtres nous échappe toutes les fois qu'il ne nous est pas matériellement utile de l'apercevoir. Et là même où nous la remarquons, (comme lorsque nous distinguons un homme d'un autre homme), ce n'est pas l'individualité même que notre œil saisit, c'est-à-dire une certaine harmonie tout à fait originale de formes et de couleurs, mais seulement un ou deux traits qui faciliteront la reconnaissance pratique.[3]

How many of the sensory impulses underlying our perception are utilized for the formation of memory traces? Again, a very small percentage. The tremendous amount of sensory information that reaches the brain during a day of wakefulness is therefore a largely unexploited mine from the angle of the neural processes underlying our perceptions and, still more, the formation of memory traces. The way this mine is exploited is largely related, particularly in man, to the interrelations between perception and memory, a process which is strongly influenced by the cultural background and the imagination of the individual, one that is likely to be of overwhelming importance in artistic creation.[4]

[3] Between nature and ourselves, nay, between ourselves and our own consciousness a veil is interposed: a veil that is dense and opaque for the common herd—thin, almost transparent, for the artist and the poet. What fairy wove that veil? Was it done in malice or in friendliness? We had to live, and life demands that we grasp things in their relations to our own needs. Life is action. Life implies the acceptance only of the *utilitarian* side of things in order to respond to them by appropriate reactions: all other impressions must be dimmed or else reach us vague and blurred. I look and I think I see, I listen and I think I hear, I examine myself and I think I am reading the very depths of my heart. But what I see and hear of the outer world is purely and simply a selection made by my senses to serve as a light to my conduct; what I know of myself is what comes to the surface, what participates in my actions. My senses and my consciousness, therefore, give me no more than a practical simplification of reality. In the vision they furnish me of myself and of things, the differences that are useless to man are obliterated, the resemblances that are useful to him are emphasized; ways are traced out for me in advance along which my activity is to travel. These ways are the ways which all mankind has trod before me. Things have been classified with a view to the use I can derive from them. And it is this classification I perceive, far more clearly than the color and the shape of things. Doubtless man is vastly superior to the lower animals in this respect. It is not very likely that the eye of a wolf makes any distinction between a kid and a lamb; both appear to the wolf as the same identical quarry, alike easy to pounce upon, alike good to devour. We, for our part, make a distinction between a goat and a sheep; but can we tell one goat from another, one sheep from another? The *individuality* of things or of beings escapes us, unless it is materially to our advantage to perceive it. Even when we do take note of it—as when we distinguish one man from another—it is not the individuality itself that the eye grasps, that is, an entirely original harmony of forms and colors, but only one or two features that will make practical recognition easier. (Translation by Brereton, C., and Rothwell, F., New York, Macmillan, 1924.)

[4] See A. Russi, *Poesia e realtà* [Studi di lettere, storia e filosofia pubblicati dalla Scuola Normale Superiore di Pisa, Vol. 26, 1962], for a penetrating analysis on this theme. He started from the following passage of one of the greatest Italian poets, Leopardi, a passage which should be known to the neurophysiologist: "To a sensitive and imaginative man, who would live, as I have been living for a long time, continuously feeling and imagining, the world and all objects are in a certain way double. He will see with his eyes a tower, a field; he will hear with his ears the ringing of a bell; and at the same time in his imagination he will see another tower, another field, will hear another sound. In this second sort of objects lie all the beauty and pleasure of things. Sad is that life (and life is usually so) which sees, hears and feels nothing but those simple objects, that our eyes and ears and other senses

All these considerations lead to the conclusion that the neural processes underlying learning and forgetting, storage and retrieval of memory traces are quantitatively small with respect to the background activity of the cerebrum, although the highest achievements of mankind, from artistic creation to scientific discovery, are dependent upon them. This conclusion fits the well-established notion that mental activity does not appear to be associated with an increase in the overall cerebral metabolic rate, but might be regarded as a serious objection to the hypothesis I have tried to develop in my report, namely, that sleep should be considered as the negative image of conscious activity. There are some reasons to be surprised that almost one third of our life is needed for recovery from an activity which is responsible for such a small portion of the overall energy output of the brain. The only possible explanation is that these recovery processes are extremely slow, entirely different in nature from the fast recovery from all kinds of activity related with the conduction or synaptic transmission of nerve impulses. Assuredly this is not the whole story, and Sokoloff has rightly pointed out that "in a heterogeneous organ like the brain in which so many parts are functionally inversely related, there may be simply a redistribution of the patterns of activity among the various component parts." [5]

We are once more led, therefore, to the speculations on the macromolecular activity which would be related with the plastic changes of the central nervous system. I am not going to develop these concepts, because Professor Eccles has devoted one of his reports at this symposium to a penetrating analysis of the plastic changes underlying enduring psychic memory. He has provided convincing evidence of their localization at the level of some highly specialized synapses.

Most of these macromolecular buildings are extremely labile. They are partially or totally destroyed, reconstructed, repaired, or modified every day. Sherrington's concepts on the need of sleep for the central structure which "has suffered wear and tear" seem to be particularly cogent for the synapses where plastic phenomena occur. Certainly forgetting does not necessarily imply a breakdown of labile macromolecular

---

are able to perceive" [Leopardi; *Zibaldone, 30,* XI, 1828]. In analyzing Leopardi's thought to develop his own esthetic theory, Professor Russi points out that the "second sort of objects" is the refraction of the original perception through memory, coming to the conclusion that in the whole process of aesthetic creation there are, in fact, three "towers": (a) the *tower-object* in the usual perception; (b) the *tower-memory,* which is evoked by perception in the mind of "the imaginative man"; (c) the *tower-work of art,* which results from an elaboration of the memory data. In this sense, a good percentage of men are potentially artists and able to perceive the second "tower," but only very few are capable of creating "objects" made of colors, sounds, words, etc., to express the complexity of mental experience.

[5] L. Sokoloff. Metabolism of the central nervous system in vivo, *Handbook of Physiology,* III, Sect. 1, p. 1853 [1843–1864].

buildings. Extinction and retroactive inhibition may conceal memory records, which occasionally will be brought back with the emotions the original perception evoked, following sensory stimulation, as in the famous story described by Proust in *A la recherche du temps perdu*, or during electrical stimulation of the temporal lobe, as beautifully shown by Professor Penfield.

We have dealt at length in our report with the fast and slow processes of recovery and we have made a distinction between "routine" and "learned" synapses. The learned synapses may be compared to the streets of the center of New York where old buildings are continuously destroyed while new ones are constructed. The routine synapses, which are likely to be far more numerous even within the cerebrum, may be compared to the streets of San Gimignano, which are more or less the same as they were at the time of Dante. The routine synapses may be intensively used, but always for the same tasks. They make no history.

SPERRY: The question of the extent to which the mnemonic recording of conscious experience may be complete or highly selective reminds me that Dr. Penfield's observations on the temporal lobe have been followed up recently by Mahl and Delgado, and coworkers at Yale, using electrodes chronically implanted in the temporal lobes of volunteer patients.

Instead of an exact playback or re-enactment of previous experience, their results tend to favor the hypothesis that the temporal lobe stimulation affects primarily the state of consciousness of the patient to favor hallucinatory, *déjà vu*, and dreamlike states including memory-like experiences that may consist in the main of real earlier experience or they may consist mostly of novel dream material or anything in between. They were able to change the type of recall they got from temporal stimulation by deliberate shaping of the patient's mental set and associations prior to stimulation. I was wondering in this connection about the patient who heard a radio playing—if this might have been influenced by her seeing the stimulator and whether she could see the lights flash when the stimulating buttons were pressed, and so on?

PENFIELD: The answer is "no" as far as the patient, watching from underneath the sheets, is concerned. (She was not my secretary! but some one else's stenographer.) She could not see any light come on, nor was there any other way for her to know when each stimulus was applied. We are also aware of the possibility of suggestion, and understand the conditions required for critical scientific conclusion.

She could see the stimulator box, of course. It looks like a gramophone. We did not know that she was supposing this to be a gramophone until later. This was the first time we had reproduced music. She never discovered what the source of that music could be until a year later. I was speaking then to the American Psychiatric Association and mentioned the case. Reporters were there and unfortunately reported it in the newspapers. Her name was not mentioned. She was living in a small town in Ontario, but she read the newspaper account of the woman who heard music. She wrote me a letter then and said "now I know how it was that I heard that music in the operating room."

Later, again, a year or so later, she wrote me a second letter. She had had no attacks, and she was very grateful. She was writing on the anniversary of the operation. She said, "I bought the music score of what I heard in the operating room, I did not know it very well, but I played it over on the piano. I can't remember where I heard it in the first place. But, in the operating room it was as though I was hearing it all over again."

COLONNIER: With respect to the concept of repair by sleep of Dr. Moruzzi, I would like to mention that in the cortex one can find many cells with invaginations of the nuclear membrane. Long tongues of cytoplasm push their way into the nucleus and seem to reach as far as the nucleolus. The number of ribosomes within these invaginations is much greater than in the rest of the cytoplasm and the number of nuclear pores along the invaginated nuclear membrane also seems greater than around the rest of the nucleus. These two facts suggest very active protein synthesis. The material I am speaking of was from cats perfused by glutaraldehyde and of course under narcosis. It would be interesting to see if these invaginations are present in cats perfused when awake. Might we not indeed find that there are significant differences at the electronmicroscopic level between animals awake and asleep. As far as I am aware only sleeping cortex has ever been described.

MORUZZI: I thank Professor Colonnier for his stimulating suggestions. His electron microscopy approach might lead to rigorously controlled results if the *same* area of the cerebral cortex of the *same* unanesthetized preparation is compared during wakefulness and during sleep. The midpontine pretrigeminal cat has a surprising tendency to remain awake. The unilateral interruption of the midbrain reticular formation will produce long-lasting patterns of EEG synchronization on the cerebral hemisphere of the same side. Of course, the syndrome produced by midbrain lesions is more similar to coma than to natural, synchronized sleep. But to compare the same areas of the two cerebral hemispheres under conditions which are so strikingly different is actually advisable in a preliminary attempt with a technique whose sensitivity has not yet been assessed for these physiological tasks.

HINSHELWOOD: In connection with these wonderful phenomena of plasticity which Professor Moruzzi has talked of, I wonder if neurophysiologists have considered the suggestions they might get from the behavior of many of the adaptive enzymes which play a part in even simple forms of lifelike bacteria. These enzymes very rapidly develop in new media in response to need, and when no longer needed, they diminish again. At first the production and disappearance of the enzyme are very rapid, according to whether the need is present or not. But if the enzyme has been repeatedly induced and maintained for a long time, it tends to persist indefinitely, even in the absence of the need. This may have suggestive analogies for neurology, especially, perhaps, when it is borne in mind that quite a number of these adaptive enzymes play a part in selective permeability phenomena.

MORUZZI: This is an extremely interesting suggestion. Thank you.

BREMER: I wish to know if the findings of neurochemical changes in epileptical mirror images of the primary focus have been confirmed and extended.

GRANIT: At an earlier date we used to think that spontaneous activity is very essential for maintaining memory, and you all know that this idea was ill founded, at least for long-term memory, where we do not believe in the necessity for continued activity. However, if you do not have a circuit, I don't see how the memory would be recalled. So I believe that the basic factor of memory must always be some new neural configuration. And if you accept this idea, the problem is how this specific circuitry is to be maintained. The difficulty is merely that we just now are so badly informed on the specificity of the excitatory and inhibitory circuits. This is the work on which emphasis ought to be put because it seems to me there must be an enormous number of specific neural circuits of which we have no idea. We like to think too much of specific substances. Then there is the plasticity that Moruzzi spoke of, the enormous resources of memory, and also growth and development due to specific chemical substances that comes into the same problem. But without circuits I don't think we can have any memory.

JASPER: I would like to reply to Professor Bremer's question. I think there is a danger for us to accept the story of plasticity which is popular at the moment, and also the RNA changes that people have been speaking so much of; and we tend to forget many other changes that have been demonstrated in the past in the neural tissue under these same conditions. Many years ago it was shown in our laboratories that this epileptic mirror focus not only displays more activity, but, if it continues for three months as a mirror focus and the primary focus be then removed, it will continue firing for as long as nine months, and then it gradually runs down, in our experiments, at least. What maintains the state for the nine months, which is quite a long time? The first thing we thought of was some cholinergic mechanism, and so intracellular cholinesterase was measured by a delicate method. There was a very significant increase in cholinesterase, and this makes me think that the whole cell metabolism should not be overlooked in the story of learning. We have got, as Dr. Granit says, a whole series of other chemical changes, which we are in process of studying, gamma amino butyric acid and enzymes, and I think rather that before accepting conclusions on RNA we should wait until we have surveyed a much larger number of substances which do change with activity.

SCHAEFER: I should like to ask Dr. Moruzzi how far he believes that feedback processes could play a role in sleep and wakefulness. I feel that this would completely fit into his theory of inhibition. I start phenomenologically from the experience of some onset of sleep. If you, for example, are driving a car, this may happen so swiftly that sometimes you scarcely can stop your car so that you avoid an accident. And this suggests to me that there must be some sort of a feedback process. I am deeply convinced that you are right in assuming that inhibition plays a role, so the onset of sleep might be some sort of a shifting over from a predominantly excitatory to a predominantly inhibitory state. I have no idea how that could be, but I just raise the question.

There is one process which most probably plays a role in such a feedback, and this is the blood pressure. I am not sure how far this influence goes, but what we observed in cats is that as soon as you raise the blood pressure slightly you get an arousal reaction.

If you lower the blood pressure again, you get then again a normal alpha EEG with human beings; I would say that little is known about blood pressure changes in falling asleep, especially in these sudden processes of falling asleep. But there are very nice investigations of blood pressure changes on waking, when suddenly the blood pressure rises with very high velocity. We know from the clinical point of view that all these states of dystonias which I mentioned this morning are accompanied by a comparatively low blood pressure.

It has been shown that there are certain types of cells in the posterior hypothalamus and in the reticular formation which seem to be extremely sensitive to an increased blood pressure, and this, of course, could bring some feedback mechanism into that whole story. So my main question would be: could you imagine any feedback process which might give an explanation for these sudden onsets of sleep?

MORUZZI: The important comments of Professor Schaefer concern (i) the problem of the sudden onset of sleep, and (ii) the relation of blood pressure to sleep.

Concerning the first point, I fully agree with Professor Schaefer. Active inhibition, possibly of the ascending reticular system, rather than reticular deactivation, is a more likely explanation of the sudden onset of sleep. The synchronizing structures of the lower brain stem might be involved in these active inhibitory processes, and their influence might be controlled by the cerebral cortex (sleep occurring during conditioning procedures) or by the receptors (sleep induced by monotonous sensory stimulations).

I am coming now to the interrelations between blood pressure and sleep. The Heidelberg group [*EEG J.*, *15*, 63, 1963] has shown that the arousal induced by adrenaline is caused by increased blood pressure, and not by a direct action of the drug; the increase of blood pressure would act directly on neurons of the ascending reticular system. On the other hand, Candia et al [*Arch. Ital. Biol*, *100*, 216, 1962] have shown that blood pressure is tonically decreased during desynchronized sleep, while a phasic fall of blood pressure (frequently associated with brady-cardia) coincides with the appearance of the rapid eye movements [Gassel et al, *Arch. Ital. Biol.*, *102*, 530, 1964]. This fall of arterial pressure becomes dramatic after bilateral sinoaortic deafferentation [Guazzi and Zanchetti, *Science*, *148*, 397, 1965].

It would be important to know whether the ascending reticular system is excited only by the sudden increase of blood pressure produced by adrenaline, or if a tonic excitatory influence is exerted also by the normal blood pressure. If the second hypothesis is true, the fall of blood pressure occurring during desynchronized sleep would lead to reticular deactivation.

SCHAEFER: Do you mean that this bradycardia is an excitation of vagus or merely an inhibition of sympathetic action?

MORUZZI: Gassel et al [*Arch. Ital. Biol.*, *102*, 530, 1964] have suggested that phasic bradycardia during the rapid eye movements may be due to short-lasting inhibition of the vagal cardio-inhibitory tone. However, for technical reasons the hypothesis has not been controlled in the chronically vagotomized cat.

ANDERSEN: When we are looking for a possible morphological basis for plasticity apart from the obvious place to look—the efficiency of synaptic transmission—I think there are a few other places to look also; and one is axonal growth. The axonal growth could be so great that it could give new branches and new synapses. We know, for example, that just after the birth of the animal the Purkinje dendrites have a great many proliferating branches. Only those dendrites that get in contact with a synaptic terminal are going to be developed, all the others are pulled into the cell. This brings me to the second possibility for plastic neuronal changes, which is the geometry of the cell. I think that cells may change their shape very much during their life. And if the cell is changing its shape, this change may increase or decrease the possibility of transfer of information from one part of the cell to another.

Finally, I would like to mention a finding of Dr. Ward in Seattle. He found cells in an experimental epileptic focus did not respond to synaptic excitation. When they took the focus out and stained the cells with the Golgi technique, they were absolutely devoid of spines. Very paradoxically, cells that were hyperactive were absolutely refractory for synaptic excitation!

CREUTZFELDT: In the context of Professor Moruzzi's statement that only part of the available input is "used" by the brain, I should like to draw the attention to the experiments of Maturana [6] and colleagues [1960] on the frog. This seems to be a very good example: The frog's retina reduces the available information considerably, so that only some parameters of the stimulus are transmitted into the midbrain. Here a further reduction of information takes place. Thus these animals apparently "see" only a few forms, but much movement. Correspondingly, the animal will mainly react to movement and less to a complex "Gestalt." The reduction of the physical world through nervous mechanisms and the exclusion of certain aspects of the outer world by the limited capability of receptors and central nervous "analyzers" of an animal thus also limit its image of the outer world and even its freedom of choice between several perceived objects. In following up this idea we get an approach as to what "conscious perception" may mean in an animal, especially in a lower animal.

HEYMANS: I would like to point out that the carotid sinus pressoreceptors not only regulate reflexly and in a homeostatic way the systemic arterial pressure, but also that these pressoreceptors also regulate reflexly the blood supply and blood flow between the extracranial and intracranial (brain) circulations. If the arterial pressure falls, the carotid sinus pressoreceptors induce, indeed, a reflex vasoconstriction and thus an increase of the peripheral resistance in the extracranial and thyroid circulations and, thus, shift the arterial blood supply from these areas to the brain. One of the first symptoms in a case of fall of arterial pressure and fainting is, indeed, pallor of the face. This is an active reaction induced by means of the carotid sinus pressoreceptors provoking a reflex vasoconstriction in the skin and other extracranial tissues in order to shift the blood to the brain. Experiments showed, however, that the carotid sinus pressoreceptors do not act directly on the activity of the cortical motor areas of the brain, but indirectly by means of the changes of blood supply to the brain that these pressoreceptors may induce reflexly.

[6] H. R. Maturana, J. Y. Lettvin, W. S. McCulloch, and W. H. Pitts. Anatomy and physiology of vision in the frog (*Rana pipiens*), *J. Gen. Physiol.*, 43/2, 129–175 [1960].

CHAIRMAN: We have had a most illuminating discussion on the most important theme of the plastic reactions of the brain, and in particular we have greatly enjoyed Professor Moruzzi's wise and thoughtful introduction.

I now call on Professor MacKay to introduce the discussion on the conscious control of action.

Conscious Control of Action

MAC KAY: May I begin by mentioning what seem to me two basic principles to be followed in formulating the problem of free action:

First, we must identify the *level* at which any question is raised before we try to answer it. Take the example of a computing machine set up to solve an equation, and suppose the solution turns out to be unstable. To ask "Why?" would be ambiguous. At a mathematical level, the explanation might be in terms of "ill-conditioning" in the equations. But quite another answer might be given by an electronic engineer who looks into the works and says "I can explain all this behavior in purely *electronic* terms."

Now the point I am making is that if you mix these two levels of discussion about the computer you make nonsense. If you ask "How does the equation exercise a physical force on the electronics in the circuits?" you create a pseudoproblem. But if you stick to one level at a time, either mathematical or electronic, then you can get a sensible answer on either level. I suggest that the same is true in our discussion of consciousness and action: that the level at which you pose your problem must be stuck to until you have come out at the other end with the answer. If you carelessly jump about from one to the other, you only make nonsense.

This leads to the second point. When we try to *correlate* descriptions at the brain level and the personal level, I think it is important to concentrate on expressions for *events* and *activities*, such as having-an-idea, contemplating-an-action, perceiving-an-object. These are hyphenated expressions, and it is a good rule not to break up the hyphens until we can justify doing so. With these suggestions, let me turn to our experience of free action.

As human beings, our first datum is that we have a range of experience which shades from "undergoing" or "suffering," to "doing." Some things happen *to* us; others, we bring about. In the domain of thought, the same gradation holds. Sometimes an idea "just strikes us"; but often we face an option and must decide it soberly by deliberate mental effort. Of course, taking a deliberate step may not necessarily mean that we were aware of an option. A criminal who strikes somebody on the head probably does not first contemplate the range of alternatives, but we would still call it a deliberate step and a responsible act. This in turn can be distinguished from what may be termed *following through,* as for example, in walking, where each leg movement may be almost unconscious, though the decision to walk was voluntary and we call walking voluntary activity. (We recognize it as such by the fact that if it were prevented, then we would do something about it.)

Our question, as Professor Eccles has put it, is not can we believe in our freedom on the basis of what we know of physiology, but quite the other way round: Do these facts of our experience create an embarrassment for theoretical physiology? Take first "having-an-idea" or "getting-an-inspiration." Here the element of control is minimal. Inspiration is something that *happens* to me. I take credit for it only in the sense that I was the lucky one who was hit, not in any sense that I have consciously created it. No embarrassment here, then, for physiology, because we have no evidence in this experience to contradict the suggestion that what happened to us had a physical cause. For all we know the cause might sometimes be the kind of indeterminate chain mesh of events to which Professor Eccles alluded in his Wayneflete Lectures, with a Heisenberg indeterminate happening as their origin. We have just no idea, but at any rate, as physiologists we can cheerfully pursue our calling without feeling that this is a skeleton in the cupboard.

Facing an option, on the other hand, we have to *do* something. We may try to decide by mentally or physically tossing a coin. In that case I suggest that our experience partakes as much of "undergoing" as of "doing," but it is just on the borderline. Here again, we have no grounds in our experience as human beings to worry us as physiologists, because nothing in our experience of a mental tossup says anything either way as to whether or not the outcome had a physical cause. It is merely something that happened to us, whose form we did not determine in any deliberate fashion.

But now we come to the domain of responsible choice, and responsible act. Here there might be an objection to our mechanistic physiology, that we are neglecting a fact of experience; because when we take a deliberate step, one of our data is that we *face an option:* More than one possibility is open to us. We must therefore make sure that our physiological way of thinking does not deny the reality of this fact. Here we come then to the question of the "belief worthiness" of our physiological science, or physical science as applied to the brain. Commonly we would describe this as the question whether it is "true" or "false," but this is an oversimplification, as we will see; because as I mentioned earlier, it is possible for some propositions to be valid for one person but not for another, so that they have no unique truth value. Here an important distinction must be observed between beliefs in *general* and beliefs in *particular*. By this I mean that a general statement of the sort, "everybody's brain is made up of a network of physically interlocking, active elements obeying physical laws," is one thing; but the particular statement, "the action that you are about to decide upon will be of such a form, because your brain is . . . , etc.," has a status which may be quite different.

The general statements of science are like blank checks or checks that are uncashed. Reducing them to particular predictions is like the operation of cashing a check, and we have to make sure that they can stand up to examination not only in their "uncashed" but in their "cashed" form. Let us ask then about the predictions of physiology in relation to free action. The scientific "check" written by theoretical physiology (at least pre-Heisenberg) says, in general, that for any action, whether we call it free or not, given the external and internal data, observers can in principle write a detailed prediction of the action. In this *general* form I see no grounds for objection in our experience.

We have no data from experience to contradict the general statement that observers in principle might be able to tell what we are going to do. But when we come to the question: does the physiological check written in general terms admit of encashment by me? does it mean that there exists a prediction belief-worthy by me? does it entail a contradiction of what I believe and indeed know to be a fact, namely, that I am facing an undetermined option? then as I showed earlier, we face this curious logical dilemma that the conditions on which the thing is valid in general, and valid for nonparticipant observers, would be violated by your trying to cash it. So it is not for you. It is something you would be wrong to believe: something not logically belief-worthy by you; and, therefore, your belief (which in fact is based on your experience) *does not contradict and is not contradicted* by the physiological story. You yourself can accept it in general as applying even to yourself; but in relation to the kinds of action we have been discussing, it has no "cash value" in particular, when applied to yourself.

Finally, let me remind you of the additional quirk which comes in when we consider *dialogue* about a free action. The question whether an action is free or not is normally relevant to the responsibility—(that is) *answerability to others*—of the agent. The point I would like to make is that in this situation our own theoretical deterministic model leads to the conclusion that agents in dialogue become indeterminate *to one another* for the same reason as to themselves. With two people in dialogue, the cause-effect relations between their two systems form a single reciprocal "figure-of-eight" information flow structure for purposes of prediction. In order to establish a determinative prediction of the state of either, you would have to determine the state of the other; and therefore for neither agent can such a determinative prediction be belief-worthy. You and I in dialogue cannot on the basis of our mechanistic physiology regard one another as fully determinate systems, in the sense of believing that there exists now a definitive prediction of your (or my) action which you and I would be right to believe, whether we know it or not, or like it or not.

Once again, we find ourselves in line with our common experience. Suppose we meet someone whom we can see to be on the point of an action that we would deplore. If we maintained isolation, we might in principle be certain that he would do this. But does this generate the conviction that the outcome is therefore already settled? Of course not. On the contrary, we recognize that we now have an option as to whether or not the outcome shall take exactly the form that we have envisaged. If once we engage in dialogue with the agent, we know, as well as he, that for us both the outcome is indeterminate until we have argued it out.

In other words, what I am trying to make clear is that the concept of free action is not purely a private one, but also a social one; and that our conviction that the physiological game is worth playing is in no way negatived by our experience of free action, either in ourselves or in those with whom we are in dialogue.

SPERRY: Among the many attempts to solve this old problem of *determinism versus free will* I know of no better suggestions, and at points I was thinking that I might go home with a feeling of freedom. However, I am still not sure that I would really want to feel that my choices were being made with no antecedent cause.

In order to avoid confusions on these matters I think that we must in principle divorce the problem of prediction from that of causal determinism. Concentrating on the problem of determinism now, I gather that according to your argument, my behavior is causally determined so long as I do not believe someone's prediction about it. In the case of two or more people, does each person's behavior fit entirely with the principle of causal determinism, provided no one starts communicating predictions or believing predictions about himself? I suppose this means that all animal behavior fits into the old scheme of causal determinism; that is, science is still in business as far as the animals go, and also, probably, as far as people go up to some future point when they can start communicating reasonable predictions about one another's choices.

But there is another point here relating to the insertion of a prediction into a person's behavior at a choice point. This is in itself an impossibility unless the prediction takes into account the prediction and its effects; it is like the story within a story, that goes forever and can never be complete. It seems like a purely logical difficulty in the realm of prediction rather than a contradiction of causal determinism, but maybe I still do not properly understand.

MAC KAY: I think it is important to distinguish between predictability (the possibility that a prediction could be *made*) and the stronger notion of determinateness, and I would like to stick to determinateness. I take the claim that an act is determinate to mean that there exists now, before it takes place, a determinative specification or prediction of it, whether anyone knows it or not, or likes it or not (that is, regardless of whether anyone can in fact *make* the prediction). What I am suggesting is that in the case of a choice you have not yet made, no such determinative specification exists, which you would be right to believe whether you know it or not, or like it or not.

This is the point; it is not a case of experimentally having to go and give you the prediction. What I am saying is that when you look into what would be the necessary physical condition of your believing such a prediction, you find that the prediction would not be valid for you. It would be self-nullifying. So this is a "nonexistence theorem" which does not hinge on our actually communicating the prediction to you.

SPERRY: You would agree, I gather, that the concept of causal determinism would apply to an organism by itself, and to a society without an observer? Is that correct so far?

MAC KAY: Predictions could certainly be belief-worthy by nonparticipant observers. As long as we are outside a particular group, then in principle, on a physiological basis we can validly form expectations of what the group will do.

SPERRY: So far, I am unable to see a clear contradiction of causal determinism in all this. You keep referring to belief-worthiness and this logical difficulty, but where is the flaw in the concept of causal determinism? Aren't you concerned here mainly with the attitude of the person faced with a prediction of his behavior and whether he should believe in it or not?

MAC KAY: It is not a matter of his attitude. I am talking about whether or not we, who are outside his system, can say that what we believe is something that he ought (that is, would be correct) to believe, whatever his attitude is to it. And I am saying that even a determinate causal model could not justify this, because in fact the agent would be in error if he believed us, even if his brain were as mechanical as clockwork. In other words, I am questioning a common but fallacious assumption as to the logical consequences of deterministic physiology.

LIBET: Do I have this straight, that this is one way of looking at the problem of free will—that you really assume physical determinism, but this still permits the primary feeling of free will in the system?

In any case there are other possible ways of looking at the feeling or fact of free will: for example, that there is no necessary or complete physical determinism.

This could be done without violating observations that there are (or may be) physiological correlates of free choice making. Even if we accept the assumption that there will be found a complete correspondence or correlation between physical states of brain and mental states or activities, this does not necessarily force one to accept complete physical determinism of mental activity or of free-choice behavior. Interaction between "separable" cerebral and mental states, each capable of affecting the other, would also result in such a correspondence. In this case one would have to assume that the effect of any given mental state on cerebral processes is "produced" consistently, if any observable correlation is to be maintained, and it would thereby in principle be predictable. But completely new mental influences might appear which could not be predicted by any external observer of cerebral processes, unless and until such a mental activity has already appeared at least once.

MAC KAY: Yes, it is always possible to have a theory which denies the axioms of mechanistic physiology, and this would lead to the assumption that even in taking a deliberate step, my decision could not be predicted by anybody. The difficulty is to draw the line there between "doing" and "suffering." I would say that that kind of unpredictability would be something I suffered from, rather than something I could take credit for.

THORPE: I think I understand the essence of your idea, because I do happen to know that paper of Popper about calculating machines. I think that your argument is very closely comparable, if not actually identical, with his. Please correct me if I am wrong. But what I am wondering is whether it is, in any sense, the same kind of formulation which Polanyi is making when he speaks, for instance, of biology being a science which "explains" living things in terms of mechanisms founded on the laws of physics and chemistry but not determined by them. He is arguing that the operational principles of living beings are embodied in the parameters left *undetermined* by physics and chemistry. That is, he argues that borderline conditions are left open by the operations of sciences at a lower level (in this case, physics and chemistry), enabling the higher level (in the case of man-made machines, the aims of the designer) to control these borderline conditions which are left open by the laws governing inanimate matter. Thus he recognizes that living beings, even when represented as machines, comprise at least two levels of existence in which the higher may rely on the lower without interfering with the laws governing the lower. This distinction that Polanyi makes between the different kinds of sciences seems to me very similar to that which Pantin makes when he speaks of the "restricted" and "unrestricted" sciences. My question then is: Is your argument essentially that neurophysiology leaves open certain boundary conditions or circumstances which the will can then determine without, of course, ever violating the laws of physiology or, indeed, of physics and chemistry or any of the sciences lower in the hierarchy?

MAC KAY: I think that it is a different point, because neurophysiology in principle regards itself as based on physics, and in pre-Heisenberg physics, at least, there *existed* a determinative specification for any configuration in the future, whether people knew it or not. Even though it would not therefore claim to have said all that there was to be said, physiology would claim to say all there was to be said predictively at the level of observable physical behavior, which is enough, of course, to create the traditional apparent problem for the freedom of the will, that is, if one does not see the fallacy I have indicated.

Popper's argument (reference to Popper [1950] in my paper) confines itself to proving the impossibility of predicting the situation. This is open to the objection people have been raising, that this only means the chap is ignorant of the truth. I am trying to carry the argument a stage further, by proving the *nonexistence* of a universally binding determining specification, which is something a little different.

CHAGAS: I would just like to ask Dr. MacKay if I can understand from what he has said that machines built to copy the human mind would prove exactly that the two are not adequately comparable.

MAC KAY: If I had to decide, I would say that if we were able to replicate in some other material exactly the kind of information flow map that a human brain has, and if as a result the "artificial person" became an accepted member of our human community, I would ask for good evidence before regarding "him" as unconscious and irresponsible. It would, I think, be safer to treat this as the artificial begetting of a real person.

But, of course, it is a matter of commitment, and as I indicated earlier, we cannot have any conclusive deductive grounds for this. I must say that I am skeptical of our ever being able to produce such a person; but I think I would hesitate, for example, to feel free to dismantle someone whom one had known over a period of years, even if his body were made of metal! But I am not sure what is at issue here. We do not doubt, do we, that the embryological process itself is susceptible of mechanistic explanation, so that the mechanical origin of a person's body should not in principle be the deciding factor?

BREMER: I am not willing nor prepared to enter a metaphysical discussion like this one. I would simply ask Dr. MacKay if the introduction of the concept of belief does not mean introduction of introspection in the problem and if it is possible to proceed in its analysis in using introspective data. Is it not a closed circuit?

MAC KAY: Not in this case. We are considering the mechanical correlate of belief, imagining that one day physiology has discovered what are the physical correlates of a change of belief from A to B. And we are simply asking ourselves, what would be the logical consequences of this man's going through that change, if my prediction of his action depended on his *not* going through that change? The end product of science is meant to be that people believe things, and I am only insisting that in brain science we have to take this end event into account, with the same kind of paradoxical results as in quantum theory, where people had to face the fact that you have to disturb things in order to observe them. You also have to disturb people's brains in order that they should believe.

SPERRY: I wonder how you treat the old example of the posthypnotic suggestion in which a person is told to do something specific at some time about a week later and to forget the suggestion and the whole trance situation. A week later he carries out the specified act, and when you ask him why, he has lots of good reasons that he rationalizes for himself. The subject feels quite certain and convinced that he did this on his own free will. All of us, however, who were in on the experiment knew what he was going to do from the beginning.

MAC KAY: I think one says of him that to the extent that our prediction of his action was belief-worthy by him before he made the decision, to that extent he had diminished responsibility. In principle you could measure this; if you knew enough about the process of posthypnotic suggestion, which we do not, you could measure the extent to which this earlier manipulation of his brain has rendered him irresponsible for the act, by making it predictable for him whether he knows it or not, or likes it or not.

SPERRY: But you would agree in this case that his action and his choice followed the laws of causal determinism, and that your scheme probably does not apply. And similarly, you would probably group most of the animals, and perhaps even people who have not reached the point where they have a belief in the predicted outcome, or whether they are free to choose or not. Well, I am not sure just what you mean by belief, but, if it is a very precise statement in terms of causal determinism as an exact event, you could not say any precise prediction of this sort, and we will not have it for generations to come. You have to predict not only the individual but the surroundings. So do we have to put off application of this scheme to choices until we reach a state where we can begin to introduce prediction of this precise kind?

MAC KAY: The argument I have sketched grants the determinist the whole of the process you suggest. But it applies *a fortiori* now, if we lack the evidence to make a determinative prediction even for a nonparticipant. My argument is that even at the end of the road, where our knowledge might produce a prediction that a nonparticipant might be right to believe, we still could not claim that this was a determinative prediction that the *agent* would be right to believe.

CHAIRMAN: Thank you Dr. MacKay for the very skillful parrying of the whole barrage that you have received. Of course, as a neurophysiologist I keep on thinking that this is fine as a first-level discourse, but that ultimately one will have to face up to the problem in terms of neural responses in the cerebral cortex. How can free choices achieve expression in the medium of the dynamic operation of the neuronal mechanisms of the cortex?

Convergences, Divergences, Lacunae

by H.-L. Teuber

Your introduction, Professor Eccles, reminds me once again of the "thinking" horse of Elberfeldt—the famous horse that has been alluded to in earlier sessions. The horse turned out to do little thinking but was able to respond to barely perceptible signs. And so, I hope, I will be able to do that, although at the end of a full week it may be difficult to react to signs, whether obvious or barely perceptible.

When I first started out in this field as a beginning graduate student, I went up to Karl Lashley after the first seminar he had given us and asked him a question about pattern perception. Lashley listened patiently to my question, laughed a bit and said, "Let's make a contract. I will tell you about that next week if you, in turn, can tell me by then how I (Lashley) can do this." And he flexed three fingers of his right hand, one after the other. I must have replied, "Oh, that's easy to explain! I am going to look it up." Whereupon Lashley smiled his puckish smile and said, "Good luck!"

A week later, I went up to him after class and flexed my fingers, in sequence, as he had done, and said, "Sorry, Professor Lashley, I have no idea." He smiled again, saying, "As long as you cannot explain serial patterns of movement—voluntary movement—I won't have to explain to you anything about pattern perception."

From that day on, we would greet each other by making that private gesture.

What Karl Lashley had conveyed in this case to a beginning graduate student and impressed upon him for life was this: that there seems to be a logical analogy in the difficulty of coming to terms with problems of patterning in perception and patterning of serially coordinated movements, and while neurophysiology may have gotten closer to an answer to the first question, that of pattern perception, it has not gotten much farther in those 25 years toward a solution of the other, the question of coordinated movement.

With this in mind, I would like to go over the four topics that have recurred over and over again in our discussions this week. I put on the blackboard the problems of neural correlates of *perception, action, retention,* and *awareness.* On the other side of the blackboard, I shall now try to list in three columns, next to each of these four topics, some of those instances where the opinions over the last week seemed to converge, where they seemed to diverge, and lastly, where there were obvious gaps.

Perception

To begin with perception, may I propose that there seems to be an impressive amount of general agreement running through all of the presentations and through the discussions that followed them, an agreement on the proposition that a major step forward has in fact been made. Different participants have described this advance in different ways. Professor Granit has given a thorough review of recent developments, particularly for the visual system, and has referred many times to the work of Hubel and Wiesel, as have many others at this meeting. Professor Colonnier has described the columns in the visual cortex of the cat as anatomical structures which he believes correspond to the Mountcastelian columns; that is, the columnar arrangement first discovered by electrophysiologic means by Professor Mountcastle in the somatic-sensory cortex.

We thus begin to realize that at the level of sensory cortex in the visual or somatosensory system, the perceptual input is already categorized to an amazing extent. In the visual system, for instance, the cortical units can abstract direction of lines and of movement, lengths of lines, edges, and possibly more complex qualities, and all that on the basis of elementary principles of excitatory and inhibitory interaction within a given receptor field.

I should add that if we had similarly convergent data for the next two topics, for the understanding of action or of retention, not to speak of awareness, we would still be farther along, but we clearly are not. But to return to perception. One might put the essence of the new findings a bit differently by saying that we are beginning to discover the stimulus. At least this is how psychologists might put it. They should have pointed out all along (but usually did not) that the stimuli used by neurophysiologists in trying to understand information processing, especially in the visual and auditory systems, were singularly inadequate, unphysiologic stimuli; for instance, a flood of uniform light filling the entire visual field, a mode of visual stimulation known to the psychologist as "Ganzfeld," as something that destroys perceptual organization in three dimensions, leading in the normal onlooker to a loss of perceived distance, depth, and texture; or, at the other extreme, a single dot of light known to psychologists as another inadequate stimulus, since its perceptual qualities in a dark surrounding, for a normal human observer, consist of rapidly increasing erratic movements, an instability of localization called autokinetic movement. Nor is the auditory system built to receive bursts of noise, or for that matter, pure tones, but must have built-in predilections for certain species-specific patterns.

Our divergence begins perhaps at the point where we are trying to discuss how the Hubel-Wiesel units in the visual system compare or contrast with the exquisitely specific units discovered by Professor Mountcastle and his colleagues at thalamic and cortical levels in the somaticsensory system, or when we attempt to find further analogues for a similar kind of sequential stimulus-processing in the auditory system.

But the major lacuna, the gap on which we all agree, lies probably elsewhere, between any of these sensory systems and the classical motor system. It is here that I believe our knowledge is as rudimentary and "primitive" as Professor Eccles indicated a short while ago. Lashley once compared this extreme difficulty (of finding a transition from the sensory inputs to the patterning of motor output) with a magnificent bridge across a chasm. He had been invited to attend the inauguration, together with many others who had gathered at one end of the new bridge. The ribbon was cut, the elect company walked across and were trapped on the other side of the bridge by "impenetrable virgin forests." How do we make the transition from the receptor-field theory to the problems of coordinated action?

Action

In expressing many doubts about a workable approach to the problem of sensory-motor relations, I do not wish to detract from the modelling of these processes in terms of meta-organizing systems. Professor MacKay himself has said that these have to be found in the brain in order to be clothed in protoplasm. Perhaps our opinions show maximal convergence if we focus on these primitive "releasing" stimuli described by Professor Thorpe, particularly the famous example he did not mention, though Professor Schaefer did, I believe: the "innate fear of the hawk-shape" and similar ethological observations. Here we have a configurational stimulus which will elicit fairly specific motor patterns. Certain young birds, at least in some laboratories under some conditions, flutter and crouch when this particular stimulus complex appears. This particular releasing effect might fit quite nicely into the Hubel-Wiesel story; the schematic hawk-shape moving above the barnyard, with the broad edge leading, might conceivably appeal to pre-designed receptor fields, so as to release the pattern of escape.

Perhaps a clearer example of a rather direct coupling between releasing stimulus and fixed action pattern is the behavior of male jumping spiders, the salticids, with their exquisite image-forming eyes. Here the male, as so often among insects, is small and rather homely and in great danger of being eaten by the female, who bears two parallel rows of dots on her back—landing markers, so to speak. The male stalks the female and, when lined up properly with these markers, takes a flying leap. If he misses, he gets eaten before he can mate, but if he alights properly, he can see to it that salticids will propagate, and gets eaten only afterwards. There is thus an enormous selection pressure for adequate linkage between the look and the leap, with the releasing pattern on the female's back acting as specific releaser, essentially in lock-and-key fashion.

Perhaps the crucial difference between species is the distance between the look and the leap. In higher forms, the release of action by particular configurations of inputs is much less direct. When Tinbergen first described the reaction to the hawk-shape in young goslings, he spoke of "innate fear" and there definitely seems to be an "inner" aspect to the release of action, an emotional *im*pression, even though all we permit ourselves to talk about is the patterned *ex*pression of this emotional state. Yet it would be most artificial, as Professor Thorpe pointed out, if we were to deny that there is emotion in the animal that displays all of the outward signs of fright.

But here and elsewhere, we run into a serious divergence of views. Many of the participants here stressed in their papers and in the discussions that one of the best ways of recording receptor fields is under anesthesia, and yet this is clearly a state in which a human perceiver would not only be unemotional about his sensory input but altogether unaware of it. Professor Jasper pointed this out in his presentation: how can we go from the behavior of units under deep anesthesia to their role in the waking state? Undoubtedly, current methods permit registration of unit activity without anesthesia, and at varying stages of narcosis and sleep, as Dr. Creutzfeldt and others have done, but the crucial question on which there was much disagreement concerns the role of the non-specific systems (and it certainly should be a plural), in this respect. Do we need a duplicity-theory of conscious perception, in which the specific and non-specific systems have to interact? Scepticism about the presumed role of non-specific systems has been expressed by Professor Bremer, and again, quite recently in these discussions, by Professor Mountcastle. But the fact remains that there is here a crucial gap in our understanding. We must find out how specific and non-specific systems mesh, a question also raised by Professor Moruzzi.

Perhaps this lacuna will be filled in some day, if we think seriously enough about how the central nervous system acts back, so to speak, upon its own perceptual inputs. On the whole, this question is one that tends to be overlooked, because we are so accustomed to entering upon the analysis of central nervous system action from the stimulus-side, and it is then, I would suggest, that we find it almost impossible to cross the bridge to the motor end. Yet Professor MacKay's information-flow diagrams certainly suggest an inverse direction for one's analysis—from motor to sensory.

It is the problem of how the animal or the human observer manages to maintain the order of his perceptions in the face of continual self-produced movements.

As von Holst and Mittelstaedt, and quite independently, Professor Sperry, have pointed out, an organism which moves has to take its own movements into account. While looking into the world, he must be able to distinguish those movements of the environment that are environmentally produced from those movements that are consequences of the organism's own action. I suspect that self-awareness may largely depend on an elaboration of this very capacity, yet physiologically speaking, we are encountering here one of the largest lacunae in our understanding of perception as well as action, even though Professor Jasper hinted at some possibly relevant recent disclosures on this score. Perhaps we have to admit that the fundamental problems of action, perception, and awareness are not as separable as they might have seemed, that we can understand as little of perceptual mechanisms without taking motor mechanisms into account, as vice-versa.

All the magnificent physiologic information gathered on motor maps in the neocortex, beginning with the discoveries by Lord Adrian, in experimental animals, and extended to man by Professor Penfield and his colleagues, sets the stage for asking the questions about coordinated movements. I am sure we would agree that we do not know how serially-patterned, coordinated movement comes about. Is the motor cortex, in the restricted sense of the precentral gyrus in primates, a system for programming movements, or rather an area of confluence of facilitatory or inhibitory pathways playing upon more central and more vital mechanisms, as Professor Penfield has so often suggested? Perhaps the work of Professor Phillips and that of Dr. Edward Evarts, to whom Professor Phillips and others have referred, holds promise of extending to the motor cortex some of the analyses used for the visual system by Hubel and Wiesel.

Yet I cannot help but feel that we are not asking the questions of the action system quite in the way we should. We may not be able to fill the biggest lacuna, that of finding a physiologic correlate of self-produced motion, until we consider the possibility of a continual inter-action between the sensory and motor systems not only, as traditionally accepted, from sensory to motor, but in the reverse direction, from motor to sensory. If we accept, for a moment, the postulate of a corollary discharge, a flow of impulses from the motor system directly, centrally, to the sensory areas, during every efferent discharge, we would have a mechanism for two things at once: for the way in which the organism can take into account those environmental motions that result from its own movements (because these motions of the environment are centrally "expected"), and we would have a physiologic marker, so to speak, for the "voluntariness" of self-produced motion. Here lies a major lacuna, then, for our understanding of action, but in recognizing the gap, we might come closer to filling it. Thus, to summarize what might be said about *action*, I think the convergence lies in our agreement that the motor cortex, as now approached, still hides, rather than reveals, the answer to a physiology of patterned movement. Our divergence con-cerns the ways in which we hope to bridge the gap between sensory and motor functions, and our biggest lacuna lies at this juncture, between sensation and action, or, differently put, within the problem of voluntary movement.

Retention

You will see how the task of summarizing gets simpler as we move down my list from perception and action towards retention and aware-ness, because the farther down we go, the less there is known to us, and hence the less to summarize. With respect to retention, our most general agreement comes in the form of a confession of persisting ignorance. We agree that we do not know how the nervous system remembers a single thing, and, I am afraid, we hold divergent views about the best strategy for finding a neural basis for retention.

Professor Eccles insists that it ought to turn out to be a synaptic change, in line with the classical concepts of Cajal, while Professor Hinshelwood has pointed out that adaptive enzymes are, after all, quite convincing biological models of learning.

In fact, there were several people around this table who spoke, from time to time, in favor of what was, in this symposium, a minority view, the notion of a macromolecule as the basic memory mechanism, in spite of the serious difficulties with this view which were mentioned by Professor Eccles in his second paper. He warned against precipitous acceptance of Hydén's proposal, and it is certainly true that the experi-mental evidence, so far, is unconvincing.

Perhaps we can come closer to a resolution by exploiting the rapid developments in our knowledge of those structures that in man, at least, appear to play a crucial role in certain aspects of retention. Interference with basal temporal structures, as has been shown by Brenda Milner, by William Scoville, and by Professor Penfield and others, can have devastating effects on a patient's ability to go from short-term to long-term retention. The very special structure of the hippocampus may yield some clues, together with the fact that retention is temporarily blocked by the application of agents that interfere with protein synthesis at that level.

Further clues might come from quite different sources, from considerations of the nature of those inputs that can or cannot be stored, or can or cannot be transmitted from one part of the central nervous system to another. Professor Sperry's disclosures of the two central hemispheres' partial isolation from each other are even more beautiful by virtue of the demonstration that some types of input, e.g., those concerning luminous flux, can leak across, from one side to the other, even after the transection of all forebrain commissures, while other kinds of input, e.g., those concerned with certain visual patterns, cannot.

There is a fascinating corollary to these observations in some recent work of one of our post-doctoral fellows, David Ingle, who has studied interocular and intraretinal transfer of sensory information in goldfish. In one of these experiments, the goldfish learns to swim forward, and thus avoids an electric shock, when shown a vertical line as opposed to an oblique line, inclined by, say, 30 degrees from vertical. If the fish "knows" this with the anterior part of his retina, he will remember it with the posterior part to which these patterns had not been exposed. Yet if his task involves distinguishing a vertical from a very slightly inclined oblique, say 15 degrees, he will learn this nearly as fast with the anterior region of his retina but fail to swim forward and avoid the electric shock when these hard-to-distinguish patterns are exhibited to the untutored posterior portion of his retina. Yet under these conditions, when the proper skeletal response is absent, his heart rate will nevertheless show a characteristic change, as though he "knew" in his heart that one of the patterns meant danger but fails to know what to do about it. Dissociations of this type were first discovered by McCleary whose methods Ingle has adopted. They suggest degrees or levels of learning and remembering which our physiologic interpretations may have to take into account.

Awareness

Again, my comments on the preceding topic, on retention, have shaded into those next in line, the problems of awareness, its degrees or levels, and its possible physiologic bases. Perhaps the most obvious region of convergent opinion here might be found in the fact that a group composed primarily of neurophysiologists should be willing to discuss the topic of awareness at all. Only ten or fifteen years ago, many of our colleagues might have thought that awareness could not be a proper topic for serious exploration. By contrast, most of us here seemed to think it good and proper when we came, and all of us think so still, by the end of this week. What made this consensus possible? Perhaps it was a collective readiness to forego any definition of conscious awareness.

Certainly we are all agreed that the units which categorize sensory inputs—the units which decide that a visual vertical is vertical, or that a finger joint has been moving up or down—these units may be necessary at some early stage for conscious awareness, but they cannot be sufficient.

Yet every conceivable divergence of opinion seemed to arise when we tried to delineate the systems or mechanisms that might be necessary for consciousness. We were not even quite sure, if we follow Professor Thorpe's lead, as to how we might decide what consciousness is for. Nor were we in complete agreement about the possible role of centrencephalic structures, although we tended to agree on the notorious sensitivity of these structures to anesthetics and were impressed by Dr. Creutzfeldt's observations on these differential susceptibilities at the single-cell level. He, as well as Professors Jasper and Moruzzi, reminded us of the unsolved problems of sleep, and although Professor Mountcastle reiterated his doubts about the supposed role of non-specific systems in maintaining the waking state, many of us still felt that some form of interaction between primary and non-specific systems might hold important clues. In this connection we should not forget Professor Bremer's fundamental demonstration that not only can the reticular core "awaken" the cortex, but the cortex, in turn, can arouse the reticular formation in the brain stem. Not enough is known, in any case, to justify that we assign empirical weights to the relative roles of an "upward" and "downward" drive. In the end, we do agree that the problem of awareness remains a gap in our understanding of the nervous system.

But rather than close on this obvious note, let me draw attention once more to the issue of specific versus general or non-specific systems, a point also touched upon by Professor Mountcastle in his closing discussion. In my own paper, I stressed a number of extremely specific changes in conscious perception after variously localized lesions of the human brain. There is nothing I would want to retract, but there is something I would like to add, if only to vindicate Lashley.

Besides all those tasks which, in our hands, brought out exceedingly focal and specific effects of localized brain lesions, there was one obviously simple and straightforward test that was performed amazingly poorly by patients with lesions in any lobe—frontal, parietal, temporal or occipital, right, left, or bilateral. This task involved the visual analysis of line patterns, in which a simpler pattern was concealed by surrounding and overlapping contours. Thus, this hidden-figure task brought out a general or non-specific deficit in the same population of patients in which other tasks had disclosed extremely specific symptoms. I submit that this coexistence of specific and general symptoms, in the same cases of selective cerebral lesions, suggests that general and specific mechanisms do interact in perception and conscious awareness.

This sort of formulation is hopelessly vague and does not yield any real understanding of problems of consciousness. We obviously are still far from being able to go from our incipient understanding of the functions of individual neurons and synapses to the functions of the neural masses in the brain when it controls perception and action and retention and awareness.

But I also think that we need not make any excuse for having dared to ask these questions. As George Wald said, "The great questions are those an intelligent child asks and, getting no answers, stops asking. That is known as growing up." Yet the growth of any field demands that we ask these questions and do not stop.

Index